The Shoulder

Edited by

CHARLES A. ROCKWOOD, JR., M.D.

Professor and Chairman Emeritus
Department of Orthopaedics
The University of Texas
Health Science Center at San Antonio
San Antonio, Texas

FREDERICK A. MATSEN III, M.D.

Professor and Chairman
Department of Orthopaedics
University of Washington
School of Medicine
Seattle, Washington

VOLUME 2

1990

W.B. SAUNDERS COMPANY

Harcourt Brace Jovanovich, Inc.

Philadelphia   London   Toronto   Montreal   Sydney   Tokyo

W. B. SAUNDERS COMPANY
Harcourt Brace Jovanovich, Inc.

The Curtis Center
Independence Square West
Philadelphia, PA 19106

Library of Congress Cataloging-in-Publication Data

The Shoulder/[edited by] Charles A. Rockwood, Jr., Frederick A. Matsen III.

p. cm.

ISBN 0–7216–2828–1 (set).

1. Shoulder—Diseases.   I. Rockwood, Charles A., 1936–
II. Matsen, Frederick A.
[DNLM: 1. Shoulder.   2. Shoulder Joint.   WE 810 S55861]

RC939.S484   1990

617.5′72–dc20

DNLM/DLC   89–24221

Editor: Lewis Reines
Designer: Karen O'Keefe
Production Manager: Carolyn Naylor
Manuscript Editor: Tom Gibbons
Illustration Coordinators: Brett MacNaughton and Ceil Kunkle
Indexer: Ann Cassar
Cover Designer: Ellen Bodner

ISBN 0–7216–2829–x Volume 1
0–7216–2830–3 Volume 2
0–7216–2828–1 Set

THE SHOULDER

Printed in the United States of America.

Last digit is the print number: 9   8   7   6   5   4   3   2

We dedicate these volumes to Anne, Patsy, and our families who support us

and

To all the past, present, and future generations of clinicians and investigators interested in unraveling the mysteries of the shoulder.

Contributors

David W. Altchek, M.D.
Assistant Professor of Surgery (Orthopaedics), Cornell University Medical College; Assistant Attending Orthopaedic Surgeon, The Hospital for Special Surgery, New York, New York

Kai-Nan An, Ph.D.
Professor of Bioengineering, Mayo Medical School; Consultant, Orthopedic Biomechanics Laboratory, Mayo Clinic, Rochester, Minnesota

Gunnar B. J. Andersson, M.D., Ph.D.
Professor of Orthopedic Surgery, Rush Medical College; Senior Attending and Associate Chairman, Department of Orthopedic Surgery, Rush-Presbyterian–St. Luke's Medical Center, Chicago, Illinois

Steven P. Arnoczky, D.V.M.
Associate Professor of Surgery (Comparative Orthopaedics), Cornell University Medical College; Director, Laboratory for Comparative Orthopaedic Research, The Hospital for Special Surgery, New York, New York

Craig T. Arntz, M.D.
Acting Instructor, Department of Orthopaedics, University of Washington School of Medicine, Seattle, Washington; Associate Staff, Valley Medical Center, Renton, Washington

Louis U. Bigliani, M.D.
Assistant Professor of Orthopaedic Surgery, College of Physicians and Surgeons; Assistant Attending of Orthopaedic Surgery, Columbia Presbyterian Medical Center, New York, New York

Desmond J. Bokor, M.B.
Clinical Fellow, University of Western Ontario, London, Ontario, Canada; Honorary Surgeon, University of Sydney; Orthopaedic Surgeon, Westmead Hospital, Sydney, Australia

Ernest M. Burgess, M.D.
Clinical Professor, Department of Orthopaedics, University of Washington School of Medicine; Attending, University and Affiliated Hospitals of University of Washington, Seattle, Washington

Wayne Z. Burkhead, Jr., M.D.
Clinical Assistant Professor, The University of Texas Health Science Center, Southwestern Medical School; Chief of Shoulder Service, Dallas Veterans Hospital; Attending Physician, W. B. Carrell Memorial Clinic; Associate Attending, Baylor University Medical Center, Dallas, Texas

Kenneth P. Butters, M.D.
Clinical Assistant Professor, University of Oregon Orthopedic Teaching Program; Orthopedic Surgeon, Sacred Heart Hospital, Eugene, Oregon

Michael A. Caughey, M.B., Ch.B.
Consultant Orthopaedic Surgeon, Middlemore Hospital, Auckland, New Zealand

Robert H. Cofield, M.D.
Professor of Orthopedics, Mayo Medical School; Consultant in Orthopedics, Mayo Clinic, Rochester, Minnesota

Ernest U. Conrad III, M.D.
Assistant Professor, Department of Orthopaedic Surgery, University of Washington School of Medicine; Director of Division of Musculoskeletal Oncology, University of Washington; Director of Bone Tumor Clinic, Children's Hospital and Medical Center, Seattle, Washington

Edward V. Craig, M.D.
Associate Professor of Orthopaedic Surgery, University of Minnesota Medical School; Attending Surgeon, University of Minnesota Hospital; Consultant, Veterans Administration Hospital, Minneapolis, Minnesota

Ralph J. Curtis, Jr., M.D.
Clinical Assistant Professor of Orthopaedics, Department of Orthopaedics, The University of Texas Health Science Center at San Antonio, San Antonio, Texas

Anthony G. Gristina, M.D.
Professor, Bowman Gray School of Medicine; Attending, North Carolina Baptist Hospital, Winston-Salem, North Carolina

Richard J. Hawkins, M.D.
Professor, University of Western Ontario; Attending, University Hospital, London, Ontario, Canada

Christopher M. Jobe, M.D.
Assistant Professor, Department of Orthopaedics, Loma Linda University School of Medicine; Staff, Loma Linda University Medical Center and Loma Linda Community Hospital; Consulting Staff, Veterans Administration Hospital, Loma Linda, California

Frank W. Jobe, M.D.
Clinical Professor, Department of Orthopaedics, University of Southern California School of Medicine, Los Angeles, California; Associate, Kerlan-Jobe Orthopaedic Clinic; Staff, Centinela Hospital Medical Center, Inglewood, California

Gordon Kammire, M.D.
Private Practice, Lexington, North Carolina; Formerly Chief Resident in Orthopedic Surgery, Bowman Gray School of Medicine/North Carolina Baptist Hospital, Winston-Salem, North Carolina

Stephen P. Kay, M.D.
Clinical Instructor, Division of Orthopedic Surgery, UCLA Center for Health Sciences; Attending Staff, Century City Hospital and Cedars-Sinai Medical Center, Los Angeles, California

Ronald S. Kvitne, M.D.
Assistant Clinical Professor, Department of Orthopaedics, University of Southern California School of Medicine, Los Angeles, California; Assistant Clinical Instructor, Sports Medicine and Reconstructive Service, Rancho Los Amigos Hospital, Downey, California; Staff, Centinela Hospital Medical Center, Inglewood, California; Staff, Rancho Los Amigos Hospital, Downey, California

Robert D. Leffert, M.D.
Associate Professor of Orthopaedic Surgery, Harvard Medical School; Chief of the Surgical Upper Extremity Rehabilitation Unit and the Department of Rehabilitation Medicine, Massachusetts General Hospital, Boston, Massachusetts

James V. Luck, Jr., M.D.
Associate Clinical Professor, Department of Orthopaedics, University of Southern California School of Medicine; Medical Director and Chief Operating Officer, Orthopaedic Hospital, Los Angeles, California

Leonard Marchinski, M.D.
Staff, Reading Hospital, Reading, Pennsylvania

Frederick A. Matsen III, M.D.
Professor and Chairman, Department of Orthopaedics, University of Washington School of Medicine; Chief, Shoulder and Elbow Service, University of Washington Medical Center, Seattle, Washington

Bernard F. Morrey, M.D.
Professor of Orthopedics, Mayo Medical School; Chairman, Department of Orthopedics, Mayo Clinic, Rochester, Minnesota

J. Patrick Murnaghan, B.Sc., M.D.
Assistant Professor, Division of Orthopaedic Surgery, University of Ottawa; Staff Orthopaedic Surgeon, Ottawa Civic Hospital; Consultant, Royal Ottawa Hospital and Ottawa Cancer Foundation, Ottawa, Ontario, Canada

Stephen J. O'Brien, M.D.
Assistant Professor of Surgery (Orthopaedics), Cornell University Medical College; Assistant Attending Orthopaedic Surgeon—HSS Assistant Scientist, The Hospital for Special Surgery; Assistant Attending Orthopaedic Surgeon, The New York Hospital, New York, New York

L. Brian Ready, M.D.
Associate Professor of Anesthesiology, University of Washington School of Medicine; Chief, Division of Regional Anesthesia, and Director, Acute Pain Service, University Hospital, Seattle, Washington

Charles A. Rockwood, Jr., M.D.
Professor and Chairman Emeritus, Department of Orthopaedics, The University of Texas Health Science Center at San Antonio, San Antonio, Texas

Robert L. Romano, M.D.
Clinical Professor, University of Washington School of Medicine; Staff, Providence Hospital, Swedish Hospital, and Children's Orthopedic Hospital, Seattle, Washington

S. Robert Rozbruch, B.A.
Cornell University Medical College, New York, New York

Kiriti Sarkar, M.D.
Professor, Department of Pathology, University of Ottawa, Ottawa, Ontario, Canada

Michael J. Skyhar, M.D.
Assistant Clinical Professor, University of California, San Diego; Assistant Attending Orthopaedic Surgeon, Scripps Memorial Hospital, San Diego, California

Elizabeth A. Szalay, M.D.
Active Staff, St. Elizabeth Hospital and Baptist Hospital of Southeast Texas, Beaumont, Texas; Courtesy Staff, Beaumont Medical and Surgical Hospital, Beaumont, Texas; Clinical Staff, Shriners Hospital for Crippled Children, Houston Unit, Houston, Texas

Steven C. Thomas, M.D.
Shoulder Fellow, Department of Orthopaedics, University of Washington School of Medicine; Shoulder Fellow, University of Washington Medical Center, Seattle, Washington

James E. Tibone, M.D.
Clinical Associate Professor of Orthopaedics, University of Southern California, Los Angeles, California; Staff, Centinela Hospital Medical Center, Inglewood, California

Hans K. Uhthoff, M.D.
Professor and Chairman, Division of Orthopaedic Surgery, University of Ottawa; Active Staff, Ottawa General Hospital, Ottawa, Ontario, Canada

Anna Voytek, M.D.
Private Practice, Greensboro, North Carolina; Formerly Chief Resident in Orthopedic Surgery, Bowman Gray School of Medicine/North Carolina Baptist Hospital, Winston-Salem, North Carolina

Russell F. Warren, M.D.
Professor of Orthopaedic Surgery, Cornell University Medical College; Attending Orthopaedic Surgeon and Chief, Sports Medicine and Shoulder Services, The Hospital for Special Surgery; Attending Orthopaedic Surgeon, The New York Hospital, New York, New York

Lawrence X. Webb, M.D.
Associate Professor, Bowman Gray School of Medicine; Attending, North Carolina Baptist Hospital, Winston-Salem, North Carolina

Peter Welsh, M.B., Ch.B.
Assistant Professor, Department of Surgery, University of Toronto; Deputy Chief of Staff, Orthopaedic and Arthritic Hospital; Staff Orthopaedic Surgeon, The Wellesley Hospital; Consultant Orthopaedic Surgeon, Hillcrest Hospital and Riverdale Hospital, Toronto, Ontario, Canada

Kaye E. Wilkins, M.D.
Clinical Professor of Orthopaedics and Pediatrics, The University of Texas Health Science Center at San Antonio; Staff, Santa Rosa Children's Hospital and Southwest Texas Methodist Hospital, San Antonio, Texas

Virchel E. Wood, M.D.
Chief, Hand Surgery Service, and Professor of Orthopaedic Surgery, Loma Linda University School of Medicine; Staff, Loma Linda University Medical Center, Loma Linda Out-Patient Surgery Center, and Loma Linda Community Hospital, Loma Linda, California

D. Christopher Young, M.D.
Staff Orthopaedic Surgeon, Brooke Army Medical Center, San Antonio, Texas

Foreword

It is a privilege to write the Foreword for *The Shoulder* by Drs. Charles A. Rockwood, Jr., and Frederick A. Matsen III. Their objective when they began this work was an all-inclusive text on the shoulder that would also include all references on the subject in the English literature. Forty-six authors have contributed to this text.

The editors of *The Shoulder* are two of the leading shoulder surgeons in the United States. Dr. Rockwood was the fourth President of the American Shoulder and Elbow Surgeons, has organized the Instructional Course Lectures on the Shoulder for the Annual Meeting of the American Academy of Orthopaedic Surgeons for many years, and is a most experienced and dedicated teacher. Dr. Matsen is President-Elect of the American Shoulder and Elbow Surgeons and is an unusually talented teacher and leader. These two men, with their academic know-how and the help of their contributing authors, have organized a monumental text for surgeons in training and in practice, as well as one that can serve as an extensive reference source. They are to be commended for this superior book.

CHARLES S. NEER II, M.D.
Professor Emeritus, Orthopaedic Surgery,
Columbia University; Chief, Shoulder Service,
Columbia-Presbyterian Medical Center, New York

Preface

The past twenty years have witnessed a huge surge in interest and new knowledge concerning the shoulder. The shoulder is now recognized as one of the principal sites of pathology in sports injuries, work-related injuries, arthritis, and age-related degeneration. We find ourselves in an age of discovery of the mechanisms of shoulder stability and rotator cuff degeneration and about basic mechanics of the shoulder.

Our primary goal at the outset of this project was to develop a text that would become the definitive work on the management of shoulder problems in children and in adults, encompassing developmental anatomy, biomechanics, fractures, dislocations, tumors, infections, amputations, and other related areas. The contributors, each of whom is a recognized authority in his or her field, were challenged to present an in-depth review of the current available knowledge about the shoulder for their chapters, and this they have done. Each chapter follows a logical pattern and, where applicable, contains a historical review, anatomy, classification, radiographic findings, open versus closed treatment, and finally, and of importance, the author's preferred method of treatment. In addition, each chapter includes extensive references on the subject.

We realize that it is risky to put down in print the state of the art of such a rapidly moving field: new knowledge is appearing literally every day. On the other hand, it seems important to consolidate the platform of knowledge as it exists today so that it can serve as the foundation for the addition of the knowledge of tomorrow. It is our hope that *The Shoulder* will be that foundation.

To the readers we offer our best wishes in your studies of the shoulder. It is a fascinating joint! To the contributors we express our deepest gratitude; the book would not have been possible without you. We offer our sincere appreciation and thanks to our teacher, Charles S. Neer II, M.D., of New York City. We thank Rita Mandoli and Sarah Sato at the University of Washington School of Medicine and Natalie Merryman and Carol Cafiero at the University of Texas School of Medicine in San Antonio for their unfailing energy and devotion to this work. Their perseverance and attention to detail ensured that this book would be of the highest quality.

We also acknowledge the help we received from our Shoulder Fellows, Doug Harryman and Steve Thomas from the University of Washington and Jerry Williams and Mike Wirth from the University of Texas.

CHARLES A. ROCKWOOD, JR., M.D.
FREDERICK A. MATSEN III, M.D.

Contents

CHAPTER 5

X-ray Evaluation of Shoulder Problems 178

Charles A. Rockwood, Jr., M.D. • Elizabeth A. Szalay, M.D. • Ralph J. Curtis, Jr., M.D.
D. Christopher Young, M.D. • Stephen P. Kay, M.D.

CHAPTER 6

Biomechanics of the Shoulder 208

Bernard F. Morrey, M.D. • Kai-Nan An, Ph.D.

CHAPTER 7

Anesthesia for Shoulder Procedures 246

L. Brian Ready, M.D.

CHAPTER 8

Shoulder Arthroscopy 258

David W. Altchek, M.D. • Russell F. Warren, M.D. • Michael J. Skyhar, M.D.

CHAPTER **9**

Fractures of the Proximal Humerus 278

Louis U. Bigliani, M.D.

CHAPTER **10**

The Scapula 335

Kenneth P. Butters, M.D.

CHAPTER **11**

Fractures of the Clavicle 367

Edward V. Craig, M.D.

CHAPTER 12

Disorders of the Acromioclavicular Joint 413

Charles A. Rockwood, Jr., M.D. • D. Christopher Young, M.D.

CHAPTER 13

Disorders of the Sternoclavicular Joint 477

Charles A. Rockwood, Jr., M.D.

CHAPTER 14

Glenohumeral Instability 526

Frederick A. Matsen III, M.D. • Steven C. Thomas, M.D. • Charles A. Rockwood, Jr., M.D.

VOLUME 2

CHAPTER **15**

Subacromial Impingement 623
Frederick A. Matsen III, M.D. • Craig T. Arntz, M.D.

CHAPTER **16**

Rotator Cuff Tendon Failure 647
Frederick A. Matsen III, M.D. • Craig T. Arntz, M.D.

CHAPTER **17**

Degenerative and Arthritic Problems of the Glenohumeral Joint 678
Robert H. Cofield, M.D.

CHAPTER **18**

Neurological Problems
Robert D. Leffert, M.D.

CHAPTER **19**

Calcifying Tendinitis
Hans K. Uhthoff, M.D. • Kiriti Sarkar, M.D.

CHAPTER **20**

The Biceps Tendon
Wayne Z. Burkhead, Jr., M.D.

CHAPTER 21

Frozen Shoulder 837

J. Patrick Murnaghan, M.D.

CHAPTER 22

Muscle Ruptures Affecting the Shoulder Girdle 863

Michael A. Caughey, M.B. • Peter Welsh, M.B

CHAPTER 23

Tumors and Related Conditions 874

Ernest U. Conrad III, M.D.

CHAPTER **24**

Sepsis of the Shoulder: Molecular Mechanisms and Pathogenesis 920

Anthony G. Gristina, M.D. • Gordon Kammire, M.D. • Anna Voytek, M.D.
Lawrence X. Webb, M.D.

CHAPTER **25**

Amputations and Prosthetic Replacement 940

Robert L. Romano, M.D. • Ernest M. Burgess, M.D.

CHAPTER **26**

The Shoulder in Sports 961

Frank W. Jobe, M.D. • James E. Tibone, M.D. • Christopher M. Jobe, M.D.
Ronald S. Kvitne, M.D.

Subacromial Impingement

Frederick A. Matsen III, M.D.
Craig T. Arntz, M.D.

Ay, there's the rub.

HAMLET, III. i. 47, SHAKESPEARE

Definition and Historical Review

In this chapter, "impingement" is defined as the encroachment of the acromion, coracoacromial ligament, coracoid process, and/or acromioclavicular joint on the rotator cuff mechanism that passes beneath them as the glenohumeral joint is moved, particularly in flexion and rotation.

Pettersson has provided an excellent summary of the early history of subacromial pathology. Because of its completeness, his account is quoted here.[157]

As already mentioned, the tendon aponeurosis of the shoulder joint and the subacromial bursa are intimately connected with each other. An investigation on the pathological changes in one of these formations will necessarily concern the other one also. A historical review shows that there has been a good deal of confusion regarding the pathological and clinical observations on the two.

The first to observe morbid processes in the subacromial bursa was Jarjavay,[95] who on the basis of a few cases gave a general description of subacromial bursitis. His views were modified and elaborated by Heineke[85] and Vogt.[205] Duplay[57] introduced the term "periarthritis humeroscapularis" to designate a disease picture characterized by stiffness and pain in the shoulder joint following a trauma. Duplay based his observations on cases of trauma to the shoulder joint and on other cases of stiffness in the shoulder following dislocation, which he had studied at autopsy. The pathological foundation for the disease was believed by Duplay to lie in the subacromial and subdeltoid bursa. He thought that the cause was probably destruction or fusion of the bursa.

Duplay's views, which were supported by his followers, Tillaux[201] and Desché,[50] were hotly disputed. His opponents, Gosselin and his pupil Duronea[58] and Desplats,[51] Pingaud and Charvot,[158] tried to prove that the periarthritis should be regarded as a rheumatic affection, neuritis, etc.

In Germany, Colley[41] and Küster[109] were of practically the same opinion regarding periarthritis humeroscapularis as Duplay. Roentgenography soon began to contribute to the problem of humeroscapular periarthritis. It was not long before calcium shadows began to be observed in the soft parts between the acromion and the greater tuberosity.[149] The same finding was made by Stieda,[193] who assumed that these calcium masses were situated in the wall and in the lumen of the subacromial bursa. These new findings were indiscriminately termed "bursitis calcarea subacromialis" or "subdeltoidea." The term "bursoliths" was even used by Haudek[78] and Holzknecht.[89] Later, however, as the condition showed a strong resemblance to humeroscapular periarthritis, it became entirely identified with the latter.

In America, Codman[35] made a very important contribution to the question when he drew attention to the important role played by changes in the supraspinatus in the clinical picture of subacromial bursitis. Codman was the first to point out that many cases of inability to abduct the arm are due to incomplete or complete ruptures of the supraspinatus tendon.

With Codman's findings it was proved that humeroscapular periarthritis was not only a disease condition localized in the subacromial bursa, but that pathological changes also occurred in the tendon aponeurosis of the shoulder joint. This theory was further supported by Wrede,[217] who, on the basis of one surgical case and several cases in which roentgenograms had revealed calcium shadows in the region of the greater tuberosity, was able to show that the calcium deposits were localized in the supraspinatus tendon.

More and more disease conditions in the region of the shoulder joint have gradually been distinguished and separated from the general concept, periarthritis humeroscapularis. For example, Sievers[185] drew attention to the fact that arthritis deformans in the acromioclavicular joint may give a clinical picture reminiscent of periarthritis humeroscapularis. Bettman[20] and Meyer and Kessler[129] pointed to the occurrence of deforming changes in the intertubercular sulcus, the canal in which the biceps tendon glides. Payr[152] attempted to isolate the clinical picture which appears when the shoulder joint without any previous trauma is immobilized too long in an unsuitable position. Julliard[102] demonstrated apophysitis in the coracoid process (coracoiditis) as forming a special subdivision of periarthritis. Wellisch[212] described apophysitis at the insertion of the deltoid muscle on the humerus, giving it the name of "deltoidalgia." Schär and Zweifel[182] described deforming changes in connection with certain cases of os acromiale.

A number of authors recognized subacromial impingement as a cause of chronic disability of the shoulder (Codman,[35] Armstrong,[4] Hammond,[76, 77] McLaughlin,[124] Moseley,[133] Smith-Petersen and colleagues,[190] and Watson-Jones[207]). These authors proposed complete acromionectomy[4, 52, 76, 77, 207] and lateral acromionectomy[124, 190] for relief of these symptoms. The term "impingement syndrome" was popularized by Charles Neer in 1972.[136] In 100 dissected scapulae, Neer found evidence of mechanical impingement in 11 with a "characteristic ridge of proliferative spurs and excrescences on the undersurface of the anterior process (of the acromion), apparently caused by repeated impingement of the rotator cuff and the humeral head, with traction of the coracoacromial ligament . . . Without exception it was the anterior lip and undersurface of the anterior third that was involved." Neer emphasized that the supraspinatus insertion to the greater tuberosity and the bicipital groove lie anterior to the coracoacromial arch with the shoulder in the neutral position and that with forward flexion of the shoulder these structures must pass beneath the arch, providing the opportunity for impingement. He introduced the concept of a continuum in the impingement syndrome from chronic bursitis and partial tears to complete tears of the supraspinatus tendon, which may extend to involve rupture of other parts of the cuff. He pointed out that the physical and plain radiographic findings were not reliable in differentiating chronic bursitis and partial tears from complete tears. Importantly, he emphasized that patients with partial tears seemed more prone to increased shoulder stiffness and that surgery in this situation was inadvisable until the stiffness had resolved. He described the temporary relief of pain resulting from subacromial injection of lidocaine, which is helpful in substantiating the diagnosis and in predicting the effectiveness of surgical decompression.

Neer described three different stages of the impingement syndrome. In Stage 1, reversible edema and hemorrhage are present in a patient under 25 years of age. In Stage 2, fibrosis and tendinitis affect the rotator cuff of a patient typically in the 25- to 40-year age group. Pain often recurs with activity. In Stage 3, bone spurs and tendon ruptures are present in the individual over 40 years of age. He emphasized the importance of nonoperative management of cuff tendinitis. If surgery was performed, Neer pointed out the need to preserve a secure acromial origin of the deltoid, smooth resection of the undersurface of the anteroinferior acromion, careful inspection for other sources of impingement (such as the undersurface of the acromioclavicular joint), and careful postoperative rehabilitation.[136, 137, 139]

Anatomy

The anatomy relative to the impingement syndrome includes the coracoacromial arch, the subacromial–subdeltoid bursa, the cuff tendons, the long head of the biceps, and the upper surface of the humerus (Fig. 15–1). The coracoacromial arch includes two scapular processes—the coracoid and the acromion. The coracoacromial ligament connects these processes and is continuous with the less dense clavipectoral fascia. Passage of the cuff tendons and proximal humerus under this arch is facilitated by the subacromial–subdeltoid bursa, which normally is not a space but rather two serosal surfaces (one on the undersurface of the acromion and deltoid and the other on the cuff) lubricated by synovial fluid to slide easily on each other. Deep to the bursa lies the rotator cuff, with tendinous components of the subscapularis, supraspinatus, infraspinatus, and teres minor along with its subjacent capsular component (Fig. 15–2). The ten-

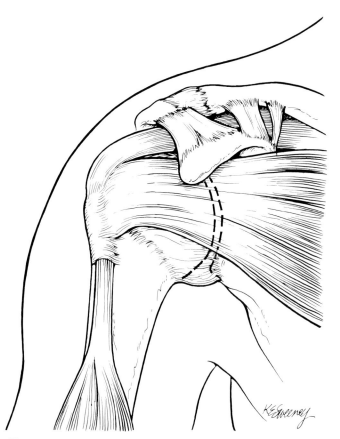

Figure 15–1. Anatomy relative to the impingement syndrome. The supraspinatus tendon is seen passing beneath the coracoacromial arch.

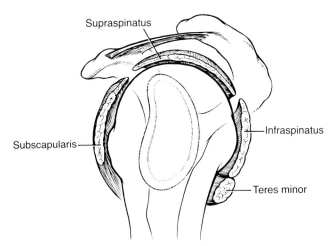

Figure 15-2. Sagittal view of the normal shoulder. Note the close anatomical relationship between the coracoacromial arch and underlying supraspinatus tendon.

dons of these muscles blend and fuse with one another as they cross the joint; they attach to the lesser tuberosity, the greater tuberosity, and the transverse humeral ligament that bridges the bicipital groove. The long head tendon of the biceps penetrates the rotator cuff between the subscapularis and supraspinatus tendons at the rotator interval, which is bridged in part by the coracohumeral ligament. The cuff itself is continuous in the form of a sheath around the biceps tendon. As described by Neer, the supraspinatus insertion along with the subjacent biceps tendon and upper infraspinatus pass beneath the coracoacromial arch with most normal use of the shoulder.

The functions of the rotator cuff include (1) stabilizing the shoulder, for example, against the actions of the prime movers (e.g., the deltoid and pectoralis major), preventing excessive anterior, posterior, inferior, or superior motion, and (2) adding power to the motions of glenohumeral rotation and elevation. A proposed third function of the rotator cuff is containing the synovial fluid, thereby enhancing joint cartilage nutrition.[136]

TENDON VASCULARITY

Lindblom[114] proposed that the rotator cuff is hypovascular or avascular near the supraspinatus attachment to the greater tuberosity, the "critical zone"[35] where many cuff lesions occur. Moseley and Goldie[134] used microradiography and histology to study the vascular supply of the cuff in cadaver subjects ranging in age from 33 to 70. They concluded that the critical zone is not significantly less vascular than the remainder of the cuff, but rather that this area corresponds to the zone of anastomoses between the osseous and tendinous vessels. The morphology of this vascular pattern did not appear to change with age. The major vessels contributing to the cuff blood supply are the anterior humeral circumflex, the suprascapular, and the subscapular arteries. Iannotti and coworkers[90] have

detected substantial blood flow in the critical zone of the rotator cuff using the laser Doppler.

Two mechanisms for compromise of supraspinatus blood flow have been proposed: (1) Rathbun and Macnab[168] found in their injection studies that glenohumeral adduction puts the supraspinatus tendon under tension and "wrings out" its vessels. (2) Sigholm and colleagues[186] used a micropipette infusion technique to measure the effect of active shoulder flexion on subacromial pressure. They found that the normal resting pressure of 8 mm Hg was elevated to 39 mm Hg by flexion to 45 degrees and to 56 mm Hg by the addition of a 1-kg weight to the hand in the elevated position. If sustained, these pressures are sufficiently high to substantially reduce the tendon microcirculation.[122] However, since the shoulder is frequently moved, it is unclear whether either of these mechanisms could produce ischemia of sufficient duration to cause tendon damage.

THE ACROMION

The acromion arises from three separate centers of ossification—a preacromion, a mesoacromion, and a meta-acromion.[31, 135, 180a] These centers of ossification are usually united by age 22. When these centers fail to unite, the united portion is referred to as an os acromiale. This condition may have been first recognized by Schär and Zweifel[182] in 1936, as was mentioned by Pettersson.[157] Grant[70] found that 16 of 194 cadavers aged over 30 years demonstrated incomplete fusion of the acromion; the condition was bilateral in 5 subjects and unilateral in 11 subjects. In a large review of 1000 radiographs, Liberson[111] found unfused acromia in 2.7 per cent; of these, 62 per cent were bilateral. Most commonly the lesion is a failure of fusion of the mesoacromion to the meta-acromion. He found the inferosuperior view (now known as the axillary view) to be most helpful in revealing the condition. Impingement may arise from both the downward hinging of the acromion and from spurs or soft tissue proliferation at the nonunion site. The size of the unfused fragment may be substantial—up to 5 × 2 cm.[136] Resection of a fragment this large creates a serious challenge for deltoid reattachment. Norris and coworkers[146] and Bigliani and associates[22] have pointed to the association of impingement syndrome and unfused acromial epiphysis. Mudge and coworkers[135] found that of 145 shoulders identified as having cuff tears, 9 of them, or 6 per cent, had an os acromiale. This figure is higher than that obtained by Liberson[111] for unselected scapulae (2.7 per cent).

Variations of acromial shape are commonly observed in patients with impingement and cuff tears (Fig. 15–3).[22, 136] Bigliani and colleagues[21] studied 140 shoulders in 71 cadavers. The average age was 74.4 years. They identified three types of acromion: Type I (flat) in 17 per cent, Type II (curved) in 43 per cent, and Type III (hooked) in 40 per cent. Fifty-eight per cent of the

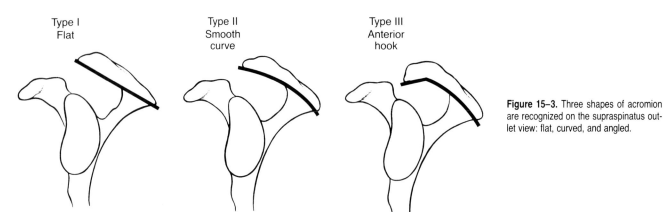

Figure 15-3. Three shapes of acromion are recognized on the supraspinatus outlet view: flat, curved, and angled.

cadavers had the same type of acromion on each side. Thirty-three per cent of the rotator cuffs had full-thickness tears, of which 73 per cent were seen in the presence of Type III acromions, 24 per cent in Type II, and 3 per cent in Type I. The anterior slope of the acromion with cuff tears was 28.7 degrees, whereas the slope of the acromion without cuff tears was 22.7 degrees. Morrison and Bigliani[132] reviewed 200 modified lateral scapular views in a series of patients with shoulder problems. Eighty per cent of patients with rotator cuff tears had hooked acromia; the remaining 20 per cent had curved acromia. Patients with a clinical picture of impingement but without cuff tears had a normal distribution of acromial shapes (only 30 to 40 per cent hooked acromia). Finally, in 50 patients having open acromioplasties, 70 per cent with full-thickness cuff tears had hooked acromia.

Although these data indicate a strong association between cuff tears and hooked acromia, it cannot be determined if the acromial shape was caused by or resulted from the cuff tear. If the acromial slope is measured to the most anterior part of the acromial undersurface, secondary proliferative spurs and excrescences on the undersurface of the anterior acromion could yield a measurement indicating a greater slope. Is "hooking" of the acromion a cause of impingement, a result of impingement, or both?

The anterior extension of the acromion beyond the extrapolated anterior contour of the clavicle may contribute to impingement with the shoulder in the flexed position. Resection of this anterior prominence is illustrated in Neer's original article.[136]

A final anatomical feature of importance is the acromial branch of the thoracoacromial artery. This artery runs in close relation to the coracoacromial ligament and usually is transected in the course of an acromioplasty and coracoacromial ligament section.

Classification

It is evident that in the normal shoulder the cuff mechanism is intimately applied to the coracoacromial arch, separated only by the thin lubricating surfaces of the bursa. Compression and friction can be minimized by several factors—a shape of the coracoacromial arch that allows unimpaired passage of the subjacent cuff mechanism, a normal undersurface of the acromioclavicular joint, a normal bursa, the normal function of the humeral head depressors (the rotator cuff musculature and biceps tendon), normal capsular laxity, and a smooth upper surface of the cuff mechanism.

A number of factors may alter this normal mechanism, thereby increasing the encroachment, impingement, or wear of the coracoacromial arch on the cuff mechanism. Some of these are listed in Table 15-1. The importance of such a list lies in pointing out the complexity of the subacromial and cuff mechanisms and the wide variety of factors that can adversely affect them.

Incidence and Mechanisms of Injury

Neer[136] noted that elevation of the arm, particularly in internal rotation, causes the critical area of the cuff to pass under the coracoacromial arch. In cadaver dissections he found that 11 of 100 scapulae (age unknown) showed alterations attributable to mechanical impingement. These changes included a characteristic ridge of proliferative spurs and excrescences on the undersurface of the anterior process. It is significant to note that Neer proposed that these changes were "*caused* by repeated impingement of the rotator cuff and humeral head, with traction on the coracoacromial ligament" (italics added). He also pointed out that at 80 degrees of abduction, "excrescences on the undersurface of the anterior margin of the acromion may impinge on the cuff."

In the Shoulder Clinic at the University of Washington, afflictions of the cuff tendons account for almost one-third of our new patient visits. Of patients with cuff tendon involvement, about one-third relate the onset of their symptoms to their work. Certain occupations seem to be particularly problematic, including tree pruning, fruit picking, nursing, grocery clerking,

Table 15-1. FACTORS POTENTIALLY INCREASING ROTATOR CUFF IMPINGEMENT

Structural

Acromioclavicular joint
    Congenital abnormality
    Degenerative spurs

Acromion
    Unfused (bipartite acromion)
    Abnormal shape (flat or overhanging)
    Degenerative spur
    Nonunion of fracture
    Malunion of fracture

Coracoid
    Congenital abnormality
    Post-traumatic or postsurgical change in shape or location

Bursa
    Primary inflammatory bursitis (e.g., rheumatoid arthritis)
    Chronic thickening from previous injury/inflammation/injection
    Pins, wires, sutures, and other foreign materials projecting into the bursal space

Rotator cuff
    Thickening related to chronic calcium deposits
    Thickening from retraction of partial-thickness tears
    Flaps and other irregularities of upper surface due to partial or complete tearing
    Postoperative or post-traumatic scarring

Humerus
    Congenital abnormalities or fracture malunions producing relative or absolute prominence of the greater tuberosity
    Abnormally inferior position of a humeral head prosthesis producing relative prominence of the greater tuberosity

Functional

Scapula
    Abnormal position
        Thoracic kyphosis
        Acromioclavicular separation
    Abnormal motion
        Paralysis (e.g., of trapezius)
        Fascioscapulohumeral muscular dystrophy
        Restriction of motion at the scapulothoracic joint

Loss of normal head depression mechanism
    Rotator cuff weakness (e.g., suprascapular nerve palsy or C5–C6 radiculopathy)
    Rotator cuff tear (partial- or full-thickness)
    Constitutional or post-traumatic rotator cuff laxity
    Rupture of long head of biceps

Tightness of posterior shoulder capsule forcing the humeral head to rise up against the acromion during shoulder flexion

Capsular laxity

---

longshoring, warehousing, carpentry, and painting.[117] Another one-third relate the onset to some type of athletic activity such as throwing, tennis, skiing, and swimming. Richardson and associates[170] reviewed 137 of the best swimmers in the United States. The incidence of shoulder problems was 42 per cent. These authors calculated that the average national-level swimmer puts his or her shoulder through about 500,000 cycles per season. Although subluxation is a recognized problem in this group, many were found to have symptoms and signs suggesting impingement syndrome. The technique an athlete uses has a major relationship to the development of or freedom from

symptoms, as discussed by Richardson and coworkers,[170] Albright and colleagues,[1] Cofield and Simonet,[38] Penny and Welsh,[154] Neer and Welsh,[142] and Penny and Smith.[153] The final one-third have no recognized precipitating factor triggering the onset of their cuff tendon involvement. This third group tends to be older than the first two (averaging about 60 years).

In some of these situations, it appears that the impingement syndrome was precipitated by a definite injury. In the majority, however, it seems to represent the cumulative effect of many passages of the rotator cuff beneath the coracoacromial arch. Congenital abnormalities or degenerative alterations in the arch would increase the chances of damage to the cuff tendons. Scarring of the subacromial bursa and cuff tendons reduces the space available for the cuff tendons.

Cofield and Simonet[38] cautioned that the impingement syndrome can be confused with the "slightly frozen shoulder." Over the last several years in our shoulder clinic, we have been impressed with the common association of signs of impingement with shoulder stiffness, particularly stiffness involving the posterior capsule. With normal shoulder motion, the humeral head remains centered in the glenoid (Fig. 15–4 A). Stiffness of the posterior capsule may aggravate the impingement process by forcing the humeral head upward against the anteroinferior acromion as the shoulder is flexed (the humeral head "rolling up" on the posterior capsule like a yo-yo climbing a string) (Fig. 15–4B).

As previously noted, the rotator cuff functions to stabilize the shoulder against the actions of the deltoid and pectoralis major muscles. Cuff weakness from disuse, cervical radiculopathy, suprascapular neuropathy, or cuff fiber failure will weaken the humeral head depressor mechanism. In the presence of a weakened cuff mechanism, contraction of the deltoid causes upward displacement of the humeral head so that it squeezes the remaining cuff against the coracoacromial arch.

As shown in Figure 15–5, some of the effects of impingement may further intensify impingement, producing a self-perpetuating process. For example, muscle or cuff tendon weakness causes impingement from loss of humeral head depressor function, leading to tendon damage and disuse atrophy and additional cuff weakness. As a second example, bursal thickening causes impingement from subacromial crowding producing thickening of the bursa. Finally, posterior capsular stiffness leads to impingement, disuse, and stiffness.

With respect to prevention, the observation that patients with characteristic impingement syndrome do respond to stretching and strengthening exercises suggests that these exercises may be useful in the prevention of impingement syndrome in athletes, workers, and others. These exercises may be helpful in maintaining the strength of the humeral depressor mechanism and in preventing posterior capsular tightness.

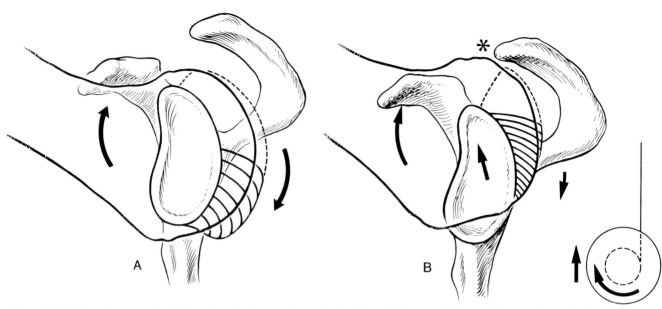

Figure 15–4. Stiffness of the posterior glenohumeral capsule is commonly associated with signs of impingement. *A,* A normally lax posterior capsule allows the humeral head to remain centered in the glenoid with shoulder flexion. *B,* Stiffness of the posterior glenohumeral capsule will aggravate the impingement process by forcing the humeral head upward against the anteroinferior acromion as the shoulder is flexed. This upward translation in association with rotation is analogous to the action of a spinning yo-yo climbing a string.

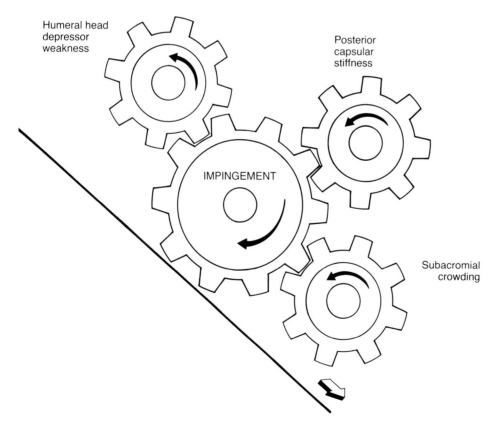

Figure 15–5. Normal shoulder function is dependent on normal function of the humeral head depressors, normal capsular laxity, and adequate subacromial space. Some of the effects of impingement (weakness of the humeral head depressors, stiffness of the posterior capsule, and crowding of the subacromial space with thickened bursa) may further intensify impingement, producing a self-perpetuating process.

Proper techniques in sport and work are additional important factors in the prevention of these shoulder problems.

Clinical Presentation

Patients with impingement syndrome usually do not present to a physician acutely but only after their shoulder symptoms have failed to resolve with time, rest, and trying to "work it out." They usually complain of functional losses due to pain, stiffness, weakness, and catching when their arm is used in the flexed and internally rotated position. Symptoms may also include difficulties in sleeping on the affected side and in carrying out routine activities of daily living, such as getting a gallon of milk out of the refrigerator. The pain is often felt down the lateral aspect of the upper arm near the deltoid insertion, over the anterior proximal humerus, or in the periacromial area.

Inspection of the shoulder may reveal deltoid or cuff atrophy, particularly if the condition has been chronic. Palpation usually reveals little if any tenderness. This is in marked contrast to the sharply localized tenderness characteristic of acute calcific tendinitis. Range of motion is often limited, particularly in internal rotation and in cross-body adduction, indicating some degree of posterior capsular tightness. Passive motion through the 60- to 90-degree arc of flexion may be accompanied by pain and crepitus, accentuated as the shoulder is moved in and out of internal rotation. Active elevation of the shoulder is usually more uncomfortable than passive elevation. Pain on maximum forward flexion is frequently seen with the impingement syndrome but is not particularly specific in that it may be associated with a tight shoulder from any cause. Strength testing of the shoulder may reveal weakness of flexion and external rotation; this weakness may be the result of disuse or of tendon damage. Pain on resisted abduction or external rotation may also indicate that the integrity of the cuff tendons is compromised. In evaluating a painful shoulder it is useful to differentiate among signs of *subacromial impingement* (subacromial crepitus on flexion and rotation), signs of *tightness* (limited range of motion), and signs of *tendon involvement* (atrophy, weakness, and pain on resisted motion).

The relief of pain on the subacromial injection of lidocaine is useful for demonstrating that the structures of the subacromial zone are a source of the patient's discomfort.[136]

ASSOCIATED CONDITIONS

The impingement syndrome may be associated with cervical radiculopathy, acromioclavicular joint arthritis, and both partial- and full-thickness rotator cuff tears as well as with various degrees of severity of stiff or "frozen" shoulder. Each of these associated conditions may modify the clinical presentation of the impingement syndrome.

Cuff Imaging Techniques

Plain radiographs may show subacromial sclerosis (the so-called "sourcil" or "eyebrow" sign) from loading of the undersurface of the acromion in the impingement process (Fig. 15–6). A true lateral view of the scapula modified by angling the beam caudally by 10 to 40 degrees may reveal variations in the shape of the undersurface of the acromion (Fig. 15–7); this is the supraspinatus outlet view described by Neer, Morrison, Bigliani, and others. Radiographs may also reveal evidence of some of the conditions associated with the impingement syndrome, such as acromioclavicular arthritis, chronic calcific tendinitis, tuberosity displacement, and the like (Figs. 15–8 to 15–11). An axillary view is helpful in visualizing a bipartite acromion. Ultrasound examination of the rotator cuff reliably demonstrates the location and extent of cuff tears over 1 cm in size.[118] Future improvements in ultrasound technique and technology may permit the reliable diagnosis of smaller tears. Shoulder arthrography demonstrates the presence of leaks in the cuff and may demonstrate partial-thickness cuff defects at the deep surface (Fig. 15–12). Owing to the fact that partial-thickness tears of the rotator cuff may produce symptoms and signs identical with those found in the impingement syndrome without cuff tear, arthrography is a valuable adjunct in the complete evaluation of patients with this syndrome. Jackson[94] has provided some preliminary evidence that the bursal volume is diminished in the impingement syndrome. This is consistent with the observation that these shoulders are frequently stiff. Arthroscopy may reveal defects of the rotator cuff involving the deep surface. As yet, no

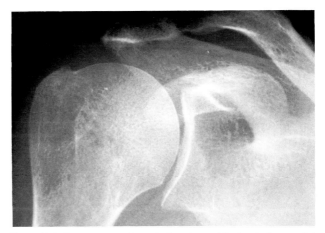

Figure 15–6. Roentgenogram demonstrating subacromial sclerosis, the so-called "sourcil" or "eyebrow" sign, from chronic loading of the undersurface of the acromion in the impingement process. Corresponding sclerosis or cystic changes involving the greater tuberosity may also occur.

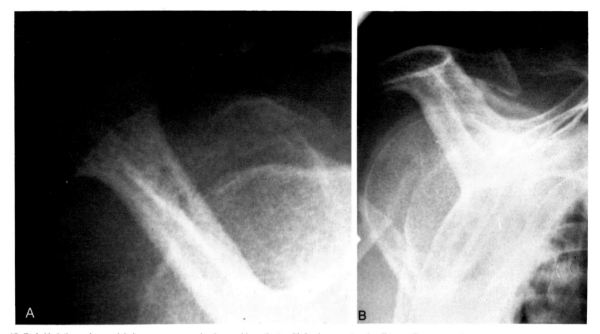

Figure 15–7. *A,* Variations of acromial shape are commonly observed in patients with impingement and cuff tears. The supraspinatus outlet view is helpful in defining this anatomy. *B,* In this arthrogram (lateral view), one can see indentation of the supraspinatus by the anteroinferior acromion.

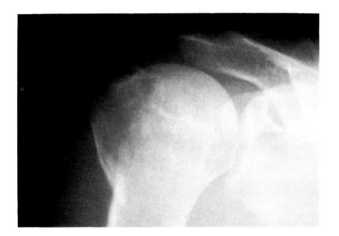

Figure 15–8. An anteroposterior roentgenogram shows malunion of a fractured greater tuberosity and malunion, which caused subacromial crowding on abduction and refractory impingement symptoms.

Figure 15–9. This patient developed refractory impingement due to the relative prominence of fracture fixation wires. The symptoms resolved upon removal of the subacromial wires.

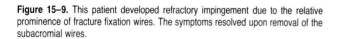

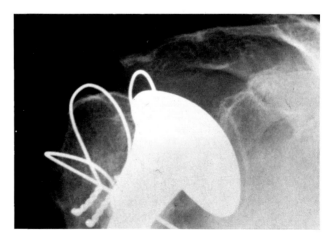

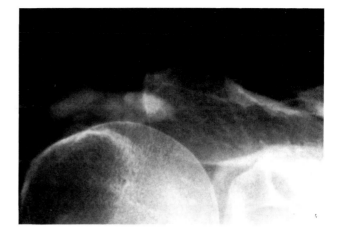

Figure 15–10. This anteroposterior roentgenogram shows chronic calcific deposits in the supraspinatus tendon. These deposits may increase the thickness of the tendon and thereby contribute to subacromial impingement.

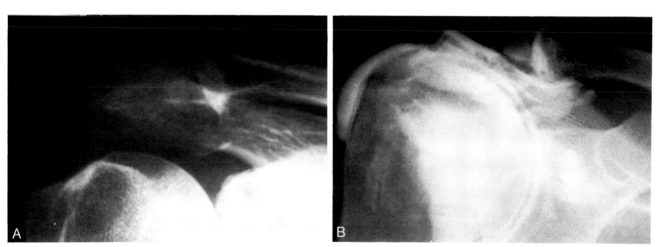

Figure 15–11. *A,* This anteroposterior roentgenogram shows acromioclavicular joint arthritis. *B,* An arthrogram in the same patient reveals dye leakage into the acromioclavicular joint ("geyser sign"), confirming the clinical suspicion of a rotator cuff tear. Note the indentation of the cuff caused by the acromioclavicular joint osteophytes.

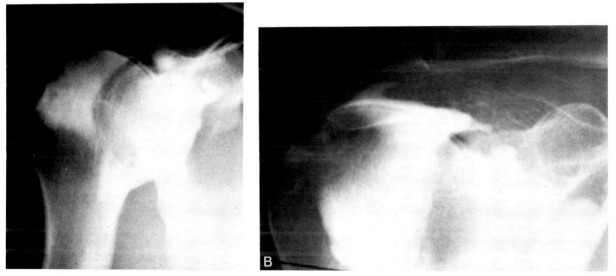

Figure 15–12. Arthrograms of two different shoulders showing partial thickness, deep surface tears of the cuff. *A,* Note the "feathered" edge of the contrast material laterally, indicating the loss of the normal insertion at the base of the tuberosity. The absence of filling of the bursa suggests that the tendon defect is not full thickness. These findings were confirmed at surgery. *B,* Another patient had a falciform-shaped deep surface tear.

nonsurgical technique demonstrates tears of the cuff midsubstance. Seeger and coworkers[184] and Kneeland and associates[108] provide initial information on the use of magnetic resonance to image the cuff; however, the sensitivity and selectivity of this method are undetermined at present. Bone scans, electromyography, and computed tomography (CT) scans may be helpful in excluding other possibilities in the differential diagnosis.

Complications

The principal complications of impingement syndrome are rotator cuff tears. Neer[137] found 95 per cent of cuff tears to be associated with impingement. The relationship between the impingement syndrome and cuff tendon fiber failure is apparent but, to a certain extent, problematic. It has been proposed that prolonged and repeated impingement "wears out" the rotator cuff and produces a cuff defect, much as the knees on a child's blue jeans wear through from months of heavy use. However, it is also true that weakness and deficiency of the rotator cuff deprives the shoulder of its normal head depression mechanism, which counterbalances the upward pull of the deltoid in motions of flexion and abduction.[159, 162] Even small amounts of weakness in this depressor mechanism may allow for some upward riding of the humerus against the acromion, exacerbating impingement and increasing cuff wear. If partial defects in the cuff or biceps tendons are managed by repeated steroid injections, persistent impingement and cuff damage may go unnoticed.

Differential Diagnosis

The differential diagnosis of impingement syndrome includes all causes of shoulder pain and dysfunction. These may be divided into (1) other afflictions of the cuff tendon and (2) causes of shoulder pain extrinsic to the cuff tendons. The first group includes tendinitis (acute or chronic tendon inflammation) from some cause other than impingement, tendon strain (minor tendon tears), or larger partial or complete tendon tears. The picture of acute *calcific tendinitis* is distinct, with local tenderness and "paralyzing pain." Chronic calcific deposits in the cuff tendons may increase the size of the tendon, predisposing the shoulder to subacromial impingement. Calcium deposits may be identified by internal and external rotation radiographs using soft-tissue technique. *Cuff tendon strain* is not detectable by imaging techniques; it must be diagnosed from a history of overuse and from the physical findings of pain on resisted motion or passive stretching of the tendon. *Cuff tears*, particularly if they are not large, may produce findings virtually identical with cuff tendinitis or cuff strain. Arthrography, ultrasonography,

bursoscopy, and arthroscopy may each help to image a substantial defect in the cuff surface, although reliably imaging small defects is difficult. Cofield and Simonet[38] reported a 19-year-old athlete who presented with impingement symptoms and who was found to have a partial-thickness cuff tear on arthrography. In that the bursa is always involved with the impingement syndrome, *bursitis* is not viewed as a separate entity unless there is primary involvement such as in septic bursitis, gouty bursitis, or rheumatoid bursitis. The long head tendon of the biceps is frequently involved in the impingement syndrome. *Biceps tendinitis* is evidenced by anterior shoulder pain on shoulder flexion and extension while the biceps is tensed (the "sawing test") and by tenderness in the bicipital groove.

Differential diagnostic possibilities for "impingement-like" pain arising extrinsic to the cuff include *cervical radiculopathy,* which often produces pain in the superolateral shoulder, especially at night or on turning of the head. This diagnosis can usually be made by the history, findings of spondylosis and radiculopathy on physical examination, and, if necessary, electromyography. Cervical spine radiographs so commonly demonstrate C5–C6 changes in the absence of symptoms that this examination lacks specificity. *Brachial neuritis* involving the suprascapular nerve or suprascapular nerve entrapment may produce shoulder pain and weakness and an impingement-type picture owing to loss of the head depressor function of the supraspinatus and infraspinatus.[6, 119, 120]

As described previously, *acromioclavicular arthritis* may both imitate and contribute to an impingement syndrome. Joint tenderness on physical examination, relief on selective lidocaine injection, and coned-down radiographs may help establish the diagnosis of acromioclavicular arthritis.

Glenohumeral instability is an important diagnosis to exclude, particularly in the young, athletic patient with symptoms suggesting impingement. Certainly a lax cuff and capsular mechanism can increase the opportunity for the humeral head to displace upward and for the cuff to be encroached upon by the coracoacromial arch. Standard tests for glenohumeral instability, particularly seeking those maneuvers that reproduce the patient's chief complaint, are helpful. Our experience suggests that the coexistence of multidirectional glenohumeral instability with a mild to moderate impingement syndrome is not unusual. Acromioplasty is probably not appropriate in this patient group. *Abnormalities of the joint surfaces* (e.g., previous intra-articular fracture or degenerative joint disease) may produce pain, stiffness, weakness, and catching but should be distinguished from impingement with routine radiographs (Fig. 15–13). As described previously, a *stiff* or *"frozen" shoulder* is a frequent concomitant of an impingement syndrome and is recognized by limitation of active and passive ranges of motion (especially in internal rotation and cross-body adduction) in the presence of normal glenohumeral joint surfaces. *Snapping scapula* may produce catching on shoulder use.

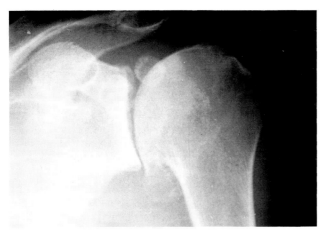

Figure 15–13. Degenerative joint disease may produce pain, stiffness, weakness, and catching. This condition can be readily diagnosed with radiographs.

In contrast to the catching and crepitus from impingement, this condition produces symptoms at the superomedial border of the scapula on shrugging the shoulder with the arm at the side.

Methods of Treatment

NONOPERATIVE MANAGEMENT

In his article on anterior acromioplasty, Neer[136] states, "Many patients . . . were suspected of having impingement, but responded well to conservative treatment." During the period covered by his report he operated on an average of only 10 shoulders a year with this diagnosis. The effectiveness of nonoperative management is worthy of emphasis!

An acute impingement syndrome (e.g., from a fall or from overuse in tennis or throwing) usually responds to a nonoperative program of time, rest, nonsteroidal anti-inflammatory medications, and general shoulder rehabilitation.[37, 137] Heat, cold, massage, pulsed electromagnetic field therapy, and acupuncture have been suggested as therapy, but it is difficult to ascertain their therapeutic effectiveness.[18, 24, 171]

It seems to be the common experience that subacromial injections of corticosteroids produce symptomatic relief in many patients with supraspinatus tendinitis.[88] However, many reports concerning steroid injections are not well controlled for the specific diagnosis or the criteria of success. Certain control studies have been carried out. Withington and coworkers[216] reported a double-blind trial of steroid injections for supraspinatus tendinitis and found no evidence of the efficacy of such treatment. Valtonen[204] found no difference between subacromial and gluteal injections of steroids in the treatment of supraspinatus tendinitis. Berry and colleagues[18] compared acupuncture, physiotherapy, steroid injections, and anti-inflammatory medications in the treatment of painful stiff shoulder and found no

difference among these treatments. It is likely that steroid injections in or near the cuff and biceps tendons may produce tendon atrophy or may reduce the ability of damaged tendon to repair itself. Such changes have been well documented in other tissues.[116, 173, 202] Ford and DeBender[65] reported 13 patients who developed 15 ruptured tendons subsequent to injection of steroid in or about tendons; two of these were supraspinati. Other authors have reported spontaneous ruptures of the Achilles tendon and patellar tendon after steroid injection.[14, 92, 110, 126, 189] The harmful effects of repetitive intra-articular injection of steroids have been noted by several investigators, including Behrens and colleagues[15] Cruess and associates,[45] Mankin and Conger,[121] Salter and coworkers,[179] and Sweetnam.[196] Although Matthews and colleagues[123] failed to find a deleterious effect of corticosteroid injections on rabbit patellar tendons, Kennedy and Willis[103] found a substantial effect in the rabbit Achilles tendon. They concluded that physiological doses of local steroid placed directly in a *normal* tendon weaken it significantly for up to 14 days following the injection. This weakening was attributed to collagen necrosis. In the context of the impingement syndrome, in which one of the consequences is rupture of damaged tendons, the risk-to-benefit ratio of each steroid injection must be carefully weighed.[46, 103] In this light, one can appreciate the potential hazard of making a diagnosis of "bursitis" or "bicipital tendinitis" and treating the situation with repeated steroid injections until the reality of a major cuff or tendon rupture becomes inescapable.

Although most authors describe the importance of conservative or nonoperative management, the optimal nonoperative protocol has not been defined. In his original article on the impingement syndrome in 1972,[136] Neer stated that patients were advised not to have an acromioplasty until the stiffness of the shoulder had disappeared and the disability had persisted for at least nine months. Neviaser and coworkers[145] described a nonoperative program that consists of moist heat, anti-inflammatory medication, restricted exercise, and avoidance of the overhead position. If nonoperative treatment produces no response within six weeks, Neer[136] recommended the use of arthrography to evaluate the possibility of a full-thickness cuff tear. If arthrography is positive, surgery is advised. Jobe and Moynes[98] have described a comprehensive rehabilitation program for cuff injuries, and Kerlan and coworkers[105] have outlined a rehabilitation program for throwers. Pappas and associates,[150, 151] Richardson and coworkers[170] and Fowler[66] have described other rehabilitation approaches for athletes. Hawkins and Kennedy[84] and Cofield and Simonet[38] emphasized the importance of nonoperative treatment in athletes. It seems to be particularly important to avoid repeated motions of the shoulder in which the humerus makes a greater than 10-degree angle above the scapular spine. Higher angles of glenohumeral elevation bring the acromion and humerus into close proximity. Expert throwers achieve the "overhead" motion by tilting the thorax to the opposite side, thereby avoiding impingement. Expert swimmers use proper body roll and shoulder extension.[1, 5] The low success rate in returning athletes to competition after surgical decompression[200] tends to reinforce the importance of nonoperative management in this population. Stretching, strengthening, and technique modification are the most effective methods for managing impingement in the athlete. Similar comments apply to workers who are required to use their shoulders in positions aggravating impingement: "exercises and job modification before acromion modification."

SURGICAL DECOMPRESSION

In 1972 Neer[136] described the indications for surgical decompression as (1) long-term disability from chronic bursitis and partial tears of the supraspinatus tendon or (2) complete tears of the supraspinatus. He pointed out that the physical and roentgenographic findings in these two categories were indistinguishable, including crepitus and tenderness over the supraspinatus with a painful arc of active elevation from 70 to 120 degrees and pain at the anterior edge of the acromion on forced elevation. Neer's 1983 report[137] listed the indications for acromioplasty as (1) a positive arthrogram (the acromioplasty to be done at the time of the cuff repair), (2) patients older than 40 years with negative arthrograms but persistent disability for one year despite adequate conservative treatment (including efforts to eliminate stiffness), provided that the pain can be temporarily eliminated by the subacromial injection of lidocaine, (3) certain patients under 40 with refractory Stage II impingement lesions, and (4) patients undergoing other procedures for conditions in which impingement is likely (such as total shoulder replacement in patients with rheumatoid arthritis or old fracture). The purpose of acromioplasty was to relieve mechanical impingement, preventing wear at the critical area of the rotator cuff. Surgery was not considered until any stiffness had resolved and until the disability had persisted for at least nine months. Subacromial injection of lidocaine provided a "useful guide of what the procedure would accomplish." Even in patients who had had a previous lateral acromionectomy with continuing symptoms, Neer considered anterior acromioplasty, having found that many still had problems related to subacromial impingement. His indications for resection of the lateral clavicle included (1) arthritis of the acromioclavicular joint, (2) exposure of more of the supraspinatus in a cuff repair, and (3) nonarthritic enlargement of the acromioclavicular joint resulting in impingement on the supraspinatus (in this situation only the undersurface of the joint was resected).[137] Finally, Neer found that the rare patient with an irreparable tear in the rotator cuff can be made more comfortable and can gain surprising function if impingement is relieved and if the deltoid remains strong.[137]

Various surgical approaches have been recommended for treatment of the impingement syndrome. In his classic article, Neer[136] described approaching the shoulder through a 9-cm incision made in Langer's lines from the anterior edge of the acromion to a point just lateral to the coracoid. The deltoid is split for 5 cm distal to the acromioclavicular joint in the direction of its fibers. It is then dissected from the front of the acromion and the acromioclavicular joint capsule. The stump of the deltoid's tendinous origin is elevated upward and preserved for the deltoid repair. Using an osteotome, a wedge-shaped piece of bone .09 cm × 2.0 cm is resected from the anterior undersurface of the acromion, along with the entire attachment of the coracoacromial ligament. If acromioclavicular osteophytes are present, the distal 2.5 cm of the clavicle are also excised along with the prominences on the acromial side of the joint. If supraspinatus tears are found, they are repaired to humeral bone near the greater tuberosity. The deltoid is carefully repaired to the acromioclavicular joint capsule, the trapezius, and its tendon of origin.

Findings at surgery, according to Neer,[136] include proliferative bursitis, prominence of the coracoacromial ligament and the anterior third of the acromion, acromial excrescences, irregularities in the greater tuberosity, minor calcium deposits, bicipital tendinitis, and acromioclavicular arthritis.

When impingement is associated with an unfused acromial epiphysis, Neer[137] recommends resection of small unfused centers. He internally fixes larger centers so that the acromion is tilted up to avoid impingement.

Other approaches to cuff decompression include coracoacromial ligament section,[84, 94, 106, 154] resection arthroplasty of the acromioclavicular joint,[106] extensive acromionectomy,* and combined procedures such as acromioplasty, incision of the coracoacromial ligament, acromioclavicular resection arthroplasty, and excision of the intra-articular portion of the biceps tendon with tenodesis of the distal portion of the bicipital groove.[73, 145, 164] Comparison of the results of these procedures is difficult owing to the heterogenous patient groups and varying methods of evaluation. Currently emphasis has been placed on performing anteroinferior acromioplasty with coracoacromial ligament section and preserving the deltoid origin.

The results of open surgical decompression indicate a high percentage of improvement. In 16 patients with chronic bursitis with fraying or partial tear of the supraspinatus, Neer[136] found that 15 attained satisfactory results (no significant pain, less than 20 degrees of limitation of overhead extension, and at least 75 per cent of normal strength). Thorling and coworkers[199] found good to excellent results in 33 of 51 patients following acromioplasty (11 required resection of the acromioclavicular joint as well).

Arthroscopic acromioplasty has been performed, and techniques are being developed for controlling the

---

*See references 4, 52, 76, 77, 124, 130, 133, 190, 207.

adequacy of this procedure. Ellman[61] presented the initial results on 50 consecutive cases of arthroscopic acromioplasty for Stage II impingement without cuff tear (40 cases) and for full-thickness cuff tear (20 cases). Eighty-eight per cent of the patients had excellent or good results, and the rest were unsatisfactory at a one- to three-year follow-up. He pointed out that the technique was technically demanding. We have seen the effect of the learning curve: on one hand grossly inadequate arthroscopic acromioplasties and on the other hand a virtually total arthroscopic acromioplasty leaving a major compromise of the deltoid origin. Gartsman[68] reported his series of 100 arthroscopic subacromial decompressions. At an average of 18.5 months' follow-up, 85 shoulders were improved and 15 were failures, of which 9 required subsequent open acromioplasty. The procedure took longer than open acromioplasty and did not speed the patient's return to work or sport. Morrison[131] reported a series of arthroscopic acromioplasties in which the quality of the result was closely correlated with the conversion of a curved or hooked acromion (Types II or III) to a flat undersurface (Type I).

In every series of open surgical decompression there are patients who do not improve, even if the technique of the procedure seems appropriate. The incidence of these failures ranges from 3 to 11 per cent.[136, 160, 165, 199] In Post and Cohen's series, 11 per cent continued to have significant pain after surgery.[160, 161] Fifty-six per cent of those with weakness before surgery still had weakness postoperatively; 29 per cent of those with preoperative limitations of motion still had limitation of motion after surgery. The rate of return to high-level athletics or challenging occupations is lower. Tibone and colleagues[200] found that of 35 athletes having impingement syndrome treated by anterior acromioplasty, 20 per cent still had moderate to severe pain, and 9 per cent had pain at rest and with activities of daily living. Only 43 per cent returned to their preinjury level of competitive athletics, and only 4 of 18 returned to competitive throwing. Hawkins and coworkers[83] have shown that it is difficult for patients injured on the job to return to their original occupations following acromioplasty.

Why is this? Failure to achieve complete relief of symptoms through acromioplasty may indicate (1) incorrect diagnosis, (2) incomplete decompression, (3) failure of deltoid reattachment, (4) excessive removal of the acromion, (5) irreversible cuff pathology (partial-thickness tears, intratendinous scarring), (6) postoperative complications such as dense scarring between the cuff and the acromion, or (7) failure of rehabilitation. Many of these problems can leave the patient more symptomatic than before the surgery (Fig. 15–14).

Radical acromionectomy may worsen a patient's comfort and function. This procedure removes the origin of the deltoid muscle and facilitates scar formation between the deltoid muscle and the rotator cuff. Neer and Marberry have pointed out that a radical acromionectomy may seriously compromise shoulder

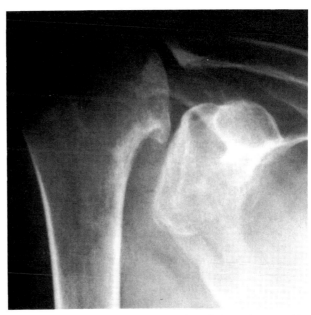

Figure 15–14. Anteroposterior roentgenogram after radical acromionectomy. This procedure removes the origin of the deltoid muscles and may fail to provide complete subacromial decompression. This patient's symptoms were much more severe after surgery than before.

function without achieving subacromial decompression.[140] In their series of 30 patients, all had marked shoulder weakness and almost all had persistent pain. In the 20 shoulders reoperated upon, all had a retracted and scarred middle deltoid that was adherent to the cuff and humerus. Fifteen of the patients had residual cuff tears. Attempts to reconstruct these severely damaged shoulders were disappointing. The effects of loss of the deltoid attachment and the permanent contracture could not be reversed. In addition, these authors observed a high incidence of wound problems and infections following the radical acromionectomy, which further complicated their attempts at revision.

To help understand some of the other causes of unsuccessful acromioplasty, Flugstad and coworkers[64] reviewed 19 patients referred to the University of Washington Shoulder Clinic because of persistent pain and stiffness after open acromioplasty performed elsewhere. The average age was 42; 16 were male. Eleven patients had a traumatic onset of their shoulder problem; eight of these were work related. The average time of postoperative immobilization was four weeks. At the time of presentation to our clinic, the patients complained of pain and stiffness. Physical examination revealed an average of 126 degrees of forward flexion and 36 degrees of external rotation and internal rotation so that the thumb could touch T12. In 13 of these patients we performed revision surgery after an exercise program failed to improve their symptoms. The average interval between the initial surgery and revision surgery was 15 months. At the revision surgery, 10 patients had prominent anterior acromia that had continued to impinge on the rotator cuff. In the site of the previous acromioplasty, five patients had distinct spurs protruding from the lateral or medial acromion;

eight patients had large amounts of subacromial scarring in which heavy bands of cicatrix connected the undersurface of the acromion to the rotator cuff. Three patients had acromioclavicular joint spurs, one had a large ununited acromial fragment, and another had an os acromiale. Although no patient had a full-thickness cuff tear, the incidence of partial-thickness deep surface or midsubstance cuff tears is unknown. The revision surgical procedure included excision of scar tissue, revision of the acromioplasty to assure adequate resection of the anterior and inferior acromion, resection of acromioclavicular spurs, inspection of the rotator cuff, and careful deltoid repair. Immediately after surgery, gentle range-of-motion exercises were initiated to minimize restriction from postoperative scar. Follow-up at an average of 10 months postoperatively revealed substantial although incomplete improvement in comfort, range of motion, and ability to work.

This report emphasizes the importance of adequate resection of the anterior and inferior acromion as well as of the undersurface of the acromioclavicular joint. Before closure of any subacromial decompression, meticulous visual and tactile exploration of the subacromial zone is necessary to assure adequate passage of the rotator cuff beneath the coracoacromial arch as the shoulder is flexed and rotated. Furthermore, it is apparent that acromioplasty creates an opportunity for substantial scarring between the cuff and acromion and the raw undersurface of the acromion after the hypertrophic bursa has been resected. The primary strategy for avoiding this scarring is to institute assisted motion immediately after surgery rather than waiting (e.g., for the one-month period averaged by the patients in this series of unsuccessful acromioplasties). Finally, it is important to assure a complete and accurate diagnosis before performing acromioplasty. Three of the patients failing acromioplasty had unrecognized acromioclavicular joint degeneration. Unrecognized acromioclavicular joint problems were responsible for five failures in Post's series, constituted a "frequent cause of failure of surgical treatment" in the series of Penny and Welsh,[154] and were the only unsatisfactory result in Neer's series. In their series of patients having persisting problems after acromioplasty, Hawkins and colleagues[83] reported that 45 per cent of the patients had a diagnosis other than continuing impingement, including acromioclavicular joint problems, cervical spondylosis, reflex sympathetic dystrophy, rotator cuff tear, thoracic outlet syndrome, glenohumeral osteoarthritis, and glenohumeral instability. Thirty-three per cent were thought to have continuing impingement. The striking finding in this series was the relative lack of improvement in patients on workmen's compensation after revision acromioplasty. Even in these authors' series of primary acromioplasties, only 78 per cent of the workmen's compensation cases had a satisfactory result, compared with 92 per cent of non–workmen's compensation cases.[82] Post and Cohen[161] also observed that worse results were obtained from surgery performed for work-related impingement syndrome. This inability to return to work may be due to unhealed partial-thickness cuff tears, residual tendon scarring, and residual weakness. Post and Cohen emphasized the need for recovery of muscle strength before the laborer is returned to work; otherwise, recurrence can be anticipated. The difficulty of returning workers to their jobs after acromioplasty is reminiscent of the problems described by Tibone and coworkers[200] in returning athletes to a competitive level of function. The common feature may be that acromioplasty does not restore the tendons to a state where they can withstand the daily demands of high-performance sports or heavy work.

The foregoing review indicates that some major challenges exist in the diagnosis and treatment of the impingement syndrome.

1. How can the integrity of the cuff be reliably determined preoperatively (to include the diagnosis of partial-thickness cuff tears)?

2. What is the best nonoperative program for impingement syndrome, and how can it be determined that the patient has given it an adequate try?

3. How can one provide optimal surgical decompression with minimal compromise of the deltoid origin?

4. Should resection arthroplasty of the acromioclavicular joint be routinely performed or reserved for those cases in which there is obvious degenerative change with osteophytic encroachment on the rotator cuff?

5. How should partial-thickness cuff tears be managed? Does acromioplasty prevent progression of fiber failure in these instances?

6. How should the throwing or swimming athlete with a picture of impingement be managed? What if nonoperative management fails?

7. What is the optimal postoperative management of patients who have had surgical decompression?

8. What are the best diagnostic and therapeutic approaches to patients with continuing symptoms after surgical decompression?

Authors' Preferred Method of Treatment

NONOPERATIVE MANAGEMENT

In our approach to the impingement syndrome, we recognize the important interplay between weakness of the humeral head depressor mechanism, stiffness of the posterior capsule, tendon fiber damage, and subacromial wear. Most patients with the syndrome of pain on forward elevation and shoulder tightness can be managed nonoperatively. We refer to our nonoperative approach to cuff tendinitis as the Jackins Program (in honor of Sarah Jackins, who has been the Physical Therapist for the University of Washington Shoulder Clinic since its inception in 1975). This treatment regimen is analogous to one that would be used for managing a tennis elbow or Achilles tendinitis and includes (1) avoidance of repeated injury, (2) restoration of normal flexibility, (3) restoration of normal strength, (4) aerobic exercise, and (5) modification of work or sport. The emphasis is on simple, low-tech exercises that the patient can perform unassisted. Key elements in this program are informing the patients (what their problem is, why the exercises will help, and how to do the exercises) and giving them regular, positive feedback on their progress.

The Jackins Program

Step 1: Avoidance of Repeated Injury

Although it seems obvious that an injured tendon must be rested, we see patients each week who are trying to continue vigorous overhead work or swimming miles per week in the presence of impingement symptoms. It is difficult to treat a tendinitis when the affected structure is being repeatedly injured. Therefore, just as with Achilles tendinitis, activities often need to be modified—light duty, reducing mileage, less throwing, using the kickboard for a major part of the workout rather than continuing to try to "swim through" the problem, or working on the forehand and footwork rather than beating away at the serve.

Step 2: Restoration of Normal Flexibility

The goal of Step 2 is to stretch out all directions of tightness. Shoulders with cuff tendinitis are usually stiff, especially in the posterior capsule (Fig. 15–15). This stiffness limits forward flexion, internal rotation, and cross-body adduction. The range of forward flexion is measured with the patient supine as the angle between the humerus and thorax while the patient's arm is passively elevated. Internal rotation is recorded

by the name of the vertebral spine that can be touched with the extended thumb of the internally rotated affected arm (e.g., L2 or T7). The range of cross-body adduction is recorded by having the patient lie supine with the arm in maximum cross-body adduction and measuring the minimum distance between the antecubital fossa and the contralateral coracoid process.

The range of the normal shoulder is used as the goal of the flexibility program. The patient is taught that *gentle, sustained* stretching against all directions of tightness repeated five times per day is the most effective method for regaining normal motion. We particularly emphasize internal and external rotation, cross-body adduction, and flexion. Regaining normal motion is essential to restoration of shoulder comfort and function. Positive feedback is provided by keeping a chart of the patient's motions and showing him or her the improvement on successive visits.

Step 3: Restoration of Normal Strength

When near-normal passive flexibility of the shoulder is restored, the patient starts rotator muscle strengthening. As with the flexibility exercises, the patient is given the responsibility for strengthening the shoulder. Internal and external rotator–strengthening exercises are carried out with the arm at the side to strengthen the anterior and posterior humeral head depressors without the potential for subacromial grinding that exists with exercises in abduction and flexion (Fig. 15–16). These exercises are most conveniently performed against the resistance of rubber tubing, sheet rubber, bike inner tubes, or springs. It is convenient if the resistance device can be carried in pocket or purse for frequent use through the day. Feedback is given during successive visits by measuring the strength manually

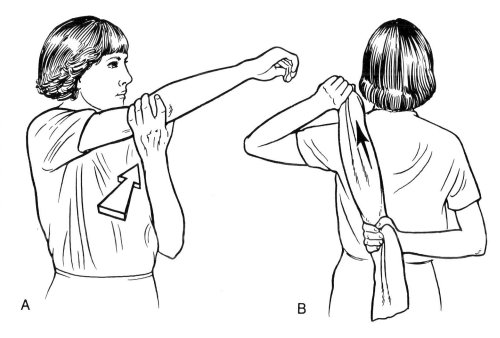

Figure 15–15. Restoration of normal flexibility is an important part of nonoperative management of the impingement syndrome. Shoulders with cuff tendinitis are usually stiff, especially in the posterior capsule, and most patients demonstrate limitation of cross-body adduction and internal rotation. Gentle static stretching exercises in cross-body adduction (*A*) and internal rotation (*B*) are effective in reducing this stiffness.

A

B

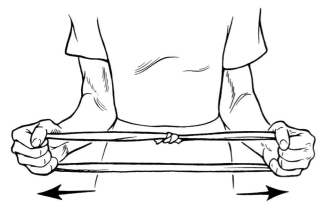

Figure 15–16. Strengthening of the anterior and posterior humeral head depressors is conveniently performed against the resistance of rubber tubing. These exercises are carried out with the arm positioned at the side to avoid subacromial irritation.

with spring scales or with more sophisticated techniques, if available. Progress is recognized by advancing the patient to more resistance: thicker tubing, tougher rubber sheets, or more springs. Athletes are not returned to full activity until the shoulder has full mobility and strength.

Step 4: Aerobic Exercise

We observe that major shoulder dysfunction frequently takes patients out of the mainstream of their usual activities, an event that leads to their becoming out of shape, overweight, depressed, and recreation starved. As a result, we emphasize to patients that regular (at least three times a week) aerobic exercise (sufficient to raise their heart rate above 120 beats per minute for 30 minutes) will help keep them in shape, raise their pain threshold, improve their flexibility, and improve their sense of well-being. Brisk walking may be the safest and most effective type of aerobic exercise, but other suitable forms include jogging, biking, stationary biking, and so on. Aerobic calisthenics as usually defined must be carefully reviewed to ensure that they do not involve much arm use in the impingement positions of flexion and abduction. The patient's progress with the aerobic program is reviewed at each visit. Increments in time, distance, and speed are rewarded with positive feedback.

Step 5: Modification of Work or Sport

Obviously, the purpose of the program is to return patients to the comfortable pursuit of their normal activities. Not infrequently this requires some analysis of their working and recreational techniques. Occasionally this is as simple as having the short grocery clerk stand on a platform at work. The technique of swimmers is reviewed to ensure, for example, adequate roll on the freestyle stroke. Throwers are taught the importance of leaning the body and rotator strength. Adequate knee bend and lumbar extension is reinforced in the execution of the tennis serve. If the

patient has an occupation that requires vigorous or repeated use of the shoulder in the impingement position, vocational rehabilitation to a different job may be required if cuff tendon involvement is refractory. We prefer to modify the job *before* considering modifying the acromion.

What does one do if the nonoperative program fails to produce results? As long as the patient is improving with the Jackins program, we encourage him or her to remain on it. If six weeks on this program produce no improvement (unusual) or if major symptoms persist after three months, we become concerned that some other problem may be involved. We then perform an ultrasound or arthrogram to look for evidence of a partial- or full-thickness cuff tear. Ultrasonography or arthrography is used earlier in patients with evidence of tendon damage: pain on resisted external rotation, shoulder weakness, or spinatus atrophy. If the result of the ultrasound or arthrogram is positive, we discuss with the patient the option of cuff repair with acromioplasty. If the result is negative, the patient is reassured concerning the absence of a major cuff tear and advised to continue the Jackins program for a total of six months before considering surgery. After this trial of nonoperative management, a patient with painful subacromial crepitus on flexion, abduction, and rotation is informed of the option of subacromial decompression. At this point, transient relief of pain by the subacromial injection of lidocaine provides assurance to the patient and surgeon that at least part of the patient's problem lies in the subacromial zone.

In our experience, the results of subacromial decompression are likely to be good in the following circumstances: (1) a well-motivated patient over 40, (2) absence of posterior capsular stiffness, (3) presence of subacromial crepitus, (4) pain relieved by the subacromial injection of lidocaine, and (5) a condition that is unrelated to the patient's occupation. Poor prognostic signs include: (1) age less than 40, (2) stiffness, (3) absence of subacromial crepitus, (4) lack of relief by subacromial injection, (5) attribution of problem to occupation, (6) concomitant evidence of glenohumeral instability, and (7) neurogenic cuff muscle weakness.

SURGICAL TREATMENT OF IMPINGEMENT REFRACTORY TO NONOPERATIVE MANAGEMENT

Surgery is considered only in those patients who have put forth an excellent nonoperative effort, who have explored vocational rehabilitation if appropriate, and who continue to have substantial impingement symptoms. Ultrasonography or arthrography is routinely obtained preoperatively. This is because tears of the rotator cuff may produce symptoms and signs identical with those found in the impingement syndrome without cuff tear, yet the presence of these cuff tears may alter the surgical procedure and postoperative course.

We use an open subacromial decompression, removing the anteroinferior surface of the acromion and the coracoacromial ligament through a "deltoid-on" approach. This approach provides excellent exposure and control over the adequacy of the resection in less time and with greater assurance than can be accomplished arthroscopically. We emphasize providing complete subacromial decompression with minimal disruption of deltoid, cuff, or biceps function. The deltoid-on approach virtually eliminates the need for postoperative immobilization.

The acromion is exposed by an incision in the tendon separating the lateral and anterior deltoid, which arises from the anterolateral corner of the acromion. This incision is carried up on the acromion itself (Fig. 15–17). The deltoid origin is sharply elevated from the acromion in continuity with the acromial periosteum and the trapezius insertion (Fig. 15–18). Great care is taken to create a strong flap medially and laterally that can be closed side to side, restoring the deltoid origin. The deltoid tendon is split in line with its fibers, and the split is deepened under direct vision until the bursa is entered (Fig. 15–19). The deltoid split is limited to 4 to 5 cm from the anterolateral corner of the acromion to protect the axillary nerve. Rotating the humerus provides easy differentiation between the deltoid (which does not move with humeral rotation) and the superficial surface of the cuff (which does). The sub-

acromial subdeltoid bursa is palpated for any evidence of adhesions, which are released. The anterior acromion is squared off with a rongeur. A thin-bladed osteotome is used to resect the anterior undersurface of the acromion (Fig. 15–20). This osteotomy is oriented in line with the extrapolated undersurface of the posterior acromion (identified by palpation and direct vision). Care is taken that the osteotomy does not continue into the posterior acromion or scapular spine. The coracoacromial ligament is resected along with the acromial fragment. The undersurface of the acromion is then smoothed using a "pine cone" power bur, taking care that no spurs are left laterally in the deltoid origin or medially at the acromioclavicular joint (Fig. 15–21). The shoulder is thoroughly irrigated to remove all bone fragments. Inferiorly directed acromioclavicular osteophytes are resected. The lateral 1.5 cm of the clavicle is resected if substantial acromioclavicular degenerative change exists. The rotator cuff is thoroughly explored for evidence of superior surface blisters, partial tears, thinning, or full-thickness defects. Gentle rotation of the arm facilitates inspection of the critical zone (Fig. 15–22). Careful palpation of the cuff is an important part of this examination. The "dye test" (Fukuda) is used to evaluate shoulders with suspicious cuff integrity. In this test a 20 per cent methylene blue solution is injected into the glenohumeral joint to determine the extent and location of cuff thinning.

The biceps is left undisturbed unless it appears to be seriously inflamed, obviously unstable, or doomed to imminent rupture, in which case we perform a tenodesis to the proximal humerus.

Before final closure, the undersurface of the acromion is palpated to ensure that no bony prominences remain either medially or laterally in the acromion. The shoulder is passively elevated and rotated to ensure ample clearance for the cuff and tuberosities below the coracoacromial arch, including the acromioclavicular joint. Finally, the shoulder is gently manipulated through its full range of motion. A secure deltoid reconstitution is essential so that early postoperative motion may be instituted. The deltoid is repaired by side-to-side closure of the medial and lateral flaps using No. 2 nonabsorbable suture (Fig. 15–23). If these flaps are not secure, two drill holes are placed in the acromion. Suture from the medial hole is passed through the lateral part of the deltoid tendon and suture from the lateral hole is passed through the medial part of the deltoid tendon to effect a crisscross closure. This avoids the "telltale V" defect that reveals a poor deltoid closure.

Postoperative Program

Postoperatively the patient is started on an assisted range-of-motion program on the day of surgery. This is facilitated if the procedure is performed under brachial plexus block, which lasts from 12 to 18 hours. These exercises are already familiar to the patient,

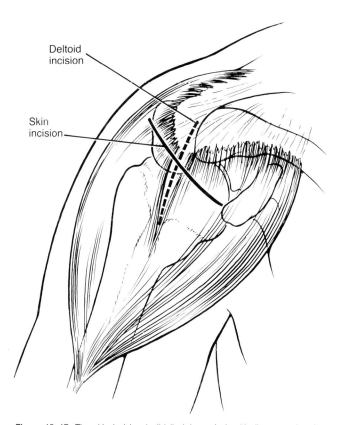

Figure 15–17. The skin incision (*solid line*) is made in skin lines crossing the anterior corner of the acromion. The acromion is exposed by an incision in the tendon between the anterior and lateral deltoid (*dotted line*).

Deltoid incision

Skin incision

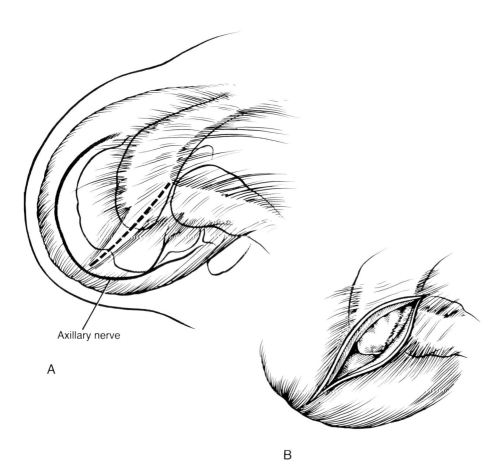

Axillary nerve

A

B

Figure 15–18. *A,* The incision is centered on the anterolateral corner of the acromion and carried medially on the superior surface of the acromion. *B,* The deltoid origin is sharply elevated from the acromion in continuity with the acromial periosteum and trapezius insertion. Care is taken to create strong flaps that can be securely repaired, restoring the deltoid origin.

Figure 15–19. The "deltoid-on" approach offers excellent exposure to the coracoacromial arch and the underlying rotator cuff. The *dotted line* indicates the anterior extent of the acromion to be removed.

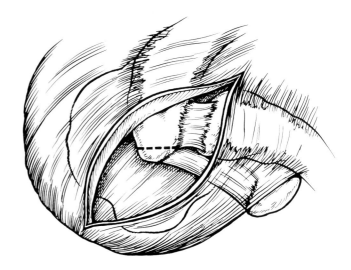

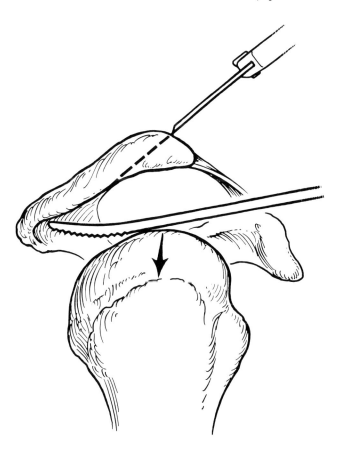

Figure 15–20. A thin-bladed osteotome is used to resect the anteroinferior surface of the acromion. The coracoacromial ligament is resected along with the acromial fragment. The osteotomy is oriented in line with the extrapolated undersurface of the posterior acromion. Exposure and access are facilitated by employing a Darrach retractor to gently depress the humeral head.

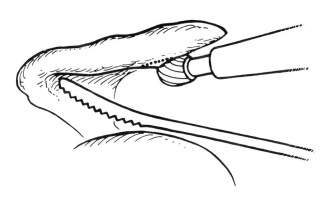

Figure 15–21. Any irregularities remaining on the undersurface of the acromion are smoothed using a "pine cone" bur. The undersurface of the entire acromion and the acromioclavicular joint are carefully inspected to ensure that no troublesome spurs or osteophytes remain and that the cuff passes beneath the coracoacromial arch without contact.

Figure 15–22. The underlying cuff is systematically explored and palpated. This is accomplished by rotating the arm to bring the different parts of the cuff into view (rather than by extending the incision). (Reproduced with permission from Codman EA: Rupture of the Supraspinatus Tendon and Other Lesions In or About the Subacromial Bursa. Malabar, FL: Robert E Krieger, 1984.)

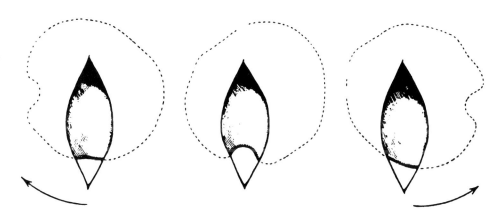

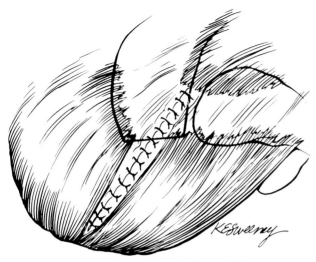

Figure 15-23. A secure deltoid reconstruction is essential so that immediate postoperative motion can be instituted.

having been performed as part of the preoperative trial of the Jackins program. The patient is allowed active use of the shoulder within the realm of comfort unless there is concern for the strength of the deltoid reattachment. Internal and external rotation–strengthening exercises are also begun immediately. Athletics are not allowed for three months after surgery and until normal motion and strength are regained.

MANAGEMENT OF "FAILED" PREVIOUS ACROMIOPLASTY

Patients who have had previous acromioplasty with unsatisfactory results are evaluated to determine if the primary problem is (1) pain, (2) stiffness, or (3) weakness. Those patients with pain or stiffness are placed on the Jackins program described earlier. Those with definite weakness and those who do not improve after the Jackins program are evaluated with ultrasonography or arthrography and by electromyography. Vocational rehabilitation is essential for many of these patients.

Reoperation is considered in well-motivated patients with evidence of residual impingement or postoperative scarring. Often these patients note more pain and less motion after their initial procedure than before. In contrast to primary acromioplasty, we are willing to reoperate on patients with refractory stiffness because often the problem in failed acromioplasty seems to be subacromial scarring. A careful history will usually indicate that motion was not initiated immediately after the first procedure. Radiographs, including the supraspinatus outlet view, are taken to seek for evidence of bone spurs, acromioclavicular osteophytes, and inadequate resection. Our revision procedure is identical with our primary acromioplasty described earlier.

We have been fortunate in that over 80 per cent of the patients on whom we have reoperated after previous acromioplasty have experienced substantial improvement in comfort and function after as many as four previous "acromioplasties."

References

1. Albright JA, Jokl P, Shaw R, and Albright JP: Clinical study of baseball pitchers: correlation of injury to the throwing arm with method of delivery. Am J Sports Med 6:15–21, 1978.
2. Alexeeff M: Ligament patellae rupture following local steroid injection. Aust NZ J Surg 56:681–683, 1986.
3. Apoil A, Dautry P, Koechlin P, and Hardy J: The surgical treatment of rotator cuff impingement. In Bayley I, and Kessel L (eds): Shoulder Surgery. Berlin: Springer-Verlag, 1982, pp 22–26.
4. Armstrong JR: Excision of the acromion in treatment of the supraspinatus syndrome: report of ninety-five excisions. J Bone Joint Surg 31B:436–442, 1949.
5. Atwater AE: Biomechanics of overarm throwing movements and of throwing injuries. Exerc Sport Sci Rev 7:43–85, 1979.
6. Bacevich BB: Paralytic brachial neuritis. J Bone Joint Surg (Am) 58A:262, 1976.
7. Balasubramaniam P, and Prathap K: The effect of injection of hydrocortisone into rabbit calcaneal tendons. J Bone Joint Surg 54B:729, 1972.
8. Barnes DA, and Tullos HS: An analysis of 100 symptomatic baseball players. Am J Sports Med 6(2):62–67, 1978.
9. Basmajian JV, and Bazant FJ: Factors preventing downward dislocation of the adducted shoulder joint: an electromyographic and morphological study. J Bone Joint Surg 41A:1182–1186, 1959.
10. Basmajian JV: Muscles Alive: Their Functions Revealed by Electromyography, 2nd edition. Baltimore: Williams & Wilkins, 1967.
11. Basmajian JV: The surgical anatomy and function of the armtrunk mechanism. Surg Clin North Am 43:1471, 1963.
12. Bateman JE: The Shoulder and Neck, 2d ed. Philadelphia: WB Saunders, 1978, pp 280, 286.
13. Bayley JC, Cochran TP, and Seldge CB: The weight-bearing shoulder: the impingement syndrome in paraplegics. J Bone Joint Surg 69A:676–678, 1987.
14. Bedi SS, and Ellis W: Spontaneous rupture of calcaneal tendon in rheumatoid arthritis after local steroid injection. Ann Rheum Dis 29:494, 1970.
15. Behrens F, Shepherd N, and Mitchell N: Alteration of rabbit articular cartilage by intra-articular injections of glucocorticoids. J Bone Joint Surg 57A1:70, 1975.
16. Bennett GE: Shoulder and elbow lesions of the professional baseball pitcher. JAMA 117:510–514, 1941.
17. Bennett GE: Shoulder and elbow lesions distinctive of baseball players. Ann Surg 126:107–110, 1947.
18. Berry H, Fernandes L, Bloom B, et al: Clinical study comparing acupuncture, physiotherapy, injection and oral anti-inflammatory therapy in shoulder-cuff lesions. Curr Med Res Opin 7(2):121–126, 1980.
19. Berquist TH, McCough PF, Hattrup SH, and Cofield RH: Arthrographic analysis of rotator cuff tear size. Paper presented at American Shoulder and Elbow Surgeons 4th meeting, Atlanta, 1988.
20. Bettman: Monatsschr Unfallheilk, p. 14, 1926.
21. Bigliani LU, Morrison D, and April EW: The morphology of the acromion and its relationship to rotator cuff tears. Orthop Trans 10:228, 1986.
22. Bigliani LU, Norris TR, Fischer J, et al: The relationship between the unfused acromial epiphysis and subacromial impingement lesions. Orthop Trans 7(1):138, 1983.
23. Bigliani LU, Perez-Sanz JR, and Wolfe IN: Treatment of trapezius paralysis. J Bone Joint Surg 67A:871–877, 1985.
24. Binder A, Parr G, Hazleman B, and Fitton-Jackson S: Pulsed electromagnetic field therapy of persistent rotator cuff tendinitis. Lancet 1:695–698, 1984.
25. Bosworth DM: An analysis of twenty-eight consecutive cases

of incapacitating shoulder lesions, radically explored and repaired. J Bone Joint Surg 22:369–392, 1940.

26. Bosworth DM: The supraspinatus syndrome—symptomatology, pathology, and repair. JAMA 117:422, 1941.

27. Brems JJ, and Wilde AH: Surgical management of cuff tear arthropathy. Paper presented at American Shoulder and Elbow Surgeons 4th meeting, Atlanta, 1988.

28. Brewer BJ: Aging of the rotator cuff. Am J Sports Med 7:102–110, 1979.

29. Brown JT: Early assessment of supraspinatus tears: procaine infiltration as a guide to treatment. J Bone Joint Surg 31B:423, 1949.

30. Carter SL, Miller SH, and Graham WP III: An evaluation of the local effects of triamcinolone acetonide on normal soft tissues in monkey digits. Plast Reconstr Surg 39(3):407–410, 1977.

31. Chung SMK, and Nissenbaum MM: Congenital and developmental defects of the shoulder. Orthop Clin North Am 6:382, 1975.

32. Clancy WG Jr (ed): Symposium: shoulder problems in overhead-overuse sports. Am J Sports Med 7:138–144, 1979.

33. Codman EA: Obscure lesions of the shoulder, rupture of the supraspinatus tendon. Boston Med Surg J 196:381, 1927.

34. Codman EA: The pathology of the subacromial bursa and of the supraspinatus tendon. In The Shoulder: Rupture of the Supraspinatus Tendon and Other Lesions In or About the Subacromial Bursa. Malabar, FL: Robert E Krieger, 1984, supplement edition, pp 65–107.

35. Codman EA: Rupture of the supraspinatus tendon. In The Shoulder: Rupture of the Supraspinatus Tendon and Other Lesions In or About the Subacromial Bursa. Malabar, FL: Robert E Krieger, 1984, supplement edition, pp 123–177.

36. Cofield RH: Arthroscopy of the shoulder. Mayo Clin Proc 58:501–508, 1983.

37. Cofield RH: Current concepts review rotator cuff disease of the shoulder. J Bone Joint Surg 67A:974–979, 1985.

38. Cofield RH, and Simonet WT: Symposium on sports medicine: Part 2, the shoulder in sports. Mayo Clin Proc 59:157–164, 1984.

39. Colachis SC Jr, and Strohm BR: Effect of suprascapular and axillary nerve blocks and muscle force in upper extremity. Arch Phys Med Rehabil 52:22, 1971.

40. Colachis SC Jr, Strohm BR, and Brechner VL: Effects of axillary nerve block on muscle force in the upper extremity. Arch Phys Med Rehabil 50:647, 1969.

41. Colley F: Die Periarthritis humeroscapularis. Deutsche Zeitschrift für Chirurgie. Rose E, and Helferich von FCW (eds): Leipzig: Vogel, 1899.

42. Cone RO III, Resnick D, and Danzig L: Shoulder impingement syndrome: radiographic evaluation. Radiology 150:29, 1984.

43. Cowan MA, and Alexander S: Simultaneous bilateral rupture of Achilles tendons due to triamcinolone. Br Med J 1:1658–1659, 1961.

44. Crenshaw AH: Campbell's Operative Orthopedics, 5th ed, vol 2. St. Louis: CV Mosby, 1971.

45. Cruess RL, Blennerhassett J, MacDonald FR, et al: Aseptic necrosis following renal transplantation. J Bone Joint Surg 50A:1577, 1968.

46. Darlington LG, and Coomes EN: The effects of local steroid injection for supraspinatus tears. Rheumatol Rehabil 16:172–179, 1977.

47. DePalma AF: Surgery of the Shoulder, 2nd ed. Philadelphia: JB Lippincott, 1973, pp 206–210, 229, 234–235.

48. DePalma AF, Gallery G, and Bennett CA: Variational anatomy and degenerative lesions of the shoulder joint. In American Academy of Orthopaedic Surgeons Instr Course Lect 6:255–281, 1949.

49. DePalma AF, White JB, and Callery G: Degenerative lesions of the shoulder joint at various age groups which are compatible with good function. In AAOS Instructional Course Lectures. St. Louis: CV Mosby, 1950, p 168.

50. Desché: Contribution à l'étude et au traitement de la périarthrite scapulohumérale. Thèse, Paris, 1892.

51. Desplats H: De L'atrophie musculaire dans la péri-arthrite scapulo humérale. Gazette Hebdomadaire de Médicine et de Chir 24:371, 1878.

52. Diamond B: The Obstructing Acromion. Springfield, IL: Charles C Thomas, 1964.

53. Dines D, Warren RF, and Inglis AE: Surgical treatment of lesions of the long head of the biceps. Clin Orthop 164:165–171, 1982.

54. Dominguez RH: Shoulder pain in age group swimmers. Int Ser Sports Sci 6:105–109, 1978.

55. Donovan WH, and Kraft GH: Rotator cuff tear vs. suprascapular nerve injury. Arch Phys Med Rehabil 55:424, 1974.

56. Drez D: Suprascapular neuropathy in the differential diagnosis of rotator cuff injury. Am J Sports Med 4:43, 1976.

57. Duplay: Arch gén de méd 2:513, 1872.

58. Duronea: Essai sur la scapulalgie. 1873.

59. Ellis DG: Cross-sectional area measurements for tendon specimens: a comparison of several methods. J Biomech 2:175, 1968.

60. Ellman H: Arthroscopic subcromial decompression: a preliminary report. Paper presented at American Shoulder and Elbow Surgeons First Open Meeting, Las Vegas, NV, January 23, 1985.

61. Ellman H: Arthroscopic subacromial decompression: analysis of one- to three-year results. J Arthroscopic Rel Surg 3(3):173–181, 1987.

62. Elmslie RC: Calcareous deposits in the supraspinatus tendon. Br J Surg 20:190, 1932.

63. Ferguson LK: Lesion of the subacromial bursa and supraspinatus tendon. Am J Surg 105:243–256, 1937.

64. Flugstad D, Matsen FA, Larry I, and Jackins SE: Failed acromioplasty and the treatment of the impingement syndrome. Paper presented at ASES. 2nd Open Meeting, New Orleans, 1986.

65. Ford LT, and DeBender J: Tendon rupture after local steroid injection. South Med J 72(7):827–830, 1979.

66. Fowler P: Swimmer problems. Am J Sports Med 7(2):141–142, 1979.

67. Gainor BJ, Piotrowski G, Puhl J, et al: The throw: biomechanics and acute injury. Am J Sports Med 8:114–118, 1980.

68. Gartsman GM: Arthroscopic treatment of Stage II subacromial impingement. Paper presented at ASES. 4th Meeting, Atlanta, 1988.

69. Godsil RD, and Linscheid RL: Intratendinous defects of the rotator cuff. Clin Orthop 69:181–188, 1970.

70. Grant JCB: Grant's Atlas of Anatomy, 6th ed. Baltimore: Williams & Wilkins, 1972.

71. Grant JCB, and Smith CG: Age incidence of rupture of the supraspinatus tendon (abstract). Anat Rec 100:666, 1948.

72. Ha'eri GB: Ruptures of the rotator cuff. Can Med Assoc J 123:620–627, 1980.

73. Ha'eri GB, Orth MC, and Wiley AM: Shoulder impingement syndrome. Clin Orthop 168:128–132, 1982.

74. Ha'eri GB, and Wiley AM: An extensile exposure for subacromial derangements. Can J Surg 23(5):458–461, 1980.

75. Halverson PB, McCarty DJ, Cheung HS, and Ryan LM: Milwaukee shoulder syndrome: eleven additional cases with involvement of the knee in seven (basic calcium phosphate crystal deposition disease). Semin Arthritis Rheum 14:36–44, 1984.

76. Hammond G: Complete acromionectomy in the treatment of chronic tendinitis of the shoulder. J Bone Joint Surg 44A(3):494–504, 1962.

77. Hammond G: Complete acromionectomy in the treatment of chronic tendinitis of the shoulder. A follow-up of ninety operations of eighty-seven patients. J Bone Joint Surg 53A:173–180, 1971.

78. Haudek: Wien klin Wochenschr p. 43, 1911.

79. Hawkins RJ: Impingement syndrome. Orthop Trans 3:274, 1979.

80. Hawkins RJ: The rotator cuff and biceps tendon. In Evarts CM (ed): Surgery of the Musculoskeletal System. New York: Churchill Livingstone, 1983.

81. Hawkins RJ, and Abrams JS: Impingement syndrome in the absence of rotator cuff tear (Stages 1 and 2). Orthop Clin North Am 18(3):373–382, 1987.

82. Hawkins RJ, and Brock RM: Anterior acromioplasty: early results for impingement with intact rotator cuff. Orthop Trans 3(3):274, 1979.

83. Hawkins RJ, Chris AD, and Kiefer G: Failed anterior acromioplasty. Paper presented at ASES 3rd Meeting, San Francisco, 1987.

84. Hawkins RJ, and Kennedy JC: Impingement syndrome in athletes. Am J Sports Med 8(3):151–158, 1980.

85. Heineke: Die Anatomie und Pathologie der Schleimbeutel und Sehnenscheiden. Erlangen, 1868.

86. Herberts P, Kadefors R, Hogfors C, and Sigholm G: Shoulder pain and heavy manual labor. Clin Orthop 191:166–178, 1984.

87. Hill JA: Epidemiologic perspective on shoulder injuries. Clin Sports Med 2:241–246, 1983.

88. Hollingworth GR, Ellis RM, and Hattersley TS: Comparison of injection techniques for shoulder pain: results of a double blind, randomized study. Br Med J 287:1339–1341, 1983.

89. Holzknecht G: Über Bursitis mit Konkrementbildung. Wiener Medizinische Wochenschrift 43:2757, 1911.

90. Iannotti JP, Swiontkowski M, Esterhai J, and Boulas HJ: Intraoperative assessment of rotator cuff vascularity using laser Doppler flowmetry. Abstract presented to AAOS 1989 Meeting, Las Vegas, 1989.

91. Inman VT, Saunders JB de CM, and Abbott LC: Observations on the function of the shoulder joint. J Bone Joint Surg 26A:1–30, 1944.

92. Ismail AM, Balakishnan R, and Rajakumar MK: Rupture of patellar ligament after steroid infiltration. J Bone Joint Surg 51B:503, 1969.

93. Jackson DW, and Graf BJ: Decompression of the coroacromial arch. In Shoulder Surgery in the Athlete (Techniques in Orthopaedics). Rockville MD: Aspen Publications, 1985.

94. Jackson DW: Chronic rotator cuff impingement in the throwing athlete. Am J Sports Med 4(6):231–240, 1976.

95. Jarjavay JF: Sur la luxation du tendon de la longue portion du muscle biceps humeral; sur la luxation des tendons des muscles peroniers latéraux. Gazette Hebdomadaire de Médecine et de Chir 21:325, 1867.

96. Jobe FW: Symposium: shoulder problems in overhead-overuse sports. Am J Sports Med 7(2):139–140, 1979.

97. Jobe FW: Painful athletic injuries of the shoulder. Clin Orthop 173:117–124, 1983.

98. Jobe FW, and Moynes DR: Delineation of diagnostic criteria and a rehabilitation program for rotator cuff injuries. Am J Sports Med 10:336–339, 1982.

99. Jobe FW, Tibone JE, Perry J, and Moynes DR: An EMG analysis of the shoulder in throwing and pitching: a preliminary report. Am J Sports Med 11:3–5, 1983.

100. Jobe FW, Yocum LA, Moynes DR, et al: Shoulder and Arm Exercises for Baseball Players. Inglewood, CA: Centinela Hospital Medical Center, 1982.

101. Johansson JE, and Barrington TW: Coracoacromial ligament division. Am J Sports Med 12:138–141, 1984.

102. Julliard: La coracoidite. Revue Médicale de la Suisse Romande 12:47, 1933.

103. Kennedy JC, and Willis RB: The effects of local steroid injections on tendons: a biomechanical and microscopic correlative study. Am J Sports Med 4:11–21, 1976.

104. Kennedy JC, Hawkins R, and Krissoff WB: Orthopaedic manifestations of swimming. Am J Sports Med 6:309–322, 1978.

105. Kerlan RK, Jobe FW, Blazina ME, et al: Throwing injuries of the shoulder and elbow in adults. In Ahrstrom JP Jr (ed): Current Practice in Orthopedic Surgery, Vol. 6. St. Louis: CV Mosby, 1975, Chap 6.

106. Kessel L, and Watson M: The painful arc syndrome. Clinical classification as a guide to management. J Bone Joint Surg 59B(2):166–172, 1977.

107. Keyes EL: Anatomical observations on senile changes in the shoulder. J Bone Joint Surg (Am) 17:953, 1935.

108. Kneeland JB, Middleton WD, Carnera GF, et al: MR imaging of the shoulder: diagnosis of rotator cuff tears. AJR 149:333–337, 1987.

109. Küster E: Ueber habituelle Schutter Luxation. Verb Dtsch Ges Chir 11:112–114, 1882.

110. Lee HB: Avulsion and rupture of the tendo calcaneus after injection of hydrocortisone. Br Med J 2:395, 1957.

111. Liberson F: Os acromiale—a contested anomaly. J Bone Joint Surg 19:683–689, 1937.

112. Lie S, and Mast WA: Subacromial bursography: technique and clinical application. Tech Dev Instrum 144(3):626–630, 1982.

113. Lilleby H: Shoulder arthroscopy. Acta Orthop Scand 55:561–566, 1984.

114. Lindblom K: On pathogenesis of ruptures of the tendon aponeurosis of the shoulder joint. Acta Radiol 20:563, 1939.

115. Linge B, and Mulder JD: Function of the supraspinatus and its relation to the supraspinatus syndrome. An experimental study in man. J Bone Joint Surg 45B:750, 1963.

116. Lund IM, Donde R, and Knudsen EA: Persistent local cutaneous atrophy following corticosteroid injection for tendinitis. Rheumatol Rehabil 18:91–93, 1979.

117. Luopajärvi T, Kuorinka I, Virolainen M, and Holmberg M: Prevalence of tenosynovitis and other injuries of the upper extremities in repetitive work. Scand J Work Environ Health 5(3):48–55, 1979.

118. Mack LA, Matsen FA III, Kilcoyne RF, et al: Ultrasound: US evaluation of the rotator cuff. Radiology 157:205–209, 1985.

119. Macnab I: Rotator cuff tendinitis. Ann Roy Coll Surg 53:271–287, 1973.

120. Macnab I, and Hastings D: Rotator cuff tendinitis. Can Med Assoc J 99:91–98, 1968.

121. Mankin HJ, and Conger KA: The acute effects of intra-articular hydrocortisone on articular cartilage in rabbits. J Bone Joint Surg 48A:1383, 1966.

122. Matsen FA III: Compartmental Syndromes. San Francisco: Grune & Stratton, 1980.

123. Matthews LS, Sonstegard DA, and Phelps DB: A biomechanical study of rabbit patellar tendon: effects of steroid injection. J Sports Med 2(6):9, 1974.

124. McLaughlin HL: Lesions of the musculotendinous cuff of the shoulder. I. The exposure and treatment of tears with retraction. J Bone Joint Surg 26:31–51, 1944.

125. McLaughlin HL: The selection of calcium deposits for operation: the technique and results of operation. Surg Clin North Am 43:1501, 1963.

126. Melmed EP: Spontaneous bilateral rupture of the calcaneal tendon during steroid therapy. J Bone Joint Surg 47B:104, 1965.

127. Meyer AW: Further evidence of attrition in the human body. Am J Anat 34:241, 1924.

128. Meyer AW: The minute anatomy of attrition lesions. J Bone Joint Surg 13A:341, 1931.

129. Meyer and Kessler: Strassbourg méd 2:205, 1926.

130. Michelsson JE, and Bakalim G: Resection of the acromion in the treatment of persistent rotator cuff syndrome of the shoulder. Acta Orthop Scand 48:607–611, 1977.

131. Morrison DS: The use of magnetic resonance imaging in the diagnosis of rotator cuff tears. Paper presented at ASES 4th Meeting, Atlanta, 1988.

132. Morrison DS, and Bigliani LU: The clinical significance of variations in acromial morphology. Paper presented at ASES 3rd Open Meeting, San Francisco, 1987.

133. Moseley HF: Shoulder Lesions, 3rd ed. Edinburgh and London: E and S Livingstone, 1969.

134. Moseley HF, and Goldie I: The arterial pattern of the rotator cuff of the shoulder. J Bone Joint Surg 45B:780, 1963.

135. Mudge MK, Wood VE, and Frykman GK: Rotator cuff tears associated with os acromiale. J Bone Joint Surg 66A(3):427–429, 1984.

136. Neer CS II: Anterior acromioplasty for the chronic impingement syndrome in the shoulder. A preliminary report. J Bone Joint Surg 54A:41–50, 1972.

137. Neer CS II: Impingement lesions. Clin Orthop 173:70–77, 1983.

138. Neer CS II, Bigliani LU, and Hawkins RJ: Rupture of the long head of the biceps related to subacromial impingement. Orthop Trans *1*:111, 1977.

139. Neer CS II, Flatow EL, and Lech O: Tears of the rotator cuff. Long term results of anterior acromioplasty and repair. Paper presented at ASES 4th Meeting, Atlanta, 1988.

140. Neer CS, and Marberry TA: On the disadvantages of radical acromionectomy. J Bone Joint Surg *63A*(3):416–419, 1981.

141. Neer CS II, and Poppen NK: Supraspinatus outlet. Paper presented at ASES 3rd Open Meeting, San Francisco, 1987.

142. Neer CS, and Welsh RP: The shoulder in sports. Orthop Clin North Am *8*(3):583–591, 1977.

143. Neviaser J: Arthrography of the Shoulder: The Diagnosis and Management of the Lesions Visualized. Springfield, IL: Charles C Thomas, 1975.

144. Neviaser RJ: Lesions of the biceps and tendinitis of the shoulder. Orthop Clin North Am *11*(2):343, 1980.

145. Neviaser TJ, Neviaser RJ, Neviaser JS, and Neviaser JS: The four-in-one arthroplasty for the painful arc syndrome. Clin Orthop *163*:107–112, 1982.

146. Norris TR, Fischer J, Bigliani LU, et al: The unfused acromial epiphysis and its relationship to impingement syndromes. Orthop Trans *7*(3):505, 1983.

147. Norwood LA, Del Pizzo W, Jobe FW, and Kerlan RK: Anterior shoulder pain in baseball pitchers. Am J Sports Med *6*(3):103–106, 1978.

148. Noyes FR, DeLucas JL, and Torvik PJ: Biomechanics of anterior cruciate ligament failure: an analysis of strain-rate sensitivity and mechanisms of failure in primates. J Bone Joint Surg *56A*:236–253, 1974.

149. Painter: Boston Med Surg J *156*:345, 1907.

150. Pappas AM, Zawacki RM, and McCarthy CF: Rehabilitation of the pitching shoulder. Am J Sports Med *13*(4):223–235, 1985.

151. Pappas AM, Zawacki RM, and Sullivan TJ: Biomechanics of baseball pitching. A preliminary report. Am J Sports Med *13*:216–222, 1985.

152. Payr E: Gelenk "Sperren" und "Ankylosen;" über die "Schultersteifen verschiedener Ursache und die sogenannte "Periarthrities humero-scapularis," Ihre Behandlung. Zbl f Chir *58*:2993–3003, 1931.

153. Penny JN, and Smith C. The prevention and treatment of swimmer's shoulder. Can J Appl Sport Sci *5*:195–202, 1980.

154. Penny JN, and Welsh RP: Shoulder impingement syndromes in athletes and their surgical management. Am J Sports Med *9*(1):11–15, 1981.

155. Peterson CJ, and Gentz CF: Ruptures of the supraspinatous tendon—the significance of distally pointing acromioclavicular osteophytes. Clin Orthop *174*:143, 1983.

156. Petersson CJ, and Redlund-Johnell I: The subacromial space in normal shoulder radiographs. Acta Orthop Scand *55*:57–58, 1984.

157. Pettersson G: Rupture of the tendon aponeurosis of the shoulder joint in antero-inferior dislocation. Acta Chir Scand (Suppl.) *77*:1–187, 1942.

158. Pingaud and Charvot: Scapulalgie. *In* Dechambre: Dictionaire Encyclopédique des Sciences Médicales, Vol II. Paris: 1879, p 232.

159. Poppen NK, and Walker PS: Normal and abnormal motion of the shoulder. J Bone Joint Surg *58A*:195, 1976.

160. Post M, and Cohen J: Impingement syndrome—a review of late Stage II and early Stage III lesions. Proceedings of the ASES First Open Meeting, 1985.

161. Post M, and Cohen J: Impingement syndrome. Clin Orthop *207*:126–132, 1986.

162. Post M, and Jablon M: Constrained total shoulder arthroplasty; long-term follow-up observations. Clin Orthop *173*:109–116, 1983.

163. Priest JD, and Nagel DA: Tennis shoulder. Am J Sports Med *4*:28–40, 1976.

164. Pujadas GM: Coraco-acromial ligament syndrome. J Bone Joint Surg *52A*:1261–1262, 1970.

165. Raggio CL, Warren RF, and Sculco T: Surgical treatment of impingement syndrome: a four year follow-up. Proceedings of the ASES First Open Meeting, 1985.

166. Rask MR: Suprascapular nerve entrapment: a report of two cases treated with suprascapular notch resection. Clin Orthop *123*:73–75, 1977.

167. Rask MR: Suprascapular axonotmesis and rheumatoid disease. Clin Orthop *134*:266–267, 1978.

168. Rathbun JB, and Macnab I: The microvascular pattern of the rotator cuff. J Bone Joint Surg *52B*:540, 1970.

169. Rengachary SS, Neff JP, Singer PA, and Brackett CE: Suprascapular entrapment neuropathy: a clinical, anatomical, and comparative study. Neurosurgery *5*(4):441–446, 1979.

170. Richardson AB, Jobe FW, and Collins HR: The shoulder in competitive swimming. Am J Sports Med *8*(3):159–163, 1980.

171. Rocks JA: Intrinsic shoulder pain syndrome. Phys Ther *59*(2):153–159, 1979.

172. Rockwood CA: The role of anterior impingement to lesions of the rotator cuff. J Bone Joint Surg *62B*(2):274, 1980.

173. Rostron PK, Orth MCH, Wigan FRCS, and Calver RF: Subcutaneous atrophy following methylprednisolone injection in Osgood-Schlatter epiphysitis. J Bone Joint Surg *61A*(4):627–628, 1979.

174. Rothman RH, and Parke WW: The vascular anatomy of the rotator cuff. Clin Orthop *41*:176, 1965.

175. Rowe RG: Brush up your medicine; sporting injuries of the shoulder. Med J Aust 16–18, 1978.

176. Saha AK: Theory of Shoulder Mechanism. Springfield, IL: Charles C Thomas, 1961, p 54.

177. Saha AK: Mechanics of elevation of glenohumeral joint: its application in rehabilitation of flail shoulder in upper brachial plexus injuries and poliomyelitis and in replacement of the upper humerus by prosthesis. Acta Orthop Scand *44*:668, 1973.

178. Sahlstraud T, and Save-Soderbergh J: Subacromial bursitis with loose bodies as a cause of refractory painful arc syndrome. A case report. J Bone Joint Surg *62A*(7):1194, 1980.

179. Salter RB, Gross A, and Hall JH: Hydrocortisone arthropathy: an experimental investigation. Can Med Assoc J *97*:374, 1967.

180. Salter RB, and Murray D: Effects of hydrocortisone on musculo-skeletal tissues. J Bone Joint Surg (Br) *51B*:195, 1969.

180a. Samilson RL: Congenital and developmental anomalies of the shoulder girdle. Orthop Clin North Am *11*(2):219–231, 1980.

181. Schaer H: Ergebn d Chir u Orthop *29*:211, 1936.

182. Schar W, and Zweifel C: Das os acromiale und seine klinische Bedeutung. Bruns Beiträge zur Klinischen Chir. Breitner B, and Nordmann O (eds). Berlin: Urban & Swarzenberg, 1936, p 101.

183. Schneider JE, Adams OR, Easley KJ, et al: Scapular notch resection for suprascapular nerve decompression in 12 horses. JAMA *187*(10):1019–1020, 1985.

184. Seeger LL, Gold RH, Bassett LW, and Ellman H: Shoulder impingement syndrome: MR findings in 53 shoulders. AJR *150*:343–347, 1988.

185. Sievers: Verh dtsch Ges Chir 43. Kongr., p 243, 1914.

186. Sigholm G, Styf J, Körner L, and Herberts P: Pressure recording in the subacromial bursa. J Orthop Res *6*(1):123–128, 1988.

187. Silvij S, and Nocini S: Clinical and radiological aspects of gymnast's shoulder: Note 1. J Sports Med *22*:49–53, 1982.

188. Skinner HA: Anatomical considerations relative to rupture of the supraspinatus tendon. J Bone Joint Surg *19A*:137, 1937.

189. Smaill GB: Bilateral rupture of Achilles tendon. Br Med J *1*:1657, 1961.

190. Smith-Petersen MN, Aufranc OE, and Larson CB: Useful surgical procedures for rheumatoid arthritis involving joints of the upper extremity. Arch Surg *46*:764–770, 1943.

191. Solheim LF, and Roaas A: Compression of the suprascapular nerve after fracture of the scapular notch. Acta Orthop Scand *49*:338–340, 1978.

192. Stamm TT: A new operation for chronic subacromial bursitis. J Bone Joint Surg *45B*:207, 1963.

193. Sticda A: Zur Pathologie der Schulter gelenkschlembeutel. *In* Archiv für Klinische Chirurgie. Langenbeck B (ed). Berlin: Verlag von August Hirschwald, 1908, p 910.

194. Strizak AM, Danzig L, Jackson DW, et al: Subacromial bur-

sography: an anatomic and clinical study. J Bone Joint Surg *64A*(2):196, 1982.

195. Sutek L, and Mast WA: Subacromial bursography: technique and clinical application. Tech Dev Instrum *144*(3):626–630, 1982.

196. Sweetnam R: Corticosteroid arthropathy and tendon rupture. J Bone Joint Surg *51B*:397, 1969.

197. Tamai K, and Ogawa K: Intratendinous tear of the supraspinatus tendon exhibiting winging of the scapula. Clin Orthop *194*:159–163, 1985.

198. Taylor GM, and Tooke M: Degeneration of the acromioclavicular joint as a cause of shoulder pain. J Bone Joint Surg *59B*:507, 1977.

199. Thorling J, Bjerneld H, Hallin G, et al: Acromioplasty for impingement syndrome. Orthop Scand *56*:147–148, 1985.

200. Tibone JE, Jobe FW, Kerlan RK, et al: Shoulder impingement syndrome in athletes treated by an anterior acromioplasty. Clin Orthop *198*:134–140, 1985.

201. Tillaux: Traité de la chirurgie clinique. Paris, 1888.

202. Uitto J, Teir H, and Mustakallio KK: Corticosteroid induced inhibition of the biosynthesis of human skin collagen. Biochem Pharm *21*:2161, 1972.

203. Unverferth LJ, and Olix ML: The effects of local steroid injections on tendon. J Sports Med *1*:31–37, 1973.

204. Valtonen EJ: Double acting betamethasone (Celestone Chronodose) in the treatment of supraspinatus tendinitis: a comparison of subacromial and gluteal single injections with placebo. J Int Med Res *6*:463–467, 1978.

205. Vogt: Deutsche Chirurgie Lief 64, 1881.

206. Watson M: The refractory painful arc syndrome. J Bone Joint Surg *60B*:544–546, 1978.

207. Watson-Jones R: Fractures and Joint Injuries, 4th ed. Baltimore: Williams & Wilkins, 1960, pp 449–451.

208. Watters WB, and Buck R: Scanning electron microscopy technique. J Microscopy *94*:185–187, 1971.

209. Weaver HL: Isolated suprascapular nerve lesions. Injury: Br J Accident Surg *15*(2):117–126, 1983.

210. Weiner DS, and Macnab I: Superior migration of the humeral head. A radiological aid in the diagnosis of tears of the rotator cuff. J Bone Joint Surg *52B*(3):524–527, 1970.

211. Weiss JJ: Intra-articular steroids in the treatment of rotator cuff tear: reappraisal by arthrography. Arch Phys Rehabil *62*:555–557, 1981.

212. Wellisch: Wien med Wschr p. 974, 1934.

213. Welsh P, Penny N, and Mcnab I: Proceedings of the Canadian Orthopaedic Association. J Bone Joint Surg *61B*(2):243, 1979.

214. Wiley AM, and Older MWJ: Shoulder arthroscopy. Am J Sports Med *8*:31–38, 1980.

215. Wilson CL: Lesions of the supraspinatus tendon: degeneration, rupture and calcification. Arch Surg *46*:307, 1943.

216. Withrington RH, Girgis FL, and Seifert MH: A placebo-controlled trial of steroid injections in the treatment of supraspinatus tendinitis. Scand J Rheumatol *14*:76–78, 1985.

217. Wrede L: Ueber Kalkablagerungen in der Umgebung des Schultergelenks und ihre Beziehungen zur Periarthritis. *In* Archiv für Klinische Chir. Berlin: Verlag von August Hirschwald, 1912, p 259.

218. Wrem RN, Goldner JL, and Markee JL: An experimental study of the effect of cortisone on the healing process and tensile strength of tendons. J Bone Joint Surg *36A*:588, 1954.

Rotator Cuff Tendon Failure

Frederick A. Matsen III, M.D.
Craig T. Arntz, M.D.

A stitch in time saves nine

Historical Review

It is often difficult to tell where concepts actually begin. It is certainly not obvious who first used the term *rotator* or *musculotendinous cuff*. Credit for first describing ruptures of this structure is often given to J. G. Smith, who in 1834 described the occurrence of tendon ruptures after shoulder injury in the London Medical Gazette.[221] In 1924 Meyer published his attrition theory of cuff ruptures.[152] In 1934 Codman's classic monograph summarized his 25 years of observations on the musculotendinous cuff and its components and discussed ruptures of the supraspinatus tendon.[39] He proposed a traumatic etiology for cuff rupture. Beginning 10 years after the publication of Codman's book and for the next 20 years, McLaughlin wrote on the etiology of cuff tears and their management.[147–150] Arthrography, the definitive test for cuff tears, was first carried out by Oberholtzer in 1933.[185] He used air as the contrast medium. Lindblom and Palmer[136] used radio-opaque contrast and described their results in 1939. Using this technique, these authors described partial-thickness, full-thickness, and massive tears of the cuff.

Codman recommended early operative repair for complete cuff tears. He apparently carried out the first cuff repair in 1909.[39] Current views of cuff tear pathogenesis, diagnosis, and treatment are quite similar to those that he proposed over 50 years ago.

Anatomy and Function

The rotator cuff is generally defined as the complex of four muscles that arise from the scapula and attach to the tuberosities of the humerus, along with the subjacent capsule that blends in with these tendons near their insertion. The subscapularis arises from the anterior aspect of the scapula and attaches over much of the lesser tuberosity. It is innervated by the upper and lower subscapular nerves. The supraspinatus muscle arises from the supraspinatus fossa of the scapula, passes beneath the acromion and the acromioclavicular joint, and attaches to the upper aspect of the greater tuberosity. It is innervated by the suprascapular nerve after it passes through the suprascapular notch. The infraspinatus muscle arises from the infraspinous fossa of the scapula and attaches to the posterolateral aspect of the greater tuberosity. It is innervated by the suprascapular nerve after it passes through the spinoglenoid notch. The teres minor arises from the lower lateral aspect of the scapula and attaches to the lower aspect of the greater tuberosity. It is innervated by a branch of the axillary nerve.

The vascular anatomy of the cuff tendons has been described by a number of investigators. Lindblom[134, 135] described an area of relative avascularity in the supraspinatus tendon near its insertion. Moseley and Goldie found that the primary blood supply of the rotator cuff comes from the anterior humeral circumflex, the subscapular, and the suprascapular arteries.[166] Their histological and injection studies showed a rich vascular pattern with many anastomoses in the tendon of the supraspinatus. They concluded that the "critical zone" of the supraspinatus (prone to ruptures and calcium deposits) was not much less vascularized than other parts of the cuff. Rather, this zone is rich in anastomoses between the osseous and tendinous vessels. This interconnection between tendinous and osseous vessels may help account for the collapse of the humeral head seen with chronic massive cuff tears.[170] Rothman and Parke[207] found contributions to the cuff vessels from the suprascapular, anterior circumflex, and posterior circumflex arteries in all cases. The thoracoacromial contributed in 76 per cent of the cuff's blood supply, the suprahumeral in 59 per cent, and the subscapular in 38 per cent. These authors found the area of the supraspinatus just proximal to its insertion to be markedly undervascularized in relation to the remainder of the cuff.

Rathbun and Macnab,[201] however, found that the filling of cuff vessels was dependent on the position of the arm at the time of injection. They noted a consistent zone of poor filling near the tuberosity attachment of the supraspinatus when the arm was adducted; with the arm in abduction, however, there was almost full filling of vessels to the point of insertion. The authors suggested that tendon failure might be caused by "constant pressure from the head of the humerus which tends to wring out the blood supply to these tendons when the arm is held in the resting position of adduction and neutral rotation." Nixon and DiStefano[183] suggested that the "critical zone" of Codman corresponds to the area of anastomoses between the osseous vessels (the anterolateral branch of the anterior humeral circumflex and the posterior humeral circumflex) and the muscular vessels (the suprascapular and the subscapular vessels). Uhthoff and coworkers[235] observed relative hypovascularity of the deep surface of the supraspinatus insertion as compared with its superficial aspect. Recently, the vascularity of the supraspinatus tendon has been reconfirmed by the laser Doppler studies of Swiontkowski.[228] The laser Doppler assesses red cell motion at a depth of 1 to 2 mm. Swiontkowski found substantial flow in the "critical zone" of normal tendon and increased flow at the margins of cuff tears.

The histology of the supraspinatus insertion has been studied in some detail. Codman[39] observed that there were "transverse fibers in the upper portion of the tendon." He stated that "these are probably some of those of the infraspinatus . . . the insertion of the infraspinatus overlaps that of the supraspinatus to some extent. Each of the other tendons also interlaces its fibers to some extent with its neighbor's tendons." Clark[34] studied 22 shoulders with intact rotator cuffs and confirmed this interlacing. He found that the tendons of the four cuff muscles flare out and interdigitate as they insert into the humerus. The subscapularis and supraspinatus fuse where they cross the biceps tendon and thus form a part of the tendon's sheath. The penetration of the infraspinatus into the supraspinatus was even more extensive. All of these tendons were well supplied with blood vessels. These findings suggest that the cuff is well designed to bear tension and to resist upward displacement of the humerus. Parenthetically, when dissecting what appeared to be an intact cuff, Clark frequently encountered a deep-substance tear in which fibers were avulsed from the humerus.

Benjamin and coworkers[14] have analyzed four zones of the supraspinatus attachment to the greater tuberosity: (1) the tendon itself, (2) uncalcified fibrocartilage, (3) calcified fibrocartilage, and (4) bone. Whereas there were blood vessels in the other three zones, the zone of uncalcified fibrocartilage appeared avascular. A tidemark existed between the uncalcified and calcified fibrocartilage that was continuous with the tidemark between the uncalcified and calcified portions of articular cartilage. The collagen fibers often meet this tidemark approximately at right angles. In the tendon of the supraspinatus there is an abrupt change in fiber angle just before the tendon becomes fibrocartilaginous and only a slight change in angle within fibrocartilage. In interpreting the significance of these findings, these authors point out that the angle between the humerus and the tendon of the suprapinatus changes constantly in shoulder movement. While the belly of the muscle remains parallel to the spine of the scapula, the tendon must bend to reach its insertion. This bending appears to take place above the level of the fibrocartilage so that the collagen fibers meet the tidemark at right angles. The fibrocartilage provides a transitional zone between hard and soft tissues, protecting the fibers from sharp angulation at the interface between bone and tendon. The fibrocartilage pad keeps the tendon of the supraspinatus from rubbing on the head of the humerus during rotation, as well as keeping it from bending, splaying out, or becoming compressed at the interface with hard tissue.

The rotator cuff muscles dynamically stabilize and steer the head of the humerus. They balance the major forces applied by the prime mover muscles (the deltoid and the pectoralis major) during motions such as flexion and abduction.* This dynamic stabilization can easily be demonstrated by contrasting the anteroposterior laxity of the relaxed shoulder with that of the same shoulder while the muscles are gently contracted. Certainly contraction of the anterior deltoid, elevating the arm in a forward direction, would tend to push the head of the humerus out the back of the shoulder joint were it not for the reciprocal contraction of the infraspinatus, producing a force couple. Even minor attempts to abduct the shoulder by the deltoid benefit from the action of the supraspinatus and other humeral head depressors to prevent the head of the humerus from rising up against the coracoacromial arch (Figs. 16–1 and 16–2).

The cuff contribution to shoulder power has been evaluated by Colachis and associates,[47, 48] who used selective nerve blocks and found that the supraspinatus and infraspinatus provide 45 per cent of abduction and 90 per cent of external rotation stength. Howell and coworkers[107] measured the torque produced by the supraspinatus and deltoid muscles in forward flexion and elevation. They found that the supraspinatus and deltoid muscles are equally responsible for producing torque about the shoulder joint in the functional planes of motion.

Functionally speaking, the long head of the biceps tendon may be considered a part of the rotator cuff.

---

*See references 5, 67, 108–110, 209, 229, 241.

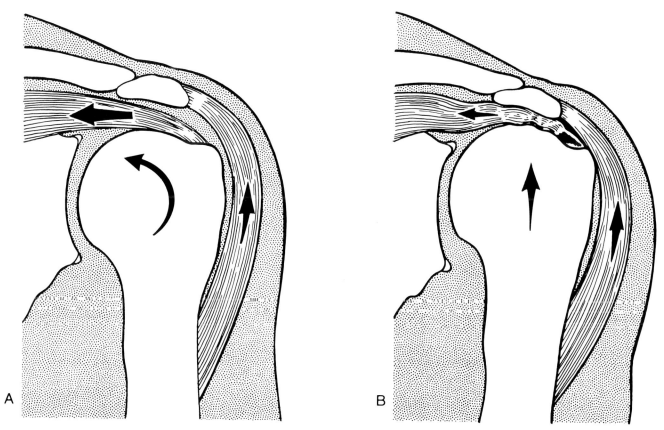

Figure 16–1. *A,* The supraspinatus helps to stabilize the head of the humerus against the upward pull of the deltoid. Here subacromial impingement is prevented by normal cuff function. *B,* Deep surface tearing of the supraspinatus weakens the ability of the cuff to hold the head of the humerus down. Impingement of the tendon against the acromion is the result.

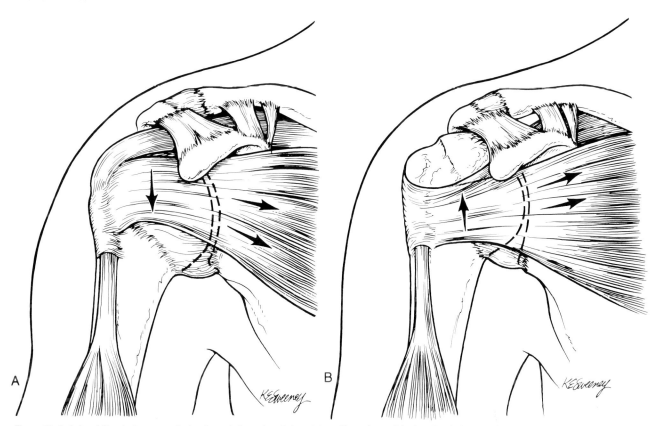

Figure 16–2. *A,* In addition to the supraspinatus, the anterior and posterior rotator cuff muscles and the long head of the biceps tendon depress the humeral head and balance the upward-directed forces applied by the deltoid muscle. *B,* Major cuff fiber failure and retraction allows the humeral head to protrude upward through the cuff defect, creating a type of "boutonniere" lesion. When the remaining cuff tendons slip below the equator of the head, their action is converted from humeral head depression to humeral head elevation.

It attaches to the supraglenoid tubercle of the scapula, runs between the subscapularis and the supraspinatus, and exits the shoulder through the bicipital groove under the transverse humeral ligament, attaching to its muscle in the proximal arm. Slätis and Aalto[220] point out that the coracohumeral ligament and the transverse humeral ligament keep the biceps tendon aligned in the groove. The long head of the biceps is positioned to act as a humeral head depressor. Furthermore, it has the potential for guiding the head of the humerus as it is elevated, the bicipital groove traveling on the biceps tendon like a monorail on its track. This mechanism helps to explain why the humerus is capable both of substantial rotation when it is adducted and of very little rotation when it is maximally abducted, in which position the tuberosities straddle the biceps tendon near its attachment to the supraglenoid tubercle. The close functional relationship between the rotator cuff and biceps tendon is emphasized by the frequency with which tears of the two structures coexist.

Classification of Injury

Many terms have been used to describe cuff tendon failure, including partial and full thickness, acute and chronic, and traumatic and degenerative. It is useful to recognize that cuff failure is almost always peripheral, near the attachment of the cuff to the tuberosities, and nearly always begins in the supraspinatus part of the rotator cuff near the biceps tendon. An important aspect of cuff tendon failure is whether the tendon defect extends all the way through from the articular surface to the bursal surface of the rotator cuff (a *full-thickness* tear) or involves only the superficial surface, midsubstance, or deep surface (a *partial-thickness* tear). *Acute* tears are those occurring suddenly, usually as a result of a definite injury. Acute cuff tears accounted for only 8 per cent of 510 candidates for cuff repair in a 24-year Mayo Clinic series.[46] *Chronic* tears are those that have existed for a long time (e.g., three months or more); they may be insidious in onset and degenerative in nature. A chronic tear is at risk for an *acute extension*—the sudden failure of additional fibers with the production of acute symptoms superimposed on those of the chronic tear. We characterize cuff tears according to the length of the detachment from the humerus, the specific tendons involved, and the state of the detached tendons (e.g., retracted, atrophic, or absent).

Incidence and Mechanism of Injury

INCIDENCE

The incidence of full-thickness tears of the rotator cuff has been measured in various series of cadaver dissections: Smith[221] found an incidence of 18 per cent; Keyes,[117] 19 per cent; Wilson,[252, 253] 20 per cent in a series of autopsy dissections and 26.5 per cent in a series of cadaver dissections; Cotton and Rideout,[52] 8 per cent; Yamanaka and coworkers,[261] 7 per cent; Fukuda and associates,[87] 7 per cent; and Uhthoff and colleagues,[235] 20 per cent. Neer found that the incidence of complete cuff tears in more than 500 cadaver shoulders was less than 5 per cent.[169]

Partial-thickness tears appear to be about twice as common. Yamanaka and coworkers[261] reported on 249 cadaver shoulders in which they found a 13 per cent incidence of partial-thickness tears; 32 per cent of shoulders over 40 had had cuff tears, whereas there were no tears seen in those under 40. The incidence of bursal side tears was 2.4 per cent. In 249 cadaveric left shoulders, Fukuda found a 13 per cent incidence of partial-thickness cuff tears; 3 per cent were on the bursal side, 7 per cent were intratendinous, and 3 per cent were on the joint side. In his studies of 96 shoulders in patients ranging in age from 18 to 74 years, DePalma found a 37 per cent incidence of partial-thickness tears of the supraspinatus and infraspinatus, a 21 per cent incidence of partial-thickness tears in the subscapularis, and a 9 per cent incidence of full-thickness tears. Uhthoff and associates[235] found a 32 per cent incidence of partial-thickness tears in 306 autopsy cases with a mean age of 59 years. Other studies report partial-thickness tears in approximately 20 to 30 per cent of cadaver shoulders.* As pointed out by Pettersson,[195] an examination that is confined to inspecting the bursal aspect of the supraspinatus will overlook the commonest form of tear—the partial-thickness tear on the deep surface. In their clinical series of partial-thickness cuff tears Fukuda and associates[86] found 9 tears on the bursal side, 11 on the joint side, and 1 intratendinous. The bursal side tears had the most severe symptoms. All of these tears were localized in the critical area of the supraspinatus tendon. Arthroscopists have reported partial-thickness articular surface tears with increasing frequency in the shoulders of athletes.[133] In the absence of a method for noninvasively assessing midsubstance tendon fiber failure, it is difficult to ascertain the incidence of such problems; however, the data of DePalma and Fukuda attest to their frequency. It is apparent that the incidence of the more difficult to observe partial-thickness tears is significantly greater than that of the obvious full-thickness tears.

The incidence of cuff tears in clinical subjects has also been studied. Age obviously correlates with the incidence. In their series of shoulder dislocations, Reeves[202] and Moseley[165] found the incidence of cuff tears among patients under 30 to be very low. These authors found that the incidence of cuff failure in dislocated shoulders rose dramatically with the age of the patient. Yamada and Evans found no cuff tears in 42 shoulders under age 40.[258] Pettersson[195] found that

---

*See references 40, 46, 52, 86, 96, 102, 117, 134–136, 235.

in patients with anteroinferior dislocations, the incidence of arthographically proven partial- or full-thickness cuff tears was 30 per cent in the fourth decade and 60 per cent in the sixth decade. Even more amazing, he found that of 27 asymptomatic, untraumatized shoulders in patients aged 55 to 85, 13 had partial- or full-thickness rotator cuff tears diagnosed arthrographically.

MECHANISM OF INJURY

The literature contains much discussion of the mechanism of cuff tendon failure. Normal tendon is exceedingly strong. The work of McMasters[151] is frequently quoted in this regard. He conducted experiments showing that loads applied to normal rabbit Achilles tendons produced failure at the musculotendinous junction, at the insertion into bone, at the muscle origin, or at the bone itself, but not at the tendon midsubstance. In his preparation, one-half of the tendon's fibers had to be severed before the tendon failed in tension. If the tendon was crushed with a Kocher clamp, pounded, and then doubly ligated above and below the injury, rupture could be produced in half of the specimens when tested over four weeks later. Normal tendon is obviously tough stuff! However, human tissues weaken as they grow older. As an example, Hollis and associates[107] showed that the anterior cruciate ligament of a 70-year-old is only 20 to 25 per cent as strong as that of a 20-year-old.*

The proposed causes of cuff tendon failure have included trauma,[38, 40] attrition,[68, 118, 152, 164] ischemia,[134–136, 166, 201, 207] and impingement. Neer,[168, 169] Neviaser and Neviaser,[180] Craig,[53] Peterson and Gentz,[194] and Watson[242] have emphasized the importance of impingement of the cuff against the overlying acromion, the coracoacromial ligament, and the acromioclavicular ligament. It is recognized that the supraspinatus insertion and the biceps lie anterior to this coracoacromial

---

*See references 39, 66, 134–136, 143, 168, 169, 183, 195, 245.

arch with the arm at the side and must pass underneath it as the arm is elevated. Neer[168] emphasized that the critical area for wear is centered on the supraspinatus tendon and long head tendon of the biceps. Variations and abnormalities of the acromion are correlated with the incidence of cuff tears. He proposed that impingement wear can lead to incomplete or complete rotator cuff tears and rupture of the long head of the biceps. He observed that cuff tears have a 95 per cent association with subacromial impingement.[169]

In a series of 47 patients with arthrographically confirmed supraspinatus tendon ruptures, Peterson and Gentz[194] found that 51 per cent had distally pointing acromioclavicular joint osteophytes. A similar incidence was found in their series of 170 autopsy specimens with cuff defects. The incidence of distally pointing acromioclavicular osteophytes in normal shoulders was 14 per cent and 10 per cent in the clinical and cadaver studies, respectively.

Nixon and DiStefano[183] remarked that the incidence of cuff lesions in athletes called into question the statement that normal tendon does not rupture. Recent arthroscopic evidence corroborates partial tendon tearing in the "normal" shoulders of throwers. Interestingly, these do not seem to be intratendinous tears but rather avulsions from the bone. This finding is actually not new and not confined to athletes. In 1934 Codman described the "rim rent" in which the deep surface of the cuff is torn at its attachment to the tuberosity (Figs. 16–3 and 16–4).[39] It is interesting to note that even his example of a "normal" supraspinatus insertion shows this lesion to a small degree: "Notice how close to the rim of the articular cartilage the fibers are attached and that a few of them in this specimen have given way at the very edge." Codman's view of the frequency of this lesion and the potential range of pathology is indicated by the following passage:

[Figure 16–3] shows an extensive tear so that the rent has come through to the most superficial fibers of the tendon. The reader should visualize this vertical section so as to understand that the rent also extends along the curve of the edge of the joint cartilage to a considerable extent, leaving the sulcus bare, perhaps for an inch or more. This condition

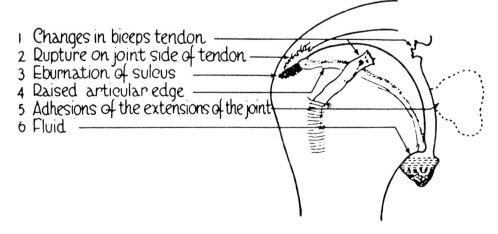

Figure 16–3. In 1934 Codman described the "rim rent" wherein the deep surface of the cuff is torn at its attachment to the tuberosity. (Reproduced with permission from Codman EA: The Shoulder: Rupture of the Supraspinatus Tendon and Other Lesions In or About the Subacromial Bursa. Malabar, FL: Robert E Krieger, 1984.)

1 Changes in biceps tendon
2 Rupture on joint side of tendon
3 Eburnation of sulcus
4 Raised articular edge
5 Adhesions of the extensions of the joint
6 Fluid

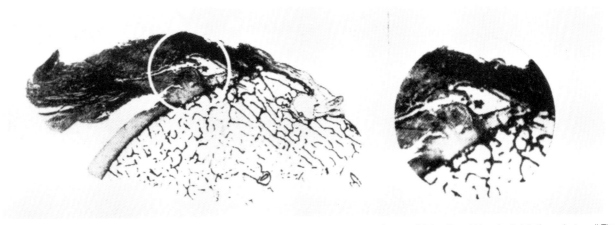

Figure 16–4. Codman's illustration of "A rim rent where all the tendon is torn away from the sulcus except the superficial portion which extends into the periosteum." These photomicrographs provide a convincing argument that cuff tears frequently begin on the deep surface and extend outward until they become full thickness defects. (Reproduced with permission from Codman EA: The Shoulder: Rupture of the Supraspinatus Tendon and Other Lesions In or About the Subacromial Bursa. Malabar, FL: Robert E Krieger, 1984.)

I like to call a "rim rent," and I am confident that these rim rents account for the great majority of sore shoulders. It is my unproved opinion that many of these lesions never heal, although the symptoms caused by them usually disappear after a few months. Otherwise, how could we account for their frequent presence at autopsy?

Codman's wonderful book contains many photomicrographs of these rim rents, providing a convincing argument that cuff tears frequently begin on the deep surface and extend outward until they become full-thickness defects (see Fig. 16–4). Codman even offers a challenge to the concept of subacromial impingement as the primary cause of these defects: "It would be hard to explain this section . . . by erosion from contact with the acromion process." Similarly, McLaughlin[147] observed that partial tears of the cuff "commonly involve only the deep surface of the cuff, so that the retracted tab of tissue may produce an internal derangement of the shoulder joint in just the same way that a mobile tab of medial meniscus produces symptoms in the knee." Wilson and Duff[253] also described partial tears near the insertion of the cuff. These occurred on the articular surface, on the bursal surface, and in the substance of the tendon. Cotton and Rideout[52] also described "slight" tears on the deep surface of the supraspinatus adjacent to the biceps tendon in their necropsy studies. DePalma described and copiously illustrated the fact that "the innermost fibers of the cuff begin to tear away from their bony insertion into the humeral head in the fifth decade."[66] Pettersson states that incomplete transverse ruptures are generally situated on the inner aspect of the aponeurosis just above the greater tuberosity.[195] The partial-thickness tears observed by Uhthoff and coworkers[235] were always on the articular side; none occurred on the bursal side in spite of the occasional presence of spurs or osteophytes on the acromion. Other authors also have described partial thickness tears.* These observations are most consistent with the

concept that the deep fibers of the cuff near its insertion to the tuberosity are vulnerable to failure, whether from heavy use in throwing or as the summation of many years of routine activities.

Most full-thickness cuff tears appear to occur in tendon that is weakened by some combination of age, repeated small episodes of trauma, steroid injections, subacromial impingement, hypovascularity of the tendon, major injuries, and previous partial tearing. In all series, the incidence of these partial-thickness tears begins to rise in the 50- to 60-year age group and peaks in the 70-year and over age group. Pettersson[195] states that "even in cases of traumatic rupture . . . the age distribution indicates that changes in the elasticity and tensile strength are prerequisites for the appearance of the rupture." Rotator cuff tears are uncommon prior to age 40 and, as noted by DePalma, even massive injuries to young healthy shoulders "seem more likely to produce glenohumeral ligament tears and fractures than ruptures of the rotator cuff." Many cuff tears occur in 50- to 60-year-old individuals who have led quite sedentary lives without a history of injury or heavy use. Neer provided evidence for a nontraumatic etiology of cuff tears:[169] (1) 40 per cent of his patients with cuff tears were "individuals who have never done strenuous physical work"; (2) there was a high percentage of bilateral cuff tears; (3) many heavy laborers never develop cuff tears; and (4) 50 per cent of his patients had no recollection of shoulder trauma. In their 1988 report to the American Shoulder and Elbow Surgeons (ASES), Neer and coworkers[171] found that of 233 patients with cuff tears, all but 8 were over 40; 70 per cent of tears occurred in sedentary individuals doing light work, 27 per cent in females, and 28 per cent in the nondominant arm.

Pettersson[195] provides an excellent summary of the early work on degenerative changes of the cuff tendons. Citing the research of Loschke, Wrede, Codman, Schaer, Glatthaar, Wells, and others, he builds a convincing case for primary, age-related degeneration of the tendon manifested by changes in cell arrangement, calcium deposition, fibrinoid thickening, fatty

*See references 17, 18, 39, 85, 87, 129, 161, 189, 225, 230, 231, 233, 259–261.

degeneration, necrosis, and rents. He states that "the degenerative changes in the tendon aponeurosis of the shoulder joint, except for calcification and rupture, give no symptoms, as far as is known at present. On the other hand the tensile strength and elasticity of a tendon aponeurosis that exhibits such degenerative lesions are unquestionably less than in a normal tendon aponeurosis." Pettersson noted that the innermost fibers of the cuff begin to tear away from their bony insertion to the humeral head in the fifth decade and that these partial-thickness tears increase in size over the next several decades. The weakening of the rotator cuff by attrition was promoted as a concept by Meyer[152, 153] and corroborated by the studies of DePalma. Uhthoff observed fibrillation, microtears, and hyalinization on light and scanning electron microscopy. Nixon and DiStefano, reviewing the literature on the microscopic anatomy of cuff deterioration,[183] found loss of the normal organizational and staining characteristics of bone, fibrocartilage, and tendon *without evidence of repair*. They summarized these degenerative changes as follows:

Early changes are characterized by granularity and a loss of the normal clear wavy outline of the collagen fibers and bundles of fibers. The structures take on a rather homogenous appearance; the connective tissue cells become distorted and the parallelism of the fibers is lost. The cell nuclei become distorted in appearance—some rounded, others pyknotic or fasiculated. Some areas of the tendon have a gelatinous or edematous appearance with loosening of fibers that contain broken, frayed elements separated by a pale staining homogeneous material.

Brewer[26] has demonstrated age-related changes in the rotator cuff. These changes include diminution of fibrocartilage at the cuff insertion, diminution of vascularity, fragmentation of the tendon with loss of cellularity and staining quality, and disruption of the attachment to bone via Sharpey's fibers. The bone at the insertion becomes thinner and prone to fracture.

All this evidence leads one to wonder if the commonly diagnosed entity of "cuff tendinitis" may actually represent failure of fibers of the rotator cuff. These fiber failures produce acute, self-limited symptoms, perhaps "responding" to ultrasound treatments, anti-inflammatory medications, and steroid injections. After these ruptures occur, however, they must leave the cuff somewhat weaker than before. The number of fibers failing may be influenced by the magnitude and direction of force applied to the tendon as well as the strength of the tendon against that direction of load. The degree to which these areas of fiber failure can heal and the degree to which fibers that remain intact may hypertrophy or strengthen to take up the function of the damaged fibers are not known.

It appears likely that repeated failure of small groups of fibers lead not only to self-limited, acute symptoms but also to progressive weakness of the rotator cuff, making it more susceptible to damage from lesser loads. This gives rise to the "creeping tendon ruptures"

described by Pettersson. If the process is slowly progressive, the shoulder may compensate in a way that minimizes symptoms and maximizes comfort and function. Pettersson[195] performed arthrography on 71 apparently healthy, asymptomatic shoulders ranging in age from 15 to 85 years. These shoulders were contralateral to shoulders exposed to dislocation (46 shoulders) or other trauma (25 shoulders). Thirteen of these shoulders were found to have positive arthrograms for partial- or full-thickness tears, all in patients aged 55 or older; most were observed between the ages of 70 and 75 years. All these shoulders were symptom free and without history of trauma. He concluded that these tears resulted from age-related degenerative changes. The observation that many massive cuff tears occur without any recognized incidence of major trauma suggests that previous minor, often subclinical, fiber failure leaves the cuff tendons unable to resist even normal loads. Repeated episodes of fiber failure lead to progressive cuff weakness but not necessarily to pain, unless the extension of the defect is acute and substantial.

Thus, cuff fiber failures are expected to start in the area of maximal load or pre-existing weakness or both. They would then be expected to propagate with less severe loads. This propagation may lead to a progressive partial-thickness tear or to a full-thickness tear, in which case an arthrogram would be positive.[66] Full-thickness tears may propagate with continued use, resulting in the progressive detachment of the supraspinatus insertion; this is followed in the posterior direction by detachment of the infraspinatus and teres minor and in the anterior direction by the transverse humeral ligament and subscapularis.

The traumatic and the degenerative theories of cuff tendon failure can be synthesized into a unified view of pathogenesis. Let us assume that the normal cuff starts out well vascularized and with a full complement of fibers. Through its life it is subjected to various adverse factors such as traction, contusion, impingement, inflammation, injections, and age-related degeneration. Each of these factors places fibers of the cuff tendons at risk. Even though laboratory studies show that normal tendon does not fail before failure of the musculotendinous junction or the tendon bone junction, in the clinical situation the cuff tendon ruptures both at its insertion to bone and in its midsubstance. With the application of loads (whether repetitive or abrupt, compressive or tensile), each fiber fails when the applied load exceeds its strength. Fibers may fail a few at a time or *en masse* (an acute tear or acute extension). Because these fibers are under load even with the arm at rest, they retract after their rupture. Each instance of fiber failure has at least three adverse effects: (1) it increases the load on the neighboring fibers (fewer fibers to share the load), (2) it detaches muscle fibers from bone (diminishing the force that the cuff muscles can deliver), and (3) it risks the vascular elements in close proximity by distorting their anatomy (a particularly important factor owing to the fact that the cuff tendons contain the anastomoses between the osseous and muscular vessels). Thus, the initially well-vascularized cuff tendon becomes progressively avascular with succeeding injuries. Although some tendons, such as the Achilles tendon, have a remarkable propensity to heal after rupture, cuff ruptures communicate with joint and bursal fluid, which removes any hematoma that could contribute to cuff healing. Even if the tendon could heal with scar, scar tissue lacks the normal resilience of tendon and is, therefore, under increased risk for failure with subsequent loading (minor or major). These events weaken the substance of the cuff, impair its function, and diminish its ability to effectively repair itself. With subsequent episodes of loading this pattern repeats itself, rendering the cuff weaker, more prone to additional failure with less load, and less able to heal.

One of the major functions of the cuff is humeral head depression—keeping the head and cuff from subacromial impingement. Cuff failure compromises this protective function and subjects the tendon to additional damage from subacromial wear (see Fig. 16–1). Subacromial wear stimulates the development of subacromial spurs, which may exacerbate impingement. With progressive loss of the depressor mechanism, the head rises higher and higher under the upward pull of the deltoid. The end stage of this process is the shoulder equivalent of a "boutonniere" lesion (see Fig. 16–2).[184] When the head protrudes upward through a major defect in the rotator cuff, the remaining cuff tendons slip below the equator of the head. Their action is converted from humeral head depression to humeral heal elevation. Just as in the boutonniere of the finger, the buttonholed cuff is victimized by the conversion of balancing forces into unbalancing forces. Fixed contractures may develop, as is recognized by the surgeon who attempts to get the humeral head to stay in its normal position after chronic superior subluxation in chronic cuff deficiency.

In summary, cuff failure from any cause results in (1) lessened cuff function (e.g., less humeral head depression), leading to more impingement and more cuff damage; (2) load concentration on remaining fibers, diminishing their ability to withstand loads and leading to additional failure; and (3) diminished local vascularity, resulting in compromised strength and compromised repair. Like a rip in nylon, cuff tendon tears tend to propagate.

Associated Pathology

Upward displacement of the humeral head results in loading of the coracoacromial arch. This loading may give rise to traction spurs extending into the coracoacromial ligament from the acromion.

Rotator cuff tears are frequently accompanied by changes in the long head tendon of the biceps. This tendon is well situated to produce humeral head depression in partnership with the cuff. When the cuff is ruptured, an additional load is borne by the biceps tendon. Ting and coworkers[234] found that the electromyographic activity and size of the long head tendon of the biceps is significantly greater in patients with cuff tears compared with the uninjured shoulder. Upward displacement of the humeral head produces greater impingement of the coracoacromial arch on the biceps as well as the cuff. Neer[168] clearly demonstrated that the proximal bicipital groove is within the impingement zone. This is consistent with the frequent coincidence of bicipital tears and cuff tears. A complete tear of the biceps tendon by itself produces no shoulder pain; thus, the patient with rupture of the long head of the biceps and shoulder pain must be suspected of having a cuff tear. In many cases of cuff tear, the biceps is seen to be hypertrophied and flattened to the contour of the humeral head—almost as if it were trying to become a substitute cuff (Fig. 16–5). Even more frequently, in large cuff tears the biceps tendon is ruptured. Finally, the biceps tendon may be dislocated medially in large cuff tears that involve the transverse humeral ligament and the subscapularis.[220]

The cartilage and bone of the proximal humerus may also be affected in chronic cuff deficiency. These changes may be the result of rubbing of the uncovered and upwardly displaced humeral head on the undersurface of the coracoacromial arch (Fig. 16–6). Neer and colleagues[170] have called attention to the phenomenon of cuff-tear arthropathy. Factors in the pathogenesis of this lesion are thought to include lack of normal joint nutrition and mechanical stability. In this condition, chronic cuff deficiency is accompanied by loss of the articular cartilage and softening of the subchondral bone of the humeral head. Loss of the articular surface of the humeral head may then lead to destruction of the glenoid articular surface.

Clinical Presentation

HISTORY

Patients with rotator cuff tears are almost always over 40 years of age. Even the asymptomatic partial- or full-thickness rotator cuff tears identified by Pettersson occurred in individuals aged 55 and older.[195] Neer and associates[171] found that all but 8 of 233 patients presenting with primary full-thickness cuff tears were over 40 years of age; 70 per cent occurred in patients who did only light work, 27 per cent were in females, and 28 per cent were in the nondominant arm. Of 55 patients with arthrographically verified cuff tears, Bakalim and Pasila[3] found only 3 who were under 40 years of age. In Hawkins and coworkers' recent series of 100 cuff repairs, only 2 patients were in their third or fourth decade.[102] Since individuals younger than 40 subject their shoulders to more violence, age-related weakening is apparently required

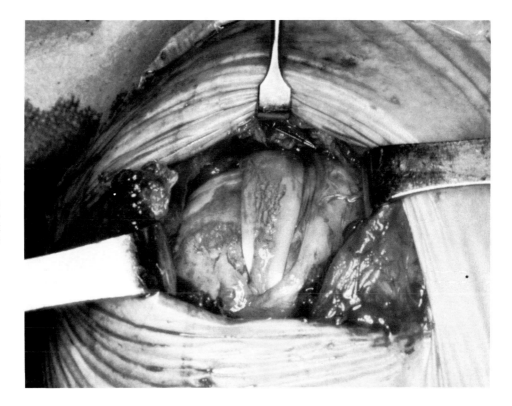

Figure 16–5. Rotator cuff tears are frequently accompanied by changes in the long head tendon of the biceps as it exits the bicipital groove within the impingement zone. In many cases the biceps is seen to be hypertrophied and flattened to the contour of the humeral head—almost as if it were trying to become a substitute cuff.

before the cuff can be torn. About half of the patients with cuff tears can recall a specific episode of shoulder use or trauma that seemed to initiate their symptoms, but this is usually not a major injury. Patients with cuff tears usually have a history of recurrent episodes of shoulder "tendinitis" or "bursitis." These episodes, which often consist of an episode of soreness following shoulder use, may become asymptomatic after a course of rest or a cortisone injection. As described in the previous section, it is likely that these episodes actually represent tendon fiber failure, the acute symptoms of which resolve.[102] As the process of tendon weakening progresses, the patient may notice more persistent shoulder discomfort, particularly on elevation and external rotation of the arm against resistance, as well as pain at night and an inability to sleep on the affected

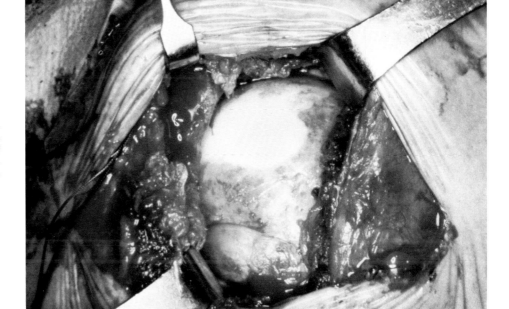

Figure 16–6. Articular surface degeneration is often seen with chronic cuff deficiency. The changes may be the result of rubbing of the uncovered and upward-displaced humeral head against the undersurface of the coracoacromial arch.

side. Full-thickness tears may produce symptoms of subacromial crepitus, particularly when the arm is put in a position where the supraspinatus origin is beneath the acromion—flexion, abduction, and internal rotation. Shoulder weakness may arise from substantial tendon fiber detachment or from disuse atrophy. At this stage patients often relate that cortisone injections "no longer help." Samilson and Binder found that the most common symptoms of cuff tears included pain, weakness in shoulder elevation, and "crackling and popping in the shoulder."[211]

Fukuda and coworkers[87] characterized patients with partial-thickness cuff tears as having pain on motion, crepitus, and stiffness. They observed that patients with bursal side tears seemed more symptomatic than those with deeper tears. In their 1987 report to the ASES, Neviaser and coworkers characterized 31 patients older than 35 years of age, all of whom were unable to elevate their arm after reduction of a shoulder dislocation.[179] Most were incorrectly presumed to have an axillary nerve injury. Eight subsequently developed recurrent anterior dislocation. All patients were found to have cuff tears involving the subscapularis. Repair was effective in preventing recurrent dislocations and in restoring elevation of the arm. Prompt diagnosis and treatment of this lesion was recommended.

PHYSICAL FINDINGS

The physical findings may be related to the lack of smooth surfaces in the subacromial zone (crepitus), loss of tendon attachment to bone (weakness of flexion, abduction, and external rotation), inability to use the cuff muscles normally (atrophy), loss of the depressor mechanism (upward riding of the humeral head upon deltoid contraction), or fluid in the bursa (a bursal effusion). Partial cuff tears may be associated with shoulder stiffness. Many patients with full-thickness cuff tears have a palpable cuff defect. Tenderness may be present over the tuberosities and bicipital groove, although this is usually mild. Patients with full-thickness cuff defects may still retain the ability to actively abduct the arm. Neviaser[176] reported 42 such cases. Brems[21] used a handheld digital strength analyzer to measure the external rotator strength in patients with cuff tears. He found that the external rotator strength was directly related to the size of the tear. Larger tears may produce gross weakness such that the range of passive motion may substantially exceed that of active motion.[102] Ruptures of the long head of the biceps are commonly associated with cuff tears. Tamai and Ogawa[233] reported a case of a horizontal intratendinous tear of the supraspinatus accompanied by nonparalytic winging of the scapula. Neither the pain nor the reflex muscle spasm was lessened by the subacromial injection of local anesthetic. The symptoms resolved after anterior acromioplasty, resection of the affected part of the tendon, and cuff repair to bone.

Imaging Evaluation

Although it may be argued that the diagnosis of a cuff tear can be reliably made from the patient's history and physical examination alone, this has not been our experience. Patients with full-thickness tears can have strong active elevation of the arm; patients without a full-thickness defect may be unable to raise their arm. Neer[169] states that "since physical signs or roentgenographic changes are not reliable, an arthrogram is required for the early recognition of complete-thickness cuff tears and to distinguish them from the other impingement lesions." Since a goal of treatment is to identify and repair a full-thickness tear while it is reparable, imaging of the cuff is important when symptoms and signs do not respond promptly to routine measures, e.g., symptoms of "tendinitis" or "bursitis" that do not respond to three months of rehabilitation or a shoulder that remains weak in flexion or external rotation six weeks after a dislocation.

Plain radiographs are usually normal in small cuff tears. Evidence of impingement may be seen on the x-rays, including bony cysts at the normal cuff insertion, concavity of the undersurface of the acromion, subacromial sclerosis, and acromial spurs (Fig. 16–7).[52, 91, 101, 128, 248] Acromioclavicular arthritis may be present. With larger tears radiographs reveal upward displacement of the head of the humerus with respect to the glenoid and acromion (Figs. 16–8 and 16–9).[39, 52, 92, 102, 113, 248] This feature can be accentuated by externally rotating the arm while the patient attempts isometric abduction. If some external rotators are intact, internal rotation may minimize upward displacement of the head.

Shoulder ultrasonography provides a noninvasive, nonradiographic method for imaging the rotator cuff. In 1982, one of us (F.A.M.) observed that even slight fetal movement enhanced the resolution of ultrasound imaging. This principle also applies to ultrasonography

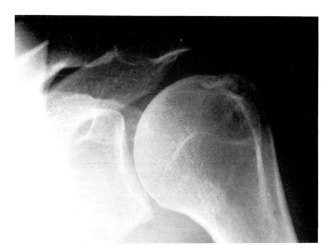

Figure 16–7. In small rotator cuff tears, radiographs may reveal evidence of chronic impingement such as bony cysts at the normal cuff insertion, subacromial sclerosis, and acromial spurs.

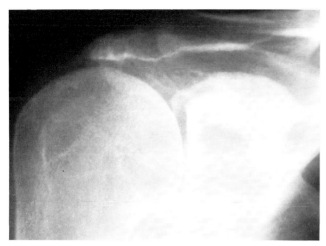

Figure 16–8 With larger cuff tears, radiographs reveal upward displacement of the humeral head with marked narrowing of the interval between the humeral head and acromion. Note the marked cystic changes and sclerosis involving the undersurface of the acromion.

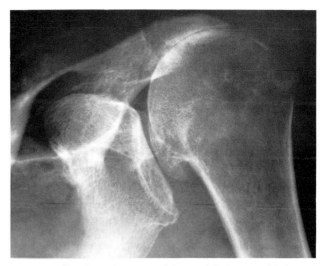

Figure 16–9. Chronic massive tears result in upward displacement of the humeral head until it articulates with the acromion. Humeral osteophytes result from abnormal glenohumeral articulation.

of the cuff: moving the shoulder through a small arc helps to distinguish the cuff tendons from the deltoid and acromion. We presented the first series of ultrasound examinations of the shoulder in 1983.[77] Since that time the criteria for diagnosing cuff lesions have evolved, as have the quality of the equipment and the technique. By careful positioning the experienced ultrasonographer can demonstrate the upper and lower subscapularis, the biceps tendon, the anterior and posterior supraspinatus, the infraspinatus, and the teres minor. Defects are revealed as absence of the normal tissue echoes and failure of the tissue to move appropriately with the appropriate humeral movements (Figs. 16–10 and 16–11). Ultrasonic differentiation of edema, scarring, partial-thickness defects and small

full-thickness tears is still difficult. Mack and coworkers[142] have provided a detailed summary of the technique. In their series of 141 patients from the University of Washington Shoulder Clinic, ultrasonography showed a specificity of 98 per cent and a sensitivity of 91 per cent when compared with surgical findings. Most of the false-negative results occurred in patients found to have tears less than 1 cm in size. Ultrasonography has the advantages of speed and safety, and it allows for comparison with the contralateral shoulder. Low cost is another feature: a bilateral shoulder ultrasound is usually half the cost of a unilateral arthrogram and one-eighth the cost of a shoulder MRI. With improvements in technology and the tech-

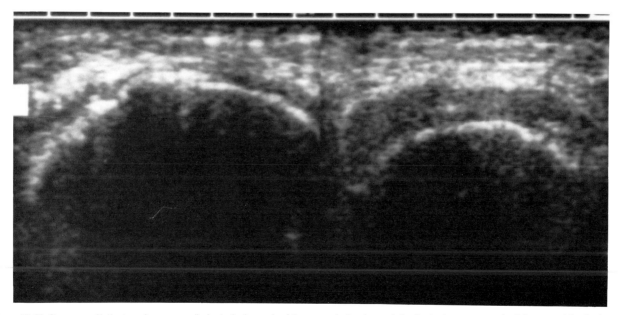

Figure 16–10. Sonogram with the transducer perpendicular to the long axis of the supraspinatus demonstrates the tendon as an arc of soft tissue overlying the humeral head on the normal side (*right*) and absent on the side with a large cuff tear (*left*).

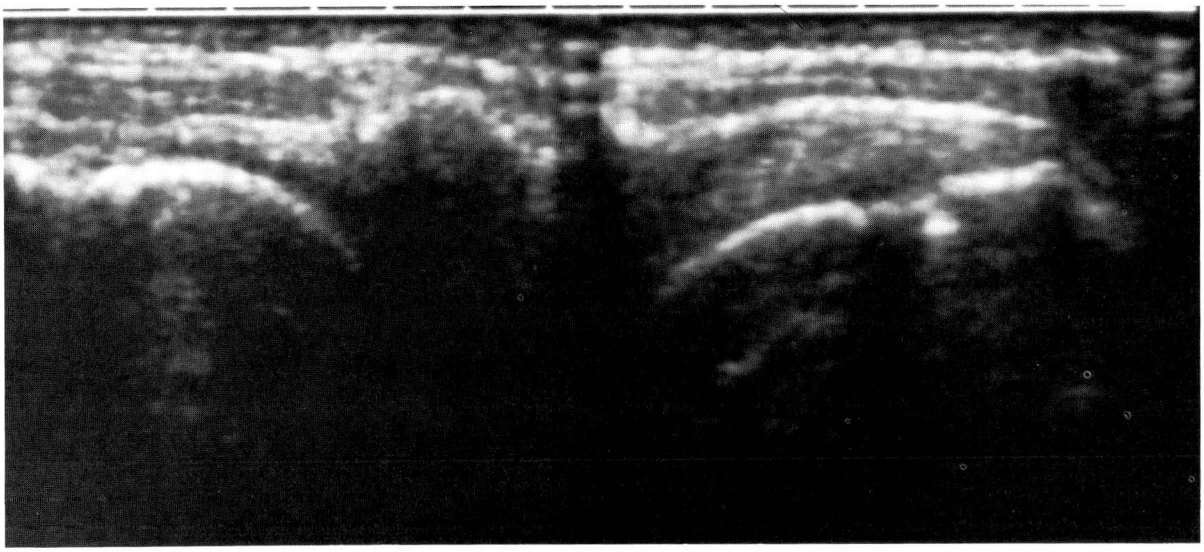

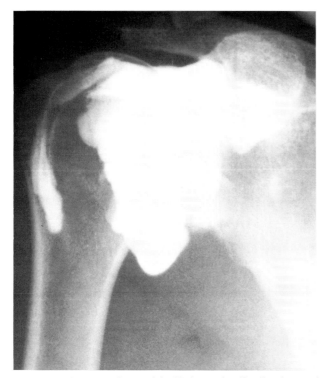

Figure 16–11. Sonogram in the plane of the supraspinatus. The normal attachment to the greater tuberosity is shown on the *right*. Absent supraspinatus insertion is shown in the shoulder with a large cuff tear (*left*).

nique of ultrasonography, the resolution may improve substantially and may in the future provide for the accurate assessment of partial-thickness lesions of the cuff.[49, 60, 156, 159, 160] Crass and Craig,[55] in a recent summary of ultrasonography, pointed to its high degree of accuracy, noninvasiveness, effectiveness in the evaluation of postoperative patients for recurrent tear,[57] and potential for diagnosing incomplete tears.[56]

For many years the shoulder arthrogram has been the standard technique for diagnosing rotator cuff tears. In this test, contrast material is injected into the glenohumeral joint; after brief exercise, radiographs are taken to reveal intravasation of the dye into the tendon or extravasation of the contrast agent through the cuff into the subacromial subdeltoid bursa (Figs. 16–12 and 16–13). In 1933 Oberholzer[185] used air as a contrast agent, injecting it into the glenohumeral joint prior to radiographic evaluation. Air contrast is still

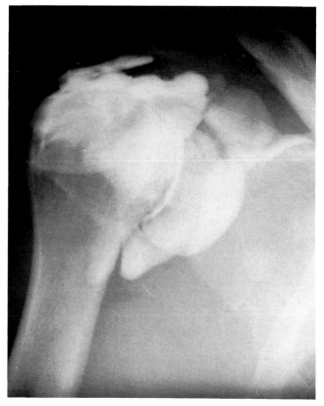

Figure 16–12. Arthrogram of a normal shoulder in neutral position. Note the normal extension of dye beneath the coracoid into the subscapularis bursa. Also note the normal extension of dye beneath the transverse humeral ligament and into the biceps sheath. The superolateral extension of dye is limited by the normal cuff attachment.

Figure 16–13. This arthrogram shows dye leakage into the subacromial space and beyond the normal cuff attachment at the greater tuberosity.

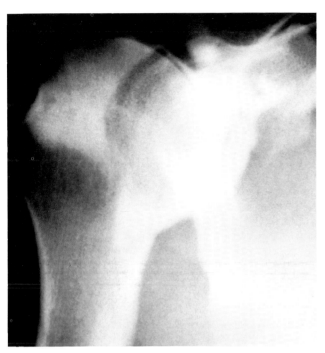

Figure 16–14. This arthrogram shows evidence of a partial thickness rotator cuff tear originating at the articular surface of the cuff. Leakage of dye is seen to extend beyond the normal deep surface cuff attachment and is restrained by the more superficial cuff fibers that insert further laterally (see Fig. 16–3). These findings were confirmed at surgery.

useful in those patients allergic to iodine. In 1939 Lindblom used contrast opaque medium.[134–136] Since then iodinated contrast media have been the standard for single-contrast arthrography. Descriptions of the refinement of this technique are provided by Kerwein and associates[113] Samilson and colleagues,[212] Killoran and coworkers,[122] Resnick,[204] Neviaser,[178] and Ahovuo and colleagues.[1] Pettersson[195] demonstrated the effectiveness of arthrography in revealing partial-thickness cuff tears (Fig. 16–14). Arthrography cannot reveal isolated midsubstance tears or superior surface tears. Craig[53] described the "geyser sign" in which dye leaks from the shoulder joint through the cuff into the

acromioclavicular joint. The presence of this sign suggests a large tear with erosion of the undersurface of the acromioclavicular joint (Fig. 16–15). Double-contrast arthrography using both air and iodinated material may enhance the resolution of arthrography.[1, 75, 89, 113] Berquist and associates[15] reported on the use of single- and double-contrast arthrograms to evaluate the size of the cuff tears seen at surgery. Their ability to accurately predict one of four cuff tear sizes (small, medium, large, and massive) was just over 50 per cent. The reported incidence of false-negative arthrograms in the presence of surgically proven cuff tears ranges from 0 to 8 per cent.* The anatomical resolution of shoulder arthrography can be enhanced to a certain degree by obtaining tomograms with the contrast material in place to give information about the size and location of the tear and the quality of the remaining tissue. Further resolution can be obtained by performing double-contrast arthrotomography.[82, 92, 93, 121] Kilcoyne and Matsen[121] used arthropneumotomography to evaluate the size of the cuff tear and the quality of the residual tissue. They found a good correlation with the surgical appearance.

The subacromial injection of contrast material (bursography) has been used to evaluate the subacromial zone and the upper surface of the rotator cuff.† Fukuda reported six patients having normal arthrograms and positive bursograms, which he defined as pooling of the subacromially injected contrast in the cuff tissue. He reported an overall accuracy for bursography of 67 per cent when compared with operative findings. Although lesions can be identified on this type of examination, criteria for making diagnoses have not been rigorously defined.

Computed tomography (CT) and magnetic resonance imaging (MRI) can image the rotator cuff, and there are some reports of the use of these techniques to judge the integrity of the cuff. The criteria for

---

*See references 102, 103, 162, 176, 198, 211, 256.
†See references 85, 87, 132, 134–136, 161, 173, 225.

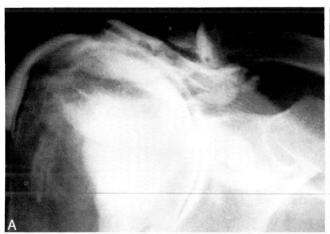
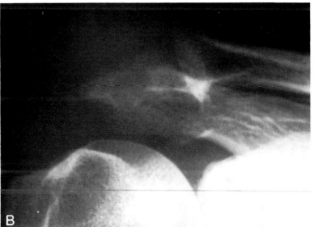

Figure 16–15. *A,* This arthrogram shows leakage of dye into the subacromial space and beyond the normal cuff attachment at the greater tuberosity. Note dye leakage into the acromioclavicular joint, the "geyser" sign. Also note the marked inferior displacement of the cuff outline caused by this arthritic acromioclavicular joint. *B,* Plain radiograph of the same joint.

diagnosing cuff tears with these techniques have yet to be defined. Crass and Craig[55] conclude that the accuracy of MRI in diagnosing cuff pathology is unknown. Kieft and associates[120] reported on 10 patients with shoulder symptoms evaluated with MRI and arthrography. Arthrography showed a tear in three patients, whereas MRI detected none of them. Seitz and coworkers[218] compared arthrography, ultrasonography, and MRI for the detection of cuff tears in 25 patients. They found that ultrasonography was the most helpful study in accurately documenting the size and location of the tear when it existed. MRI suffered from problems of image resolution. Arthrography was reliable in determining full-thickness tears, but correlation with size and location of the tear was difficult.

Complications

The principal complication of rotator cuff tearing is progression of the lesion. Progressive extension of partial- or full-thickness tears results in the progressive loss of tendon fibers, weakness of the cuff mechanism, and progressive loading of the remaining fibers. Shoulder symptoms may be reactivated by a period of overuse or by an injury, producing an acute extension of the cuff tear.

"Rotator cuff tear arthropathy" is a term coined by Neer and coworkers[170] to denote collapse of the humeral articular surface in association with a massive rotator cuff tear (Fig. 16–16). It is estimated that this complication occurs in 4 per cent of patients with full-thickness cuff tears. In their definitive report, Neer and colleagues described 26 shoulders that were surgically explored and then treated with shoulder arthroplasty. Interestingly, over 75 per cent of the patients were female. The average age was 69 years; 20 per cent had evidence of contralateral cuff arthropathy,

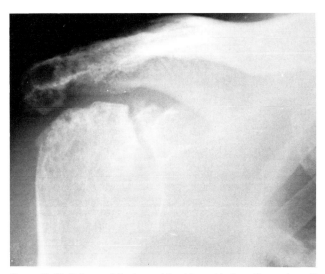

Figure 16–16. Collapse of the humeral head in combination with massive cuff deficiency—"cuff tear arthropathy."

and 75 per cent had no history of trauma. All these observations suggest a degenerative etiology of the arthropathy. The patients complained of pain and diminished use of the shoulder. Although some had had previous surgery and/or steroid injections, these did not appear to be common factors. Examination revealed the shoulder to be swollen, the muscles atrophic, and the long head biceps ruptured; passive elevation was limited to an average of 90 degrees of elevation and 20 degrees of external rotation (a degree of limitation atypical of uncomplicated cuff tears). Often the shoulder demonstrated anteroposterior instability. Collapse of the proximal humeral articular surface was a common observation. Glenoid, greater tuberosity, acromial, and lateral clavicular erosion were often observed. At surgery all patients had ruptures of the supraspinatus, and almost all had symptoms of the impingement and major biceps pathology. These authors hypothesized that the arthropathy resulted from both mechanical factors (such as anteroposterior instability and superior migration of the humeral head) and nutritional factors (such as loss of a closed joint space, lack of normal diffusion of nutrients to the joint surface, and disuse). To this list could be added the disruption of the tendinous–osseous circulation entering through the subscapular, anterior humeral circumflex, and suprascapular vessels. This condition is distinct from osteoarthritis, rheumatoid arthritis, avascular necrosis, and neurogenic arthropathy.[169] Treatment options are limited—the cuff tendons are severely weakened so that cuff repair is prone to failure; resurfacing arthroplasty without secure cuff repair has a high chance of failure,[81] fixed fulcrum prostheses are prone to loosen in this condition; and the patients are usually poor candidates for arthrodesis.[169] In a 1986 report to the ASES, Brownlee and Cofield reported on 20 surgical procedures for cuff tear arthropathy.[29] These included Neer-type total shoulder arthroplasty, total shoulder arthroplasty using a hooded glenoid, and proximal humeral replacement without a glenoid. Extensive mobilization of tendons was attempted for repair. Pain relief was substantial in each group. Active abduction was best in the group with proximal humeral replacement. Three of the glenoid components loosened.

Arntz and Matsen reviewed 10 patients having combined massive irreparable cuff defects and destruction of the glenohumeral joint surface. These shoulders were managed with humeral hemiarthroplasty (Fig. 16–17). This approach frees the patient from the inconvenience of an arthrodesis and from the risk of glenoid component loosening. Often the prosthesis articulated with the sculpted "acromiohumeral joint," providing a smooth fulcrum to resist the upward pull of the deltoid. Postoperative care emphasized early active use. All patients showed substantial improvement in function. Specifically, preoperative pain was rated as marked and disabling, whereas postoperative pain (if any) was slight in all patients. Function was improved in all patients. One patient returned to

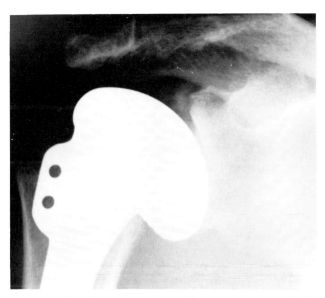

Figure 16-17. Resurfacing of the humeral head improved the comfort and function of the shoulder shown in Figure 16-16.

competitive horseshoe pitching; eight months after surgery he was pitching 50 per cent ringers.

Differential Diagnosis

Traditionally it is stated that rotator cuff tears must be differentiated from cuff *tendinitis* and *bursitis* and that tests such as arthrography or ultrasonography are necessary to make this distinction. Perhaps a more realistic view is that many of the symptoms often attributed to tendinitis and bursitis are, in actuality, episodes of acute fiber failure that cannot be detected by the usual diagnostic tests. Rotator cuff tears must be differentiated from all other causes of shoulder pain and weakness.

Patients with a *frozen shoulder* demonstrate, by definition, a restricted range of passive motion. Patients with partial-thickness cuff defects may similarly demonstrate motion restriction, whereas patients with major full-thickness defects usually have a good range of passive shoulder motion but may be limited in strength or range of active motion. An arthrogram in the case of frozen shoulder shows a diminished volume and obliteration of the normal recesses of the joint.

Cervical spondylosis involving the fifth and sixth cervical nerve route may produce pain in the same areas as rotator cuff involvement as well as weakness on flexion, abduction, and external rotation. Cervical radiculopathy is suggested if a patient has pain on neck extension or turns the chin to the affected side. Sensory, motor, or reflex abnormalities on physical examination and electromyographic changes are additional diagnostic findings. Inasmuch as many asymptomatic patients have degenerative changes at the C5–C6 area, cervical spine radiographs may not be a

selective diagnostic tool. In cases in which this differentiation cannot be easily made we often institute a cervical spine program, including gentle neck mobility exercises, isometric neck-strengthening exercises, home traction, and protection of the neck during sleep, along with other indicated treatment for the shoulder. If the condition worsens, further evaluation is carried out.

Suprascapular neuropathy may arise from at least three causes: (1) traction injury, (2) stenosis at the suprascapular notch, and (3) brachial neuritis. Kopell and Thompson[127] first described entrapment of the suprascapular nerve. Since then, other authors have reported similar cases.* Weaver[246] has summarized many of the aspects of suprascapular nerve lesions. The syndrome that he describes is characterized by dull pain over the shoulder exacerbated by movement of the shoulder, weakness in overhead activities, wasting of the spinati, weakness of external rotation, and normal radiographic evaluation. This picture is very similar to that expected in patients with cuff tears.

Electromyography will usually reveal abnormalities of supraspinatus and infraspinatus denervation when there is substantial involvement from any of the causes listed above. In C5–C6 radiculopathy, involvement of the biceps, deltoid, and other muscles is seen as well. Suprascapular nerve conduction times may be measured and are expected to be abnormal in suprascapular nerve traction injuries, suprascapular nerve entrapment, and brachial neuritis affecting the suprascapular nerve. These latter three conditions must be differentiated essentially by the history. Traction injuries to the suprascapular nerve are usually associated with a history of downward traction on the shoulder and may be a part of a larger Erb's palsy–type injury to the brachial plexus. Suprascapular nerve entrapment may produce chronic recurrent pain and weakness aggravated by shoulder use. Finally, brachial neuritis often produces a rather intense pain lasting for several weeks, with the onset of weakness being noted as the pain subsides. None of these conditions should produce cuff defects on shoulder ultrasonography or arthrography. Suprascapular neuropathy may also result from surgical dissections, including attempts to mobilize the rotator cuff. Thus preoperative electromyography should be considered prior to revision surgery when rotator cuff weakness is present.

Snapping scapula may produce shoulder pain on elevation and a catching sensation somewhat reminiscent of the subacromial snap of a cuff tear. However, the latter can usually be elicited with the scapula stabilized while the arm is rotated in the flexed and somewhat abducted position. Scapular snaps usually arise from the superomedial corner of the scapula, producing local discomfort, and are elicited on shoulder shrugging without much glenohumeral motion.

Other conditions such as *acromioclavicular* or *gle-*

*See references 11, 27, 36, 70, 71, 73, 76, 88, 125, 127, 167, 196, 200, 203, 214, 216, 222, 226.

nohumeral arthritis and *glenohumeral instability* may also produce shoulder pain, weakness, and catching. Thoracic outlet syndrome and superior sulcus (Pancoast's) tumor may produce shoulder pain and weakness. These diagnoses can be reliably differentiated from rotator cuff disease by a careful history, physical examination, and roentgenographic analysis as described in the relevant chapters.

Methods of Treatment

It is essential to realize that cuff tears are not always symptomatic. This is best demonstrated by the data of Pettersson,[195] who performed arthrography on 71 symptom-free, healthy shoulders contralateral to a shoulder having an injury. Of these 71, 13 had positive arthrograms indicating partial- or full-thickness rotator cuff tear. Aggressive treatment is not indicated in the absence of symptoms. If the shoulder is symptomatic, the goals of treatment of rotator cuff disease should include:
1. Restoration of comfort.
2. Restoration of function.
3. Prevention of recurrence or progression.

Sometimes these therapeutic goals are in conflict. For example, the repeated subacromial administration of cortisone can make the shoulder more comfortable and more functional for a variable interval. However, there is substantial documentation of the atrophic effects of corticosteroids and of their retarding of tissue repair. Thus, they may contribute to, rather than prevent, progression of the problem of cuff weakness and fiber failure.

NONOPERATIVE TREATMENT

Nonoperative methods of treatment include physical therapy, administration of nonsteroidal anti-inflammatory medications, rest, avoidance of precipitating activities, and steroid injections. Takagishi demonstrated that 44 per cent of patients with arthrographically proven cuff tears responded to nonoperative measures; many of these respondents had small cuff defects.[232] Although Weiss[249] presented some evidence that patients with arthrographically proven cuff tears are symptomatically improved by intra-articular injections, there is little evidence for a protracted benefit from this method. Other observers found that steroid injections offered no benefit to patients with cuff tears. Coomes and Darlington,[51, 62] Lee and colleagues,[131] and Connolly[50] compared steroid and local anesthetic injections in patients with tendinitis and tendon tears. They found a small subjective benefit in relief of pain but no effect on function in the steroid-treated group. Watson[243] reviewed the surgical findings in 89 patients with major ruptures of the cuff. He found that all 7 patients who had had no local steroid injections had

strong residual cuff tissue. Thirteen of 62 patients having one to four steroid injections had soft cuff tissue that held suture poorly; 17 of the 20 patients having more than four steroid injections had very weak cuff tissue. Shoulders with weak cuff tissue had poorer results after surgical repair. These results are consistent with the findings of Uitto and colleagues,[236] who demonstrated corticosteroid-induced inhibition of the biosynthesis of collagen in human skin. The discussion in Chapter 15 on the deleterious effects of steroids on tendon indicates that steroids cannot be expected to help heal the tendon tear but rather contribute to tendon weakening. Thus any transient benefit of steroid injections in the management of cuff tears may compromise the opportunities for subsequent sound surgical repair.

Various authors have observed that patients with cuff tears will improve with nonoperative management. The incidence of such improvement was 33 per cent in Wolfgang's 1974 series[255] and varied to 90 per cent in Brown's 1949 series.[28] Takagishi[232] found good results in only 44 per cent with nonoperative treatment. The incidence of improvement with nonoperative management was 59 per cent in Samilson and Binder's 1975 series (compared with 84 per cent good to excellent results in their operative series, even though the operated series included massive tears).[211] These studies do not distinguish between acute and chronic tears, do not confirm the magnitude of the tears arthrographically, and do not provide follow-up arthrographic evidence of tendon healing. We know of no clinical series showing conversion of abnormal arthrograms to normal after nonoperative treatment or of no *post mortem* study showing evidence of "healed" cuff tears.

In interpreting reports of nonoperative management, it is essential to ensure, first, that the patients had documented cuff tears and, second, that the management program produced something more than the abatement of the acute discomfort. The evidence suggests that this abatement in discomfort represents nothing more than recovery from an acute extension of the tear and has nothing to do with tendon healing.

OPERATIVE TREATMENT

Samilson and Binder listed the following indications for operative repair:[211] (1) a patient "physiologically" younger than 60 years, (2) clinically or arthrographically demonstrable full-thickness cuff tear, (3) failure of patient to improve under nonoperative management for a period not less than six weeks, (4) patient's need to use the involved shoulder in overhead elevation in his or her vocation or avocation, (5) full passive range of shoulder motion, (6) patient's willingness to exchange decreased pain and increased external rotator strength for some loss of active abduction, and (7) ability and willingness of the patient to cooperate. The authors of this chapter consider repair of all acute tears and of chronic symptomatic tears in active, cooperative patients.

The surgical approaches to the complete cuff tear vary substantially. These include a saber cut,[38] an anterior approach through the acromioclavicular joint,[7] a posterior approach,[63] and an "extensile" approach.[98] Many authors prefer the anterior acromioplasty approach, taking care to preserve the deltoid attachment and acromial lever arm (see Chapter 15).[43, 46, 168, 172] This technique provides excellent exposure of the common sites of lesions—the anterior cuff, biceps groove, undersurface of the acromion, and acromioclavicular joint. Packer and coworkers,[191] reporting on 63 cuff repairs followed for an average of 32.7 months, found that subacromial decompression yielded more pain relief than cuff repair without decompression. If greater access to the supraspinatus is needed, the acromioclavicular joint can be excised.[169] Debeyre and associates[63] described a posterior approach with acromial osteotomy. Ha'eri and Wiley described an approach that is extensile through the acromioclavicular joint to the supraspinous fossa.[98]

Fukuda and colleagues[86, 87] described the management of six patients with partial-thickness bursal-side tears by acromioplasty and/or wedge resection with tendon repair to bone. They used an intraoperative "color test" in which dye was injected into the shoulder joint to indicate the extent of joint side tears. The results were satisfactory in 90 per cent of cases.

Operative techniques for dealing with full-thickness cuff defects include tendon-to-tendon repair and tendon advancement to bone. McLaughlin[147] described his approaches to transverse ruptures (reinsertion into bone), longitudinal rents (side-to-side repair), and tears with retraction (side-to-side repair followed by reinsertion of the retracted portion of cuff into the head wherever it will reach with ease with the arm at the side). Although many of his principles are still applied today, most authors would not concur with his use of the transacromial approach or his belief that "distinct benefits are gained by excising and discarding the outer fragment of the divided acromion."[147-150] Hawkins and colleagues used side-to-side repair for small tears and tendon-to-bone repair for larger defects.[102] Cofield has emphasized the identification of the tear pattern and the use of direct repair and flaps as indicated by the tear pattern.[44, 46]

A number of authors have described extensive tendon mobilization or advancement of major tendon flaps to repair large defects. Cofield recommended the transposition of the subscapularis for repair of large cuff defects.[44] In this technique the subscapularis and the anterosuperior capsule are freed from the anteroinferior capsule, leaving the middle and inferior glenohumeral ligaments intact. The tendon is then transferred superiorly to the anterior aspect of the greater tuberosity. Most patients required postoperative protection in an abduction splint or cast for four to five weeks. These patients, who had severe symptoms of pain and limitation of function preoperatively, had less pain and

slight improvement in active motion; 12 of 26 patients gained more than 30 degrees of active abduction, and 4 lost this amount of motion. Two patients disrupted their repair during the acute postoperative period. Of the 26, 25 were satisfied with the procedure. In less than 5 per cent of his cuff repairs, Neer[169] shifts the infraspinatus and upper half of the subscapularis superiorly to close a defect in the supraspinatus, leaving the lower half of the subscapularis, the teres minor, and the intervening capsule intact. He describes the use of a second incision posteriorly for better mobilization of the infraspinatus toward the top of the greater tuberosity. Neviaser and Neviaser[180] described the transposition of both the subscapularis and the teres minor to close the defect. Debeyre and colleagues and others described the use of a supraspinatus muscle slide to help close major cuff defects.[63, 98, 100] Ha'eri and Wiley[100] used the supraspinatus advancement technique of Debeyre; most of their 18 patients achieved satisfactory results. This technique is of interest, but in our experience isolated supraspinatus tears can usually be repaired without such an advancement. Alternatively, in large or massive tears involving the infraspinatus and/or the subscapularis, the supraspinatus slide seems to offer too little tissue to close the defect.

Some authors have used biological and prosthetic grafts to repair large cuff defects. Neviaser,[176] Bush,[30] and McLaughlin and Asherman[150] employed grafts from the long head tendon of the biceps to patch cuff defects. Ting and coworkers[234] found that the electromyographic activity and size of the long head tendon of the biceps is significantly greater in patients with cuff tears compared with the uninjured shoulder. Their study suggests that the long head of the biceps may be a greater contributor to abduction and flexion in the shoulder with cuff tear than in the normal shoulder and that sacrificing the intracapsular portion of the tendon for grafting material may not be advisable. Heikel[104] used fascia lata to close cuff defects, and both Heikel and Bateman described the use of the coracoacromial ligament. Freeze-dried rotator cuff has been used by Neviaser and coworkers[177] In this report, 16 patients with massive tears had cadaver grafts, producing decrease in nocturnal pain in all 16. The change in shoulder function and strength was not reported. Post[197] reported on preliminary results in five patients in whom a carbon fiber prosthesis was used to manage massive cuff deficiencies. Three had excellent to good results and two failed, one because of possible infection. The author states that these results are no better than with conventional repairs. Finally, synthetic cuff prostheses have been used by Ozaki and colleagues[188] and Post.[197] The former found that of 168 shoulders with cuff tears (almost all of which were "chronic" and "massive"), 25 could not be repaired by standard surgical techniques. Their defects were typically 6 × 5 cm. These patients had cuff reconstruction with Teflon fabric, Teflon felt, or Marlex mesh. This procedure was followed by a structured postoperative program, including the use of an abduction orthosis to keep the arm elevated in the plane of the scapula for two to three months and continued rehabilitation for three to six months. At an average of 2.1 years follow-up, 23 of 25 patients gained 120 to 160 degrees of abduction (the other 2 having had axillary nerve injury). Whereas 20 had reported continual or intolerable pain preoperatively, pain was absent in 23 patients at follow-up. The authors found that results were better with the thicker felt and now recommend the use of 3- to 5-mm-thick Teflon felt in their patients with massive defects.

The prescribed postoperative management is variable. Some authors recommend postoperative immobilization in an abduction splint,[3, 7, 63, 104] while others advise against this.[149, 183]

Results

Neer and coworkers[171] reported the results of 233 primary cuff repairs with an average follow-up of 4.6 years. Results were excellent (essentially normal), in 77 per cent, satisfactory in 14 per cent, and unsatisfactory in 9 per cent. The unsatisfactory ratings were usually due to lack of strength rather than pain and usually occurred in patients with long-standing, neglected tears. Hawkins and coworkers found that 86 per cent of their patients had relief of pain after repair.[102] Recovery of strength was more common in patients with smaller tears.[102] In other series pain relief was reported in 58 per cent,[193] 60 per cent,[104] 66 per cent,[63] 74 per cent,[90] and 85 per cent.[211]

Gore and associates[95] reviewed the results from 63 primary cuff repairs with an average of 5.5 years' follow-up. The shoulders without a traumatic onset were repaired an average of 32 months after the onset of symptoms, whereas those with a traumatic onset were repaired an average of 6 months after the traumatic episode. The surgical approach and technique varied somewhat but usually consisted of acromioplasty and tendon repair to bone or to adjacent tendon. Six shoulders had biceps tendon grafts. Most shoulders were immobilized at the side for four to six weeks, but 12 had immobilization in abduction. Subjective improvement was seen in 95 per cent of shoulders with repaired cuffs. Flexion averaged 126 degrees actively and 147 degrees passively. Most patients had marked relief of pain and minimal or no problems with activities of daily living. Patients with tears less than 2.5 cm long had better results than those with larger tears. The superior results with repair of smaller tears is consistent with the observations of Godsil and Linscheid[90] and Post and coworkers.[198] Watson[243] found that results were worse in patients with larger cuff defects, with multiple preoperative steroid injections, and with preoperative weakness of the deltoid. Ellman and colleagues[75] reported a 3.5-year follow-up of 50 patients having rotator cuff repair. Techniques of repair included tendon-to-tendon suture, reimplantation

into bone, grafts, and tendon flaps. Comfort and function were usually improved by these procedures. Their report provides additional support for timely repair: patients with symptoms of longer standing had larger tears and more difficult repairs. Shoulders with Grade 3 or less strength of abduction before surgery had poorer results; those with an acromiohumeral interval of 7 mm or less also had poorer results. Arthrography was not consistently accurate in estimating the size of the tear.

Hawkins found that acromioplasty and cuff repair relieved the patients' pain and restored the ability to sleep on the affected side in most patients. Seventy-eight per cent were able to use the arm above shoulder level after surgery, whereas only 16 per cent were able to do so before surgery. Hawkins and coworkers[102] found that the results of cuff repair were worse in patients on workmen's compensation. Only 2 out of 14 patients unable to work because of cuff tears could return to work after surgery, whereas 8 of 9 patients not on workmen's compensation did return to work after operation. Other series of cuff repairs include those of Codman,[39] Moseley,[164] Neviaser,[176] Wolfgang,[255] Bakalim and Pasila,[3] Bassett and Cofield,[6] Earnshaw and coworkers,[72] Packer and associates,[191] Post and colleagues,[198] Samilson and Binder,[211] and Weiner and Macnab.[247] Cofield[46] averaged the results of many reports in the literature and found that pain relief occurred in 87 per cent (range 71 to 100 per cent), and patient satisfaction averaged 77 per cent (range 72 to 82 per cent).

The importance of continued postoperative exercises is emphasized by the data of Walker and associates,[241] who measured the isokinetic strength of the shoulder after cuff repair. They found a significant increase in strength between 6 and 12 months after surgery. One year after operation, abduction was 80 per cent of normal and external rotation was 90 per cent of normal. Brems[21] found that the strength of external rotation after cuff repair averaged 20 per cent at three months, 38 per cent at six months, 57 per cent at nine months, and 71 per cent at one year.

An analysis of the results of cuff repair is hampered by lack of a uniform description based on the following criteria: the magnitude and location of the cuff defect, the quality of the remaining tissue, and the outcome in terms of anatomical integrity, comfort, and function. The need for correlation of anatomical and functional outcomes is demonstrated by the results of cuff debridement for irreparable tears. Neer,[168] Rockwood,[205] and others have reported that in certain cases of a massive cuff defect, comfort and function may be enhanced by debridement of the shreds of residual cuff and subacromial decompression followed by muscle strengthening and range-of-motion exercises. The realization that patients may have surprisingly good function and comfort in the presence of major cuff defects makes the definition of "success" after a cuff repair difficult. Interestingly, there have been few follow-up studies of cuff repairs with rigorous attempts to determine the integrity of the cuff using techniques such as arthrography or ultrasonography. Lundberg[138] followed 21 cuff repairs with arthrography and found leakage in 7. The results in the leaking cuffs were not as good as in those with sealed cuffs. By contrast, Calvert and associates[31] performed double-contrast arthrograms in 20 patients at an average of 30 months after operative repair of a torn cuff. In 17 of 20 shoulders the contrast leaked into the bursa, indicating a cuff defect. These defects were estimated to be small in 8, medium in 8, and large in 2. However, 17 patients had complete relief of pain, 15 had a full range of shoulder elevation, and 10 felt that they had regained full function. The authors suggest that a completely watertight closure is not essential for a good functional result and that arthrography may not be helpful in the investigation of failure of repair. Mack and coworkers[141] have made some preliminary investigations of the accuracy of ultrasonography in this regard. In a group of symptomatic postoperative shoulders that were subsequently reoperated, ultrasonography accurately diagnosed recurrent cuff tears in 25 of 25 cases and correctly confirmed cuff integrity in 10 of 11.

A number of authors have reported the results of decompression and debridement of the cuff (as opposed to surgical repair). Bakalim and Pasila[3] found that acromial excision alone gave relief of night pain in certain cases. Rockwood[205] has demonstrated some dramatic improvements in comfort and function with debridement of ratty cuff tissue and subacromial decompression in carefully selected patients in whom repair was technically impossible. It is apparent that more studies correlating the integrity of the cuff with the surgical results are necessary if we are to fully understand the elements essential to the treatment of cuff problems.

With respect to acute tears, Bakalim and Pasila reviewed their series of 55 patients with arthrographically verified rupture of the cuff tendons treated surgically.[3] Whereas only half of the workers were able to return to their previous work, all workers operated upon within one month of a traumatic rupture of the cuff were able to return to their jobs. Bassett and Cofield[6] presented a series of 37 patients having surgical repair within three months of cuff rupture. At an average follow-up of seven years, active abduction averaged 168 degrees for those having repair within 3 weeks and 129 degrees for those having repair within 6 to 12 weeks after injury. Patients with small tears averaged 148 degrees and those with large tears averaged 133 degrees of elevation. The authors concluded that surgical repair must be considered within 3 weeks of injury to obtain maximal return of shoulder function.

The results of surgery for failure of previous cuff repairs are inferior to those of primary repair. DeOrio and Cofield[65] reviewed their experience with rerepairs. At a minimum of two years' follow-up (average four years), 76 per cent of patients had substantial diminution of pain; however, 63 per cent still had moderate or severe pain. Only seven patients gained more than 30 degrees of abduction, and only four patients were felt to have a good result. The authors suggest that the main benefit of repeat cuff surgery is likely to be a reduction in discomfort.

Authors' Preferred Method of Treatment

THEORY

A cuff tear is the failure of muscle attachment to bone. Our treatment of cuff tears is based on the theory that this failure may occur in many patterns, ranging along a continuum from single fiber failure to sudden avulsion of an entire tendon. When only a few fibers fail, the resulting clinical picture may suggest tendinitis or bursitis. The repeated application of moderate loads may overwhelm the weakest of the remaining fibers or those bearing the greatest part of the load. The sudden application of large loads may abruptly tear larger numbers of fibers. Because the failure of a fiber places an additional load on its intact neighbor, tendon tears tend to propagate—partial-thickness tears become full-thickness tears, and small full-thickness tears become larger by extending anteriorly or posteriorly. Fiber failure (aggravated, perhaps, by secondary muscle atrophy) lessens the strength of the humeral depressors, subjecting the remaining cuff tissue to pressure and rubbing under the coracohumeral arch. Finally, we suggest that ruptured cuff fibers do not have much potential to become whole again. Rupture is accompanied by retraction; the intra-articular environment does not favor the rebuilding of new fibers; the tear itself compromises the tendon's blood supply. Pathological specimens have not shown evidence of fiber healing with nonoperative management. This set of observations leads us to the concept that early diagnosis and prompt surgical treatment of symptomatic cuff tears are important if cuff integrity is to be restored.

EVALUATION

Patients are evaluated by careful history to elucidate the time and circumstances of onset of symptoms, their duration, and previous treatment (with particular reference to the number and spacing of steroid injections). On physical examination we seek evidence of cuff tears, such as bursal effusion, palpable cuff defects, muscle atrophy, pain on shoulder elevation, less active than passive range of motion, and subacromial crepitus. We document external rotator strength by having the patient push outward isometrically against the examiner's hand with his or her arm in 90 degrees of elbow flexion and neutral shoulder rotation. This standardized position has proved most effective in comparing external rotator strength among shoulders. We have found loss of external rotator strength to be one of the most sensitive indicators of the magnitude of the tear. The history and physical examination also seek to exclude other diagnoses such as cervical radiculopathy and suprascapular neuropathy, which may mimic cuff pathology.

Plain radiographs (an anteroposterior view in internal and external rotation and an axillary view) are obtained to exclude joint surface changes and other bony abnormalities. The acromiohumeral interval also gives some indication of the size of the tear. Certainly, if the acromion and humeral head are in contact, the humeral head has "buttonholed" through a substantial cuff defect.

NONOPERATIVE TRIAL

Patients with the *chronic* syndrome of lateral shoulder pain worsened by elevation and external rotation against resistance receive a trial of "tendinitis treatment": rest, administration of nonsteroidal anti-inflammatory medication, and gentle rotator cuff stretching as well as internal and external rotator strengthening exercises. This program is often bypassed in active patients with acute cuff tears—surgical repair is usually the preferred approach.

Rest. The patient is taught which activities stress the cuff tendons. If work or sport requires such actions, modifications are suggested. For example, a short grocery clerk may stand on a platform to permit use of the shoulder at a lower level. Tennis players may temporarily abstain from serving and backhands, devoting the time to practicing the forehand. Swimmers may use a kickboard.

Medication. There is little documentation of a therapeutic effect for medication in cuff tears. Nevertheless, we frequently suggest the use of aspirin, ibuprofen, or another nonsteroidal anti-inflammatory medication as a therapeutic trial. We try to avoid steroid injections, even in the bursa, because of concern that they may contribute to further weakening of an already damaged cuff.

Stretching. The shoulder is stretched gently but persistently against all directions of tightness. These commonly include forward flexion, cross-body adduction, and internal rotation up the back. The patient is taught these exercises by the therapist and is asked to do them in five five-minute sessions per day. Stretching after aerobic exercise or a hot bath is encouraged as well.

Strengthening. The internal and external rotators are *gently* strengthened by patient-conducted exercises. These begin with isometrics and progress to rotation against the resistance of small rubber tubing, elastic bands, or light weights. The patient is instructed not to overdo these exercises lest the cuff problem be aggravated. Any soreness from the exercises must subside within a few minutes of their cessation. Strengthening exercises with the arm above 60 degrees of elevation are avoided to prevent excessive loading

of the tendons and tendon wear under the coracoacromial arch.

Patients are informed that this program may take approximately six weeks to yield improvement—it should not be abandoned if the shoulder is not better after a few days! If there is no improvement in two months, cuff imaging is performed. If there are signs of atrophy, weakness, or suspicious circumstances (such as a recent shoulder dislocation in someone over 40 or weakness after a shoulder injury), cuff imaging is obtained without delay.

CUFF IMAGING

If an experienced diagnostic ultrasonographer is not available, single-contrast shoulder arthrography is the cuff imaging procedure of choice. After the injection of contrast, the shoulder is vigorously exercised. Radiographs are then obtained in the following positions: an axillary view and an anteroposterior view in the plane of the scapula with the humerus in both internal and external rotation. The technique is adjusted to slightly underpenetrate the area of the cuff insertion to facilitate the identification of partial-thickness tears on the articular side. Partial-thickness tears near the supraspinatus insertion are more easily identified with the arm held in slight passive abduction and external rotation; this slackens the tendon and facilitates filling of the defect with contrast medium.

In our Shoulder Clinic we enjoy the partnership of an experienced ultrasonographic team. In their hands dynamic ultrasonography provides a specific, noninvasive test. However, even in expert hands this test has the disadvantage of missing some tears smaller than 1 cm. Thus a normal ultrasound in a persistently symptomatic patient should be followed up with arthrography to exclude a small tear. One of the advantages of shoulder ultrasonography is that the opposite shoulder can be conveniently imaged. The routine examination of the contralateral shoulder indicates a high incidence of bilateral involvement.

If ultrasonography or arthrography indicates an intact cuff, patients are advised to continue working on the exercise program for another six weeks before other options such as additional work-up or acromioplasty are considered. Patients with persistent symptoms are examined frequently and should not be lost to follow-up; otherwise, they may come back a year later with an irreparable cuff tear.

RETURN TO ACTIVITIES

If the patient improves and is prepared to go back to the activities that may have caused the problem, these activities are carefully reviewed in an attempt to minimize situations that will unnecessarily challenge the cuff mechanism. For the athlete, attention is directed toward the techniques of his or her activity, such as pitching, tennis serving, or swimming. Mistakes include the use of the arm in excessive elevation (inadequate body lean) in throwing and serving and insufficient body roll in swimming. "Fitness" programs are reviewed to ensure that exercises are not done with the arms in abduction and that weightlifting is directed at achieving a high number of repetitions with reasonable resistance rather than using massive weights for only a few repetitions. The workplace environment is reviewed to minimize the use of the arm in flexion and abduction.

WHEN TO REPAIR A TORN CUFF

Acute tears are repaired acutely (within three weeks), if possible, before retraction, scarring, tendon edge degeneration, and muscle atrophy can occur to a substantial degree.

We recommend that active patients with symptomatic chronic cuff tears consider surgical treatment. Patients are informed of the natural history of untreated cuff tears, the risks of surgery, and the anticipated outcome of surgery based on the preoperative assessment of tear size, tendon quality, and rehabilitation potential. Surgery for chronic tears may be indicated to improve comfort and function and to prevent subsequent extensions of the cuff defect. We attempt to present a realistic assessment of the patient's chances for improvement after attempted cuff repair. Factors suggesting the presence of good-quality cuff tissue amenable to sound surgical repair include (1) an acute onset of shoulder symptoms without a history of prior cuff problems, (2) an onset of symptoms related to an injury, (3) physiological age of less than 60 years, (4) good strength of external rotation (Grade 4 or better), and (5) normal radiographs (normal joint space, normal acromiohumeral interval). In such a situation, the surgeon will usually find a reparable defect with strong cuff tissue that can be securely implanted in bone. The patient with these signs is told that repair provides a good chance for improvement in function as well as comfort. Factors suggesting deficiency in the quantity and quality of cuff tissue that will make a sound repair more difficult include (1) an insidious, atraumatic onset of cuff pathology, (2) Grade 3 or less strength of external rotation, (3) physiological age over 60 years, (4) upward displacement of the humeral head relative to the glenoid and acromion, and (5) a history of multiple steroid injections. In the presence of these characteristics, the patient is told that a vigorous attempt will be made to mobilize and repair the cuff but that the quality of the tissue may limit the possibilities for repair—the surgeon may find that the cuff tendons have all the strength of wet Kleenex. Even in these circumstances, however, patients are informed that they may experience pain relief from the removal of debris and irregularities from the subacromial space.

PROCEDURE

The goals of surgical repair of full-thickness defects are (1) to achieve solid fixation of good-quality cuff tendon to the humerus, (2) to have the site of fixation be as nearly anatomical as possible, (3) to place the tendon under physiological tension, (4) to prevent postoperative subacromial impingement through adequate decompression, and (5) to permit postoperative rehabilitation that will minimize unwanted scar.

Exposure

The patient is positioned in a semisitting (beach chair) position. Both the anterior and posterior aspects of the chest and the arm are prepared to allow access to the back of the shoulder and full motion of the arm. The shoulder is entered through an acromioplasty "deltoid-on" approach as described in detail in Chapter 15 (Fig. 16–18 A–C). Particular attention is paid to preserving the deltoid integrity at its origin from the acromion. A standard acromioplasty is performed to decompress the repair and to enhance exposure of the tendons. Resection of the lateral 1.5 cm of the clavicle is carried out only when acromioclavicular arthritis exists or, occasionally, if greater exposure to the supraspinatus is required. Hypertrophic bursa is cleared away, carefully dissecting it from the subjacent cuff. If a cuff tear is not obvious, the cuff tendons are inspected for hyperemia and palpated for a change in the thickness of the cuff, which may indicate a deep surface or midsubstance tear. A 25 per cent methylene blue solution is injected into the joint, as described by Fukuda,[86] to facilitate the identification of partial-thickness lesions. Substantial partial-thickness tears are treated by excising the area of cuff weakness and reattaching the residual tendon to bone. We have made some shoulders more comfortable by arthroscopically debriding the ends of deep-surface partial-thickness cuff tears, although this obviously does nothing to restore the strength of the remaining tendon fibers and may do little to alter the long-term course of the shoulder.

If a full-thickness tear is identified, its margins are clearly identified before repair is attempted. "Ratty" borders of the cuff tendon are conservatively debrided back to tissue that is capable of holding suture. Tendon fragments remaining on the tuberosities are rarely useful in the repair and are usually debrided.

Mobilization

Retracted tendon is freed from the acromion, deltoid, glenoid, and coracoid as needed. In small cuff defects with minimal loss of tissue, extensive cuff mobilization is not necessary. Mobilization of the retracted cuff from the deltoid is accomplished with a probing finger or blunt dissector gently passed over the supraspinatus and infraspinatus muscles. During these maneuvers, care must be exercised to avoid injury to

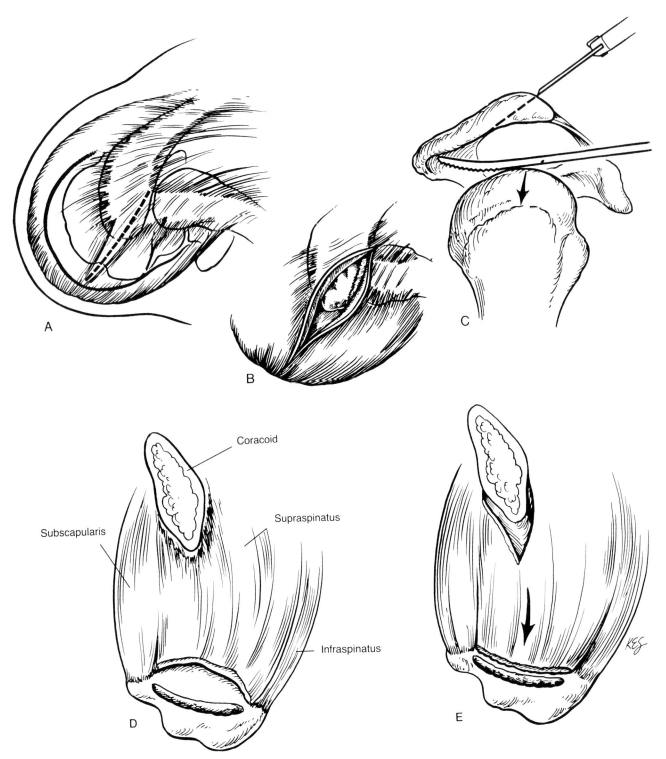

Figure 16–18. Surgical approach to rotator cuff repair. *A,* The shoulder is entered through an acromioplasty approach as described in detail in Chapter 15. *B,* The "deltoid-on" approach offers excellent exposure to the coracoacromial arch and the underlying rotator cuff while maintaining the integrity of the deltoid origin. *C,* A standard acromioplasty is performed to enhance exposure and to decompress the cuff repair. *D,* The supraspinatus and subscapularis muscles have fascial attachments to the coracoid base via the coracohumeral ligament. *E,* Lateral mobilization of the retracted cuff is facilitated by release of these attachments.

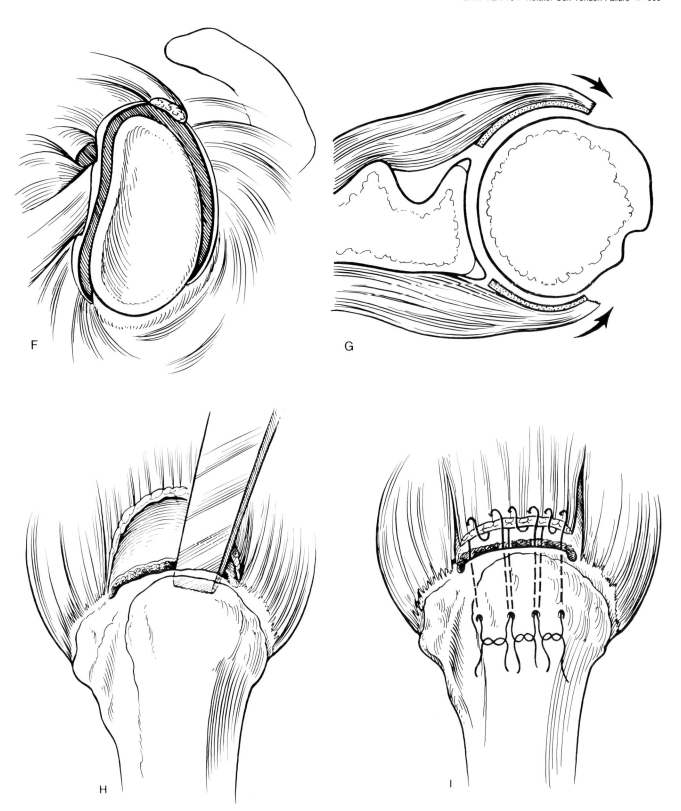

Figure 16–18 *Continued F, G,* Substantial lateral advancement of the cuff can be achieved by freeing the capsule from the glenoid. This is accomplished by sharply incising the capsule at its insertion to the glenoid labrum as shown. Care is taken to avoid injury to the long head tendon of the biceps and to the labrum itself. *H,* A beveled bony trough is created in the sulcus just lateral to the articular surface. This trough extends into the well-vascularized cancellous bone to optimize tendon/bone healing. *I,* The cuff has been fully mobilized and a beveled bony trough has been created. Drill holes for sutures are made connecting the base of the trough to the lateral aspect of the greater tuberosity. These holes are sufficiently low so that the tied knots will be out of the impingement area. A double loop suture technique is used to achieve an optimal bite on the tendon edge and facilitate delivery deep into the bony trough.

Illustration continued on following page

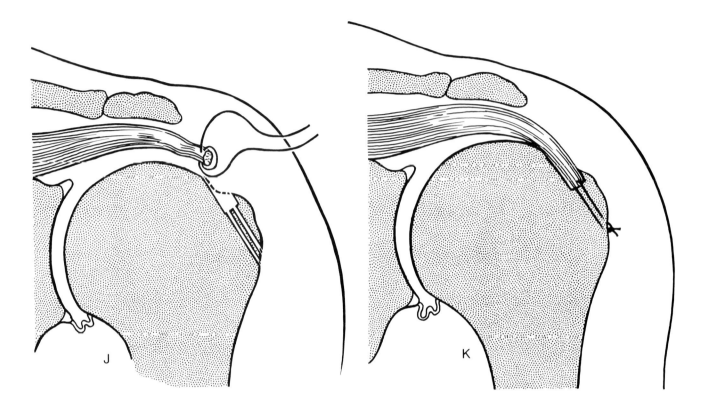

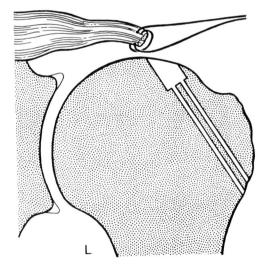

Figure 16–18 *Continued J, K,* The sutures are passed through the appropriately placed bony holes, and the cuff edge is drawn deep into the trough. Adequate cuff mobilization is required to permit good quality cuff tissue to reach the sulcus under physiological tension when the arm is at the patient's side. This technique provides fixation to bone that is sufficiently secure to allow early passive motion. *L,* Where major amounts of cuff have been lost, it may be necessary to create a trough in the articular surface of the head, more medial than the anatomical attachment site. The trough must be positioned to leave the cuff at physiological tension when the arm is at the patient's side. This technique is not a substitute for complete cuff mobilization.

the suprascapular nerve as it runs along the spinoglenoid notch. The supraspinatus and subscapularis have fascial attachments to the coracoid base via the coracohumeral ligament, which when sharply released allow further tissue mobility (Fig. 16–18 *D, E*). In larger defects, further cuff mobilization is achieved by freeing the cuff from the glenoid by incising the capsule at its insertion to the glenoid labrum (Fig. 16–18 *F, G*). This release permits substantial lateral advancement of the cuff, which is usually sufficient to manage a tear with moderate loss of cuff tissue. An adequate mobilization has been achieved when traction on the tendon produces a bouncy, muscular resistance, free from constraint by adhesions or capsule. A final step (used very rarely) that may be used in cuff mobilization involves making a separate posterior incision over the scapular spine, dissecting into the supraspinatus and infraspinatus fossae to identify and free up the retracted ends of these tendons. In this approach attention must be paid to the suprascapular nerve, which is at risk. If cuff mobilization permits good-quality cuff tissue to reach the sulcus between the tuberosity and the articular surface with the arm at the side and if each tendon approaches its normal attachment site, we will achieve a "near anatomical" repair.

The Repair

A trough is created in the sulcus just lateral to the articular surface, extending into cancellous bone to optimize tendon–bone healing (Fig. 16–18 *H*). This trough is beveled at its medial edge to prevent excessive bending of the cuff as it enters the trough. Drill holes for suture are made connecting the base of the trough to the lateral aspect of the tuberosity, sufficiently low that the knots will be out of the impingement area. We use No. 2 nonabsorbable suture for the cuff repair. A double-loop suture technique is used to achieve an optimal bite on the tendon edge and facilitate delivery of the tendon edge deep into the bony trough (Fig. 16–18 *I*). After the sutures have been passed through the appropriate bony holes, the cuff edge is drawn deep into the trough, leaving the cuff under physiological tension when the arm is at the side (Fig. 16–18 *J, K*). Splits in the tendons in the direction of their fibers are repaired side to side with a buried knot technique to minimize suture rubbing under the acromion. This technique provides fixation of the cuff to bone that is sufficiently secure to allow early passive motion.

When major amounts of cuff tissue have been lost, an anatomical repair is not possible. If thoroughly mobilized cuff will reach within 1 to 1.5 cm of the sulcus with the arm at the side, a trough is made in the articular surface of the head of the humerus for attachment (Fig. 16–18 *L*). The trough must be positioned to leave the cuff under physiological tension when the arm is at the side. In situations in which this advancement is required, the cuff defect is, by definition, large, and the articular surface in the new area of cuff implantation is often devoid of articular carti-

lage owing to rubbing on the undersurface of the acromion.

The cuff tendons come under substantial loads when the shoulder is actively elevated. Therefore, when secure reattachment of good cuff tendon to bone cannot be accomplished, we question the advisability of a "precarious repair" in which flimsy tissue is insecurely reattached so that "protection" for a prolonged period of time in abduction is required. By analogy with the internal fixation of fractures, the cuff and its fixation must be secure enough for early passive motion. We do not attach greater importance to achieving a "watertight" closure, believing that the top priority is to re-establish the connection of muscle to bone through tendon.

Massive Cuff Tears

Rarely, in the presence of massive cuff defects, we have used subscapularis flaps to enhance the quality of tissue in the area normally occupied by the supraspinatus, as described by Cofield.[44] The challenge here is that in its transferred position the subscapularis comes under great tension with the shoulder in elevation and external rotation. We have not used devitalized tissues such as grafts or prostheses to replace missing tendon, relying instead on the implantation of mobilized cuff tendon into bleeding cancellous bone as the optimal method of repair. We prefer to leave the long head of the biceps if it is intact and not subluxated—this tendon provides humeral head depression and is often hypertrophied in chronic cuff tears. If the tendon is irretrievably destroyed or dislocated, biceps tenodesis and sectioning of the tendon at its glenoid attachment may provide a viable graft to reinforce a cuff repair.

Before final closure, complete decompression of the newly repaired cuff is confirmed. The shoulder is gently manipulated through a wide range of motion to ensure ample clearance of the cuff beneath the coracoacromial arch. Finally, a secure deltoid repair is essential so that early postoperative motion may be instituted.

Postoperative Management

After surgery, cuff repairs are protected with a sling during daily activities. Massive tendon repairs may be protected from maximum adduction by an abduction bolster, not because the arm will not reach to the side (the ability of the arm to reach the side must be ensured at the operating table) but in order to avoid early tension on the repaired tendon (for the same reason that hand surgeons protect flexor tendon repairs from maximum extension). Early (second day) assisted mobilization in flexion and external rotation is initiated to avoid adhesions, disuse atrophy, and disruption of the repair upon delayed mobilization. During the first three postoperative months, the cuff repair will not be stronger than it is immediately after surgery. The repair is likely to be weakest at three weeks, when the healing process is under way but no enhancement of tensile strength has occurred. In the mobilization program we emphasize forward flexion and external rotation in a range comfortable for the patient (the limit of these motions is determined at surgery upon completion of the cuff repair).

At six weeks we begin gentle, external rotation isometric exercises within the limits of comfort. At this point the patient is allowed to perform gentle activities of daily living with the elbow at the side. At 12 weeks the patient may begin more active use of the shoulder, avoiding sudden, heavy, and jerky movements. Recognizing that the tension in the normal rotator cuff is large and learning from the experience with knee ligament repair, we advise that such connective tissue reconstructions should be protected from large loads for six months to one year after repair. We inform patients that premature heavy use may excessively challenge the repair.

Results

Dr. Douglas Harryman followed 112 shoulders with rotator cuff repairs from the University of Washington Shoulder Clinic for an average of 4.7 years.[101a] Experienced sonographers (Dr. Laurence Mack and Dr. Keith Wang) determined the cuff integrity at follow-up: 80 per cent of the tears involving only the supraspinatus were intact, whereas only 50 per cent of tears involving all of the infraspinatus or the subscapularis were intact. Sarah Jackins, a registered physical therapist, determined the shoulder comfort and function. Active arm elevation correlated with cuff integrity (by ultrasound); intact shoulders averaged 122 degrees, those with retear confined to the supraspinatus averaged 110 degrees, and those with retear involving the subscapularis averaged 80 degrees. Over 80 per cent of the patients experienced good pain relief. The degree of pain relief was relatively independent of the postoperative cuff integrity.

Causes of Failure

Rotator cuff repair may fail to yield a satisfactory result for many reasons, including infection, deltoid denervation, deltoid detachment, loss of the acromial lever arm, subacromial–subdeltoid adhesions, inadequate subacromial decompression, denervation of the cuff, failure of the cuff repair, failure of abnormal tendon in a new site different from the repaired area, failure of grafts to "take," and failure of rehabilitation. Effective treatment of these failures depends on the establishment of the proper diagnosis. Superficial *infection* requires culture-specific antibiotics and irrigation and drainage if purulence is present. A prompt definitive approach may prevent extension of the process into the joint. Acute *failure of the deltoid reattachment* requires prompt repair before muscle retraction becomes fixed. Chronically painful and functionally limiting *postoperative scarring* often responds to gentle,

frequent stretching at home. Shoulder manipulation in this situation is, in our opinion, contraindicated because of the risk of cuff damage. However, in certain shoulders that are refractory to rehabilitation, substantial improvement in comfort and function can be achieved by an open lysis of adhesions, revision of the acromioplasty, and smoothing of roughness of the upper surface of the cuff, followed by early assisted motion. *Weakness* of shoulder elevation often responds to gentle, progressive strengthening of the anterior deltoid and external rotators. Persistent weakness requires evaluation for possible neurological injury or cuff failure. *Denervation of the deltoid* is diagnosed by selective electromyography of the anterior muscle fibers. In selected cases, anterior deltoid denervation is treated by anterior transfer of the origin of the middle deltoid with closure to the clavicular head of the pectoralis major. *Denervation of the supraspinatus and infraspinatus or subscapularis* is diagnosed by selective electromyography and is difficult to manage (we have no experience with transfers of the teres major, latissimus, or trapezius for this condition). *Postoperative cuff failure* may be difficult to diagnose. Failure of the patient to regain strength of external rotation or elevation of the shoulder, subacromial snapping, and upward instability of the humeral head are all consistent with failure of the cuff repair or failure of the cuff in a new location. In this situation arthrography may not be reliable; false-negative results from scarring or false-positive results from inconsequential leaks reduce the diagnostic accuracy. Ultrasonography of the shoulder in motion provides more specific data on cuff thickness and integrity, although diagnostic guidelines for the postoperative shoulder are still in evolution. When cuff failure is suspected, repeat cuff exploration and repair is considered, using the same techniques as for the primary repair, if there is reason to believe that a better job of surgery and rehabilitation could be carried out and if the patient is a good candidate for another procedure. When a shoulder has been devastated by infection, deltoid detachment or denervation, intractable cuff failure or denervation, and/or acromionectomy (rather than acromioplasty), consideration is given to shoulder arthrodesis. Our experience is that this procedure is usually successful when the primary indication is refractory weakness and somewhat less dependable when performed for refractory shoulder pain.

There are several conditions in which the orthopedist is faced with a combination of glenohumeral joint surface destruction and massive cuff deficiency. These include (1) cuff arthropathy[170] and (2) Milwaukee shoulder.[146] Our approaches to these conditions share some common features. For example, these joints are usually aspirated for gram stain, culture and sensitivity, cell examination, and crystal examination. Neuropathic arthropathy is excluded by a thorough neurological examination that includes sensitivity to pain. If this test reveals abnormalities, further evaluation may include electromyography, screening tests for diabetes, and an MRI of the cervical spinal cord to look for syringomyelia.

Patients with severe, combined deficiencies of the cuff and joint surface must be individually assessed. Each patient has an individual combination of pain and functional losses. Patients with mild pain are managed with mild analgesics and gentle, function-maintaining exercises. For patients with more severe pain and functional losses, shoulder arthrodesis is considered; because these patients are often older, however, this option may not be very attractive. Constrained total shoulder arthroplasty is an option, but the failure rate is high when associated with large cuff deficiencies. Secure cuff reconstruction with unconstrained total shoulder arthroplasty is difficult and frequently impossible owing to massive cuff tissue deficiency. Unconstrained arthroplasty without a secure cuff repair carries a high incidence of glenoid component failure resulting from the mechanical instability of the humeral head, which rides upward because of the unopposed pull of the deltoid.[81] Our current preference for patients with substantial pain and limited function from joint surface destruction in the presence of an unreconstructable cuff includes the following steps: (1) assuring a smooth coracoacromial arch (usually already created by the process itself), avoiding acromioplasty and coracoacromial ligament section, which destroys the superior constraint of the humeral head; (2) debriding useless fragments of cuff and bursa; and (3) replacing the destroyed humeral articular surface with a humeral endoprosthesis sufficiently large to articulate with the coracoacromial arch but sufficiently small to allow 50 per cent posterior translation of the head and internal rotation of at least 60 degrees. Our early results with this technique indicate improved comfort and function without the worry of glenoid loosening.

References

1. Ahovuo J, Paavolainen P, and Slätis P: The diagnostic value of arthrography and plain radiography in rotator cuff tears. Acta Orthop Scand 55:220–223, 1984.
2. Alexeeff M: Ligamentum patellae rupture following local steroid injection. Aust NZ J Surg 56:681–683, 1986.
3. Bakalim G, and Pasila M: Surgical treatment of rupture of the rotator cuff tendon. Acta Orthop Scand 46:751–757, 1975.
4. Bankart ASB, and Cantab MC: Recurrent or habitual dislocation of the shoulder joint. Br Med J 2:1132–1133, 1923.
5. Basmajian JV, and Bazant FJ: Factors preventing downward dislocation of the adducted shoulder joint: an electromyographic and morphological study. J Bone Joint Surg 41A:1182–1186, 1959.
6. Bassett RW, and Cofield RH: Acute tears of the rotator cuff. The timing of surgical repair. Clin Orthop 175:18–24, 1983.
7. Bateman JE: The diagnosis and treatment of ruptures of the rotator cuff. Surg Clin North Am 43(6):1523–1530, 1963.
8. Bateman JE: The Shoulder and Neck. Philadelphia: WB Saunders, 1972.
9. Bateman JE: Cuff tears in athletes. Orthop Clin North Am 4(3):721–745. 1973.
10. Bateman JE, and Welsh RP (eds): Surgery of the Shoulder. Philadelphia: BC Decker, 1984.
11. Bauer B, and Vogelsang H: Die Lähmung des N. Suprascapularis als Taumafloge. Unfallheilkunde 65:461–465, 1962.
12. Bayley JC, Cochran TP, and Sledge CB: The weight-bearing shoulder: the impingement syndrome in paraplegics. J Bone Joint Surg 69A(5):676, 1987.
13. Beltran J, Gray LA, Bools JC, and Zuelzer W: Rotator cuff lesions of the shoulder: evaluation by direct sagittal CT arthrography. Radiology 60(1):161–165, 1986.
14. Benjamin M, Evans EJ, and Copp L: The histology of tendon attachments to bone in man. J Anat (Br) 149:89–100, 1986.
15. Berquist TH, McCough PF, Hattrup SJ, and Cofield RH: Arthrographic analysis of rotator cuff tear size. Paper delivered to the American Shoulder and Elbow Surgeons, Atlanta, GA, February, 1988.
16. Bigliani LU, Norris TR, Fischer J, et al: The relationship between the unfused acromial epiphysis and subacromial impingement lesions. Orthop Trans 7(1):138, 1983.
17. Bosworth DM: An analysis of twenty-eight consecutive cases of incapacitating shoulder lesions, radically explored and repaired. J Bone Joint Surg 22:369–392, 1940.
18. Bosworth DM: The supraspinatus syndrome. Symptomatology, pathology and repair. JAMA 117:442, 1941.
19. Bosworth DM: Muscular and tendinous defects of the shoulder and their repair. In American Academy of Orthopaedic Surgeons: Lectures on Reconstruction Surgery of the Extremities. Ann Arbor, MI: JW Edwards, 1944, pp 380–390.
20. Braun KA, and Lemons JE: Effects of electromagnetic fields on the recovery of circulation in mature rabbit femoral heads. Trans Orthop Res Soc 7:313, 1982.
21. Brems JJ: Digital muscle strength measurement in rotator cuff tears. Paper presented at the ASES 3rd Open Meeting, San Francisco, January 1987.
22. Brems JJ: Rotator cuff tear: evaluation and treatment. Orthopaedics 11(1):69–81, 1988.
23. Brems JJ, Wilde AH, Borden LS, and Boumphrey FRS: Glenoid lucent lines. Paper presented at ASES 2nd Open Meeting, New Orleans, 1986.
24. Brems JJ, and Wilde AH: Surgical management of cuff tear arthropathy. Paper delivered to the American Shoulder and Elbow Surgeons, Atlanta, GA, February, 1988.
25. Bretzke CA, Crass JR, Craig EV, et al: Ultrasonography of the rotator cuff: normal and pathologic anatomy. Invest Radiol 20:311–315, 1985.
26. Brewer BJ: Aging of the rotator cuff. Am J Sports Med 7(2):102–110, 1979.
27. Brogi M, Laterza A, and Neri C: Entrapment neuropathy of the suprascapular nerve. Riv Neurobiol 25(3):318, 1979.
28. Brown JT: Early assessment of supraspinatus tears, procaine infiltration as a guide to treatment. J Bone Joint Surg 31B(3):423–425, 1949.
29. Brownlee C, and Cofield MD: Shoulder replacement in cuff tear arthropathy. Paper presented at ASES meeting, New Orleans, 1986.
30. Bush LF: The torn shoulder capsule. J Bone Joint Surg (Am) 57A:256–259, 1975.
31. Calvert PT, Packer NP, Stoker DJ, et al: Arthrography of the shoulder after operative repair of the torn rotator cuff. J Bone Joint Surg (Br) 68B(1):147–150, 1986.
32. Carol EJ, Falke LM, Kortmann JHJPM, et al: Bristow-Latarjet repair for recurrent anterior shoulder instability; an eight-year study. Neth J Surg 37(4):109–113, 1985.
33. Carter SL, Miller SH, and Graham WP: An evaluation of the local effects of triamcinolone acetonide on normal soft tissues in monkey digits. Plast Reconstr Surg 39(3):407–410, 1977.
34. Clark JC: Fibrous anatomy of the rotator cuff. Abstract presented to the American Academy of Orthopaedic Surgeons, 1988.
35. Clark KC: Positioning in Radiography. 2nd ed. London: William Heinemann, 1941.
36. Clein LJ: Suprascapular entrapment neuropathy. J Neurosurg 43:337–342, 1975.
37. Clein LJ: The droopy shoulder syndrome. Can Med Assoc J 114:343–344, 1976.
38. Codman EA: Complete rupture of the supraspinatus tendon. Operative treatment with report of two successful cases. Boston Med Surg J 164:708–710, 1911.

39. Codman EA: The Shoulder, Rupture of the Supraspinatus Tendon and Other Lesions in or about the Subacromial Bursa. Boston: Thomas Todd, 1934.

40. Codman EA: Rupture of the supraspinatus—1834–1934. J Bone Joint Surg 19:643–652, 1937.

41. Codman EA: Rupture of the supraspinatus. Am J Surg 42:603–626, 1938.

42. Codman EA, and Akerson TB: The pathology associated with rupture of the supraspinatus tendon. Ann Surg 93:354–359, 1911.

43. Cofield RH: Tears of rotator cuff. Instr Course Lect 30:258–273, 1981.

44. Cofield RH: Subscapular muscle transposition for repair of chronic rotator cuff tears. Surg Gynecol Obstet 154:667–672, 1982.

45. Cofield RH: Arthroscopy of the shoulder. Mayo Clin Proc 58:501–508, 1983.

46. Cofield RH: Current concepts review rotator cuff disease of the shoulder. J Bone Joint Surg 67A:974–979, 1985.

47. Colachis SC, Strohm BR, and Brechner VL: Effects of axillary nerve block on muscle force in the upper extremity. Arch Phys Med Rehabil 50:647–654, 1969.

48. Colachis SC, and Strohm BR: The effect of suprascapular and axillary nerve blocks and muscle force in the upper extremity. Arch Phys Med Rehabil 52:22–29, 1971.

49. Collins RA, Gristina AG, Carter RE, et al: Ultrasonography of the shoulder. Orthop Clin North Am 18(3):351, 1987.

50. Connolly JF: Humeral head defects associated with shoulder dislocations—their diagnostic and surgical significance. Instr Course Lect 21:42, 1972.

51. Coomes EN, and Darlington LG: Effects of local steroid injection for supraspinatus tears: controlled study. Ann Rheum Dis 35:943, 1976.

52. Cotton RE, and Rideout DF: Tears of the humeral rotator cuff. A radiological and pathological necropsy survey. J Bone Joint Surg (Br) 46B:314–328, 1964.

53. Craig EV: The geyser sign and torn rotator cuff: clinical significance and pathomechanics. Clin Orthop 191:213–215, 1984.

54. Crass JR: Current concepts in diagnostic imaging of the rotator cuff. CRC Crit Rev Diagn. Imaging 1988 (in press).

55. Crass JR, and Craig EV: Noninvasive imaging of the rotator cuff. Orthopaedics 11(1):57–64, 1988.

56. Crass JR, Craig EV, Bretzke C, et al: Ultrasonography of the rotator cuff. Radiographics 5:941–953, 1985.

57. Crass JR, Craig EV, and Feinberg SB: Sonography of the postoperative rotator cuff. AJR 146:561–564, 1986.

58. Crass JR, Craig EV, and Feinberg SB: The hyperextended internal rotation view in rotator cuff ultrasonography. J Clin Ultrasound 15:415–416, 1987.

59. Crass JR, Craig EV, and Feinberg SB: Ultrasonography of rotator cuff tears: a review of 400 diagnostic studies (abstract). Presented at American Roentgen Ray Society Annual Meeting, Miami Beach, Florida, 1987.

60. Crass JR, Craig EV, Thompson RC, and Feinberg SB: Ultrasonography of the rotator cuff: surgical correlation. JCU 12:487–493, 1984.

61. Cronkite AF: The tensile strength of human tendon. Anat Rec 64:173–186, 1936.

62. Darlington LG, and Coomes EN: The effects of local steroid injection for supraspinatus tears. Rheumatol Rehabil 16:172–179, 1977.

63. Debeyre J, Patte D, and Emelik E: Repair of ruptures of the rotator cuff with a note on advancement of the supraspinatus muscle. J Bone Joint Surg 47B:36–42, 1965.

64. deDuca CJ, and Forrest WJ: Force analysis of individual muscles acting simultaneously on the shoulder joint during isometric abduction. J Biomech 6:385–393, 1973.

65. DeOrio JK, and Cofield RH: Results of a second attempt at surgical repair of a failed initial rotator cuff repair. J Bone Joint Surg 66A:563–567, 1984.

66. DePalma AF: Surgery of the Shoulder, 2nd ed. Philadelphia: JB Lippincott, 1973.

67. DePalma AF, Cooke AJ, and Prabhakar M: The role of the subscapularis in recurrent anterior dislocations of the shoulder. Clin Orthop 54:35, 1967.

68. DePalma AF, Gallery G, and Bennett CA: Variational anatomy and degenerative lesions of the shoulder joint. Instr Course Lect 6:255–281, 1949.

69. DeSmet AA, and Ting YM: Diagnosis of rotator cuff tear on routine radiographs. J Can Assoc Radiol 28:54–57, 1977.

70. Donovan WH, and Kraft GH: Rotator cuff tear vs. suprascapular nerve injury. Arch Phys Med Rehabil 55:424, 1974.

71. Drez D Jr: Suprascapular neuropathy in the differential diagnosis of rotator cuff injuries. Am J Sports Med 4:43–45, 1976.

72. Earnshaw P, Desjardins D, Sarkar K, and Uhthoff HK: Rotator cuff tears: the role of surgery. Can J Surg 25(1):60–63, 1982.

73. Edeland HG, and Zachrisson BE: Fracture of the scapular notch associated with lesion of the suprascapular nerve. Acta Orthop Scand 46:758–763, 1975.

74. Ellis VH: The diagnosis of shoulder lesions due to injuries of the rotator cuff. J Bone Joint Surg 35B:72–74, 1953.

75. Ellman H, Hanker G, and Bayer M: Repair of the rotator cuff: end-result study of factors influencing reconstruction. J Bone Joint Surg 68A(8):1136–1144, 1986.

76. Esslen E, Flachsmann H, Bischoff A, et al: Die Einklemmungsneuropathie des N. Suprascapularis: Eine Klinisch-Therapeutische Studie. Nervenarzt 38:311–314, 1967.

77. Farrer IL, Matsen FA III, Rogers JV, et al: Dynamic sonographic study of lesion of the rotator cuff (Abstract). Paper presented at the American Academy of Orthopedic Surgeons 50th Annual Meeting, Anaheim, CA, March 10–15, 1983.

78. Ferguson LK: Suture of ruptured supraspinatus tendon four days after surgery. J Surg 29:384–386, 1935.

79. Ford LT, and DeBender J: Tendon rupture after local steroid injection. South Med J 72(7):827–830, 1979.

80. Fowler EB: Rupture of the spinati tendons and capsule: repair by a new operation. Ill Med J 61:332, 1932.

81. Franklin JL, Barrett WP, Jackins SE, and Matsen FA III: Glenoid loosening in total shoulder arthroplasty; association with rotator cuff deficiency. J Arthroplasty 3(1):39–46, 1988.

82. Freiberger RH, Kaye JJ, and Spiller J: Arthrography. New York: Appleton-Century-Crofts, 1979.

83. Froimson AI, and Oh I: Keyhole tenodesis of biceps origin at the shoulder. Clin Orthop 112:245–249, 1975.

84. Fukuda H, Ogawa K, and Mikasa M: Rotator cuff injury with special reference to "intraoperative color test." J Jpn Orthop Assoc 52:1243–1244, 1978.

85. Fukuda H: Rotator cuff tears. Geka Chiryo (Osaka) 43:28, 1980.

86. Fukuda H, Mikasa M, Ogawa K, et al: The partial thickness tear of rotator cuff. Orthopaedic Transactions 7(1):137, 1983.

87. Fukuda H, Mikasa M, and Yamanaka K: Incomplete thickness rotator cuff tears diagnosed by subacromial bursography. Clin Orthop 223:51–58, 1987.

88. Gelmers HJ, and Buys DA: Suprascapular entrapment neuropathy. Acta Neurochir (Wien) 38:121–124, 1977.

89. Ghelman B, and Goldman AB: The double contrast shoulder arthrogram: evaluation of rotary cuff tears. Radiology 124:251–254, 1977.

90. Godsil RD Jr, and Linscheid RL: Intratendinous defects of the rotator cuff. Clin Orthop 69:181–188, 1970.

91. Golding FC: The shoulder—the forgotten joint. Br J Radio 35:149–158, 1962.

92. Goldman AB, Dines DM, and Warren RF: Shoulder Arthrography: Technique, Diagnosis and Clinical Correlation. Boston: Little, Brown and Company, 1982, pp 1–3.

93. Goldman AB, and Gehlman B: The double-contrast shoulder arthrogram. Radiology 127:655–663, 1978.

94. Goodship AE, and Cooke P: Biocompatibility of tendon and ligament prostheses. CRC Crit Rev Biocompatibility, 2(4):303, 1986.

95. Gore DR, Murray MP, Sepic SB, et al: Shoulder-muscle strength and range of motion following surgical repair of full-thickness rotator cuff tears. J Bone Joint Surg 68(2):266–272, 1986.

96. Grant JCB, and Smith CG: Age incidence of rupture of the supraspinatus tendon [abstract]. Anat Rec *100*:666, 1948.

97. Ha'Eri, GB: Ruptures of the rotator cuff. Can Med Assoc J *123*:620–627, 1980.

98. Ha'Eri GB, and Wiley AM: An extensile exposure for subacromial derangements. Can J Surg *23*(5):458–461, 1980.

99. Ha'Eri GB, and Wiley AM: "Supraspinatus slide" for rotator cuff repair. Int Orthop *4*:231–234, 1980.

100. Ha'Eri GB, and Wiley AM: Advancement of the supraspinatus muscle in the repair of ruptures of the rotator cuff. J Bone Joint Surg *63A*:232–238, 1981.

101. Harrison SH: The painful shoulder. Significance of radiographic changes in the upper end of the humerus. J Bone Joint Surg *31B*:418–422, 1949.

101a. Harryman DT II, Wang KA, Mack LA, et al: Functional results of rotator cuff repair: Correlation with tear size and cuff integrity. Presented at the meeting of the American Academy of Orthopaedic Surgeons, New Orleans, February, 1990.

102. Hawkins RJ, Misamore GW, and Hobeika PE: Surgery of full thickness rotator cuff tears. J Bone Joint Surg *67A*(9):1349–1355, 1985.

103. Hazlett JW: Tears of the rotator cuff. *In* Proceedings of the Dewar Orthopaedic Club. J Bone and Joint Surg *53B*(4):772, 1971.

104. Heikel HVA: Rupture of the rotator cuff of the shoulder. Experiences of surgical treatment. Acta Orthop Scand *39*:477–492, 1968.

105. Hollingworth GR, Ellis RM, and Hattersley TS: Comparison of injection techniques for shoulder pain: results of a double blind, randomised study. Br Med J *287*:1339–1341, 1983.

106. Hollis JM, Lyon RM, Marcin JP, et al: Effect of age and loading axis on the failure properties of the human ACL. *In* Transactions of 34th Annual Meeting, Orthopedic Research Society, Atlanta, Georgia, *13*:83, 1988.

107. Howell SM, Imobersteg AM, Segar DH, and Marone PJ: Clarification of the role of the supraspinatus muscle in shoulder function. J Bone Joint Surg *68*(3):398–404, 1986.

108. Inman VT, Saunders JB de CM, and Abbott LC: Observations on the function of the shoulder joint. J Bone Joint Surg *26A*:1–30, 1944.

109. Jens J: The role of the subscapularis muscle in recurring dislocation of the shoulder (abstract). J Bone Joint Surg *34B*:780, 1964.

110. Joessel D: Über die Recidine der Humerus-Luxationen. Deutsch Ztschr Chir *13*:167–184, 1880.

111. Kaplan PE, and Kernahan WT Jr: Rotator cuff rupture management with suprascapular neuropathy. Arch Phys Med Rehabil *65*:273–275, 1984.

112. Kerwein GA: Roentgenographic diagnosis of shoulder dysfunction. JAMA *194*:1081–1085, 1965.

113. Kerwein GH, Rosenburg B, and Sneed WR: Arthrographic studies of the shoulder joint. J Bone Joint Surg *39A*:1267–1279, 1957.

114. Kessel L: Early diagnosis of ruptures of the rotator cuff of the shoulder joint., Proc R Soc Med *65*:1030, 1972.

115. Kessel L, and Watson M: The painful arc syndrome: clinical classification as a guide to management. J Bone Joint Surg *59B*:166–172, 1977.

116. Kessel L, and Watson M: The transacromial approach to the shoulder for ruptures of the rotator cuff. Int Orthop *1*:153–154, 1977.

117. Keyes EL: Observations on rupture of supraspinatus tendon. Based upon a study of 73 cadavers. Ann Surg *97*:849–856, 1933.

118. Keyes EL: Anatomical observations on senile changes in the shoulder. J Bone Joint Surg *17A*:953–960, 1935.

119. Kieft GJ, Bloem JL, Oberman WR, et al: Normal shoulder: MRI. Radiology *159*:741–745, 1986.

120. Kieft GJ, Bloem JL, Rozing PM, and Obermann WR: Rotator cuff impingement syndrome: MR imaging. Radiology *166*:211–214, 1988.

121. Kilcoyne RF, and Matsen FA III: Rotator cuff tear measurement by arthropneumotomography. AJR *140*:315–318, 1983.

122. Killoran PJ, Marcove RC, and Freiberger RH: Shoulder arthroscopy. Am J Roentgenol *103*:658–668, 1968.

123. Kneeland JB, Carrera GF, Middleton WD, et al: Rotator cuff tears: preliminary application of high resolution MRI with counter-rotating loop gap resonators. Radiology *160*:695–699, 1986.

124. Knese KH, and Biermann H: Die Knochenbildung an Sehnen und Bandansätzen im Bereich ursprünglich chondraler Apophysen. Z Zellbiol Mikro Anat *49*:142–187, 1958.

125. Komar J: Eine Wichtige Urasache des Schulterschmerzes: Incisurascapulae-Syndrom. Fortschr Neurol Psychiatr *44*:644–648, 1976.

126. Kopell HP, and Thompson WAL: Pain and the frozen shoulder. Surg Gynecol Obstet *109*:92–96, 1959.

127. Kopell HP, and Thompson WAL: Suprascapular nerve. *In* Peripheral Entrapment Neuropathies. Baltimore; Williams & Wilkins, 1963, pp 130–142.

128. Kotzen LM: Roentgen diagnosis of rotator cuff tear. Report of 48 surgically proven cases. Am J Roentgenol Radium Ther Nucl Med *112*:507–511, 1971.

129. Kutsuma T, Akaoka K, Kinoshita H, et al: The results of surgical management of rotator cuff tear. The Shoulder Joint *6*:136, 1982.

130. Laing PG: The arterial supply of the adult humerus. J Bone Joint Surg *38A*:1105–1116, 1956.

131. Lee PN, Lee M, Haq AMMM, et al: Periarthritis of the shoulder. Ann Rheum Dis *33*:116–119, 1974.

132. Lie S, and Mast WA: Subacromial bursography: technique and clinical application. Tech Dev Instrum *144*(3):626–630, 1982.

133. Lilleby H: Shoulder arthroscopy. Acta Orthop Scand *55*:561–566, 1984.

134. Lindblom K: Arthrography and roentgenography in ruptures of the tendon of the shoulder joint. Acta Radiol *20*:548, 1939.

135. Lindblom K: On pathogenesis of ruptures of the tendon aponeurosis of the shoulder joint. Acta Radiol *20*:563–577, 1939.

136. Lindblom K, and Palmer I: Ruptures of the tendon aponeurosis of the shoulder joint—the so-called supraspinatus ruptures. Acta Chir Scand *82*:133–142, 1939.

137. Lund IM, Donde R, and Knudsen EA: Persistent local cutaneous atrophy following corticosteroid injection for tendinitis. Rheumatol Rehabil *18*:91–93, 1979.

138. Lundberg BJ: The correlation of clinical evaluation with operative findings and prognosis in rotator cuff rupture. *In* Bayley I, and Kessel L(eds): Shoulder Surgery. Berlin: Springer-Verlag, 1982, pp 35–38.

139. Mack LA, Gannon MK, Kilcoyne RF, et al: Sonographic evaluation of the rotator cuff: accuracy in patients without prior surgery. Clin Orthop *234*:21–28, 1988.

140. Mack LA, Matsen FA III, Kilcoyne RF, et al: US evaluation of the rotator cuff. Radiology *157*:205–209, 1985.

141. Mack LA, Nuberg DS, Matsen FA III, et al: Sonography of the postoperative shoulder (abstract). Paper presented at American Roentgen Ray Society Annual Meeting, Miami Beach, Florida, 1987.

142. Mack LA, Nyberg DA, Kilcoyne RF, et al: Sonography of the post-operative shoulder. AJR *150*:1089–1094, 1988.

143. Macnab I: Rotator cuff tendinitis. Ann Roy Surg Engl *53*:4, 1973.

144. Macnab I, and Hastings D: Rotator cuff tendinitis. Can Med Assoc J *99*:91–98, 1968.

145. Mayer L: Rupture of the supraspinatus tendon. J Bone Joint Surg *19A*:640–642, 1937.

146. McCarty DJ, Haverson PB, Carrera GF, et al: "Milwaukee shoulder"—association of microspheroids containing hydroxyapatite crystals, active collagenase, and neutral protease with rotator cuff defects. I. Clinical aspects. Arthritis Rheum *24*(3):353–354, 1981.

147. McLaughlin HL: Lesions of the musculotendinous cuff of the shoulder. The exposure and treatment of tears with retraction. J Bone Joint Surg *26*:31–51, 1944.

148. McLaughlin HL: Rupture of the rotator cuff. J Bone Joint Surg *44A*:979–983, 1962.

149. McLaughlin HL: Repair of major cuff ruptures. Surg Clin North Am *43*:1535–1540, 1963.

150. McLaughlin HL, and Asherman EG: Lesions of the musculo-tendinous cuff of the shoulder IV: some observations based upon the results of surgical repair. J Bone Joint Surg 33A:76–86, 1951.
151. McMasters PE: Tendon and muscle ruptures: clinical and experimental studies on the causes and location of subcutaneous ruptures. J Bone Joint Surg 15A:705–722, 1933.
152. Meyer AW: Further evidence of attrition in the human body. Am J Anat 34:241–267, 1924.
153. Meyer AW: The minute anatomy of attrition lesions. J Bone Joint Surg 13A:341, 1931.
154. Michelsson JE, and Bakalim G: Resection of the acromion in the treatment of persistent rotator cuff syndrome of the shoulder. Acta Orthop Scand 48:607–611, 1977.
155. Middleton WD, Edelstein G, Reinus WR, et al: Ultrasonography of the rotator cuff: technique and normal anatomy. J Ultrasound Med 3(12):549–551, 1984.
156. Middleton WD, Edelstein G, Reinus WR, et al: Sonographic detection of rotator cuff tears. AJR 144:349–353, 1985.
157. Middleton WD, Kneeland JB, Carrera GF, et al: High resolution MRI of the normal rotator cuff. AJR 148:559–564, 1987.
158. Middleton WD, Macrander S, Lawson TL, et al: High resolution surface coil magnetic resonance imaging of the joints: anatomic correlation. Radiographics 7:645–682, 1987.
159. Middleton WD, Reinus WR, Melson GL, et al: Pitfalls of rotator cuff sonography. AJR 146:555–560, 1986.
160. Middleton WD, Reinus WR, Totty WG, et al: Ultrasonographic evaluation of the rotator cuff and biceps tendon. J Bone Joint Surg 68A:440–450, 1986.
161. Mikasa M: Subacromial bursography. J Jpn Orthop Assoc 53:225, 1979.
162. Mink JH, Harris E, and Rappaport M: Rotator cuff tears: evaluation using double-contrast shoulder arthrography. Radiology 153:621–623, 1985.
163. Morrison DS, and Burger P: The use of magnetic resonance imaging in the diagnosis of rotator cuff tears. Paper delivered to the American Shoulder and Elbow Surgeons Fourth Meeting, Atlanta, GA, February, 1988.
164. Moseley HF: Ruptures to the Rotator Cuff. Springfield IL: Charles C Thomas, 1952.
165. Moseley HF: Shoulder Lesions, 3rd ed. Edinburgh and London: E. & S. Livingstone, 1969.
166. Moseley HF, and Goldie I: The arterial pattern of the rotator cuff of the shoulder. J Bone Joint Surg 45B(4):780–789, 1963.
167. Murray JWG: A surgical approach for entrapment neuropathy of the suprascapular nerve. Orthop Rev 3(2):33–35, 1974.
168. Neer CS II: Anterior acromioplasty for the chronic impingement syndrome in the shoulder. J Bone Joint Surg 54A:41, 1972.
169. Neer CS II: Impingement lesions. Clin Orthop 173:70–77, 1983.
170. Neer CS II, Craig EV, and Fukuda H: Cuff-tear arthropathy. J Bone Joint Surg 65A:1232–1244, 1983.
171. Neer CS II, Flatow EL, and Lech O: Tears of the rotator cuff: long term results of anterior acromioplasty and repair. Paper presented at the American Shoulder and Elbow Surgeons Fourth Meeting, Atlanta, GA, February, 1988.
172. Neer CS, and Marberry TA: On the disadvantages of radical acromionectomy. J Bone Joint Surg 63A(3):416–419, 1981.
173. Nelson DH: Arthography of the shoulder. Br J Radiol 25:134, 1952.
174. Neviaser JS: Ruptures of the rotator cuff. Clin Orthop 3:92–98, 1954.
175. Neviaser JS: Arthrography of the shoulder joint: a study of the findings in adhesive capsulitis of the shoulder. J Bone Joint Surg 44A:1321–1330, 1962.
176. Neviaser JS: Ruptures of the rotator cuff of the shoulder. New concepts in the diagnosis and operative treatment of chronic ruptures. Arch Surg 102:483–485, 1971.
177. Neviaser JS, Neviaser RJ, and Neviaser TJ: The repair of chronic massive ruptures of the rotator cuff of the shoulder by use of a freeze-dried rotator cuff. J Bone Joint Surg 60A:681–684, 1978.
178. Neviaser RJ: Tears of the rotator cuff. Orthop Clin North Am 11(2):295–306, 1980.
179. Neviaser RJ: The relationship of rotator cuff tears to primary and recurrent anterior shoulder dislocation in the older patient. Paper presented at ASES 3rd Open Meeting, San Francisco, 1987.
180. Neviaser RJ, and Neviaser TJ: Transfer of subscapularis and teres minor for massive defects of rotator cuff. In Bayley I, and Kessel L (eds): Shoulder Surgery. Berlin: Springer-Verlag, 1982, pp 60–63.
181. Neviaser RJ, and Neviaser TJ: Reconstruction of chronic tears of the rotator cuff. In Bateman JE, and Welsh RP (eds): Surgery of the Shoulder. Philadelphia: BC Decker, 1984, pp 172–179.
182. Niebauer JS: Acromial splitting incision for repair of the shoulder capsule. J Bone Joint Surg 45A:66, 1963.
183. Nixon JE, and DiStefano V: Ruptures of the rotator cuff. Orthop Clin North Am 6:423–447, 1975.
184. Norris TR, Fischer J, Bigliani LU, et al: The unfused acromial epiphysis and its relationship to impingement syndromes. Orthop Trans 7(3):505, 1983.
185. Oberholtzer J: Die Arthropneumoradiographe bei habitueller Schulterluxation. Röntgenpraxis 5:589–590, 1933.
186. Olsson O: Degenerative changes in the shoulder joint and their connection with shoulder pain. A morphological and clinical investigation with special attention to the cuff and biceps tendon. Acta Chir Scand (Suppl) 181:1–130, 1953.
187. Ozaki J, Fujimoto S, Masuhara K, et al: Reconstruction of chronic massive rotator cuff tears with synthetic materials. Clin Orthop 202:173–183, 1986.
188. Ozaki J, Fujimoto S, and Masuhara K: Repair of chronic massive rotator cuff tears with synthetic fabrics. In Bateman JE and Welsh RP (eds): Surgery of the Shoulder. Philadelphia: BC Decker, 1984, pp 185–191.
189. Ozaki J, Fujimoto S, Tomita K, et al: Non-perforated superficial surface cuff tears associated with hydrops of the subacromial bursa. Katakansetsu (Fukuoka) 9:52, 1985.
190. Packard AG: Management of large tears of the rotator cuff of the shoulder. Clin Orthop 44:279–280, 1966.
191. Packer NP, Calvert PT, Bayley JIL, and Kessel L: Operative treatment of chronic ruptures of the rotator cuff of the shoulder. J Bone Joint Surg (Br) 65B:171–175, 1983.
192. Patte D, Debeyre J, and Goutallier D: Rotator cuff repair by muscle advancement. In Bayley I, and Kessel L, (eds): Shoulder Surgery. Berlin: Springer-Verlag, 1982, p 49.
193. Peterson C: Long-term results of rotator cuff repair. In Bayley I, and Kessel L (eds): Shoulder Surgery. Berlin: Springer-Verlag, 1982, pp 64–69.
194. Peterson CJ, and Gentz CF: Ruptures of the supraspinatous tendon—significance of distally pointing acromioclavicular osteophytes. Clin Orthop 174:143, 1983.
195. Pettersson G: Rupture of the tendon aponeurosis of the shoulder joint in anterior inferior dislocation. Acta Chir Scand (Suppl.) 77:1–184, 1942.
196. Picot C: Neuropathie canalaire du nerf sus-scapulaire. Rhumatologie 21:73–75, 1969.
197. Post M: Rotator cuff repair with carbon filament: a preliminary report of five cases. Clin Orthop 196:154–158, 1985.
198. Post M, Silver R, and Singh M: Rotator cuff tear: diagnosis and treatment. Clin Orthop 173:78, 1983.
199. Rask MR: Suprascapular axonotmesis and rheumatoid disease: report of a case treated conservatively. Clin Orthop 134:266–267, 1978.
200. Rask MR: Suprascapular nerve entrapment: a report of two cases treated with suprascapular notch resection. Clin Orthop 123:73–75, 1977.
201. Rathbun JB, and Macnab I: The microvascular pattern of the rotator cuff. J Bone Joint Surg (Br) 52(3):540–553, 1970.
202. Reeves B: Arthrography of the shoulder. J Bone Joint Surg 48B:424–435, 1966.
203. Rengachary SS, Neff JP, Singer PA, and Brackett CE: Suprascapular entrapment neuropathy: a clinical, anatomical and comparative study. Neurosurgery 5(4):441–446, 1979.
204. Resnick D: Shoulder arthrography. Radiol Clin North Am 19:243–252, 1981.
205. Rockwood CA: Personal communication, 1983 and 1987.
206. Rostron PK, Orth MCh, Wigan FRCS, and Calver RF: Subcutaneous atrophy following methylprednisolone injection in

Osgood-Schlatter epiphysitis. J Bone Joint Surg 61A(4):627–628, 1979.

207. Rothman RH, and Parke WW: The vascular anatomy of the rotator cuff. Clin Orthop 41:176–186, 1965.
208. Rowe CR: Ruptures of the rotator cuff. Selection of cases for conservative treatment. Surg Clin North Am 43:1531–1540, 1963.
209. Saha AK: Dynamic stability of the glenohumeral joint. Acta Orthop Scand 42:491–505, 1971.
210. Salter RB, and Murray D: Effects of hydrocortisone on musculo-skeletal tissues. J Bone Joint Surg (Br) 51B:195, 1969.
211. Samilson RL, and Binder WF: Symptomatic full thickness tears of the rotator cuff: an analysis of 292 shoulders in 276 patients. Orthop Clin North Am 6(2):449–466, 1975.
212. Samilson RL, Raphael RL, Post L, et al: Arthrography of the shoulder. Clin Orthop 20:21–31, 1961.
213. Samilson RL, Raphael RL, Post L, et al: Shoulder arthrography. JAMA 175:773–776, 1961.
214. Schilf E: Über eine Einseitige Lähmung des Nervus Suprascapularis. Nervenarzt 23:306–307, 1952.
215. Schneider H: Zur Struktur der Sehnenansatzzonen. Z Anat Entwicks 119:431–456, 1956.
216. Schneider JE, Adams OR, Easley KJ, et al: Scapular notch resection for suprascapular nerve decompression in 12 horses. JAMA 187(10):1019–1020, 1985.
217. Seeger LL, Ruskowski JT, Bassett LW, et al: MR imaging of the normal shoulder: anatomic correlation. AJR 148:83–92, 1987.
218. Seitz WH Jr, Abram LJ, Froimson AI, et al: Rotator cuff imaging techniques: a comparison of arthrography, ultrasonography and magnetic resonance imaging. Paper presented at the American Shoulder and Elbow Surgeons 3rd Open Meeting, San Francisco, CA, January, 1987.
219. Skinner HA: Anatomical consideration relative to ruptures of the supraspinatus tendon. J Bone Joint Surg (Am) 19A:137–151, 1937.
220. Slätis P, and Aalto K: Medial dislocation of the tendon of the long head of the biceps brachii. Acta Orthop Scand 50(1):73–77, 1979.
221. Smith JG: Pathological appearances of seven cases of injury of the shoulder joint with remarks. London Med Gazette 14:280, 1834. (Reported in Am J Med Sci 16:219–224, 1834.)
222. Solheim LF, and Roaas A: Compression of the suprascapular nerve after fracture of the scapular notch. Acta Orthop Scand 49:338–340, 1978.
223. Solonen KA: A method for reconstruction of the rotator cuff after rupture. In Bayley I, and Kessel L (eds): Shoulder Surgery. Berlin: Springer-Verlag, 1982, p 46.
224. Solonen KA, and Vastamäki M: Reconstruction of the rotator cuff. Int Orthop 7:49, 1983.
225. Strizak AM, Danzig M, Jackson DW, and Greenway G: Subacromial bursography. An anatomical and clinical study. J Bone Joint Surg 64A:196, 1982.
226. Strohm BR, and Colachis SC Jr: Shoulder joint dysfunction following injury to the suprascapular nerve. Phys Ther 45:106–111, 1965.
227. Sudmann E: Repair of ruptures of the cuff of the shoulder joint using a postero-superior acromion-splitting approach. J Bone Joint Surg 47B:36–42, 1965.
228. Swiontkowski M: Personal communication, 1987.
229. Symeonides PP: The significance of the subscapularis muscle in the pathogenesis of recurrent anterior dislocation of the shoulder. J Bone Joint Surg 54B:476–483, 1972.
230. Tabata S, and Kida H: Diagnosis and treatment of partial thickness tears of rotator cuff. Orthop Traumatol Surg (Tokyo) 26:1199, 1983.
231. Tabata S, Kida H, Sasaki J, et al: Operative treatment for the incomplete thickness tears of the rotator cuff. Katakansetsu (Fukuoka) 5:29, 1981.
232. Takagishi N: Conservative treatment of the ruptures of the rotator cuff. J Jpn Orthop Assoc 52:781–787, 1978.
233. Tamai K, and Ogawa K: Intratendinous tear of the supraspinatus tendon exhibiting winging of the scapula. A case report. Clin Orthop 194:159–163, 1985.
234. Ting A, Jobe FW, Barto P, et al: An EMPG analysis of the lateral biceps in shoulders with rotator cuff tears. Paper presented at ASES 3rd Open Meeting, San Francisco, 1987.
235. Uhthoff HK, Loehr J, and Sarkar K: The pathogenesis of rotator cuff tears. In Proceedings of the Third International Conference on Surgery of the Shoulder, Fukuora, Japan, October 27, 1986.
236. Uitto J, Teir HJ, and Mustakallio KK: Corticosteroid induced inhibition of the biosynthesis of human skin collagen. Biochem Pharmacol 21:2161, 1972.
237. Van Linge B, and Mulder JD: Function of the supraspinatus muscle and its relation to the supraspinatus syndrome. An experimental study in man. J Bone Joint Surg 45B:750–754, 1963.
238. Vastamaki M: Factors influencing the operative results of rotator cuff rupture. Int Orthop 10(3):177–181, 1986.
239. VonMeyer AW: Chronic functional lesions of the shoulder. Arch Surg 35(1):646–674, 1937.
240. Walker PS: Human Joints and Their Artificial Replacements. Springfield IL. Charles C Thomas, 1977, p 87.
241. Walker SW, Couch WH, Boester GA, and Sprowl DW: Isokinetic strength of the shoulder after repair of a torn rotator cuff. J Bone Joint Surg 69(7):1041–1044, 1987.
242. Watson M: The refractory painful arc syndrome. J Bone Joint Surg 60B:544–546, 1978.
243. Watson M: Major ruptures of the rotator cuff: the results of surgical repair in 89 patients. J Bone Joint Surg 67B(4):618–624, 1985.
244. Watson-Jones R: Fractures and Joint Injuries, 4th ed. Baltimore: Williams & Wilkins, 1962.
245. Watson-Jones R: Injuries in the region of the shoulder joint. Capsule and tendon injuries. Br Med J 2:29–31, 1961.
246. Weaver HL: Isolated suprascapular nerve lesions. Br J Accident Surg 15:117–126, 1983.
247. Weiner DS, and Macnab I: Ruptures of the rotator cuff: follow-up evaluation of operative repairs. Can J Surg 13:219–227, 1970.
248. Weiner DS, and Macnab I: Superior migration of the humeral head: a radiological aid in the diagnosis of tears of the rotator cuff. J Bone Joint Surg (Br) 52B:524–527, 1970.
249. Weiss JJ: Intra-articular steroids in the treatment of rotator cuff tear: reappraisal by arthrography. Arch Phys Med Rehabil 62:555–557, 1981.
250. Weiss JJ, Thompson GR, Doust V, and Burgener F: Rotator cuff tears in rheumatoid arthritis. Arch Intern Med 135(4):521–525, 1975.
251. Wiley AM, and Older MWJ: Shoulder arthroscopy. Am J Sports Med 8:31–38, 1980.
252. Wilson CL: Lesions of the supraspinatus tendon: degeneration, rupture, and calcification. Arch Surg 46:307–325, 1943.
253. Wilson CL, and Duff GL: Pathologic study of degeneration and rupture of the supraspinatus tendon. Arch Surg 47:121–135, 1943.
254. Wilson PD: Complete rupture of the supraspinatus tendon. JAMA 96:433–438, 1931.
255. Wolfgang GL: Surgical repair of tears of the rotator cuff of the shoulder, factors influencing the result. J Bone Joint Surg 56A:14–26, 1974.
256. Wolfgang GL: Rupture of the musculotendinous cuff of the shoulder. Clin Orthop 134:230–243, 1978.
257. Wrede: Arch f Chir 99:259, 1912.
258. Yamada H, and Evans F: Strength of Biological Materials. Baltimore: Williams & Wilkins, 1972, pp 67–70.
259. Yamamoto R: Rotator cuff rupture. J Joint Surg 1:93, 1982.
260. Yamanaka K, and Fukuda H: Histological study of the supraspinatus tendon. The Shoulder Joint 5:9, 1981.
261. Yamanaka K, Fukuda H, Hamada K, and Mikasa M: Incomplete thickness tears of the rotator cuff. Orthop Traumatol Surg (Tokyo) 26:713, 1983.

Degenerative and Arthritic Problems of the Glenohumeral Joint

Robert H. Cofield, M.D.

Historical Review

In 1893, over a century ago, a curious and dramatic prosthetic shoulder replacement was performed by the French surgeon Péan.[133] A platinum and rubber total joint and proximal humeral implant was inserted in a man with tuberculous arthritis of the shoulder (Fig. 17–1). It remained in place for approximately two years and at that time was removed for uncontrollable infection. This was one of the first attempts to replace any joint with a prosthesis and merits our recognition. Alternative surgical treatment methods of osteotomy, debridement, resection, arthrodesis, or amputation were otherwise the treatment methods of choice for severe joint afflictions.

In 1953, Neer presented the option of replacement of a fractured humeral head with a Vitallium prosthesis.[147] Use of this prosthesis (Fig. 17–2) was next applied to patients with irregular articular surfaces as a result of fracturing and osteonecrosis.[148] Approximately a decade later, the same author noted that this prosthesis—designed as an articular replacement for the humeral head—had been applied to the treatment of patients with traumatic, degenerative, and arthritic conditions in the shoulder (Table 17–1). Then, in 1971 and 1974, Neer published additional materials fully describing the results of the use of this proximal humeral implant for patients with rheumatoid arthritis and osteoarthritis of the glenohumeral joint.[150, 151] The article describing the method of care for the osteoarthritic shoulder contains an illustration (Fig. 17–3) and information on the use of a high density polyethylene glenoid placed at the time of surgery, a total shoulder replacement. Also in 1974, Kenmore and associates published a brief article reporting on the development of a polyethylene glenoid liner for use with a Neer

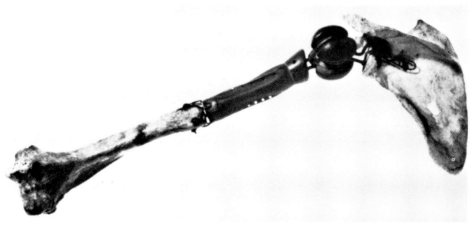

Figure 17–1. The first total shoulder arthroplasty, an artificial joint composed of platinum and rubber inserted by the French surgeon Péan in the late 1800s. (Reproduced with permission from Lugli T: Artificial shoulder joint by Péan (1893). The facts of an exceptional intervention and the prosthetic method. Clin Orthop 133:215–218, 1978.)

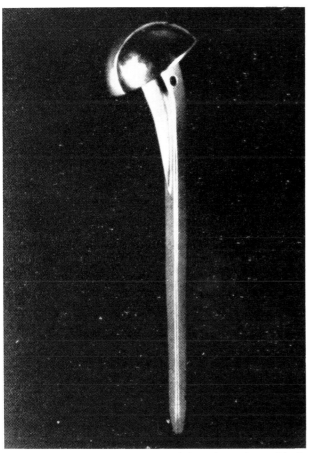

Figure 17–2. The early design of the Neer articular surface replacement for the proximal humerus. This implant was initially used in the care of patients with severely comminuted fractures of the humeral head. (Reproduced with permission from Neer CS, Brown TH Jr, and McLaughlin HL: Fracture of the neck of the humerus with dislocation of the head fragment. Am J Surg 85:252–258, 1953.)

humeral replacement in the treatment of degenerative joint disease of the shoulder.[119]

The early descriptions of the use of a prosthesis for the treatment of shoulder conditions include the 1951 article by Krueger reporting on the use of a custom-

Table 17–1. INDICATIONS FOR HUMERAL REPLACEMENT ARTHROPLASTY (1953–1963)

Diagnosis	No. Shoulders
Arthritides	
Osteoarthritis	9
Traumatic arthritis	9
Rheumatoid arthritis	2
Radiation necrosis	1
Sickle cell infarction	1
Ochronosis	1
Trauma	
Fracture-dislocation	26
"Head-splitting" fracture	4
Displaced "shell fragment" with retracted tuberosities	2
Previous humeral head resection	1

(Adapted from Neer CS II: Articular replacement of the humeral head. J Bone Joint Surg 46A:1607–1610, 1964.)

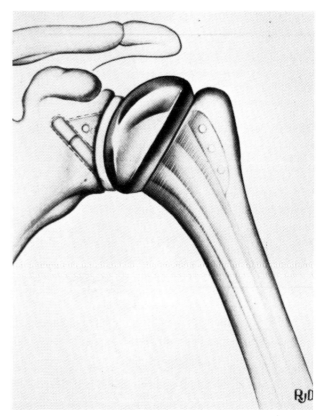

Figure 17–3. The first illustration depicting the use of a high density polyethylene glenoid component in conjunction with a proximal humeral prosthesis—a total shoulder arthroplasty. (Reproduced with permission from Neer CS II: Replacement arthroplasty for glenohumeral arthritis. J Bone Joint Surg 56A:1–13, 1974.)

made Vitallium arthroplasty of the shoulder for the treatment of osteonecrosis of the proximal humerus[128] and the 1952 article by Richard, Judet, and René presenting an acrylic prosthesis for use in the proximal humerus[180] (Fig. 17–4).

Upon this background, plus with the recognition that a significant number of patients would benefit from prosthetic arthroplasty of the shoulder, was thrust the opportunity of implant fixation to bone by polymethyl methacrylate. This stimulated many orthopedic surgeons to study further biomechanics of the shoulder and the pathology of shoulder diseases and to design total shoulder implants. The resulting designs were made to satisfy the requirements for replacement surgery posed by the patients' diseases and yet to incorporate as best as possible what was known about shoulder anatomy, arcs and patterns of movement, and forces at the joint. A number of important considerations emerged, but foremost among these were the following recognitions and beliefs: (1) The quantity of bone in the scapula was small; it would be difficult to fix a part securely. (2) The rotator cuff was almost always severely affected by the diseases causing glenohumeral joint destruction; stability greater than present in the normal shoulder articular surfaces should be included in the prosthetic design. (3) The range of motion in the shoulder is very large; a standard, single ball-in-socket design may not suffice.

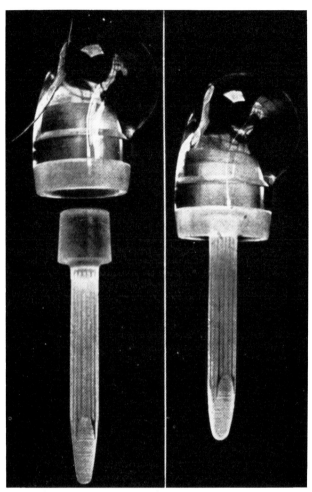

Figure 17–4. An acrylic prosthesis developed for the treatment of severe fracture-dislocations of the proximal humerus. (Reproduced with permission from Richard A, Judet R, and René L: Acrylic prosthetic reconstruction of the upper end of the humerus for fracture-luxations. J Chir *68*:537–547, 1952.)

Many designs were constructed. A few were fundamental, mirroring the implants used by Neer in the past. Included in this group were the St. Georg[70] (Fig. 17–5) and the Bechtol[13] total shoulders. However, most were not so simple. Almost all designs included a captive ball-in-socket unit to replace the stabilizing functions of the rotator cuff and shoulder capsule. Implants of this construction included the Wheble-Skorecki,[221] the Zippel[226] (Fig. 17–6), the Bickel[38] (Fig. 17–7), the Stanmore,[131] the Liverpool shoulder replacement,[15, 16] the Kölbel,[125, 126] the endoprosthesis designed by Reeves,[178] the "floating socket" total shoulder replacement,[29] the implant designed by Fenlin,[77] the Michael Reese total shoulder replacement,[169–171] the total shoulder prosthesis designed by Gerard and associates,[88] and the Kessel total shoulder arthroplasty.[122] Of these, many included complex and extensive attachments to the scapula by stems (Fig. 17–8), wedges (Fig. 17–9), a screw (Fig. 17–10), and bolted flanges (Fig. 17–11). The Bickel implant (see Fig. 17–7) was cemented entirely within the glenoid. To create more

movement in the articulation, Reeves suggested the reverse ball-in-socket configuration—attaching the ball part of the implant to the glenoid.[178] This need for more movement was expanded on by designers incorporating two ball-in-socket units; the floating-socket[29] (Fig. 17–12) and the trispherical[91] (Fig. 17–13) total shoulder prostheses are examples.

A few investigators sought a compromise between the minimal amount of constraint created by those implants mimicking, as best as possible, normal articulating surfaces and those with captured ball-in-socket units. These designs had a hood on the glenoid component, which was an attempt to prevent upward humeral subluxation associated with rotator cuff weakness or absence. Systems incorporating this modification were the Neer[155] (Fig. 17–14), the "St. Georg,"[70] the Dana,[3–5] the English-Macnab,[142] and the nonretentive prosthesis of Mazas[139] (Fig. 17–15).

By the mid-1970s, there were so many implant systems, each with its own benefits and detriments, that some order seemed necessary. It appeared best to categorize the systems as anatomical or unconstrained, semiconstrained (a hooded glenoid component), or constrained (a ball-in-socket unit) (Fig. 17–16) (Table 17–2). Behind these many designs stood theory, some intuition, and often little practical patient care experience. How prosthetic arthroplasty of the shoulder would evolve would depend on two important areas of information: (1) The pathology of shoulder arthritis that would determine what aspects of an implant

Text continued on page 686

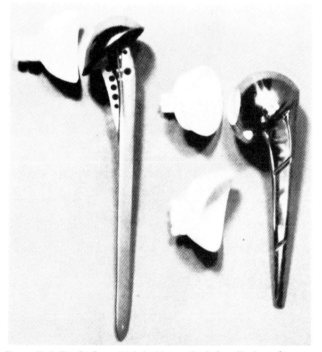

Figure 17–5. The St. Georg total shoulder prosthesis from Hamburg, Germany. Polyethylene sockets were constructed to mate with the Neer prosthesis, as shown on the left, or the St. Georg model, shown on the right. (Reproduced with permission from Engelbrecht E, and Stellbrink G: Totale Schulterendoprosthese Modell (St. Georg). Chirurg *47*:525–530, 1976.)

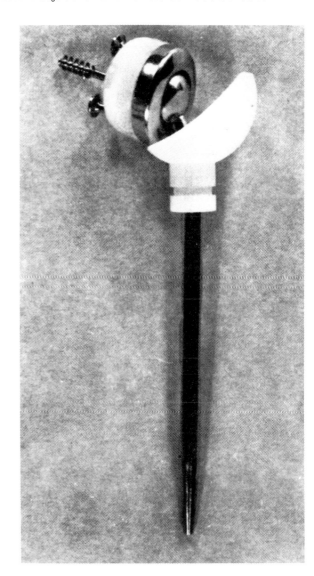

Figure 17–6. Model BME total shoulder arthroplasty designed by Zippel of Hamburg, Germany. This is an early captive ball-in-socket type of total shoulder arthroplasty. (Reproduced with permission from Zippel J: Luxationssichere Schulterendoprosthese Modell BME. Z Orthop *113*:454–457, 1975.)

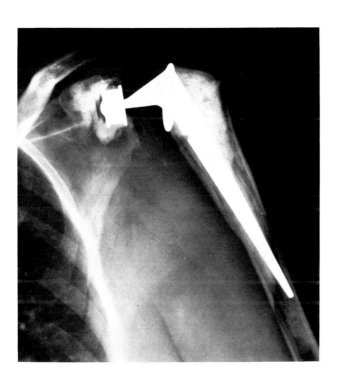

Figure 17–7. The Bickel glenohumeral prosthesis. The design included a very small ball to decrease friction between components, and the glenoid component was designed to be incorporated entirely within the glenoid cavity and, ideally, to maximize prosthesis-bone contact area. (Reproduced with permission from Cofield RH: Status of total shoulder arthroplasty. Arch Surg *112*:1088–1091, 1977.)

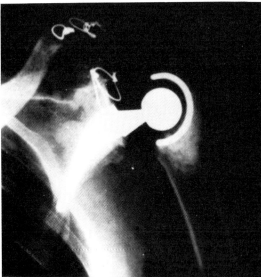

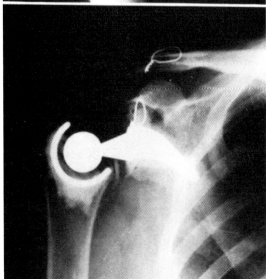

Figure 17–8. The Liverpool shoulder replacement. A reverse ball-in-socket design. The glenoid component has a stem that is inserted into the medullary cavity of the axillary border of the scapula to a depth of approximately 50 mm. (Reproduced with permission from Beddow FH, Elloy MA: Clinical experience with the liverpool shoulder replacement. *In* Bayley I, and Kessel L (eds): Shoulder Surgery. New York: Springer-Verlag, 1982, pp 164–167.)

Figure 17–9. Reverse ball-in-socket total shoulder arthroplasty designed by Fenlin. *A* shows the prosthesis assembled, and *B* shows the prosthesis disassembled. A wedge is driven into the bone of the scapula for fixation, and a column is placed down the axillary border of the scapula. (Reproduced with permission from Fenlin JM Jr: Total glenohumeral joint replacement. Orthop Clin North 6:565–583, 1975.)

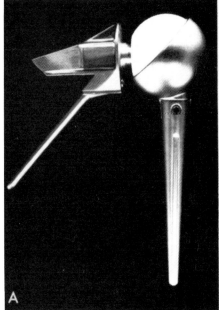

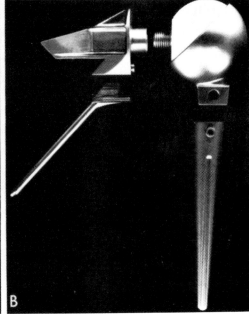

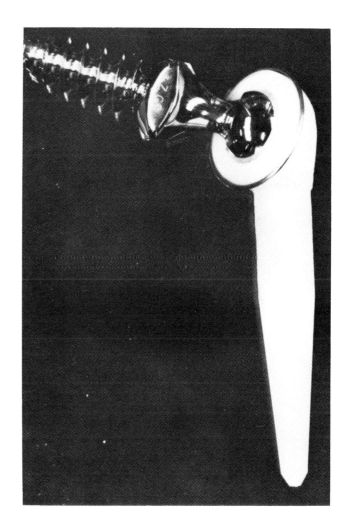

Figure 17–10. The Kessel total shoulder replacement. A reversed ball-in-socket design. The glenoid component is screwed into the glenoid, and the humeral stem is cemented in place. The components then snap together. (Reproduced with permission from Bayley JIL, and Kessel L: The Kessel total shoulder replacement. *In* Bayley I, and Kessel L (eds): New York: Springer-Verlag, 1982, pp 160–164.)

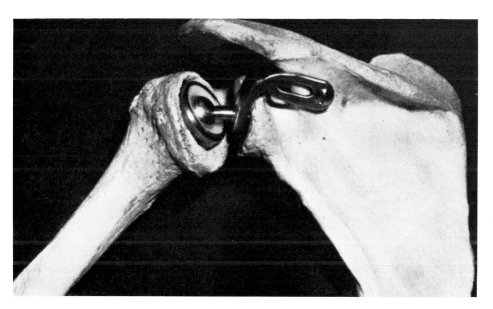

Figure 17–11. The total shoulder arthroplasty designed by Kölbel. This is a reversed ball-in-socket unit. Scapular component fixation includes a flange bolted to the base of the spine of the scapula. (Reproduced with permission from Wolff R, and Kölbel R: The history of shoulder joint replacement. *In* Kölbel R, Helbig B, and Blauth W (eds): Shoulder Replacement. New York: Springer-Verlag, 1987, pp 2–13.)

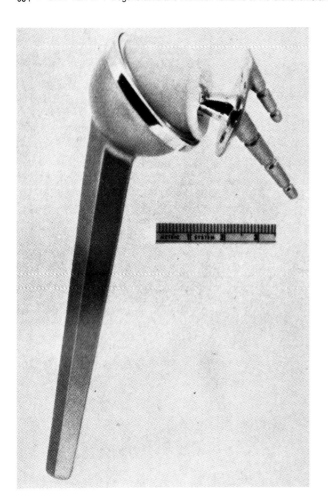

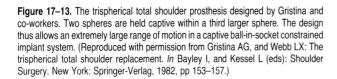

Figure 17–12. The floating socket total shoulder replacement. This implant contains a dual spherical bearing system to provide a "floating fulcrum." This configuration allows the prosthesis to have motion in excess of normal anatomical limits. (Reproduced with permission from Buechel FF, Pappas MJ, and DePalma AF: "Floating socket" total shoulder replacement: Anatomical, biomechanical, and surgical rationale. J Biomed Mat Res *12*:89–114, 1978.)

Figure 17–13. The trispherical total shoulder prosthesis designed by Gristina and co-workers. Two spheres are held captive within a third larger sphere. The design thus allows an extremely large range of motion in a captive ball-in-socket constrained implant system. (Reproduced with permission from Gristina AG, and Webb LX: The trispherical total shoulder replacement. *In* Bayley I, and Kessel L (eds): Shoulder Surgery. New York: Springer-Verlag, 1982, pp 153–157.)

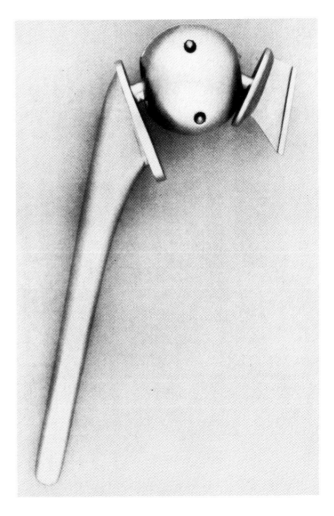

Figure 17–14. The Neer design of total shoulder arthroplasty includes a number of types of glenoid components. Five glenoid components were used in the series of patients reported in 1982. These included *(A)* the original 1973 polyethylene component; *(B)* the standard polyethylene component; *(C)* the metal-backed standard sized glenoid component; *(D)* the metal-backed 200 per cent larger glenoid component; and *(E)* the metal-backed 600 per cent larger glenoid component. These latter two hooded components were designed for additional joint constraint against superior humeral subluxation. (Reproduced with permission from Neer CS II, Watson KC, and Stanton FJ: Recent experience in total shoulder replacement. J Bone Joint Surg *64A*:319–337, 1982.)

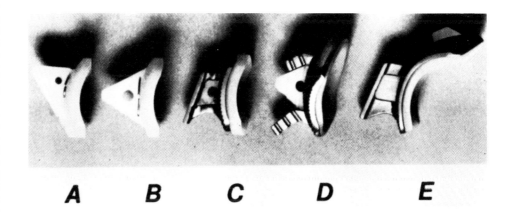

A   B   C   D   E

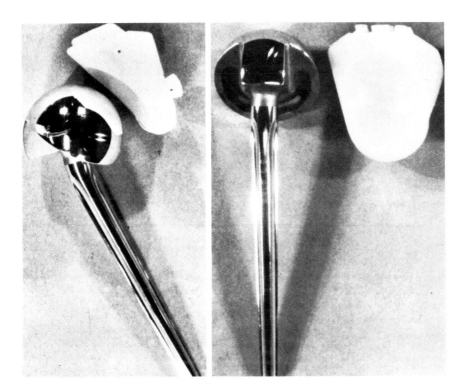

Figure 17–15. The nonretentive total shoulder arthroplasty designed by Mazas. (Reproduced with permission from Mazas F, and de la Caffinière JY: Un prothèse totale d'épaule non rétentive: A propos de 38 cas. Rev Chir Orthop *68*:161–170, 1982.)

A 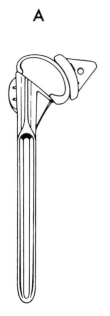   **B** 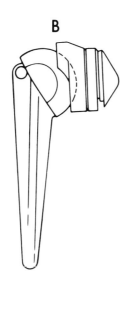   **C**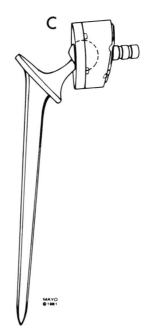

Figure 17–16. A variable amount of constraint is incorporated in the various designs of total shoulder replacement. Many implants have their articular surfaces shaped much like a normal joint surface *(A)*. The system may be partially constrained by virtue of a hooded or more cup-shaped socket *(B)*, or the components may be secured to one another as in the ball-in-socket prosthesis *(C)*. (Reproduced with permission from Cofield RH: The shoulder and prosthetic arthroplasty. In Evarts CM (ed): Surgery of the Musculoskeletal System. New York: Churchill Livingstone, 1983, pp 125–143.)

system would be needed, and (2) the results and complications experienced by the early patients undergoing joint replacement surgery. Fortunately, enough information is now available to answer many of the questions in these two important areas.

Surgical Indications

Destruction of the glenohumeral joint cartilage or distortion of the subchondral bone shape can, of course, occur for many reasons. In a historical sense, the early surgery, as we have seen, tended to concentrate on post-traumatic problems including osteonecrosis. When the explosion in the number of total joint designs occurred, early reports on patient experience

with these implants tended to focus on a single diagnosis, usually rheumatoid arthritis, or two or three diagnoses: rheumatoid arthritis, osteoarthritis, and arthritis secondary to old trauma. In 1982, Neer, in publishing on his experience with total shoulder arthroplasty, tabulated the frequency for which total shoulder arthroplasty was indicated in various diagnostic categories (Table 17–3).[155] My experience over the past 13 years has also defined the relative need for total shoulder arthroplasty among the many possible diagnostic groupings (Table 17–4). From these two tabulations of patient experience, it can be recognized that there are three diagnostic groups for which most surgery will be done. These are rheumatoid arthritis, osteoarthritis (primary or secondary), and arthritis associated with old trauma, such as fractures, fracture-dislocations, or recurrent dislocations. There are three other diagnoses accounting for the majority of the remaining patients who would require total shoulder arthroplasty. These are cuff tear arthropathy, failed

Table 17–2. VARIATIONS IN TOTAL SHOULDER ARTHROPLASTY DESIGN

Unconstrained (Anatomical)	Semiconstrained (Hooded or Cup-Shaped Glenoid)	Constrained (Ball-in-Socket)
Bechtol[13]	Dana[3–5, 68]	Bickel[37, 38]
Bipolar[11]	English-Macnab[76, 142]	Fenlin[77, 78]
Cofield[46, 47]	Mazas[139]	Floating-socket[29]
Dana[3–5]	Neer[155]	Gerard[88]
Kenmore[119]	St. Georg[70–72]	Kessel[122]
Monospherical[93]		Kölbel[125, 126]
Neer[155]		Liverpool[15, 16]
Saha[191]		Michael Reese[170–173]
St. Georg[70–72]		Reeves[178]
		Stanmore[37, 50, 131]
		Trispherical[91]
		Wheble-Skorecki[221]
		Zippel[226]
		Zimmer[225]

Table 17–3. DIAGNOSTIC INDICATIONS FOR TOTAL SHOULDER REPLACEMENT (1973–1981)

	No. Shoulders
Rheumatoid arthritis	69
Osteoarthritis (primary and secondary)	62
Old trauma	60
Prosthetic revision	32
Arthritis of recurrent dislocation	26
Cuff-tear arthropathy	16
Neoplasm	4
Congenital dysplasia	2
Glenohumeral fusion	2
Total	273

(Adapted from Neer CS II et al.: Recent experience in total shoulder replacement. J Bone Joint Surg *64A*:319–337, 1982.)

Table 17–4. DIAGNOSES IN PATIENTS REQUIRING TOTAL SHOULDER ARTHROPLASTY*

	No. Shoulders
Osteoarthritis	173
Rheumatoid arthritis	165
Traumatic arthritis	46
Cuff-tear arthropathy	42
Failed surgery	
Total	34
Proximal humeral	21
Resection	3
Fusion	4
Osteonecrosis	15
Old sepsis	5
Other	8
Total	516

*December 1965–June 1988.

previous surgery (often with a prosthesis), and osteonecrosis of the humeral head with secondary glenoid changes. Other disease categories for which total shoulder arthroplasty might be considered are quite rare. These would include such diagnoses as ancient septic arthritis, radiation necrosis, ankylosing spondylitis, various other rheumatological diseases such as lupus erythematosus, hematological diseases such as hemophilia, and various synovial diseases such as pigmented villonodular synovitis or synovial chondromatosis.

Disease Characteristics

OSTEOARTHRITIS

The pathoanatomy of osteoarthritis will, of course, include the cardinal radiographic features of osteoarthritis in any joint: joint space narrowing, subchondral sclerosis, peripheral osteophytes, and cystic changes in the subchondral-metaphyseal area. Specifics of this disease in the shoulder were detailed by Neer in 1974[151] (Fig. 17–17).

Thinning of the articular cartilage was most advanced in that area of the humeral head that is in contact with the glenoid when the arm is abducted between 60 and 100 degrees . . . the area . . . was eburnated and sclerotic. Degenerative subarticular cysts occurred just superior to the mid point of the articular surface. The largest osteophytes were located at the inferior margin of the joint where they often covered the calcar. Other marginal excrescences were found surrounding the head, obliterating the sulcus, blocking rotation, encroaching on the bicipital groove, and enlarging the diameter of the head to as much as twice the normal size.

The articular surface of the glenoid was smooth but usually consisted of eburnated bone devoid of cartilage. Marginal osteophytes . . . could be palpated within the ligaments of the glenoid, especially inferiorly, but they were rarely visible at surgery.

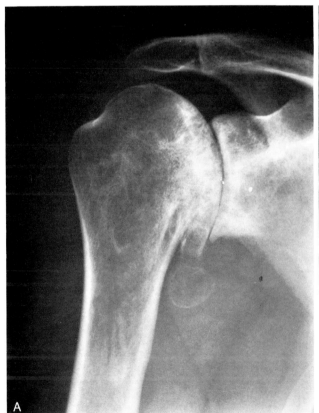

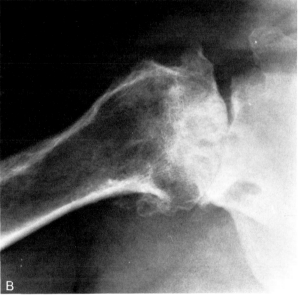

Figure 17–17. Osteoarthritis of the shoulder. *A,* A stereotypical radiographic, pathoanatomical appearance. The humeral head is somewhat enlarged and flattened. There are peripheral osteophytes, particularly prominent inferiorly. There is flattening of the humeral head with subchondral sclerosis, particularly centrally and central-superiorly. There may be intraosseous cysts. These cysts are best seen on the axillary projection, *B.* In the axillary view, one also sees asymmetrical glenoid wear with slightly greater wear of the posterior aspect of the glenoid. In addition, the glenoid is also flattened. There is a suggestion of posterior humeral subluxation, but this is not a striking feature in these radiographs.

The capsule was distended by the enlarged head and contained excess synovial fluid. . . . The majority of the joints contained one or more osteochondral loose bodies. . . . The subscapular bursa was enlarged, communicated with the joint, and at times contained loose bodies.[151]

Only one of the 48 shoulders reported had a complete-thickness rotator cuff tear; this may have been related to an injury. The subscapularis tendon usually had a fixed contracture and occasionally (4 of 48 shoulders) was lengthened.

Neer further noted in 1982[155] that the findings in osteoarthritis were remarkably consistent. Expanding on the 1974 description, advanced cases often had a flattened glenoid with posterior erosion possibly resulting in posterior subluxation of the humeral head (Fig. 17–18). Cuff tears were present in only three of 62 shoulders in this more recent series. Concomitant acromioclavicular arthritis may or may not be present.

Osteoarthritis, degenerative arthritis of the shoulder, has been studied anatomically, radiographically, and pathologically. Meachim,[143] in cadaver studies on 42 subjects with an age range from 25 to 72 years, found no thinning of the cartilage in the central portion of the joint surface of the humeral head with aging. This was confirmed in 151 dissections on 76 cadavers performed by Petersson.[165] However, degenerative changes were encountered in the soft tissues, increasing in frequency as age increased, especially after age 60. These included rotator cuff degeneration in 25 shoulders, full-thickness cuff ruptures in 23, degeneration of the long biceps tendon in 12, and rupture of the tendon in 6. When cuff degeneration or tearing was present, cartilage changes were also found. Changes were often bilateral and more frequent in women. There was little evidence to support occupation as being of major importance in the development of degenerative changes.

A radiographic study by Sillár and co-workers on both shoulder joints of 505 healthy people and random examination of 100 cases offered support to certain of Petersson's findings.[195] Radiographic changes, when occurring, tended to be multiple. Changes in left and right shoulders were equal and, when bilateral, tended to be similar. Radiographic change became more frequent with increasing age, but the frequency of changes between males and females was identical.

Kerr, Resnick, and co-workers evaluated 74 cadaveric humeri, 92 cadaveric scapulae, and 50 patients greater than age 60.[121] They noted the extent of changes to be underestimated by plain radiographs. Humeral abnormalities included osteophytes at the margin of the articular surface with greater involvement anteriorly and inferiorly, irregularities in bony surfaces at capsule and tendon attachments, and sclerosis and irregularity of the articular surface. Glenoid abnormalities included marginal osteophytes mainly along the lower two-thirds, sclerosis, and erosion, often central. Changes in the bones were associated with deterioration of the rotator cuff.

The features of osteoarthritis of the shoulder are listed in Table 17–5.

RHEUMATOID ARTHRITIS

The pathological changes seen in the shoulder with rheumatoid arthritis can be quite variable. All tissues are affected, but certain tissues are involved to a greater degree in some patients while other tissues are damaged in other patients. It has been stated that

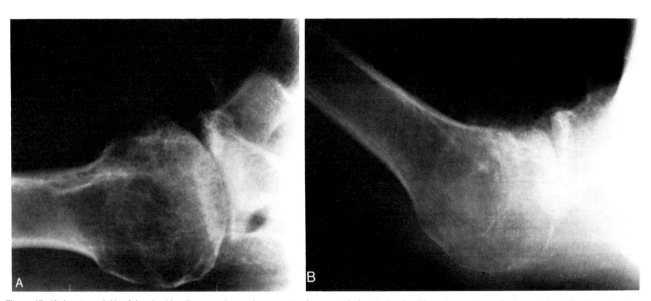

Figure 17–18. In osteoarthritis of the shoulder, there may be varying amounts of asymmetrical posterior glenoid erosion and posterior humeral instability. In A, there has been a moderate amount of asymmetrical posterior glenoid erosion and subluxation of the humeral head into the area of wear. In B, there is a lesser amount of glenoid erosion but a much larger amount of posterior humeral subluxation, suggesting significant elongation of the posterior shoulder capsule and the overlying rotator cuff. Reconstructive steps should take these changes—the glenoid erosion and the instability—into consideration.

Table 17–5. PATHOANATOMY OF GLENOHUMERAL OSTEOARTHRITIS

Humeral head
    Cartilage loss—central, superior, or complete
    Sclerosis—central, superior
    Peripheral osteophytes—most prominent inferiorly
    Increased size
    Erosion with central flattening
    Subchondral cysts
Glenoid
    Cartilage loss—central, posterior, or complete
    Sclerosis—central or posterior
    Peripheral osteophytes—lower two-thirds
    Erosion—central or posterior with flattening
    Subchondral cysts
Joint position
    Central or posterior subluxation
Capsule
    Enlarged, especially inferiorly
    Anterior contracture
Rotator cuff and biceps tendon
    Complete-thickness tearing unusual (approximately 5%)
    Degeneration or fibrosis (specially subscapularis) may be present
Loose bodies within joint or subscapularis bursa

patients with rheumatoid arthritis and shoulder involvement seldom need shoulder surgery,[33] the admonitions of pioneers in rheumatoid joint surgery notwithstanding.[198] Laine and associates of Finland defined the spectrum of shoulder disease in 277 hospitalized patients with rheumatoid arthritis.[129] Seventy-five patients (47 per cent) had glenohumeral joint arthritis; many of these also had coracoacromial arch symptoms. Thirteen other patients had rather isolated rotator cuff tendinitis; nine had bicipital tenosynovitis. Scapulocostal symptoms were present in 55 patients. Other types or areas of rheumatoid shoulder involvement included arthralgia of the glenohumeral joint without demonstrable changes in 16, frozen shoulder in 7, subacromial bursitis with hydrops in 5, calcific tendinitis in 5, sympathetic reflex dystrophy in 5, and radicular symptoms in 4. An additional nine patients had osteoarthritis of a shoulder without evidence of actual rheumatoid disease in that joint. Vainio, also working in the Rheumatism Foundation Hospital in Heinola, Finland, has subsequently defined the treatment preferences he has for these patients with these patterns of rheumatoid involvement.[214]

Petersson examined the shoulder joints of 105 patients with rheumatoid arthritis;[166] 116 shoulders in 61 patients were also evaluated radiographically. Ninety-six patients (91 per cent) reported shoulder symptoms. Patients with severe shoulder disability also usually had more widespread destructive arthritis. With an increasing duration of rheumatoid arthritis, there was progression of destructive changes. Dijkstra and co-workers used standard radiographs to evaluate the course of rheumatoid arthritis in the shoulder.[62] Over a 29-year period, 630 x-rays were taken in 286 shoulders. Gross destruction was rare. Progression of the disease was often slow or halting. Presence and progression of the disease in the glenohumeral and acromioclavicular joints followed independent courses. A similar study was done in 100 shoulder joints of 50 hospitalized patients with seropositive rheumatoid arthritis.[52] Involvement of the shoulder joint was surprisingly common. Grading the radiographs from one (no abnormalities) to five (end-stage disease), the shoulders were categorized as Grade 1 in 11 per cent, Grade 2 in 35 per cent, Grade 3 in 16 per cent, Grade 4 in 16 per cent, and Grade 5 in 22 per cent. In many patients, the shoulder caused few symptoms in spite of significant radiographic changes; however, dramatic clinical deterioration occurred in the presence of Grade 5 disease, with severe pain being present in greater than 50 per cent of those with this grade of shoulder involvement.

All of the above studies would lead us to believe that shoulder involvement is common in rheumatoid arthritis, it may manifest itself in a variety of ways, symptoms may be less than radiographs would suggest they should be, and the condition of the shoulder generally worsens with time; however, a prediction of the course for an individual may not be possible because of the sometimes halting nature of the disease. Also, when the shoulder joints are severely affected, other joints are usually not spared.[94]

Neer has classified the pattern of shoulder involvement as dry, wet, or resorptive with the possibility of low grade, intermediate, or severe changes within each group.[152] In the dry form, there is a marked tendency for loss of the joint space, periarticular sclerosis, bone cysts, and stiffness (Fig. 17–19). In the wet form, there is exuberant synovial disease with marginal erosions and intrusion of the humeral head into the glenoid

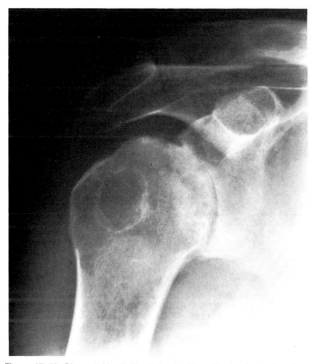

Figure 17–19. Rheumatoid arthritis of the shoulder with glenohumeral cartilage loss and joint stiffness, the so-called dry form of the disease.

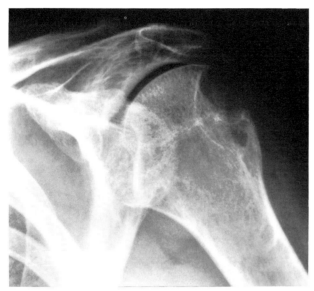

Figure 17–20. Rheumatoid arthritis in the shoulder with cartilage loss, extensive periarticular erosions, and an extremely hypertrophic synovitis, the so-called wet form of joint involvement.

(Fig. 17–20). The outstanding feature of the resorptive type is bone resorption (Fig. 17–21).

With such a large possible spectrum of shoulder involvement, it seems most logical to analyze each tissue in the shoulder for its extent of involvement. After doing so, the treatment options become much more clear (Table 17–6).

The subdeltoid-subacromial bursa may develop an isolated primary bursitis[107] (Fig. 17–22). Unfortunately, this is uncommon, for when the bursa is extensively affected, other shoulder structures usually are too, notably the rotator cuff.

Table 17–6. RHEUMATOID ARTHRITIS OF THE SHOULDER

Tissue	Type of Pathological Change
Subdeltoid bursa	Inflammation
	Fibrosis
	Synovial hypertrophy
Bone	Osteopenia
	Erosions
	Resorption
	Sclerosis
	Cysts
	Fracture
Cartilage	Loss, partial or complete
Rotator cuff	Inflammation
	Fibrosis
	Thinning, stretching
	Tearing
Synovial lining	Inflammation
	Fibrosis
	Synovial hypertrophy
Shoulder capsule	Inflammation
	Fibrosis
	Thinning, stretching
	Instability

Early in the disease, the bone about the shoulder may be normal or show only osteopenia (Fig. 17–23). With continuing synovial disease, marginal erosions develop (Fig. 17–24), and the erosions may be quite extensive (see Fig. 17–20). Further bone involvement depends first on cartilage loss (see Fig. 17–19), and then additional bony destruction or erosion can occur. Typically, some bone is resorbed from the humeral

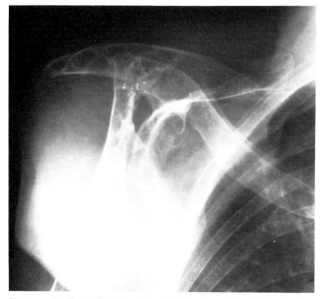

Figure 17–21. This radiograph of the shoulder of an elderly woman with long-standing rheumatoid arthritis shows extreme resorption involving the humeral head, a portion of the proximal humerus, and the lateral aspect of the scapula, including the entire glenoid.

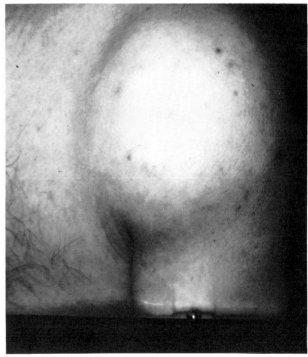

Figure 17–22. A clinical photograph of the shoulder of a young man with rheumatoid arthritis and primary rheumatoid involvement of the subacromial-subdeltoid bursa. The rotator cuff was intact, and the glenohumeral joint had minimal involvement with rheumatoid synovitis. There was a full, minimally painful range of motion in the shoulder, with excellent shoulder strength. The hypertrophic bursitis did not respond to medical management, and surgical excision of the bursa was done.

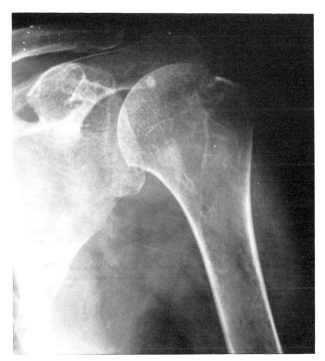

Figure 17–23. A middle-aged woman with long-standing rheumatoid arthritis and multiple joint involvement. At the time these radiographs were done she presented with severe shoulder pain and mild restriction of movement. The radiographs essentially show only osteopenia. There is maintenance of the joint space and only the slightest suggestion of marginal joint erosion. The extent of pathological changes seen here is rather mild. Unfortunately, the patient's symptoms were unresponsive to conservative management. Significant synovitis was demonstrated by arthrogram, and a shoulder synovectomy was undertaken.

head, and, in addition, a central glenoid erosion occurs (Fig. 17–25). The humeral neck may impinge on the glenoid-axillary border, causing a notable indentation. Occasionally, this area will fracture.[132]

Rarely, cartilage loss occurs without much tissue involvement except for the synovial lining (see Fig. 17–19). Usually, however, this is associated with a thinning, stretching, or fibrosis of the rotator cuff (Fig.

17–26). This may progress to frank rotator cuff tearing (Fig. 17–27), and the progression can be extensive with erosive changes affecting the acromion. This, of course, occurs following destruction of the superior aspect of the rotator cuff (Fig. 17–28). Please recall, though, that extensive rotator cuff tearing is not usual in rheumatoid arthritis. In a clinical and arthrographic study of 200 painful shoulders in patients with rheumatoid arthritis, Ennevarra found only 26.5 per cent of patients had full-thickness rotator cuff tearing.[74] In two series of patients with rheumatoid arthritis that required total shoulder arthroplasty, the rotator cuff had full-thickness tearing in 29 of 69 shoulders (42 per cent) and in 18 of 66 shoulders (27 per cent).[40, 155]

Analysis of the synovial lining may be important when symptoms are significant but x-ray changes are minor. Arthrography can define the extent of synovitis[60] (Fig. 17–29).

Rarely, the glenohumeral joint capsule may be damaged to a greater degree than adjacent structures, producing instability (Fig. 17–30). Physical examination and the usual radiographic and adjunctive evaluations done for traumatic instability can define this further.

Not rarely, an upper middle-aged person, often a woman, presents with a several year history of unilateral or bilateral shoulder pain without a history of injury or generalized arthritic disease. The rheumatoid factor may be positive. The pattern of involvement is dry in type, and Neer has termed this "the syndrome"[152] (Fig. 17–31).

Several rare complications or associations with rheumatoid arthritis in the shoulder have been reported. These include pseudothrombosis,[59] serratus anterior disruption,[145] superimposed septic arthritis,[90, 127] chylous or synovial cysts,[2, 80, 194] neuropathic arthritis secondary to cervical spine disease,[99] and suprascapular nerve damage.[177]

To reiterate, many different shoulder structures can potentially be involved in rheumatoid arthritis, each

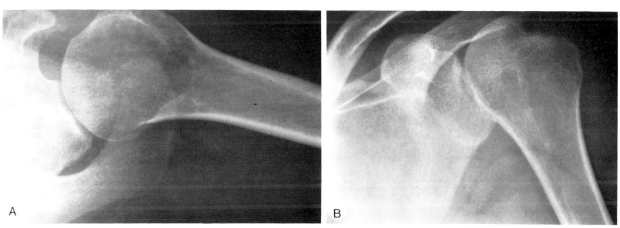

A

B

Figure 17–24. Rheumatoid arthritis involving the shoulder of a 26-year-old man with oligoarticular disease. His symptoms were moderate in extent. The radiographs show slight cartilage loss, particularly on the axillary projection (A), and erosion of the humeral head near the articular surface margin on the anteroposterior radiograph (B). Extensive synovitis was present (see Fig. 17–29).

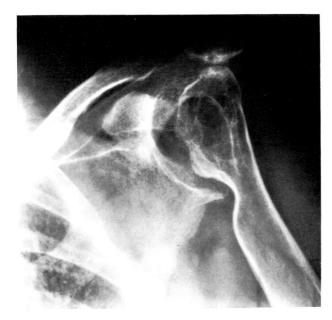

Figure 17–25. Long-standing rheumatoid arthritis of the shoulder with erosion of subchondral and adjacent bony structures. This is notable on the humeral head but most pronounced in the scapula with extreme central resorption. In patients such as this, there may not be enough remaining bone to allow placement of a glenoid component at the time of reconstructive surgery.

Figure 17–26. Rheumatoid arthritis of the shoulder. The radiograph shows a slight amount of osteopenia, cartilage loss, mild subchondral bone loss, and upward subluxation of the humeral head. In this patient, as in many with rheumatoid arthritis of the shoulder, the rotator cuff has become thin, with attrition, stretching, and fibrosis, but without full-thickness rotator cuff tearing.

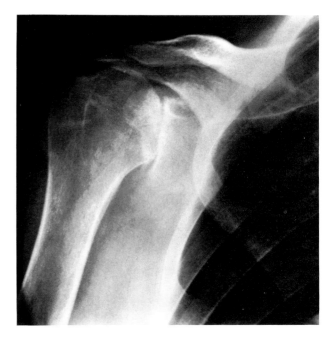

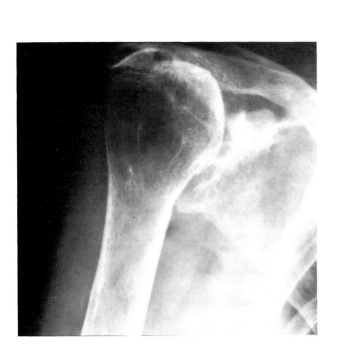

Figure 17–27. Rheumatoid arthritis of the shoulder in association with rotator cuff tearing. The radiogram shows cartilage loss, central-superior erosion of the glenoid, upward subluxation of the humeral head, and some erosion of the overlying acromion and distal clavicle. At surgery, a large rotator cuff tear was found involving the infraspinatus, supraspinatus, and subscapularis.

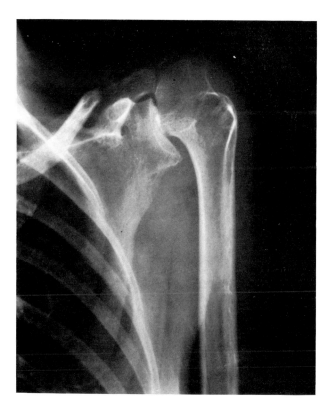

Figure 17–28. Juvenile rheumatoid arthritis with extreme rotator cuff and capsular involvement, even to the extent of acromial erosion. The humeral head is now beneath the skin across the superior aspect of the shoulder.

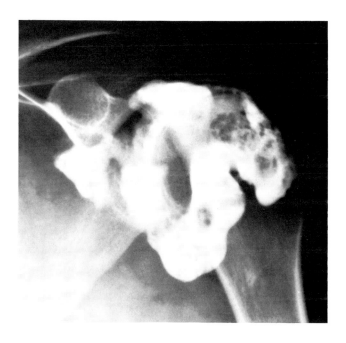

Figure 17–29. Shoulder arthrogram showing active synovitis in a patient with rheumatoid arthritis. The plain x-rays (see Fig. 17–24) showed only minor joint changes.

Figure 17–30. Axillary x-ray projection of the shoulder of a young woman with rheumatoid arthritis. Rheumatoid destruction of the anterior shoulder capsule and anterior aspect of the rotator cuff has occurred such that anterior instability now exists. Enough cartilage loss had occurred that treatment included proximal humeral prosthetic replacement, glenohumeral joint synovectomy, and anterior capsule and rotator cuff repair.

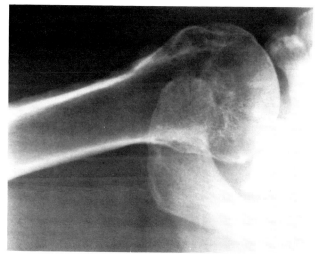

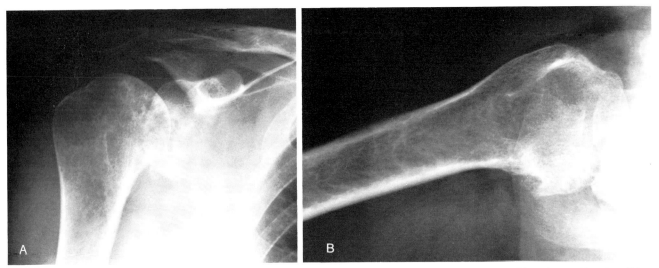

Figure 17–31. An upper-middle-aged woman with four years of progressively severe shoulder pain. She now has pain with any arm activity and at rest. There is no history of past injury nor any history of multiple joint arthritic involvement. The sedimentation rate is slightly elevated; the rheumatoid factor is negative. At surgery, the synovium exhibited histological changes of a mild chronic synovitis but was not diagnostic for a specific type of arthritic disease. As seen on the anteroposterior view, A, and the axillary view, B, this patient's disease has many of the characteristics of a nonspecific inflammatory arthritis with osteopenia, cartilage loss, granulation tissue within a cyst in the humeral head and glenoid, and minimal hypertrophic or sclerotic changes. A presentation such as this is somewhat uncommon but is not rare. Neer has labeled this presentation "the syndrome."

can be involved to a varying degree, and thus, extremely careful analysis must be done before treatment can be undertaken (see Table 17–6).

OLD TRAUMA

A number of complications from previous fractures, dislocations, or fracture-dislocations may occur that will potentially lead to the development of glenohumeral arthritis (Table 17–7). Samilson and Prieto[193] identified 74 shoulders with a history of single or multiple dislocations that exhibited radiographic evidence of glenohumeral arthritis (Fig. 17–32). The dislocations had been anterior in 62 shoulders, posterior in 11, and one had multidirectional instability. The number of dislocations was not related to the severity of the arthrosis. Shoulders with posterior instability had a higher incidence of moderate or severe arthritis, as did shoulders with previous surgery in which internal fixation devices intruded on the joint surface. Complications about the shoulder related to the use of metallic internal fixation were also described by Zuckerman and Matsen.[227] A large number of patients they studied had had operations for treatment of recurrent shoulder dislocations.

In chronic, unreduced dislocations,[102, 174, 187] the humeral head may be indented and worn. The cartilage

of the joint surfaces may be replaced with scar (Fig. 17–33), or the subchondral bone may be so weakened by bone atrophy that it will collapse after reduction, leading to an incongruous joint surface (Fig. 17–34). Hawkins and co-workers[102] have suggested hemiarthroplasty if the dislocation is greater than six months old

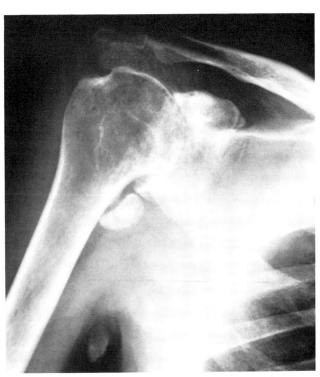

Figure 17–32. This elderly man had a five- to ten-year history of progressively severe shoulder pain and limitation of motion. As an adolescent, he had had recurrent dislocations of this shoulder, and presumably his current arthritis has developed subsequent to his recurrent instability. This sequence of events certainly can occur but is surprisingly uncommon.

Table 17–7. GLENOHUMERAL ARTHRITIS FOLLOWING TRAUMA

Potential Etiologies

Recurrent subluxations or dislocations
Chronic dislocations
Fracture malunion with joint incongruity
Osteonecrosis of the humeral head
Proximal humeral nonunion with fibrous ankylosis

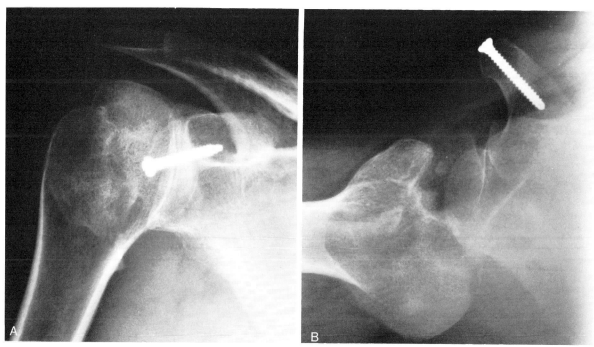

Figure 17–33. A chronic posteror shoulder dislocation in a 26-year-old man. The injury occurred approximately one year earlier. A recent previous anterior approach to the shoulder was ineffective in reducing the dislocation. At the time of the second surgical procedure, the shoulder was reduced, but the cartilage of the humeral head had been replaced with fibrous tissue. A proximal humeral prosthesis was placed as a part of the reconstructive procedure. *A* is a 40-degree posterior oblique x-ray illustrating the overlap between the humeral head and the glenoid. *B* clearly illustrates the posterior dislocation, the slight malunion between the head and shaft fragments, and the evidence of fracturing of the lesser tuberosity with healing of this tuberosity to the shaft but somewhat displaced from the humeral head segment.

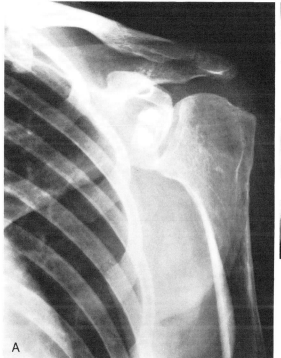

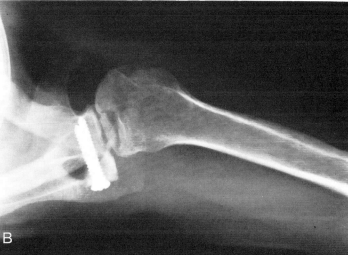

Figure 17–34. This young woman underwent open reduction of a posterior shoulder dislocation that had been unreduced for approximately two months. At the time of the reduction, the cartilage surfaces were intact; the humeral head was noted to be somewhat softened. A bone graft was added to the posterior aspect of the shoulder to substitute for an area of glenoid wear. Within the first month following open reduction, it was apparent on the anteroposterior view, *A*, and the axillary view, *B*, that the humeral head, because of its softness, had collapsed, and traumatic arthritis was developing. Subsequently a proximal humeral prosthesis was placed.

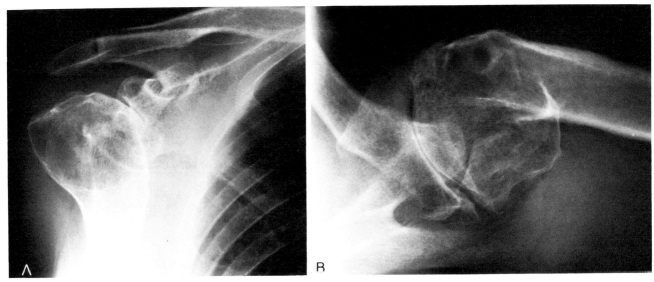

Figure 17–35. *A, B,* Traumatic arthritis with loss of glenohumeral cartilage has developed following malunion of a comminuted proximal humeral fracture.

or if the humeral head defect involves more than 45 per cent of the articular surface. If the glenoid is destroyed, a total shoulder arthroplasty will be necessary. Tanner and Cofield reviewed 28 shoulders with chronic fracture problems requiring prosthetic arthroplasty.[209] Sixteen had malunions with a joint incongruity (Fig. 17–35), eight had post-traumatic osteonecrosis (Fig. 17–36), and four had nonunion of a surgical neck fracture with a small, osteopenic head fragment.

It has been stated that in these patients with hemiarthroplasty and in those with total shoulder arthroplasty, operations following old trauma are especially difficult, and complications are more frequent.[108, 155] This may be due to a number of factors: muscle contracture, scarring, malunion requiring osteotomy, nonunion, or bone loss, especially humeral shortening.

A number of these patients also have associated nerve deficits.

CUFF TEAR ARTHROPATHY

In 1981, McCarty and co-workers described a shoulder condition: the "Milwaukee shoulder." This included significant rotator cuff disease and shoulder arthritis in older patients, often women.[86, 95, 140] The synovial fluid contained aggregates of hydroxyapatite crystals, active collagenase, and neutral protease. At that time, these authors hypothesized that the crystals within the synovial fluid were phagocytized by the macrophage-like synovial cells, and the cells in turn released enzymes, resulting in damage of the joint and

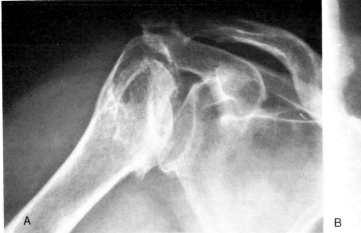
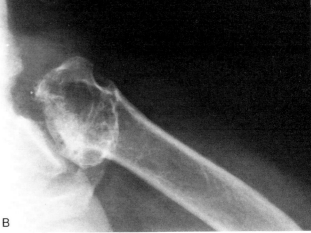

Figure 17–36. Traumatic arthritis with malunion and osteonecrosis of the head segment. Radiograph *A* shows the collapse of the head segment and the slight malunion of the greater tuberosity relative to the shaft. Radiograph *B* again shows collapse of the humeral head segment but reasonable positions of the tuberosities on this view. Damage to the glenoid articular surface is underestimated on these radiographic projections. At reconstructive surgery for situations such as this, either proximal humeral prosthetic replacement or total shoulder arthroplasty might be needed, depending on the extent of glenoid surface involvement.

joint-related structures. The inciting process could not be identified.

In 1983, the hypothesis was further refined. The crystals were identified as basic calcium phosphate (BCP).[141] It was thought these crystals would form in the synovial fluid by unknown mechanisms. They would then be phagocytosed by the synovial lining cells. These cells would then secrete the collagenase and neutral protease. This would damage the tissues and, in addition, cause the release of additional crystals. The importance of this concept may be a more universal understanding of crystal-related arthropathies and a better understanding of how multiple joint structures can be affected by an underlying problem. It is important to recall that this is a hypothesis.[96-98]

In 1983, Neer and co-workers published an article on cuff tear arthropathy describing pathological changes in 26 patients.[156] These changes included massive rotator cuff tearing, glenohumeral instability, loss of articular cartilage of the glenohumeral joint, humeral head collapse, and related bone loss (Fig. 17–37). This entity was distinctly different from osteoarthritis, which he had defined earlier. Neer felt that mechanical factors associated with extensive rotator cuff tearing played a prominent role in the creation of this problem and that secondary nutritional changes may augment the pathological changes that occur.

One should recognize that the "Milwaukee shoulder" syndrome and cuff tear arthropathy may be distinctly different problems leading to a similar end-stage, or they may, in fact, be one entity with, for example, rotator cuff damage precipitating the metabolic alterations described by McCarty.

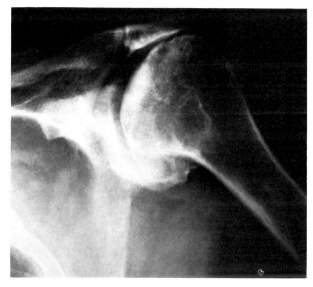

Figure 17–37. Rotator cuff tear arthropathy. The radiograph depicts the cartilage loss, mild but definite bone loss of the humeral head and glenoid, severe upward subluxation of the humeral head against the acromion with rotator cuff tearing, and some erosion of the abutting acromion. This patient has significant multi-tissue involvement: cartilage, bone, capsule, and rotator cuff. Reconstructive surgery must address all these deficiencies.

OSTEONECROSIS

Nontraumatic osteonecrosis of the subchondral bone of the humeral head is usually associated with the systemic use of steroids or is called idiopathic. Many diseases have been implicated in the etiology of osteonecrosis or at least are associated with it. Some of these conditions have required steroid use as a part of medical treatment. Implicated conditions include alcoholism, sickle cell disease, decompression sickness, hyperuricemia, Gaucher's disease, pancreatitis, familial hyperlipidemia, renal or other organ transplantation, lymphoma, and lupus erythematosus.[24, 53, 54, 184]

Staging of the process is relevant to prognosis and treatment. This has been best defined for the femoral head. Staging systems suggested by Cruess[55] based upon other previously defined staging systems will transpose to the analysis of humeral head lesions. Stage I is a preradiologic stage. The radiographs are normal, but bone scanning or magnetic resonance imaging shows changes within the humeral head. Stage II has radiologic changes of osteoporosis, osteosclerosis, or a combination of the two. There may also be a localized subchondral osteolytic lesion without fracturing and without a change in humeral head shape. Stage III has the crescent sign. This is indicative of a fracture through the abnormal subchondral bone. In the humeral head, this is located superior-centrally. There is only slight change in the contour of the head in this stage of involvement (Fig. 17–38). Stage IV includes collapse of the subchondral bone with deformity or, on occasion, a separated osteocartilaginous flap (Fig. 17–39). In Stage V, the changes on the humeral head seen in Stage IV are present, but, in addition, the glenoid shows pathological changes (Fig. 17–40).

In an analysis of 18 shoulders with steroid-induced osteonecrosis of the head of the humerus, the patients fell into three roughly equal groups.[53] One group had mild anatomical deformity and minimal symptoms. The second group had more severe deformity, but the patients' activities did not require extensive use of the shoulder and nonoperative treatment was sufficient. The third group required hemiarthroplasty because of significant deformity and persistent, severe pain. The results of surgery were gratifying, with relief of pain and nearly normal range of movement.

A similar group of patients was studied by Rutherford and Cofield.[189] Patients presenting with osteonecrosis of the humeral head were followed from two to six and one-half years. In 11 shoulders with Stage II or III disease, only two had clinical progression (Fig. 17–41). In five shoulders with Stage IV or V disease but with only moderate complaints at presentation, all symptomatically worsened with time. In ten shoulders with Stage III and IV, and early Stage V disease and severe symptoms, a hemiarthroplasty was done. Six shoulders with Stage V disease underwent total shoulder arthroplasty. Following surgery, 94 per cent of the 16 shoulders with surgery had no or slight pain, and as in Cruess' series, range of movement approached normal.

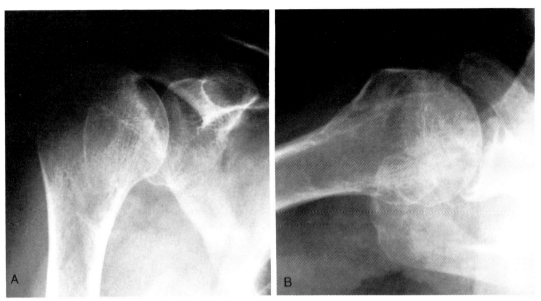

Figure 17–38. Osteonecrosis of the proximal humerus. There is an osteochondral fracture with minimal distortion of the articular surface of the humerus. This is best seen in *A*, the anteroposterior view. In *B*, the axillary view, there is a crescent sign in the anterior-central part of the humeral head.

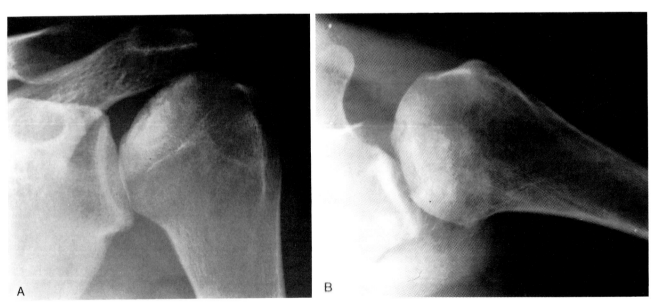

Figure 17–39. Osteonecrosis of the humeral head associated with chronic steroid use. A subchondral fracture has occurred in the past. There is distortion of the humeral articular surface shape and early glenohumeral arthritis. Symptoms were significant in this young man, and treatment with a proximal humeral prosthesis was quite effective. *A*, Anteroposterior view; *B*, axillary view.

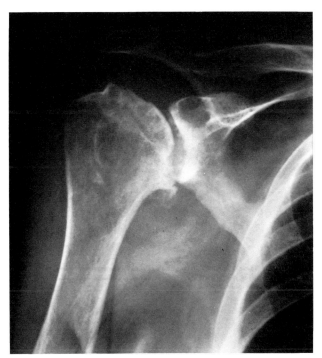

Figure 17–40. Long-standing osteonecrosis of the proximal humerus with only slight distortion of the articular surface but, unfortunately, progression to significant arthritis involving both the humeral and glenoid articular surfaces.

It appears that patients with tolerable symptoms and osteonecrosis of the humeral head should be treated nonoperatively as symptom progression may not occur (symptom progression is much more likely in Stage IV or V). Patients with substantial symptoms in association with Stage III, IV, or V disease should be considered for prosthetic arthroplasty, as this has been quite effective treatment.

INFREQUENT CAUSES OF SHOULDER ARTHRITIS

In the evaluation and care of patients with glenohumeral arthritis, it is necessary to recall that many types of systemic diseases with an associated arthritic component may affect the shoulder. Often, treatment for the systemic disease will be necessary prior to or during the time of treatment for the shoulder. Included among these disorders are the hematological conditions of hemophilia and hemachromatosis,[75, 176] primary hyperparathyroidism,[160] acromegaly,[168] amyloid arthropathy,[56] gout,[69] chondrocalcinosis,[49] ankylosing spondylitis,[81, 134] psoriasis,[81] and a new addition to the list, Lyme arthritis.[56]

Localized synovial diseases possibly leading to shoulder arthritis include pigmented villonodular synovitis[63, 64] and synovial chondrometaplasia.[104]

Radiation therapy, especially for the treatment of breast cancer, may cause a number of shoulder problems: brachial plexopathies, osteonecrosis, malignant bone tumors, and fibrous replacement of many tissues. Glenohumeral cartilage and subchondral bone are on occasion affected by these changes and may require treatment by prosthetic arthroplasty or other alternative methods (Fig. 17–42).

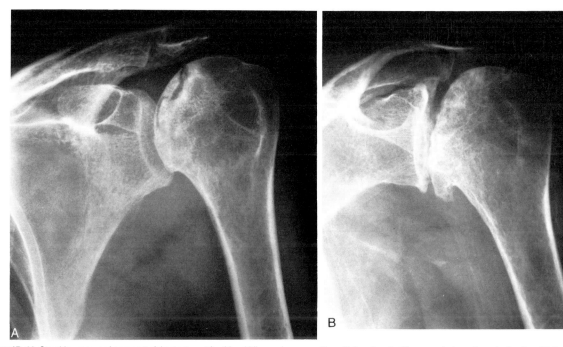

Figure 17–41. Steroids were used as a part of the treatment for this middle-aged woman with multiple sclerosis. She presented, as shown in A, with mild shoulder symptoms associated with osteonecrosis of the proximal humerus. There is minimal distortion of the articular surface shape. B shows the same shoulder about eight years later. There has been greater distortion of the articular surface shape and the development of some glenohumeral arthritis. However, the symptoms are still mild, and nonoperative treatment continues to be appropriate for this patient.

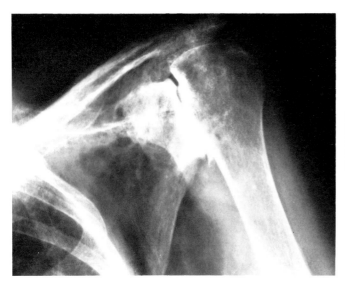

Figure 17–42. Cartilage loss, alteration of subchondral bone shape with segmental collapse, and alteration in bony texture secondary to irradiation that was done as a part of the treatment for breast cancer. Symptoms were quite significant in this elderly woman. The symptoms were effectively relieved with total shoulder arthroplasty.

DIFFERENTIAL DIAGNOSIS

Three categories of disease processes are important to recognize and differentiate from the usual evaluation and care patterns associated with glenohumeral degeneration and the other arthritides. These are shoulder problems secondary to infection, neuropathy, or neoplasia.

Septic arthritis of the shoulder is uncommon, but when it occurs, it is often in a person debilitated from a generalized disease[8, 30] or in a person who has an underlying shoulder disease process such as rotator cuff tearing[6] or rheumatoid arthritis.[127] In this latter setting, there appears to be an exacerbation of the underlying shoulder disease, and in the absence of fever or an elevated white blood count, diagnosis will depend on a high level of suspicion, joint aspiration, and bacteriological testing.

Neuropathic arthritis of the shoulder, a Charcot joint, may, contrary to most writing, present with some pain and functional limitation (Fig. 17–43). Cervical spine trauma may have occurred in the past,[179] or unrecognized syringomyelia may exist.[137, 212] Radiographically, the shoulder may have the appearance of severe degenerative joint disease or cuff tear arthropathy. Usually there is significant bone destruction and instability; an important radiographic finding is osseous debris about the joint area. Diagnosis will be by

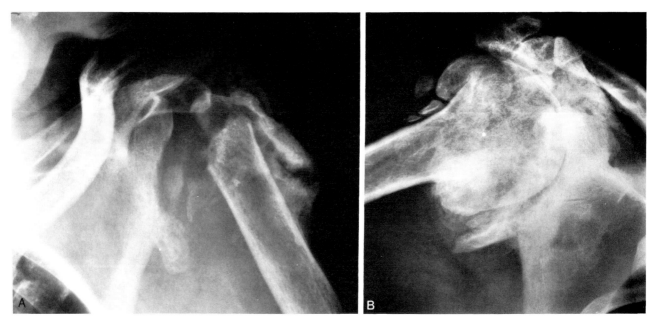

Figure 17–43. On occasion, a neuropathic arthritis can be confused with the more common forms of glenohumeral arthritis. *A* shows fragmentation of the proximal humerus with bone debris scattered throughout the joint region. *B* shows bone fragmentation also but a predominantly sclerotic response associated with the neuropathic arthritis. The underlying condition in both of these patients was syringomyelia of the cervical portion of the spinal cord.

neurological examination: electromyography, cervical spine radiographs, myelography, or in recent times, magnetic resonance. The abnormalities may be surprisingly subtle.

Neoplasia may not always be obvious in an older population with osteopenia. The tumor may incite a synovial response, further mimicking an arthritic condition[21, 144] (Fig. 17–44). The pain may be more intense than the usual arthritic pain and decidedly unresponsive to rest. Night pain is also common in shoulder arthritis and will be of little help in differentiating neoplasia from arthritis. Diagnosis will depend on knowledge of the patient's general health, routine and possibly additional health testing, high quality plain x-rays, and additional imaging modes including tomography, computerized tomographic scanning, bone scanning, or magnetic resonance imaging. Identification of the primary lesion in metastatic disease is ideal, but sometimes biopsy of the shoulder lesion will be necessary for diagnosis.

Clinical Evaluation

Evaluation of a patient with shoulder arthritis is rather straightforward, following the lines of orthopedic assessment of an individual with arthritis in any location. This is done by using the history, physical examination, radiography and adjunctive imaging modes, laboratory studies, or electromyography with nerve conduction studies when symptoms or signs suggest the need for them.

Pain is almost always the chief complaint. This is combined with some degree of functional deficit. The pain is located in the shoulder and upper arm. Less severe pain may be present in the periscapular area and in the area encompassed by the trapezius, and the pain may extend to the radial aspect of the forearm. Pain in the cervical region would lead one to also carefully study the cervical spine, and pain in the entire limb or hand would suggest neurovascular or hand disease in addition to shoulder pathology. The pain in the shoulder is worsened by use and relieved with rest but may be exacerbated by recumbency at night. A number of patients sleep in an easy chair. The usual analgesic medicines help when the arthritis is mild or moderate but are less effective when the arthritis is radiographically severe. Injections seem to offer little long-term help, except for their placebo effect. Gentle stretching, heat, massage, modification of activities, and extra warm clothing seem to offer some relief, but this relief is, of course, incomplete.

On physical examination, there may be a mild or moderate generalized muscle wasting about the shoulder. Tenderness may be present, especially at the posterior joint line. Intra-articular crepitus may be most easily appreciated at that location too. If crepitus is present anterosuperiorly, it suggests the presence of rotator cuff disease in addition to glenohumeral cartilage loss. As can be recognized from the analysis of the disease processes being considered, rotator cuff tearing is much less common than would ordinarily be expected.

Range of motion is limited in the usual patient with glenohumeral arthritis. Often, active and passive abduction are one-half to two-thirds normal. Internal rotation behind the trunk is limited to the lumbar region, and external rotation is absent or limited to 20 to 40 degrees. Strength within the limited range may be surprisingly good, but testing is often associated with pain and grating. In osteoarthritis, the shoulder contour is often altered because of posterior subluxation. The anterior aspect of the shoulder is flattened and the posterior portion more rounded than usual. In rheumatoid arthritis, the clavicle and acromion may be unusually prominent owing both to muscle wasting and central displacement of the humeral head. In cuff tear arthropathy, the shoulder may show some anterosuperior subluxation of the humeral head on the glenoid.

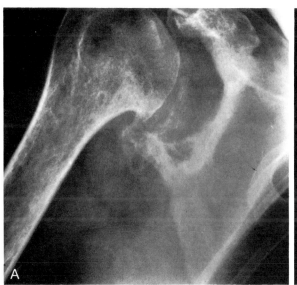
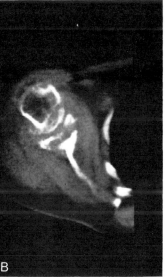

Figure 17–44. This upper-middle-aged woman presented with the gradual onset of shoulder pain and reduction of movement. The shoulder was more painful with use and was also painful at rest (often typical of shoulder arthritis). She had no known systemic illness. A shows arthritic involvement of the glenohumeral joint with some collapse of the humeral head articular surface; however, more importantly, it shows destruction of the bone of the glenoid. B, a CT image, shows this bone destruction quite well. Biopsy revealed metastatic thyroid carcinoma. A neoplastic process must always be considered in the evaluation of a patient with supposed glenohumeral arthritis.

Fluid in the subdeltoid bursa can be associated with primary bursal involvement in rheumatoid arthritis but usually indicates rotator cuff tearing with extravasation of joint fluid into the bursa. A cyst on the acromioclavicular joint is also usually indicative of glenohumeral fluid extravasation through a rotator cuff tear and subsequently through a rent in the acromioclavicular joint capsule.

The acromioclavicular joint may or may not be arthritic in association with glenohumeral arthritis. The development of arthritis in these two joints seems to be rather independent. When significant glenohumeral disease is present, acromioclavicular arthritis pales in comparison, and the joint rarely requires adjunctive treatment.

Glenohumeral arthritis has probably been under-treated in the past, as standard shoulder radiographs, anteroposterior views in internal and external rotation, are oblique to the glenohumeral joint line and will underestimate the extent of cartilage loss. Also, shoulder radiographs are non–weight-bearing views, and the lack of compressive forces across the joint may allow the surfaces to separate slightly, suggesting that some cartilage is present. Plain radiographs in internal and external rotation taken in 40 degrees of posterior obliquity, plus an axillary view, seem most accurate in defining the extent of cartilage loss.[45] Additional imaging studies are rarely necessary. Arthrography has been suggested in the past; however, in the presence of moderate or severe glenohumeral arthritis, the presence or absence of significant rotator cuff tearing is usually evident on the plain films. In rheumatoid arthritis with radiographically minor arthritic changes, a double-contrast arthrogram can nicely define the extent of synovitis. This may be helpful in the unusual patient who is a candidate for synovectomy. Also, in the patient who is suspected of having septic arthritis, an arthrogram at the time of aspiration will confirm needle position and demonstrate the presence of any fistulous tracts.

In old fractures, a lateral scapular view is helpful in further assessing tuberosity positioning. When bone deformity is present, computerized tomographic scanning may assist in understanding bony malposition and aid in operative planning.

The previous section on shoulder disease processes describes the great variety of conditions leading to glenohumeral arthritis. It is prudent to inquire about the general health of the patient, to ask about previous or current diseases, and direct specific inquiries toward other joint problems. If any concern exists, a full health assessment or rheumatological consultation is advisable. Laboratory studies such as a hematological group, chemistry group, erythrocyte sedimentation rate, rheumatoid factor, and other tests suggested by the history, physical examination, and plain radiographs are usually obtained and are always considered. It is rare that there should be an unexpected diagnosis at the time of surgery.

In the face of arthritis at the glenohumeral joint, it is often impossible to be accurate in evaluating muscle strength, as pain can prevent firm, strong muscle contraction. When an old injury or previous surgery is a component of the shoulder problem, great care should be taken in neurological evaluation because concomitant nerve injuries are not rare. It is, of course, better to know about these before a surgical procedure is done. In this setting, electromyography with nerve conduction testing is commonly considered as a part of the evaluation process. Concomitant cervical spine disease is often present in the age group with glenohumeral arthritis. This should also be investigated prior to shoulder surgery. If the shoulder arthritis is unusually severe, bony fragmentation is present, the bones are resorbing, or the shoulder is unstable, a neuropathic component to the arthritis should be considered. Evaluation would again include careful neurological assessment, electromyography, cervical spine magnetic resonance imaging, or myelography combined with computerized tomography, as assessment would indicate.

Patients with rheumatoid arthritis often have a number of joints affected by their disease. Sometimes several joints in addition to the shoulder will require surgical treatment, and a plan must be developed. Cervical spine instability may or may not require treatment. If it is associated with significant or progressing neurological symptoms, treatment of the cervical spine will certainly precede care of other joints. When walking is severely compromised by hip or knee disease, it is usually prudent to undertake total joint replacement in these areas. Joint replacement surgery is very effective and will lessen or eliminate the need for body support by the upper extremities during or following shoulder surgery. When multiple upper extremity joints are destroyed, surgery for each area should be considered on its own merit. Pain is the powerful parameter; usually the patient will direct the physician to the area first requiring surgical care. Combining surgical procedures in the rheumatoid patient initially seems attractive, particularly as it relates to hand surgery. However, unless the hand procedure is minor in time and extent, the procedures on the shoulder and in the hand are best done at separate settings. Swelling can be problematic after hand surgery, and the shoulder surgery itself or the postoperative support or positioning may intensify this. Inability to use the hand following shoulder surgery can compromise the critical early physical therapy necessary for an excellent result in prosthetic shoulder surgery. When the shoulder and elbow are severely involved, it is clear that the joint causing more pain and functional impairment should be operated on first. When the joints appear equally involved, the decision is more difficult. One group of authors favors elbow surgery before shoulder surgery, as this may result in greater functional improvement and lessen the need for later shoulder surgery.[84] However, others direct care to the shoulder first, as pain in this area is more troublesome at night and may radiate to the elbow. Restoration of arm rotation offers some protection to total elbow arthroplasty, and rehabilitation of each area will be simplified with a pain-free or minimally painful shoulder. During rehabilitation for the shoulder, a painful elbow can be splinted, if necessary.

Following careful evaluation of glenohumeral arthritis, conservative, nonoperative treatment is almost always considered. In mild to moderate disease, this is effective. In severe disease with complete cartilage loss, the effectiveness of nonsurgical care is lessened but is still entertained. Nonoperative treatment measures have been outlined earlier. When pain relief cannot be satisfactorily achieved for the patient, prosthetic shoulder surgery is the next best option in most settings. This is because of the high frequency of pain relief with this operation and the concomitant ability to be able to restore limb function. These benefits of surgery are, of course, balanced against the known complications of prosthetic arthroplasty and the possible need for revision surgery later. Several categories of previously used procedures offer additional treatment options that may seem more reasonable than prosthetic surgery, in some settings, for carefully selected patients.

Methods of Surgical Treatment

Numerous operative procedures have been suggested and used for the treatment of patients with shoulder arthritis (Table 17–8). Each technique may have some value, although endoprosthetic replacement has superseded most alternative treatment options for the majority of patients. This section will review the various treatment options and conclude with material on the most important current option—prosthetic shoulder surgery.

SHOULDER SYNOVECTOMY

A variety of diseases may produce synovial tissue hyperplasia and its attendant symptoms. Rheumatoid arthritis is the disease that most commonly does this and is the condition for which most information is available. A benchmark article on care for rheumatoid joint problems, including the shoulder, was published in 1943[198]; the article, by Smith-Peterson and co-workers, offered great insight into the surgical care of

Table 17–8. SURGICAL ALTERNATIVES FOR TREATMENT OF GLENOHUMERAL ARTHRITIS

Glenohumeral synovectomy
Resection arthroplasty
Shoulder arthrodesis
Double osteotomy
Proximal humeral prosthetic replacement
Total shoulder arthroplasty

rheumatoid patients during the preprosthetic era. These authors suggested that waiting for the disease to become quiescent prior to surgery was not always necessary or desirable, and surgery of the joint in and of itself would be unlikely to change the long-term course of the disease for the patient. When shoulder symptoms were severe and persistent, shoulder synovectomy, bursectomy when necessary, and lateral acromioplasty seemed to alleviate pain and allow the patient more normal use of the involved limb. In addition to highlighting the beneficial effects of synovectomy, these authors correctly observed that subacromial impingement in rheumatoid arthritis was usually lateral and not anterior as it is in degenerative rotator cuff disease. This lateral impingement and possible subsequent rotator cuff tearing are due to loss of glenohumeral cartilage, subchondral bone erosion, weakening of the rotator cuff, and resultant superior subluxation.

Although texts often mention synovectomy as a treatment option for rheumatoid disease in the shoulder, this operation is apparently seldom used outside of Scandinavia. In North America, most surgeons would consider shoulder synovectomy or synovectomy in any joint for a patient who has had adequate medical treatment, whose articular cartilage is still present, who has significant shoulder synovitis, and whose symptoms are severe enough and persistent enough (greater than six months is often mentioned) to warrant surgical treatment. It is postulated that early synovectomy or synovectomy and bursectomy may protect the rotator cuff from destruction, but this is not proven.

In evaluating patients for the procedure, the examiner may observe an enlarged, boggy-feeling shoulder. This indicates either primary bursal hypertrophy or rotator cuff tearing with extension of synovial tissue and fluid into the subdeltoid bursa. When the shoulder is not swollen, crepitus palpated along the posterior aspect of the joint may be indicative of synovial hypertrophy and irregularity. It is often useful in these patients to obtain a shoulder arthrogram (see Fig. 17–29). This will define the severity and extent of the synovitis and also supply information about the presence or absence of rotator cuff tearing.

Pahle and Kvarnes[164] have published an update on the application and relative effectiveness of shoulder synovectomy. Pain relief in their patients was often quite good, with significant residual pain in only 10 of 54 shoulders. Motion in these patients was slightly improved but not dramatically so. A lessening of the pain did improve limb function. In these 54 patients, approximately one-half had significant joint surface irregularity, thus suggesting that synovectomy in the shoulder may be considered for individuals who have some cartilage loss as a part of their disease process.

In approaching the shoulder surgically, Pahle and Kvarnes recommend very little or no detachment of the anterior part of the deltoid muscle, a subdeltoid and subacromial bursectomy, arthrotomy through the subscapularis, and synovectomy of all joint areas by displacement of the humeral head and the use of various straight and angled instruments. In addition, any osteophytes or other joint irregularities are removed or smoothed. If there is tenosynovial hypertrophy surrounding the long head of the biceps brachii, this tissue is also removed. Postoperatively, a light abduction pillow is placed, and exercises are commenced two to three days following surgery.

The author prefers to limit the use of synovectomy to patients with intact articular cartilage or cartilage that is at least one-half of its normal thickness. In the presence of an intact rotator cuff and the absence of bursal hypertrophy, a synovectomy may be accomplished arthroscopically (Fig. 17–45). This is facilitated by the use of at least three portals and a large motorized shaver. When bursal hypertrophy is present or a rotator cuff tear is diagnosed, open surgical treatment is usually the better option. The operative approach is through the deltopectoral interval. The subdeltoid bursal tissue is excised carefully, protecting the axillary nerve on the undersurface of the deltoid muscle. Any rotator cuff tearing is carefully identified, and the arthrotomy incision is planned. Usually, the arthrotomy will include division of the subscapularis near its insertion and division of the anterior shoulder capsule

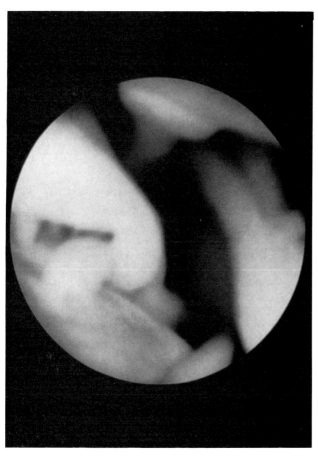

Figure 17–45. Hypertrophic synovial changes seen within the shoulder joint of a patient with rheumatoid arthritis. The synovial prominences appear drumstick-shaped. A number are whitened and fibrotic; others are erythematous with predominant vascularity.

at its humeral attachments. The capsular incision will extend up to the intra-articular portion of the long head of the biceps tendon and along this tendon to its glenoid origin. The incision will also extend inferiorly to the six o'clock position on the humeral head. Synovium is removed from the anterior portion of the shoulder and the subscapularis recess. Synovium is then removed from the inferior aspect of the joint. By preserving the fibrous layer beneath the synovial tissue, the axillary nerve will be protected. By working around the humeral head, one then removes the posterior synovial hypertrophy. Sometimes, this is facilitated by partially dislocating the joint. Following bursectomy and synovectomy, the acromion is assessed, and an inferior acromioplasty is performed, if necessary. Any rotator cuff tearing is repaired. This is accomplished by direct suturing or subscapularis transposition upward.[48] Postoperative care includes early (one to three days postoperatively) passive range of motion exercises, perhaps assisted by a passive motion machine. Active exercises are delayed for three to four weeks.

Although shoulder synovectomy seems theoretically useful for diseases other than rheumatoid arthritis, results in these disease entities are relatively unknown, and either no information or anecdotal information is available.

RESECTION ARTHROPLASTY

During preprosthetic times, resection of the humeral head was usually reserved for war injuries, severe fractures, or uncontrollable infection.[135, 202] Probably recontouring a partially excised humeral head has been done in conjunction with shoulder synovectomy in rheumatoid arthritis, but no series of patients is reported. Several authors have reported on excision of the glenoid in conjunction with synovectomy.[87, 216] This was accomplished either by an anterior or by a posterior surgical approach. Pain relief was said to be good, and motion was adequate, but motion was optimized in those with a well-preserved and round humeral head. Initially, this operation was thought to be conservative. However, resection of the glenoid will make any further reconstructive surgery extremely difficult, if not impossible. It is difficult to identify any advocacy for this procedure.

Resection arthroplasty of the shoulder may be useful as an adjunct to the care for septic arthritis of the shoulder with extensive humeral head and glenoid osteomyelitis. A joint resection will, of course, result after removal of infected or mechanically compromised implants[41, 131] (Fig. 17–46). The initial problem following resection is joint instability. Later, stiffness usually develops, and a few shoulders actually go on to bony arthrodesis.[148] Following infection and prosthetic removal, stability usually develops. Pain relief may or may not be achieved.[131] Maximum active abduction would typically be 60 to 80 degrees.[41, 131, 146, 208] However, moderate weakness persists.

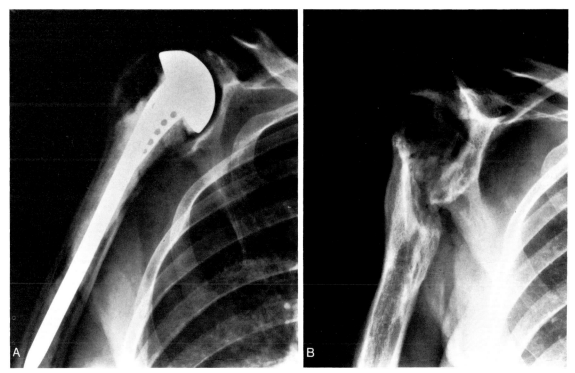

Figure 17–46. A previous proximal humeral prosthetic replacement was done in an elderly woman with multiple joint osteoarthritis. Her total knee arthroplasty became infected, and the infection spread to the proximal humeral prosthetic replacement, seen in *A*. The shoulder region was brawny and erythematous, and there was a draining sinus on the anterolateral aspect of the arm. The region was debrided, the prosthesis and cement were removed, and, after delayed primary closure, the radiographic appearance of the joint was as seen in *B*. Fortunately, the patient had only mild pain, and the shoulder was stable because of fibrosis. There was active abduction of 65 degrees and external rotation of 10 degrees.

In an attempt to improve stability and strength following resection, Jones suggested suturing the rotator cuff to the remaining portion of the upper humerus.[111, 112] Pain relief was achieved. Active motion was similar to that outlined above. The shoulders were stable, and moderate strength returned. Others, however, in following Jones' technique have not been able to improve on their results in comparison with those patients without rotator cuff suturing.[124, 147]

It would seem that there are a few, but very few, current indications for shoulder joint resection. This procedure still may be a useful adjunct to the care of a patient with chronic septic arthritis of the shoulder and humeral head osteomyelitis, to treatment for an infected shoulder implant, or to care for a rare patient with an otherwise failed implant procedure in whom another prosthesis cannot be placed for some reason or another, usually bony deficiency.

Should resection arthroplasty be undertaken, previous surgical incisions may dictate the route for approaching the joint. Usually, though, an anterior deltopectoral approach will be used. In the presence of infection, a second posteroinferior incision may promote drainage. Postoperative motion will be delayed one to two months to promote stiffness and stability. Thereafter, a gentle, active assisted range of motion program without stretching would be started. Muscle strengthening will be a prolonged process, and, of course, the return of strength will be incomplete.

SHOULDER ARTHRODESIS

Early in this decade, there were many indications for arthrodesis of the shoulder, but now there are only a few. This change is displayed in Table 17–9. The left side of the table enumerates operations done between 1950 and 1974, and the right side of the table enumerates diagnoses for those shoulder fusions done at the same institution between 1975 and 1983.[39, 44] Most shoulder fusions today are done for one of three reasons: paralysis of the deltoid and rotator cuff, infection with loss of glenohumeral cartilage, or failed reconstructive procedures. Seldom, if ever, is shoulder fusion undertaken for treatment of the more usual causes of shoulder arthritis, even in younger individuals

Table 17–9. INDICATIONS FOR SHOULDER ARTHRODESIS (AT THE MAYO CLINIC, ROCHESTER, MINNESOTA)

Diagnosis	1950–1974*	1975–1983†
Paralysis	21	20
Infection	8	15
Severe rotator cuff tearing	12	9
Traumatic or osteoarthritis	18	5
Neoplasia	0	3
Recurrent dislocations	7	0
Rheumatoid arthritis	5	0
	71	52

*Cofield RH, and Briggs BT: J Bone Joint Surg *61A*:668–677, 1979.
†Cofield RH: AAOS Instruct Course Lect *34*:268–277, 1985.

who wish to be active. An exception to this is expressed in the article by Rybka and co-workers from Finland.[190] These authors defined the results of arthrodesis in a group of patients with rheumatoid arthritis. Thirty-seven of 41 shoulders fused. Complications were few. A brace was used for postoperative support in the hope of avoiding the potential of elbow stiffness. This investigation suggested that arthrodesis was easily achieved, inexpensive, and a reliable method for the treatment of severely involved rheumatoid shoulders.

A better consensus has been reached about the desirable position of shoulder fusion. Rowe was the first to firmly state the advantages of less abduction and flexion for the surgically arthrodesed shoulder[186] (Fig. 17–47). Hawkins and Neer[103] recognized a range of acceptable positions that did not appear to compromise the eventual functional result. These authors recommended 25 to 40 degrees of abduction for the arm, 20 to 30 degrees of flexion, and 25 to 30 degrees of internal rotation. In determining arm position, the trunk is commonly used as the source of reference, with the scapula being held in the anatomical position. Other possible references to arm position exist, such as the spine of the scapula or the axillary border of the scapula, but these seem less reliable and reproducible.

There are many techniques for shoulder arthrodesis (Table 17–10). These are best classified as extra-articular, intra-articular, or a combination of the two. Extra-articular arthrodesis is of historical interest. The techniques, such as those of Putti,[175] Watson-Jones,[217] or Brittain[27] had most usefulness as adjunctive care for infection, especially tuberculosis. When performed in this manner, it was hoped to avoid the infectious focus and accomplish a fusion about the affected joint. Now, effective antimicrobial medications obviate the need for this approach.

Intra-articular fusion offers the simplest and most direct method. The joint is debrided and remaining cartilage, scar, and dense subchondral bone are removed. Cancellous bone of the humeral head and glenoid are placed against each other, and with the arm in the desired position, fixation is placed. Many forms of fixation are possible, including screws,[14, 100, 136] wires,[32] bone grafts,[105, 185] and pins.[61] Currently, the use of screws seems to be favored. A cast is usually used following this technique and is continued for three to six months. This technique still seems reasonable for the individual with an excellent rotator cuff and capsule who may later be a candidate for prosthetic replacement (Fig. 17–48).

Intra-articular fusion combined with extra-articular

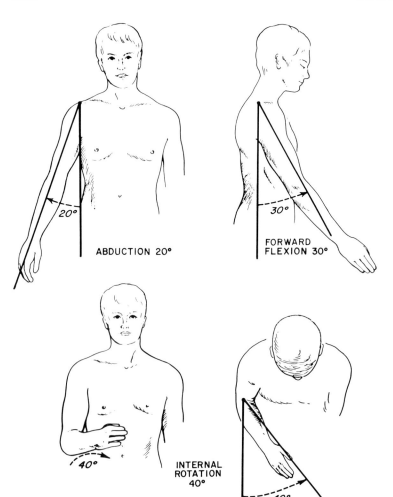

ABDUCTION 20°

FORWARD FLEXION 30°

INTERNAL ROTATION 40°

Figure 17–47. Rowe re-evaluated the position of the arm in arthrodesis of the shoulder in the adult. From his experience, he recommended that less abduction and forward flexion be incorporated into the fusion position and that internal rotation, not external rotation, was necessary. (Reproduced with permission from Rowe CR: Re-evaluation of the position of the arm in arthrodesis of the shoulder in the adult. J Bone Joint Surg *56A*:913–922, 1974.)

Table 17-10. TECHNIQUES FOR SHOULDER FUSION

Extra-articular	Intra-articular	Combined Extra- and Intra-articular
Acromion-humeral[175]	Suture[203]	Suture[89]
Spine of scapula-humeral[217]	Screws[14, 100, 136]	Screws[10, 39, 57, 138, 190, 213]
Axillary border of scapula-humeral plus tibial graft[27]	Pin[61]	Staples
	Tibial graft[185]	Wire[32]
	Bone bank graft[105]	Pins and tension band[22]
		Bone graft[18, 26]
		External fixator[34, 35, 110]
		Plate or plates[58, 73, 181, 182, 130, 183, 188, 218]

fusion is, however, the most common approach for patients who are candidates for shoulder fusion. Extra-articular bone contact is achieved by bringing the humeral head against the acromion (Fig. 17–49) or by doing this and also adding bone grafts between the humeral head or neck and the bone of the scapula adjacent to the glenoid. Fixation can be obtained by many methods, including use of screws,[10, 39, 116, 138, 190, 213] staples, bone grafts,[18, 26] external fixation,[34, 35, 110] or bone plates.[58, 130, 181, 182, 183, 188, 218] Screw fixation is the most simple but does require a cast postoperatively. Tension band wiring has been suggested for those with osteoporosis whose bone might not hold other forms of fixation[22] (Fig. 17–50). External fixation may be absolutely indicated for an individual with infection and wound problems as a part of the condition leading to arthrodesis. External fixation is somewhat awkward to apply, and nerves, especially the radial nerve, may be in jeopardy during pin placement.[34] However, fusion rate is high following the use of external fixators, and a second operation would not be required for removal of internal fixation. Figures 17–51, 17–52, and 17–53 illustrate three methods of fixator application.

Internal fixation with one or more plates has the potential to obviate the need for long-term external cast or brace support during the postoperative period. The arm position can be fixed securely in the position the surgeon wishes without worry that the arm position will change during healing. The union rate is very high using this method. Techniques of plate application are illustrated in Figures 17–54 and 17–55. Usually, narrow dynamic compression plates are used. Recently, it has been suggested that pelvic reconstruction plates are easier to apply and may be equally effective.[182]

Apparently, there is a high rate of bony fusion following many of these methods of shoulder arthrodesis (Table 17–11). Numerous complications such as infection, reflex dystrophy, acromioclavicular arthritis, and symptomatic internal fixation can occur, but all are infrequent. Fracture of the operated extremity below the fusion has seldom been studied, but when it has been, it is seen to occur more frequently than might have been expected.[44] Reoperation is commonly necessary for removal of permanent internal fixation.[44] Whether or not plates should be removed at some time after arthrodesis is uncertain since the rate of fracturing following plate removal is unknown.

No matter which position of fusion results, there will be compromised limb function (Table 17–12). This is the primary reason for avoiding fusion in individuals with such conditions as osteoarthritis, rheumatoid arthritis, or traumatic arthritis. Arm function following total shoulder arthroplasty is much better (Table 17–13).

The author prefers several fusion methods, depending on the condition being treated. When infection is quite severe or there is a large wound requiring dressing changes, an external fixator is used. An external fixator may also be advantageous when excessive bone loss is present (Fig. 17–56), as other forms of internal fixation may lack security. Screw fixation is favored when an intra-articular fusion is done or in the presence of a lesser grade of sepsis. Otherwise plate fixation is used and seems particularly advantageous in those with paralysis or failed reconstructive procedures. A single plate is almost always sufficient.

In performing the procedure, the patient is placed in a beach-chair position with the scapula draped in the field and the arm draped free. Alternatively, some surgeons prefer the lateral decubitus position. The operative approach includes an anterior incision with superior extension of the incision if plate fixation is

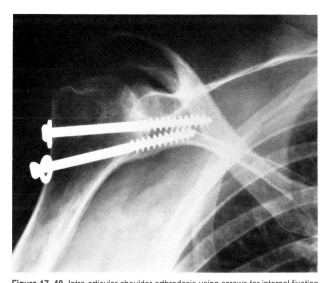

Figure 17–48. Intra-articular shoulder arthrodesis using screws for internal fixation. This young man had recurrent shoulder instability and, following anterior capsule repair, developed an infection that eventuated in cartilage loss at the glenohumeral joint. This simple form of fusion was undertaken to preserve the largely intact surrounding joint capsule and rotator cuff. His neuromuscular function is, of course, normal, and there may be a possibility in the future of reconstruction with prosthetic joint replacement.

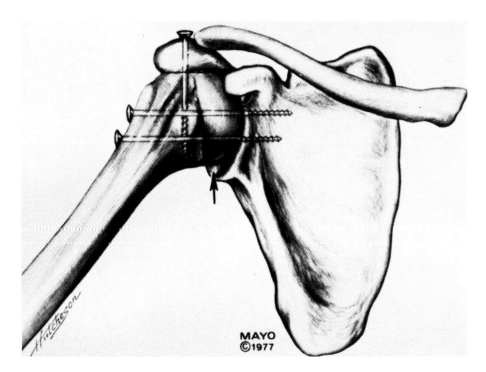

Figure 17–49. A technique of combined intra-articular and extra-articular shoulder arthrodesis using screws for internal fixation. (Reproduced from Cofield RH, and Briggs BT: Glenohumeral arthrodesis. Operative and long-term functional results. J Bone Joint Surg *61A*:668–677, 1979. By permission of Mayo Foundation.)

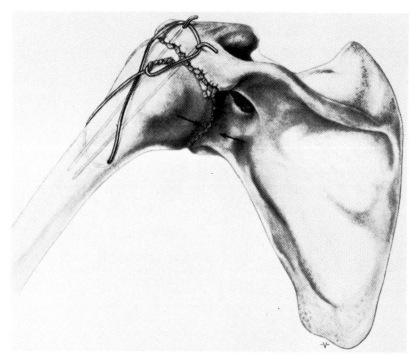

Figure 17–50. When the bones of the shoulder are extremely osteoporotic and one is attempting a shoulder arthrodesis, it has been suggested that pins and tension band wiring may be a satisfactory solution to obtaining a continuing coaptation of the joint surfaces in this situation. Supplemental fixation with a cast will be necessary. (Reproduced with permission from Blauth W, and Hepp WR: Arthrodesis of the shoulder joint by traction absorbing wire. In Chapchal G (ed): The Arthrodesis in the Restoration of Working Ability. Stuttgart: Georg Thieme, 1975, p 30.)

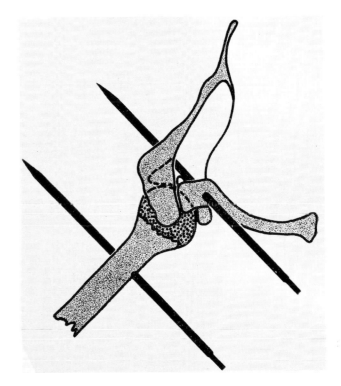

Figure 17–51. The first method of placing pins for compression arthrodesis of the shoulder as suggested by Charnley. A simple external fixator was then applied. (Reproduced with permission from Charnloy J: Compression arthrodesis of the ankle and shoulder. J Bone Joint Surg 33B:180–191, 1951.)

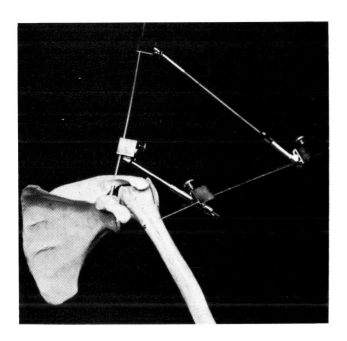

Figure 17–52. Charnley's second technique to apply pins as a part of a shoulder arthrodesis procedure so that an external fixator might be used to apply compression across the arthrodesis site. (Reproduced with permission from Charnley J, and Houston, JK: Compression arthrodesis of the shoulder. J Bone Joint Surg 46B:614–620, 1964.)

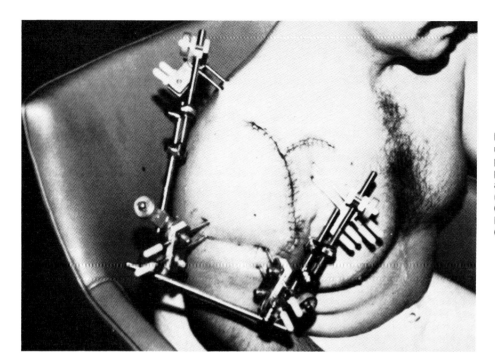

Figure 17–53. An external fixation device used for shoulder arthrodesis. Half pins are placed in the proximal humerus. The more proximal pins are inserted into the acromion and exit through the spine of the scapula. (Reproduced with permission from Johnson CA, Healy WL, Brooker AF Jr, and Krackow KA: External fixation shoulder arthrodesis. Clin Orthop 211:219–223, 1986.)

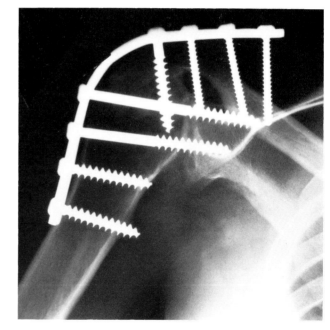

Figure 17–54. Radiographic illustration of a shoulder fusion incorporating both intra- and extra-articular bone contact. Fixation with a plate has provided immediate stability. This could preclude the use of cast support; however, a number of surgeons consider a one- to two-month period of spica cast immobilization as an adjunct to this fixation.

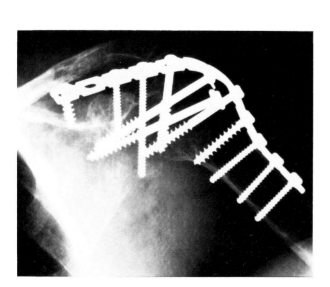

Figure 17–55. Radiograph of a shoulder arthrodesis using a pelvic reconstruction plate for internal fixation. This plate is more easily contoured than the standard DCP plate yet seems to offer enough rigidity for arthrodesis of the shoulder.[182]

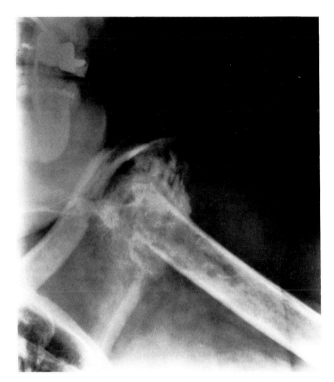

Figure 17-56. External fixation may prove to be a useful adjunct to obtaining shoulder fusion in certain patients. Certainly, patients with open wounds needing sequential debridements might be considered for this form of support for shoulder arthrodesis. This patient had had previous trauma and previous surgery, with a significant amount of bone loss. She had also lost function of her deltoid and rotator cuff. At the time of shoulder arthrodesis, pins were placed as suggested by Charnley (his revised technique). Also, iliac crest graft was placed around the junction of the remaining humerus and scapula. The patient went on to develop a solid bony fusion.

done (Fig. 17–57). If the rotator cuff is present, it can be incised in a T-shaped manner (Fig. 17–58). The joint surfaces are prepared, the arm is positioned, Steinmann pins secure the position temporarily, and, after assessment of arm position, the pins are removed and the permanent fixation is applied. Postoperatively, a cylinder cast and pelvic band are placed (Fig. 17–

Table 17-11. PSEUDOARTHROSIS FOLLOWING SHOULDER ARTHRODESIS

Series	No. Shoulders	No. Pseudoarthroses
Ten series*	87	0
Hauge (1961)[100]	34	1
Cofield and Briggs (1979)[39]	71	3
Charnley and Houston (1964)[35]	19	1
Steindler (1944)[203]	82	5
Becker (1975)[14]	47	3
Rybka and co-workers (1979)[190]	41	4
De Velasco Polo and Cardoso Monterrubio (1973)[61]	31	6
Barton[9]	10	2
AOA report	102	23
Totals	524	48

*Johnson and co-workers (1986),[110] Hucherson (1959),[105] Kalamchi (1978),[116] Matsunaga (1972),[136] May (1962),[138] Richards and associates (1985),[181] Richards and associates (1988),[182] Riggins (1976),[183] Uematsu (1979),[213] Weigert and Gronert (1974).[218]

Table 17-12. EXTREMITY FUNCTION FOLLOWING SHOULDER ARTHRODESIS*

Function	Ability to Perform Function No. (%)
Sleep on limb	46 (73)
Dress	45 (71)
Eat using limb	45 (71)
Toilet care	44 (70)
Lift 5 to 7.5 kg	43 (68)
Comb hair	28 (44)
Use hand at shoulder level	13 (21)

*No. shoulders = 63.
(Adapted from Cofield RH, and Briggs BT: J Bone Joint Surg 61A:668, 1979.)

59). One to two weeks later when the wound is healed, a plastic shoulder spica cast is applied. The cast is removed in six weeks if a single plate is used. Casting is continued for three or more months when other fixation methods, such as screws or external fixators, are used. Following cast removal, stretching is done for the scapulothoracic muscles. Strengthening exercises are added thereafter for all muscle groups surrounding the fused glenohumeral joint.

Patient satisfaction can never be perfect after such a procedure as this, but it does approach 80 per cent.[44] Some patients have shoulder girdle pain following successful bone fusion.[10, 44] This is difficult to explain, but all possible sources should be investigated. These include the acromioclavicular joint, periscapular muscles, and the brachial plexus. It used to be thought that resection of the distal clavicle would improve motion following shoulder fusion. This may be true, but motion gains are minimal, so excision of the distal clavicle would not seem indicated unless degenerative changes and pain would develop at that joint.

PERIARTICULAR OSTEOTOMY

Benjamin and associates have described the use of osteotomies adjacent to the glenohumeral joint for relief of pain in shoulder arthritis.[20, 21] In the 16 shoulders they treated with this method, all had advanced arthritic destruction. This was due to rheumatoid arthritis in 12 and osteoarthritis in 4. Average patient

Table 17-13. EXTREMITY FUNCTION FOLLOWING TOTAL SHOULDER ARTHROPLASTY*

Function	Ability to Perform Function No. (%)
Sleep on limb	64 (90)
Dress	69 (97)
Eat using limb	70 (99)
Toilet care	68 (96)
Lift 5 to 7.5 kg	60 (85)
Comb hair	56 (79)
Use hand at shoulder level	53 (75)

*No shoulders = 71.
(Adapted from Cofield RH: J Bone Joint Surg 64A:899, 1984.)

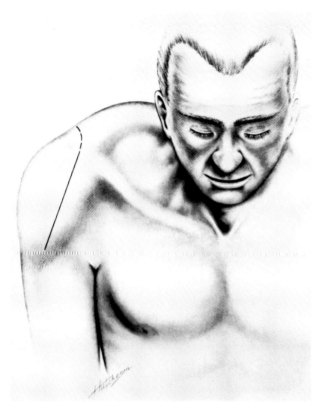

Figure 17–57. An anterior incision for shoulder arthrodesis. The incision can be extended over the superior aspect of the shoulder to expose the scapular spine if a plate is to be used for internal fixation. (Reproduced with permission from Cofield RH: Shoulder arthrodesis and resection arthroplasty. AAOS Instruction Course Lect 34:268–277, 1985.)

age was 51 years; average time to evaluation was 2 years and 11 months.

The operative technique includes a deltopectoral approach. The subscapularis muscle is either split in the line of its fibers or divided in its tendinous portion. The anterior aspect of the neck of the glenoid is exposed and an osteotomy performed 5 mm medial to the glenoid articular surface. By opening up the osteotomy, the posterior cortex of the glenoid neck is cracked and hinged without displacement. The osteotomy through the humerus is performed at the surgical neck level and is also done without bone displacement. The subscapularis is then repaired. Passive shoulder movements are started within the first postoperative week. All shoulder support is removed between one and two weeks after surgery. Physiotherapy is continued for three months.

Thirteen of the 16 shoulders had no or only mild pain postoperatively. Motion gains were seen in 13 shoulders, with an average gain of 50 degrees of abduction. All patients maintained shoulder rotation. One patient developed a nonunion of the humerus, and a second patient developed a delayed union of the humerus. By the time of follow-up evaluation, only one patient had required additional shoulder surgery for treatment of the arthritic condition.

This procedure has not been performed with any frequency and has not been reported in a large series by other surgeons.[210] This may be due to the consistency of pain relief in endoprosthetic replacement, the potential for endoprosthetic replacement to allow substantial gains in glenohumeral motion, and a low reoperation rate for the replacement procedure.

PROSTHETIC ARTHROPLASTY

Hemiarthroplasty, or proximal humeral prosthetic replacement, can be accomplished in a number of ways. These operations can best be considered in four groups. The first and most common is a metallic implant with an intramedullary stem. The second, a variation of the first, is a bipolar system. The third is cup arthroplasty, and the fourth includes a variety of plastic implant devices. When Neer developed the articular replacement for the humeral head, the appliance was designed to replace the articular surface only, to leave as much

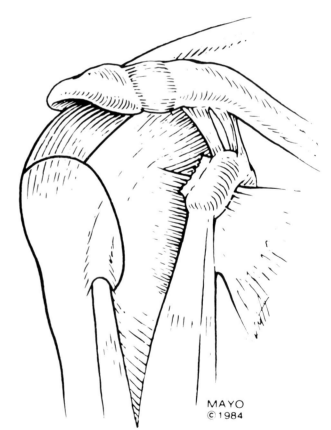

Figure 17–58. Incisions in the rotator cuff used as a part of the shoulder arthrodesis procedure. The long head of the biceps tendon either is left in position or allowed to subluxate medially. At the time of wound closure, the tendons can be partially resutured, depending on the type of internal fixation used. (Reproduced from Cofield RH: Shoulder arthrodesis and resection arthroplasty. AAOS Instruct Course Lect 34:268–277, 1985. By permission of Mayo Foundation.)

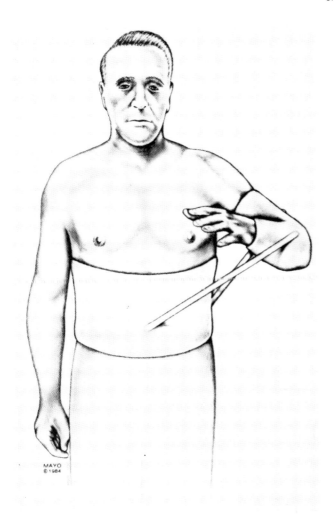

Figure 17–59. A cylinder cast and pelvic band joined together by wooden struts. This is one method of external cast support that can be used following the shoulder arthrodesis procedure. It allows observation of the wound during the early weeks following surgery. (Reproduced from Cofield RH: Shoulder arthrodesis and resection arthroplasty. AAOS Instruct Course Lect 34:268–277, 1985. By permission of Mayo Foundation.)

subchondral bone as possible, and to leave the tuberosities and their attachments undisturbed.[148] The articular portion of the implant was shaped to resemble the normal humeral head, except for flattening on the superior edge. Flanges were added to resist rotation, and stems were long to diffuse forces at the bone-implant junction. Initially, three sizes were developed (Fig. 17–60), and two more were added. In the early 1970s, the implant was redesigned to better use the alternative of cement fixation, and the articular portion was made spherical.[151] This implant has proven its versatility over time. It was initially used for acute fractures but subsequently has been shown to be effective for the care of patients with chronic fracture problems,[102, 174, 187, 209] osteoarthritis,[151, 228] rheumatoid arthritis,[150, 228] osteonecrosis,[53, 54, 189] and a variety of the more rare forms of disease affecting the shoulder joint. A number of other shoulder implant systems include a metallic humeral component that can be used without a glenoid replacement. The implant in the Cofield system is similar to the Neer design, requiring minimal

bone excision and presenting the option of use with or without supplemental cement fixation.[46, 47] The humeral components of the Dana and Monospherical systems are shaped more like the complete humeral head, require osteotomy near the anatomical head-neck junction, and are designed to be always used with polymethyl methacrylate.[3–5, 92, 93]

Bateman suggested the use of bipolar components for shoulder arthritis.[11] Swanson developed this concept further and presented a series of patients (Fig. 17–61).[206] The procedure described to place this implant includes resection of substantial bone from the upper humerus and tuberosity osteotomies with fixation. Stated advantages include provision of new joint surfaces, concentric total contact for the shoulder cavity, a spacer preventing abutment of the greater tuberosity and the acromion, self-alignment, no glenoid fixation requirement, decrease in device and glenoid wear, potential increase in range of motion, dampened stress concentrations, stability, a standard operative approach, and minimal complications; it also can be used as a salvage procedure.[206]

Observations on hip arthroplasty and on shoulder anatomy and biomechanics, including finite element analysis, suggested a cup arthroplasty might be a satisfactory alternative for prosthetic shoulder surgery.[113–114] Initially, hip cups were used,[201] and then cups were manufactured specifically for the shoulder (Fig. 17–62). One design has even incorporated the possibility of bony ingrowth.[201] The benefits of this method are somewhat unclear. As a method, it would be difficult to apply to patients with osteoporosis or shoulders with humeral head destruction.

A number of plastics and other softer materials have been used as implants. Swanson designed an all-silicon

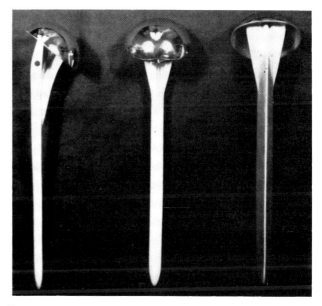

Figure 17–60. Neer replacement prosthesis for the articular surface of the humeral head. Small, medium, and large models are shown in the 1955 article. (Reproduced with permission from Neer CS II: Articular replacement for the humeral head. J Bone Joint Surg 37A:215–228, 1955.)

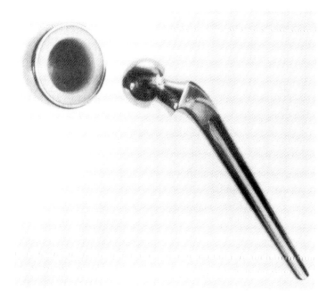

Figure 17–61. The bipolar shoulder implant system developed by Swanson. Proposed advantages include smooth concentric contact for the entire shoulder joint cavity including the coracoacromial arch as well as the glenoid, a decrease in force concentration over any one contact area, a lengthening of the glenoid joint moment arm, and avoidance of abutment of the greater tuberosity against the acromion. (Reproduced with permission from Swanson AB: Bipolar implant shoulder arthroplasty. In Bateman JE, and Welsh RP (eds): Surgery of the Shoulder. St. Louis: CV Mosby, 1984, pp 211–223.)

rubber humeral head implant in extension of the concept of flexible implants as an adjunct to resection arthroplasty.[205] Apparently, this design was used only on rare occasions, and no results are available for a series of patients. Varian reported on a clinical trial of the use of a Silastic cup in patients with rheumatoid arthritis of the shoulder.[215] Early results were promising, but another series by Spencer and Skirving described a number of complications, and the authors recommended restricted use of the device.[200]

Isoelastic shoulder implants have been used in Europe for over a decade.[31, 36, 211] The elasticity of the plastic is similar to that of bone so that, at least theoretically, stresses at the implant-bone interface are minimized. Four styles are available: a simple hemiarthroplasty, an enlarged head implant, a total shoulder system, and a head shaft prosthesis. With this variety of implants, the indications for use can be quite broad. Early reports detail pain relief and minimal complications. Return of movement and strength can be excellent but often are incomplete, with many patients being categorized as having what might be termed a "fair" result. This implant system has not been used to any extent in North America.

Within the last year, a number of total shoulder systems incorporating modular humeral head components have been introduced. The systems may reduce implant inventory. Their advantages and possible disadvantages are not defined. One would estimate though that their usefulness will parallel that of the one-piece metallic stemmed humeral head implants.

There are numerous and almost innumerable total shoulder replacement systems (see Table 17–2). Many implant systems are no longer easily available or are rarely used. This is especially true for ball-in-socket or constrained designs. The Stanmore, Michael Reese, and Trispherical total shoulder implants have limited but continuing applicability to patient care.

The Stanmore total shoulder replacement (Fig. 17–63) is a metal-on-metal implant.[50, 131] The cup-shaped socket is fixed to the glenoid with three pegs and abundant polymethyl methacrylate. The humeral implant requires limited resection of humeral bone and

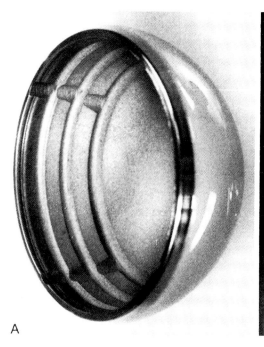

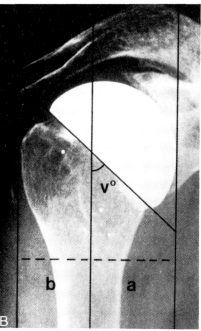

A

B

Figure 17–62. A cup arthroplasty of the shoulder. Illustrated are the cup (A) and a radiograph after implantation of a cup in a patient with rheumatoid arthritis (B). (Reproduced with permission from Jónsson E: Surgery of the rheumatoid shoulder with special reference to cup hemiarthroplasty and arthrodesis. The University Department of Orthopaedics, Lund, Sweden, 1988.)

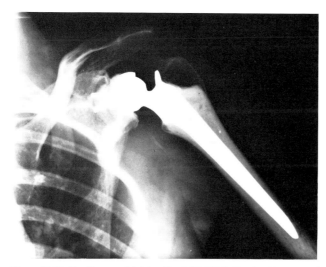

Figure 17-03. The Stanmore total shoulder replacement. The glenoid component was cemented and relied on a large amount of methyl methacrylate for support. The two components snapped together after being implanted. (Reproduced with permission from Cofield RH: Status of total shoulder arthroplast. Arch Surg 112:1088–1091, 1977.)

is cemented in place, and the two components are snapped together. One would suspect the weak links in the system to include unsnapping of the implants, instability, and glenoid component loosening. These complications have, in fact, been the most common (see below).

A tremendous amount of thought and testing went into the development of the Michael Reese prosthesis (Fig. 17–64). The key to the system was the strong scapular fixation—so strong that scapular fracturing would occur before the prosthesis-cement-bone interfaces would fail.[170] The captive ball-in-socket articulation then incorporated controlled dislocatability. If large forces were applied across the joint, the implant would dislocate rather than create a scapular fracture. The initial weak link proved to be the prosthetic humeral neck, and a number of fatigue fractures occurred. In the modified Series II design, the humeral neck was strengthened, largely eliminating this problem. However, the system then continued to have significant and variable complications: glenoid loosening, humeral loosening, and dislocation. The developer feels its use is highly selective; it is a salvage procedure in a patient with disabling pain whose rotator cuff and capsule are ineffective in maintaining shoulder stability.[172, 173]

The Trispherical total shoulder prosthesis (see Fig. 17–13) includes a glenoid component with a ball, a humeral component with a ball, and a third ball holding the two balls contained within it. This linkage incorporates a greater than normal range of motion and allows the surrounding soft tissues to act as the limiting element in movement rather than requiring this of the prosthesis. A dislocation tolerance was also designed into this system. The developers feel this implant may be useful in patients with severe pain who lack a rotator cuff or in patients with a tumor whose treatment

includes resection of periarticular bone and soft tissue.[91]

The semiconstrained total shoulder systems include a hooded glenoid component. This hood is designed to hold the humeral head in place against the prosthetic socket, preventing undesired upward subluxation of the humerus in a shoulder with unrepairable tearing of the supraspinatus tendon. This seems attractive; however, concerns arise about the increased forces transmitted to the glenoid component bone-cement junction, subluxation or dislocation adjacent to the hooded portion of the implant, and limitation of movement when compared with resurfacing designs. An early design incorporating the hooded component as an option was the St. Georg, as reported by Englebrecht and Heinert (Fig. 17–65). Unfortunately, glenoid loosening was very common (51 per cent of 152 cases).[71] Engelbrecht and coworkers have, as an alternative, chosen to continue shoulder replacement using a hemiarthroplasty. The glenoid is occasionally altered by osteotomies and bone grafts to buttress the humeral head prosthesis (Fig. 17–66).

The nonretentive prosthesis of Mazas and Caffinière also included a superiorly placed hood on the glenoid component. Of 38 shoulders operated, 9 developed instability, and 14 shoulders remained stiff after surgery.[139] A third early system including a hooded component was the English-Macnab. This system also has a nonhooded glenoid implant and incorporates porous ingrowth surfaces on the glenoid component and the humeral stem (Fig. 17–67). Early results are somewhat encouraging. Although tissue ingrowth is difficult to prove, loosening has not been a frequent clinical problem.[142] Motion gains, however, have been quite modest.[76]

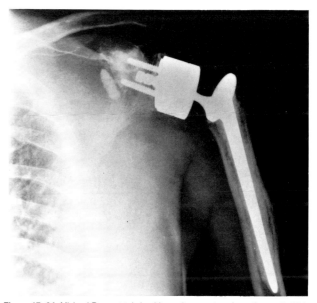

Figure 17–64. Michael Reese total shoulder replacement, perhaps the most widely used constrained total shoulder system in North America. Its placement requires resection of more proximal humerus than with many alternative prosthetic designs. (Reproduced with permission from Cofield RH: Status of total shoulder arthroplasty. Arch Surg 112:1088–1091, 1977.)

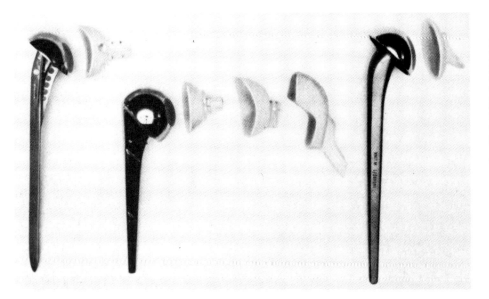

Figure 17–65. With more than 10 years' experience using unconstrained shoulder replacement, Engelbrecht and co-workers have continued to use unconstrained systems. Initially, the Neer prosthesis was used in conjunction with a high-density polyethylene component of these workers' design *(left)*. This evolved to the St. Georg implant with various glenoid components including those with rather deep hoods *(center)*. Currently, these workers have returned to a proximal humeral prosthetic replacement *(right)* with a rather simple and unconstrained polyethylene glenoid component. (Reproduced with permission from Engelbrecht E, and Heinert TK: More than ten years' experience with unconstrained shoulder replacement. *In* Kölbel R, Helbig B, and Blauth W (eds): Shoulder Replacement. New York: Springer-Verlag, 1987, pp 85–91.)

Two currently used total shoulder systems have large hooded components as an option. The Neer system includes 200 per cent and 600 per cent enlarged glenoids. The larger component precludes any possibility of reattaching the supraspinatus. These components have been used in only 12 of 273 shoulders reported.[155]

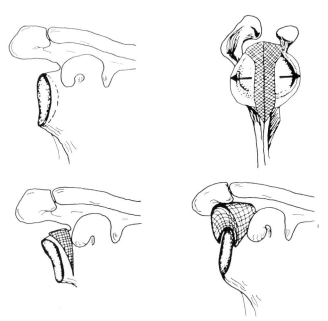

Figure 17–66. In the face of unusually frequent glenoid loosening, Engelbrecht and co-workers have tended to treat patients with shoulder arthritis with glenoid reshaping *(upper left)*, glenoid osteotomies *(upper right and lower left)*, or glenoid bone grafting *(upper right and lower left and right)* as an adjunct to proximal humeral prosthetic replacement rather than using a cemented glenoid component. (Reproduced with permission from Engelbrecht E, and Heinert TK: More than ten years' experience with unconstrained shoulder replacement. *In* Kölbel, R, Helbig B, and Blauth W (eds): Shoulder Replacement. New York: Springer-Verlag, 1987, pp 85–91.)

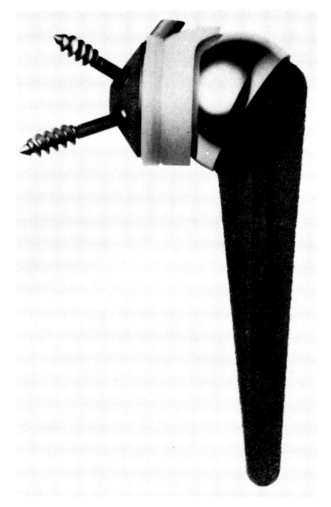

Figure 17–67. English-Macnab cementless total shoulder arthroplasty. (Reproduced with permission from Faludi DD, and Weiland AJ: Cementless total shoulder arthroplasty: Preliminary experience with 13 cases. Orthopedics 6:431–437, 1983.)

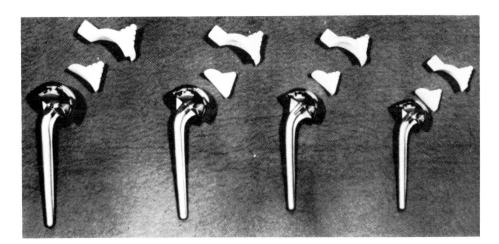

Figure 17–68. The Dana total shoulder arthroplasty. Illustrated are the four available sizes with the standard and the "hooded" glenoid components. (Reproduced with permission from Amstutz HC, Thomas BJ, Kabo JM, et al: The Dana total shoulder arthroplasty. J Bone Joint Surg 70A:1174–1182, 1988.)

suggesting that the need for them is quite uncommon. The Dana total shoulder arthroplasty (Fig. 17–68) includes a semiconstrained, hooded component designed to enhance stability in shoulders with irreparable rotator cuff tears. The hood rests against the acromion to offer additional support. Ten of 56 shoulders reported had this type of glenoid placed at the time of surgery.[5] Pain relief was obtained, and motion gains were modest. Two of ten required revision surgery. Of

the currently used implant systems, the Monospherical total shoulder also incorporates a slight hood on the glenoid component (Fig. 17–69), imparting somewhat greater stability to the articulation.[85, 93] In this design, rotator cuff repair is possible.

Experiences have been reported on four unconstrained total shoulder systems. More information is available on the Neer system than on any other (Table 17–14). The system is extensive. Components are avail-

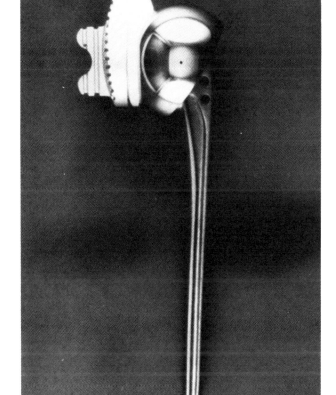

Figure 17–69. The Monospherical total shoulder replacement. A slight amount of hooding has been incorporated into the design of the glenoid component. (Reproduced with permission from Gristina AG, Romano RL, Kammire GC, and Webb LX: Total shoulder replacement. Orthop Clin North Am 18:445–453, 1987.)

Table 17–14. RESULTS OF TOTAL SHOULDER ARTHROPLASTY–NEER DESIGN

Author, Year	Mean Follow-up (yr)	Diagnosis	No. Shoulders	No or Slight Pain (%)	Average Active Elevation* (°)	Average External Rotation (°)
Neer et al, 1982[155]	3.1	Mixed	194			
Bade et al, 1984[7]	4.5	Mixed	38	93	118	
Cofield, 1984[43]	3.8	Mixed	73	92	120	48
Wilde et al, 1984[222]	3.0	Mixed	38	92		
Adams et al, 1986[1]	2.7	Mixed	33	91	96	
Hawkins et al, 1986[101]	3.0	Rheumatoid arthritis Osteoarthritis	70			
Barrett et al, 1987[12]	3.5	Mixed	50	88	100	54
Kelly et al, 1987[118]	3.0	Rheumatoid arthritis	40	88	75	40
Frich et al, 1988[83]	2.3	Mixed	50	92	58–78†	17–21†

*Elevation = abduction with 30 to 60 degrees of horizontal flexion.
†Range, depending on diagnosis.

able with two lengths of humeral head, three humeral stem diameters, and humeral stems in three different lengths—10 humeral component variations. Five different glenoids have been used by the developer in a recent series.[155] In addition, small humeral and glenoid components are available for patients with juvenile rheumatoid arthritis, and custom components have added glenoids with an angled keel or asymmetrical polyethylene thickness to the system.

The Dana shoulder was designed to best match the prosthetic component to sections of the normal humeral head. Four humeral head diameters are now available. Polyethylene glenoid components are available for each of the humeral head sizes, and these components are available in a standard and a hooded variation.[5] The Monospherical total shoulder has three humeral and two glenoid sizes.[92, 93] Preliminary experience with a bone ingrowth, unconstrained total shoulder system has been reported by Cofield.[46, 47] Three sizes of glenoid components, two humeral head lengths, four humeral stem diameters, and two humeral stem lengths are options within this system (Fig. 17–70).

Operative Techniques

The shoulder can be approached surgically from its anterior, superior, or posterior aspects, and surgical approaches for prosthetic replacement have included all of these directions. Most developers of prosthetic replacements for the shoulder have come to favor an anterior approach of some type. Three techniques will be described. This will be followed by the author's preferred method of treatment.

NEER TECHNIQUE[153, 155]

An incision is made from the clavicle over the coracoid and continued in a straight line to the anterior border of the deltoid insertion. The cephalic vein is usually ligated. The deltoid is retracted laterally. The clavipectoral fascia is incised, extending downward from the coracoacromial ligament. The subacromial space is cleared. The subscapularis tendon is divided 2 cm medial to the bicipital groove. The joint capsule is then incised anteriorly and inferiorly. A blunt elevator protects the axillary nerve. When the subscapularis is incised, one must consider that the subscapularis tendon may require lengthening, or the proximal part of it may require transfer upward to repair a tear of the supraspinatus tendon. Large tears are repaired by mobilizing and realigning the available tendons after the humeral head has been excised and before the humeral prosthesis is inserted.

The humeral head is dislocated anteriorly by an external rotation and extension of the shoulder. Osteophytes are trimmed from the humeral head. A trial prosthesis is used for sighting the proper level of humeral osteotomy. A surprisingly small amount of bone is removed. The prosthetic head should extend above the level of the greater tuberosity, and normal retroversion should usually be maintained (30 to 40 degrees). The medullary canal is prepared. The trial prosthesis is inserted, and the shoulder is reduced to assess the prosthetic height, angle of retroversion, and the thickness of the head of the prosthesis.

The arm is then abducted and supported on a bolster placed on a short arm board. The proximal end of the humerus is held posteriorly with a Fukuda retractor (MERA, Senco Medical Trading Company). Soft tissue and remaining labrum extending over the surface of the glenoid are excised. A slot the exact size of the holding device of the glenoid component is then cut into the glenoid using drills and a small curette. The prosthesis should be firmly seated within the bone, and there should be no rocking or tilting. The articular surface of the glenoid should be contoured to support the component. Uneven wear of the glenoid surface may require operative correction (Fig. 17–71). Meticulous cleansing is done to remove blood and loose fragments of bone from the depth of the glenoid. The cement is introduced with a syringe (Fig. 17–72). If there is difficulty in maintaining a dry cavity, cement

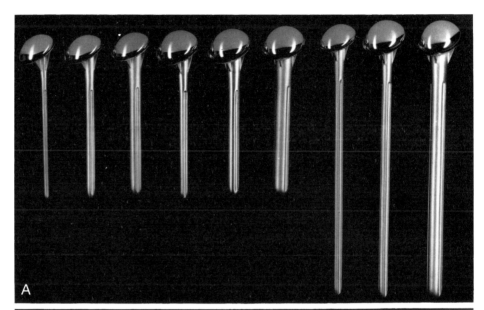

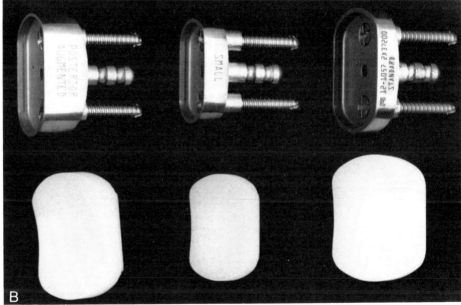

Figure 17–70. A bone ingrowth total shoulder arthoplasty. In this system, there are two humeral neck lengths, four humeral stem widths, and two humeral stem lengths *(A)*. There are two glenoid component sizes and one glenoid component with an asymmetrical construction to compensate for uneven glenoid wear *(B)*. The ingrowth material in the humeral head is only on the undersurface of the head and does not extend down onto the shaft. The ingrowth material on the glenoid component only abuts against the prepared face of the glenoid and does not extend into the scapular neck.

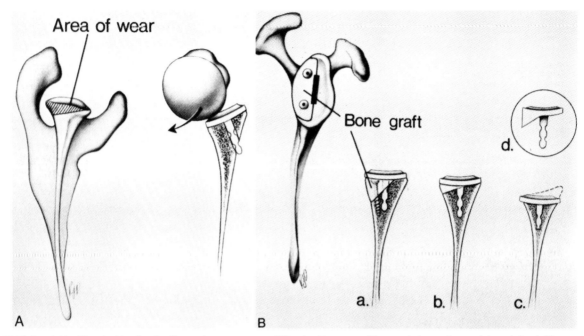

Figure 17–71. In arthritis of the shoulder, the glenoid may show uneven wear. If the glenoid component is cemented upon the remaining subchondral bone surface, as illustrated in *A,* the prosthesis may subluxate in the direction of glenoid wear and the stem of the glenoid prosthetic component may perforate the scapular neck in the opposite direction. As illustrated in *B,* this may be corrected by applying a bone graft to the area of wear, by building up the worn area with methyl methacrylate as illustrated in *b,* grinding away the prominent remaining bone in the area that has not been subject to wear as in *c,* or by using a custom-designed glenoid component as illustrated in *d.* For lesser amounts of wear, a symmetrical burring such as illustrated in *c* is generally preferred; for larger amounts of wear, bone grafting or a custom prosthesis will be necessary. Bone grafting tends to be the current preferred technique. (Reproduced with permission from Neer CS II, Watson KC, and Stanton FJ: Recent experience in total shoulder replacement. J Bone Joint Surg *64A*:319–337, 1982.)

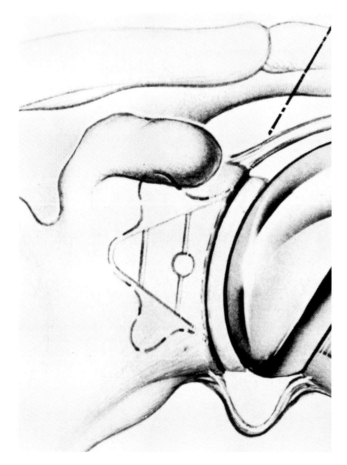

Figure 17–72. A demonstration of the cementing technique used for the Neer type total shoulder replacement. Subchondral bone is preserved except for the slot for the keel portion of the component. Soft cancellous bone is removed from beneath a portion of the subchondral plate, from the base of the coracoid process, and, to some degree, from the axillary border of the scapula. The remaining cancellous bony bed is carefully dried, and blood is removed. In this illustration, the broken line within the neck of the scapula shows the area of cancellous bone removal, which will be occupied by a prosthesis and polymethyl methacrylate. (Reproduced with permission from Neer CS II, Watson KC, and Stanton FJ: Recent experience in total shoulder replacement. J Bone Joint Surg *64A*:319–337, 1982.)

is introduced in two stages: A preliminary soft plug of cement is put into the bone, and then a second bolus of cement from the same batch is used to fill the slot in the glenoid. After the cement is hardened, the glenoid is assessed for security.

Before insertion of the permanent humeral component, anterior acromioplasty or acromioclavicular arthroplasty is done, if indicated. Large tears of the rotator cuff are repaired by mobilizing the muscles and realigning them. Drill holes and sutures are placed in the humerus prior to seating the humeral component. Methyl methacrylate is routinely used in the humerus, except in young patients with a good press-fit or when there is the possibility of prior contamination or sepsis from previous surgery. The component is cemented in 30 to 40 degrees of retroversion, judged by referencing the humeral epicondyles and the forearm with the elbow flexed. The component must extend slightly above the level of the greater tuberosity to prevent impingement of the tuberosity against the acromion. The humeral component must be of sufficient height so that the normal length of the humerus is maintained

(Fig. 17–73). Also, if there has been uneven wear on the glenoid and the glenoid component is implanted facing posteriorly, the retroversion of the humeral component must be correspondingly reduced. Alternatively, if there has been anterior wear of the glenoid and the glenoid component is placed more anteverted than usual, the humeral component must be placed in that much more retroversion.

Soft tissue repair around the implant is important. If the subscapularis was contracted, it is lengthened by a coronal Z-plasty. If there was a rotator cuff tear, the tendons should have already been mobilized so they can be reattached without tension. The long head of the biceps is not disturbed.

Suction drains are inserted. Postoperatively, the arm is placed in a sling and swathe. An abduction brace has been used when repair of the rotator cuff seems tenuous or for a shoulder that was markedly stiffened prior to surgery. A light spica cast is used to maintain stability in selected patients with preoperative instability owing to loss of bone or a long-standing dislocation.

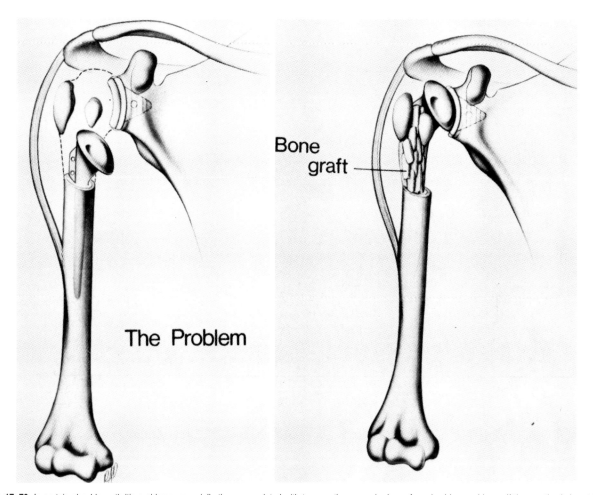

Figure 17–73. In certain shoulder arthritis problems, especially those associated with trauma, there may be loss of proximal humeral bone. If the prosthesis is set low to match the remaining bone, the prosthesis will subluxate inferiorly and the deltoid will be too long to develop any force. As illustrated on the right, the solution is to restore humeral length, setting the prosthesis opposite the glenoid and replacing deficient proximal humerus with bone graft. (Reproduced with permission from Neer CS II, Watson C, and Stanton FJ: Recent experience in total shoulder replacement. J Bone Joint Surg *64A*:319–337, 1982.)

AMSTUTZ TECHNIQUE[3, 4]

Approximate size of the implant is determined by use of templates. The patient is placed in a semi-sitting position with a roll under the scapula. The entire extremity is prepared and draped. A deltopectoral incision is made. The cephalic vein is ligated. The subscapularis is divided approximately 1.5 cm medial to the bicipital groove. The coracoacromial ligament is cut. The capsule is incised vertically. The long head of the biceps is preserved. The humerus is retracted anteriorly with the hook-shaped humeral retractor. The humeral saw guide is positioned such that the humeral head is resected at 30 degrees of retroversion and 45 degrees to the longitudinal axis of the shaft. The glenoid retractor is inserted posterior to the glenoid, holding the humerus posteriorly. The glenoid surface is freshened using a glenoid keel cutout guide. Sufficient cancellous bone for keel insertion is excavated. Additional anchorage is obtained by curetting out bone from the base of the coracoid process superiorly and along the axillary border of the scapula inferiorly. The humeral intramedullary canal is prepared with a broach and then a rasp. The glenoid and humeral trial components are fitted, and a trial reduction is done. The rotator cuff is inspected. Anterior acromioplasty or acromioclavicular arthroplasty are performed as necessary. The glenoid component is inserted after cleansing with a pulsating lavage. The acrylic bone cement is injected and pressurized in the low viscosity state. The humeral canal is plugged with a piece of bone 1 cm distal to the tip of the humeral stem. The canal is thoroughly cleansed with pulsating lavage and dried. The acrylic is again inserted in a low viscosity state using a syringe from distal to proximal. A rubber dam is placed over the proximal end of the humeral canal, and the acrylic is finger-packed. The humeral component is inserted.

The subscapularis tendon is reattached. If the rotator cuff is torn but repairable, the tendons are sutured using drill holes through the upper humerus. If the rotator cuff is not repairable, a hooded glenoid component is used. At the time of closure, a drain is placed. The extremity is positioned in a shoulder immobilizer. If there is instability, a shoulder spica cast may be used.

POST TECHNIQUE[169, 171, 196]

For placement of the Michael Reese total shoulder, the patient is positioned in a semireclining manner with a sandbag placed beneath the scapula. The extremity is draped free. The incision extends from the clavicle downward along the deltopectoral groove. Additional exposure may be obtained by elevating a portion of the deltoid from its origin on the clavicle or by osteotomizing the coracoid or transecting the tendons of the short head of the biceps and the coracobrachialis at their origin. Ordinarily, the rotator cuff is

destroyed, and no attempt is made to reattach remnants of the rotator cuff to the shaft of the humerus. Any soft tissues overlying the glenoid are excised. A glenoid guide is used to make a central hole and two eccentric holes. A reamer can be used to carefully prepare the glenoid surface; however, significant subchondral bone should not be removed.

With the arm held in anatomical position, the proximal humerus is excised at a 45-degree angle, and the cut is made so that the humeral component will be retroverted 25 degrees. The medial end of the cut bone should lie opposite or slightly inferior to the inferior aspect of the glenoid. The humeral canal is prepared.

After cleansing, methyl methacrylate is injected with a 10-ml syringe into each of the three glenoid holes. The glenoid component is inserted using the guide. Two screws are inserted into the holes. The metal humeral stem is inserted in 25 degrees of retroversion. Following cement hardening, the self-locking metal ring is placed over the humeral neck, the two-piece polyethylene socket is placed over the humeral head, and the socket is reduced into the glenoid metal cup. The metal locking ring is then tightened about the glenoid components (Fig. 17–74). The amount of passive external rotation is measured with the elbow at the side of the body. In the postoperative period, the arm should never be forced beyond this point because dislocation might occur when this motion limit is exceeded. A Velpeau bandage is used for immobilization. Passive motion within the limits determined at surgery is commenced on the second or third postoperative day. Gentle active range of motion exercises are added at 25 days.

AUTHOR'S PREFERRED METHOD OF TREATMENT

The author prefers the unconstrained type of shoulder systems for essentially all patients who would require a total shoulder arthroplasty. The Neer system has been the basic system used. Recently, this has been supplemented with the Cofield total shoulder system. Eight types of glenoid components have proved useful. These include the standard polyethylene component, the metal-backed standard component, the custom-ordered small polyethylene component, and the custom-ordered 10-degree angled keel component, all of the Neer system, the Kirschner modification of the Neer standard metal-backed component incorporating adjunctive screw fixation, and the standard, small, and posterior augmented components of the Cofield system. The Neer and Kirschner components are always secured to the glenoid with adjunctive polymethyl methacrylate fixation. The components in the Cofield system may or may not require adjunctive cement fixation. Whether or not cement fixation is used with these latter components depends on the surgeon's philosophy concerning ingrowth components, perceived patient demands, patient age, and glenoid bone quality and quantity. Cement fixation

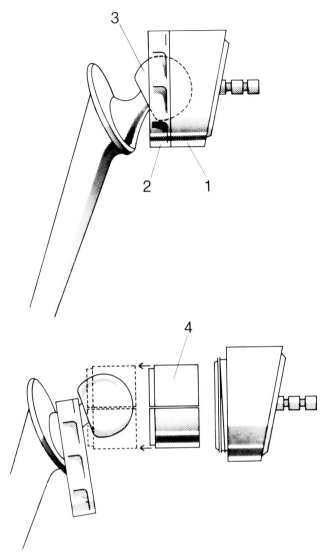

Figure 17–74. The assembly of the constrained Michael Reese total shoulder prosthesis. The components include the glenoid cup *(1)*, the locking metal ring *(2)*, the humeral component *(3)*, and the high-density polyethylene hemispheres *(4)*. (Reproduced with permission from Silver R, and Post M: Post-traumatic resection of the proximal humerus. Orthopedic Consultation 4:1–17, 1983.)

may be especially undesirable in patients who have had previous shoulder arthroplasty, component loosening, and an extensive macrophage response to fragmented polymethyl methacrylate debris.

At surgery, the patient is placed in a semireclining position and shifted to the side of the table on which the surgery is being done. The patient is positioned so the hips and knees are slightly flexed. Straps and table supports are used to hold the patient securely. One must be careful in patient positioning to avoid positions that might stretch the brachial plexus. The superior portion of the anterolateral chest, the superior portion of the posterolateral chest, the top of the shoulder girdle to the base of the neck, the axilla, the superior portion of the lateral chest wall, and the extremity down to the wrist are cleansed and prepared. The extremity is draped free, excluding the hand and forearm from the operative field (Fig. 17–75). U-drapes are helpful in exposing the shoulder for surgery and

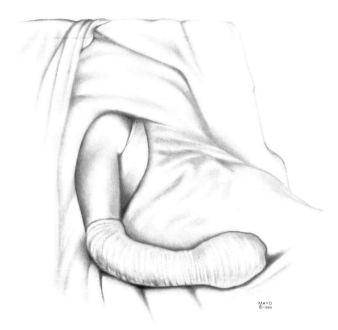

Figure 17–75. Draping in preparation for total shoulder arthroplasty. (By permission of Mayo Foundation.)

including a portion of the chest wall within the operative field. During the procedure, when the arm is at the side, it can be held to the drapes with a nonpenetrating clip. When the extremity is away from the side, it can be rested on an adjustable Mayo stand.

An anterior skin incision is made (Fig. 17–76), extending from the level of the clavicle to the anterior aspect of the insertion of the deltoid with the superior

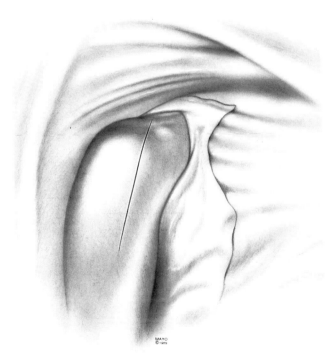

Figure 17–76. Anterior incision for total shoulder arthroplasty. The incision begins over the anterior aspect of the clavicle and extends distally to the anterior aspect of the insertion of the deltoid. (By permission of Mayo Foundation.)

aspect of the incision just lateral to the tip of the coracoid. A small medial skin and subcutaneous tissue flap is developed exposing the infraclavicular triangle and the deltopectoral groove (Fig. 17–77). The fascia overlying the superficial aspects of the pectoralis and deltoid muscles and covering the infraclavicular triangle is incised along the medial aspect of the proximal deltoid. A retractor is placed along this superior-medial edge of the deltoid, pulling the deltoid lateralward. The clavicular branch of the thoracoacromial axis is identified just distal to the clavicle and cauterized. The incision in the fascia joining the pectoralis and deltoid is continued distalward along the medial edge of the deltoid. As the incision in the fascia is made, the deltoid is pulled further lateralward. Branches from the deltoid to the cephalic vein are cauterized, and, further down the deltopectoral groove, the deltoid branch of the thoracoacromial axis is identified and cauterized. At the inferior aspect of the deltopectoral groove, the anterior one-third of the deltoid insertion is elevated from the humeral shaft. The superior 1 cm of the pectoralis major insertion is divided just medial to the bicipital groove. This exposure allows the cephalic vein to fall medially, and almost never is it necessary to ligate the cephalic vein. Should a small rent in the vein be made during exposure, this can be closed with a 6-0 vascular suture.

An incision is then made in the fascia lateral to the conjoined group of tendons, continued through the roof of the subdeltoid bursa. An elevator is placed beneath the acromion and slowly brought laterally and anteriorly, mobilizing the subacromial and subdeltoid spaces. There is often a prominent vascular connection between the anterior and posterior humeral circumflex

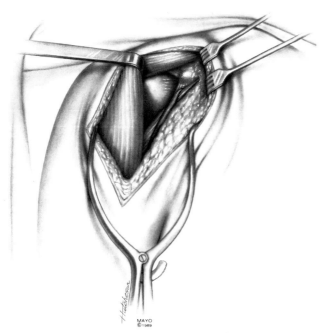

Figure 17–77. The deltopectoral groove is exposed by developing a small, medial skin and subcutaneous flap, entering the infraclavicular triangle along the medial edge of the proximal deltoid and then retracting the proximal deltoid laterally. The cephalic vein is allowed to fall medially along with the pectoralis major muscle. (By permission of Mayo Foundation.)

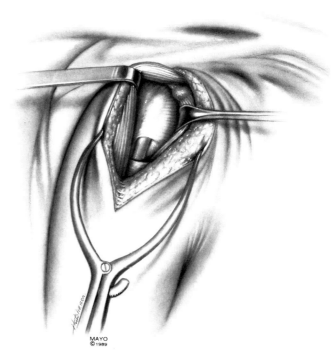

Figure 17–78. The deltoid is now fully retracted laterally, exposing the humeral head. In order to do this, it was necessary to ligate the clavicular and deltoid branches of the thoracoacromial axis and the few branches of the cephalic vein to the deltoid muscle and to elevate subperiosteally the anterior one-third of the deltoid insertion of the humeral shaft. (By permission of Mayo Foundation.)

vessels overlying the anterolateral aspect of the humeral shaft. Bleeding will be minimized if these vessels are identified and cauterized during mobilization of the subdeltoid space. A finger or blunt elevator is then slid medially over the subscapularis and under the conjoined group, freeing this space of its light bursal adhesions. The main neurovascular group, the axillary nerve, and, on occasion, the musculocutaneous nerve are then identified and protected. A large Richardson retractor is placed beneath the deltoid and over the superior-lateral aspect of the humeral head, and a short knee retractor is placed along the lateral aspect of the conjoined group to hold it medialward (Fig. 17–78).

The above exposure is ample for almost all patients who would require a total shoulder arthroplasty. There are a few who may need more extensive exposure. These include patients with previous surgery and extensive scarring, patients with inflammatory arthritides who have inflexible, scarred tissues, patients with old trauma who might require complex osteotomies of the proximal humerus, or selected patients with shoulder arthritis and large rotator cuff tears. In these situations, it may be advisable to release the deltoid from its origins on the clavicle and anterior acromion. Doing this may weaken the deltoid somewhat and, of course, subjects the patient to the possibility of the complication of deltoid detachment following surgery. When releasing the deltoid from its origins on the clavicle and anterior acromion, the incision should begin along the top of the clavicle and not at the front edge. The incision is between the attachments of the trapezius and deltoid muscles. The deltoid is then carefully stripped from the clavicle with its fibrous attachments. The incision then continues lateralward across the front of the acromioclavicular joint and along the anterior border of the acromion. By doing this carefully, fibrous attachments of the deltoid muscle are maintained with the muscle to allow firmer suture at the end of the procedure. At the time of reattachment of the deltoid, it is often necessary to sew the deltoid to the bone of the acromion, to the capsule of the acromioclavicular joint, and then to the fascia and muscle of the trapezius across the top of the clavicle.

After development of the subdeltoid and subacromial spaces, preparations are made to incise the rotator cuff and capsule and enter the joint. When the rotator cuff is intact, the incision is through the subscapularis tendon 1 to 1.5 cm medial to its insertion on the humerus (Fig. 17–79). This overlays the insertion of the capsule onto the humeral neck. The incision is continued superiorly to the anterior aspect of the intra-articular portion of the long head of the biceps tendon. Then the incision is directed superomedially along the anterior edge of this tendon to the region of the supraglenoid tubercle. The subscapularis and capsular incision is continued inferiorly along the humeral neck to the six o'clock position on the humeral head. This arthrotomy incision essentially exposes the anterior half of the joint rather than just a window through the subscapularis.

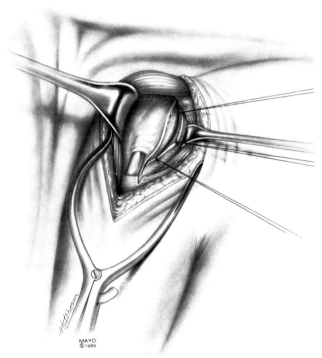

Figure 17–79. When the rotator cuff and capsule are intact, the subscapularis and anterior capsule are incised. The superior limb of the incision extends along the anterior aspect of the intra-articular portion of the long head of the biceps tendon. The central, or vertical, aspect of the incision overlies the capsular insertion on the humeral head. This is approximately 1 cm medial to the medial aspect of the bicipital groove. The inferior aspect of the incision curves toward the humeral head, and the capsular attachment on the humeral head is freed to the six o'clock position. (By permission of Mayo Foundation.)

When there is limited external rotation prior to surgery, perhaps 20 degrees or less, consideration must be given to lengthening the subscapularis tendon at the time of arthrotomy. This is most easily started by incising the interval area between the supraspinatus and subscapularis tendons just anterior to the anterior edge of the intra-articular portion of the biceps tendon. One can then place an elevator inside the joint and, by palpating outside the joint, can determine the thickness of the subscapularis tendon and capsule. If of normal thickness or thicker than usual because of scarring, the tendon and capsule can be lengthened in a medial-lateral direction by performing a Z-shaped incision through the tendon and capsule in the frontal plane. This is most easily started by incising the subscapularis at its insertion on the humerus, elevating it off the humerus to the area of the capsular attachment on the humeral neck, and then elevating two-thirds of the thickness of the subscapularis tendon off the anterior shoulder capsule and allowing the remaining posterior one-third of the thickness of the subscapularis tendon to remain with the shoulder capsule. This division of the subscapularis tendon in the frontal plane is then continued medially another 1 to 2 cm and then the incision is made in the parasagittal plane through the posterior one-third of the subscapularis tendon and capsule to enter the joint.

When there has been previous proximal humeral fracturing involving a distortion of the anatomy, it is extremely important before surgery to obtain x-rays in multiple projections, such as a shoulder trauma series, and it may be helpful also to obtain CT scanning through the area. Again, in planning arthrotomy in this situation, it is helpful to make an incision in the interval area just anterior to the intra-articular portion of the long head of the biceps. Then, by using palpation on the outer surface of the rotator cuff and an elevator on the inner surface of the rotator cuff, one can determine the positions of the lesser and greater tuberosities relative to the humeral head and shaft. If the lesser tuberosity is not malunited relative to the shaft, an incision can be made through the subscapularis as described above. If it is malunited such that it would interfere with joint function following prosthetic replacement, an osteotomy of the lesser tuberosity can be done. If the greater tuberosity is malunited such that it would interfere with joint function following placement of the arthroplasty, an osteotomy can be planned for correction and repositioning of the greater tuberosity at the time of prosthetic placement. Often this osteotomy needs to be biplanar, with one limb of the osteotomy across the top of the humeral head and a second limb of the osteotomy along the posterior aspect of the humeral head[209] (Fig. 17–80).

Having completed the arthrotomy through the soft tissue or the tuberosity osteotomy, the humerus is externally rotated and carefully extended. This delivers the humeral head anteriorly, subluxating it or dislocating it from its position against the glenoid (Fig. 17–81). Osteophytes of the humeral head are trimmed to

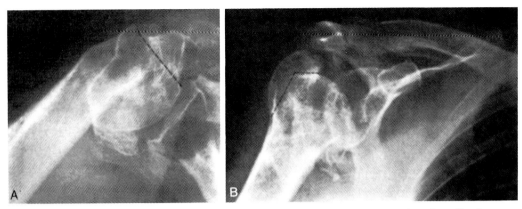

Figure 17–80. When reconstructing a malunited proximal humeral fracture, it may be necessary to perform tuberosity osteomies and reposition the osteotomized tuberosities behind a proximal humeral prosthesis. *A* shows the line of osteotomy of the lesser tuberosity. *B* shows the biplanar lines of osteotomy of the greater tuberosity. (Reproduced with permission from Tanner MW, and Cofield RH: Prosthetic arthroplasty for fractures and fracture-dislocations of the proximal humerus. Clin Orthop *179*:116–128, 1983).

eliminate any confusing distortion of proximal humeral anatomy. The osteotomy of the proximal humerus is then planned. This is assisted by sighting along the undersurface of a trial prosthesis or by using a humeral cutting guide. In the typical situation, the cut would begin on the superior-lateral aspect of the upper humerus just medial to the medial aspect of the insertion of the rotator cuff, with the cut then extending downward and medially (Fig. 17–82). In a larger person, the cut may start above this level to increase the length of the humeral neck. Rarely, however, is this necessary. Typically, the retrotorsion of the articular surface incorporated in the humeral cut will be approximately 30 degrees and is gauged by comparing the direction of the cut with the position of the flexed forearm. With the forearm flexed 90 degrees and externally rotated 30 degrees, and the cut on the humerus directed from anterior to posterior, 30 degrees of humeral retrotorsion will result (Fig. 17–82). It may be necessary to alter the amount of torsion, dependent upon glenoid wear or preoperative instability. Quite typically, an adjustment needs to be made in osteoarthritis of the shoulder, as there is a tendency for posterior glenoid wear and posterior humeral subluxation. In this circumstance, the humeral osteotomy may be made with no torsion or 10 degrees of retrotorsion built into the cut. Following upper humeral osteotomy, the upper humerus is further trimmed around its periphery such

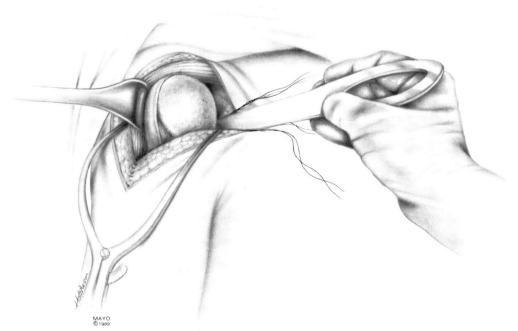

Figure 17–81. After incision of the subscapularis tendon and shoulder capsule, an elevator is placed within the glenohumeral joint. The humeral head is then externally rotated and slightly extended. This exposes the humeral head in preparation for humeral osteotomy. (By permission of Mayo Foundation.)

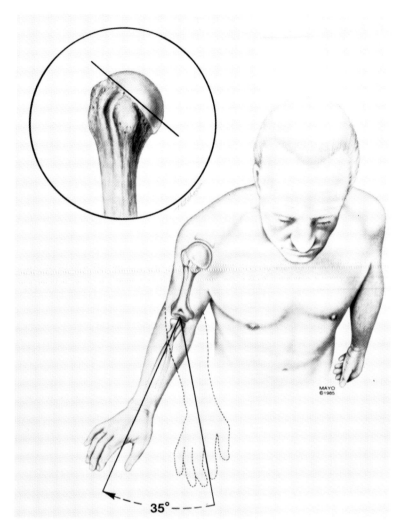

Figure 17–82. The insert shows the humeral osteotomy needed to place a Neer type of proximal humeral prosthetic replacement. Often, the remaining proximal humerus is eroded and flattened, so much less bone is removed than one might ordinarily expect. Note that the angle of the osteotomy is approximately 45 degrees to the line of the humeral shaft. This leaves some remaining humeral head and metaphyseal bone that then can be used to support the proximal humeral replacement. A portion of the remaining humeral head and bone must be trimmed to allow this to recess beneath the prosthetic humeral head. The larger portion of this illustration depicts how the flexed forearm can be used as one limb of a goniometer to determine the amount of retroversion selected for the position of the prosthesis. For example, the surgeon can position himself directly in front of the patient, as illustrated by the dotted forearm and hand. He can then rotate the flexed forearm externally 35 degrees but maintain his position. Then, by cutting directly posteriorly from his retained position at the 45-degree angle to the humeral shaft, 35 degrees of retrotorsion will be built into the osteotomy cut. (By permission of Mayo Foundation.)

that the area of exposed cancellous bone on the top of the humerus will approximate the area of the undersurface of the humeral prosthesis. Typically, this involves removal of some remaining subchondral bone from the calcar region and tapering of the remaining bone into a smooth contour with the humeral shaft.

The humeral canal is then prepared using drills and reamers (Fig. 17–83). If a press-fit is desired, it is important to obtain a tight fit of the prosthesis in the diaphyseal portion of the humerus. If cementing is planned, an appropriate thickness of the cement mantle should be determined based upon the size of the humeral canal and the size of the humeral component selected. It is important not to ream the medullary canal of the humerus too thin, for in some patients, particularly osteoporotic rheumatoid patients, this may predispose to fracturing at surgery or later. The humeral trial component is then fitted and reduced (Fig. 17–84). The soft tissues are assessed for their length in relation to the length of the prosthetic humeral neck selected, and adjustments are made in prosthetic neck length. The joint is then redislocated, and the trial humeral component is removed.

The proximal humerus is then held lateralward with a bone hook. The interior of the shoulder joint is examined. If the synovium is hypertrophic, a synovectomy is done. A Fukuda or humeral neck retractor is then placed behind the glenoid and anterior to the proximal humerus to hold the remaining humeral neck posteriorly (Fig. 17–85). This exposes the glenoid.

In certain conditions, the cartilage of the glenoid will be spared, or relatively spared, when compared with humeral articular surface wear. This is especially true in osteonecrosis or in chronic fracture-related conditions that may require the use of a prosthesis. The glenoid is inspected for its wear. If the entire surface is covered with cartilage, and there is no evidence of significant asymmetrical wear on the glenoid, a hemiarthroplasty is selected and no glenoid component is placed. In some patients with inflammatory arthritides, there may be excessive medial resorption of the glenoid bone (see Fig. 17–25). This can usually be assessed on preoperative radiographs or CT examinations. In this setting, there may not be enough bone remaining to securely place a glenoid component, and, again, a hemiarthroplasty is selected

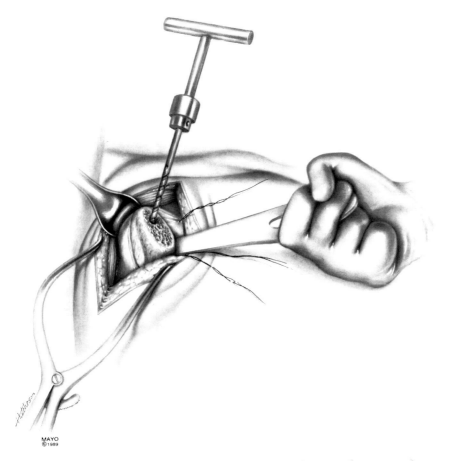

Figure 17–83. Preparation of the humeral canal. A bone awl or one-quarter-inch drill is placed through the metaphyseal bone of the proximal humerus. It is positioned so that it is central in the anteroposterior direction and is two-thirds of the distance toward the lateral aspect of the exposed metaphyseal bone in the mediolateral direction. The diaphyseal portion of the humeral canal is then drilled, or broached, to the size of the humeral component selected. Templating of the radiograph is sometimes helpful in selecting the proper prosthetic size. (By permission of Mayo Foundation.)

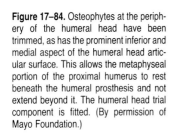

Figure 17–84. Osteophytes at the periphery of the humeral head have been trimmed, as has the prominent inferior and medial aspect of the humeral head articular surface. This allows the metaphyseal portion of the proximal humerus to rest beneath the humeral prosthesis and not extend beyond it. The humeral head trial component is fitted. (By permission of Mayo Foundation.)

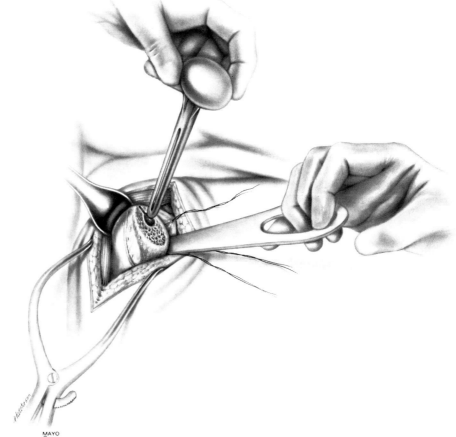

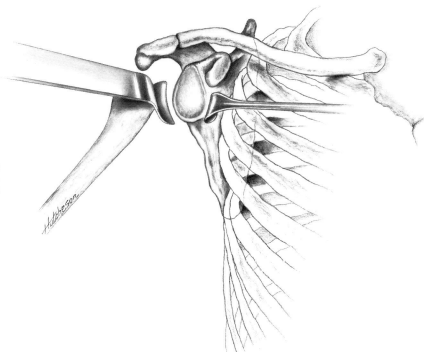

Figure 17–85. Exposure of the glenoid. The glenoid is exposed by retracting the humeral metaphysis posteriorly. Special humeral neck retractors are useful during this step of the procedure. (By permission of Mayo Foundation.)

as treatment rather than making an attempt at fixation of the glenoid component in bone significantly deficient in quantity or quality. However, in most situations involving shoulder arthritis, there will be enough glenoid bone remaining to place a glenoid component, and the surface either will be devoid of cartilage or will have asymmetrical cartilage wear. For example, in many patients with osteoarthritis, the cartilage on the anterior one-quarter to one-half of the glenoid may be relatively intact, whereas the bone on the back one-half to three-quarters may be devoid of cartilage and, in fact, the subchondral bone may be worn to a depth of 1 to 10 mm. In these situations, preparations are made for placement of a glenoid component.

Prior to carrying out the steps necessary for glenoid component placement, the soft tissues are again assessed. The superior and posterior aspects of the rotator cuff can now be palpated both on their inner and outer aspects. Their relative lengths can be ascertained. The anterior structures can also be carefully examined. Typically, the subscapularis tendon and anterior capsule may be relatively shortened compared with other aspects of the rotator cuff and capsule. When the subscapularis has been entered without lengthening, it may be advisable to gain more flexibility of the subscapularis and anterior capsule. This is most readily accomplished by incising the capsule along the glenoid rim from the position of the coracoid to the four o'clock position (when looking at the right shoulder) and then continuing the incision laterally along the upper edge of the superior band of the inferior glenohumeral ligament (Fig. 17–86). This will then free the subscapularis and anterior capsule from their attachments to the inferior capsule and the glenoid

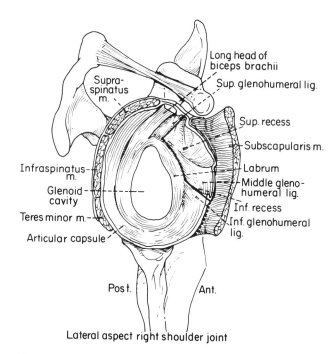

Lateral aspect right shoulder joint

Figure 17–86. A view of the right shoulder capsule and rotator cuff with the humeral head removed for clarity of illustration. At the time of total shoulder arthroplasty, the anterior capsule may be somewhat contracted, limiting later external rotation. If the contracture is not too great, this may be most easily eliminated by incising the anterior capsule at the glenoid rim from the level of the superior glenohumeral ligament to the superior edge of the inferior glenohumeral ligament and then freeing the inferior glenohumeral ligament complex from the more anterior subscapularis muscle and tendon. Thus, the subscapularis muscle and tendon along with the reinforcing anterosuperior capsule will have greater flexibility at the time of rotator cuff repair so that external rotation may be much more easily regained. By leaving the inferior glenohumeral ligament complex intact, one is left with some security that shoulder stability will be maintained. (By permission of Mayo Foundation.)

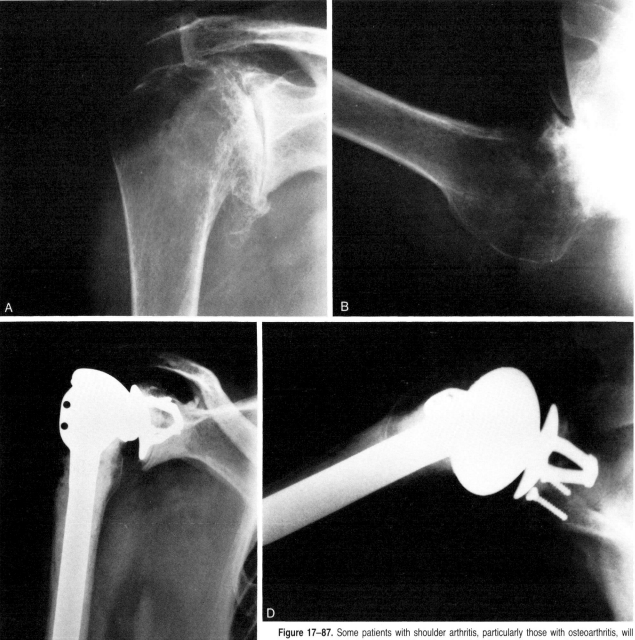

Figure 17–87. Some patients with shoulder arthritis, particularly those with osteoarthritis, will have asymmetrical glenoid wear with subluxation of the humeral head toward the area of wear. *A* is the anteroposterior view; *B* is the axillary projection, showing posterior glenoid wear and, more important, significant posterior humeral subluxation toward the area of wear. At surgery, this was addressed by lessening the amount of humeral retrotorsion—to, in effect, tighten the posterior soft tissue structure—and by placing a segment of the humeral head on the posterior aspect of the glenoid. This small segment of bone was screwed in position, and the glenoid component was positioned on top of the internally fixated bone graft resting in normal, or near normal, version (*C* and *D*).

rim. The undersurface of the subscapularis can then be teased with an elevator from its attachments on the anterior aspect of the scapula. This creates significant flexibility in the subscapularis and the attached small portion of the anterior shoulder capsule. When doing these maneuvers, one must be cognizant of the position of the axillary nerve and protect it from damage.

Now is also an ideal time to inspect the coracoacromial arch and the undersurface of the acromioclavicular joint. Sometimes, osteophytes need to be trimmed. Very rarely, an anterior acromioplasty or a distal clavicle excision is necessary.

In preparing the glenoid for placement of the prosthesis, soft tissues are incised that overlie the glenoid surface. A finger or elevator can be placed along the anterior aspect of the scapula to ascertain the direction of the neck of the scapula in a more exact fashion. Any remaining cartilage or fibrocartilage is curetted from the glenoid articular surface. When placing a keeled glenoid component, the subchondral bone of the glenoid is often recontoured to more closely approximate the shape of the face plate of the component. Care must be taken to remove only a small amount of the subchondral bone plate. The slot for the keel of the component is then constructed. Only enough bone is removed to seat the keel, being very conservative in bone removal from the scapula. The direction of the keel typically extends from the supraglenoid to the infraglenoid tubercle in a vertical manner. Soft cancellous bone is carefully removed. It is often possible to identify the anterior and posterior cortices of the glenoid neck when this preparation is being done. After enough bone has been removed to seat the keel of the trial component, additional contouring of the glenoid surface may be necessary. The undersurface of the subchondral plate is then undermined to better interlock with the cement. Should there be very slight asymmetrical wear of the glenoid, this can often be compensated for by slightly altering the angle of the keel in the glenoid neck, by slightly burring the articular surface in an asymmetrical way, or by selecting the 10-degree angled keel polyethylene component. This component will allow the keel to seat nicely in the keel slot and also allows the surface of the component to rest evenly on the subchondral bone. Should more than a minor amount of asymmetrical glenoid wear be present, the choice is usually between using a posterior augmented glenoid component or a bone graft to compensate for the glenoid wear. The latter choice is almost always preferable. A small, wedge-shaped piece of bone is removed from the osteotomized portion of the humeral head, recontoured, and held in position with two ASIF screws (Fig. 17–87). By eliminating this deficiency, the standard component will then rest flat on the surface of the glenoid, and the keel will seat properly in the glenoid neck.

The glenoid and glenoid slot are then carefully cleansed with pulsatile lavage and packed until the area is quite dry. Cement is introduced in a slightly doughy stage and forcefully packed into the keel slot. A small amount of cement may be left on the subchondral surface of the glenoid plate, and the component is forcefully impacted into position. It is held securely while the excessive cement is trimmed.

In some patients, the bone of the glenoid surface and of the scapular neck will be quite sclerotic, and, in spite of roughening these surfaces as best as possible, one gains the impression that interdigitation of the cement with this bone will be suboptimal. In this situation, it may be desirable to use the modified glenoid component that would incorporate both keel fixation using methyl methacrylate and adjunctive screw fixation superior and inferior to the glenoid keel slot (Fig. 17–88). The excellence of the results when using a glenoid component with a keel and methyl methacrylate for fixation has been recognized in a number of reports (see below).

In 1981, the author began to explore the possibility of constructing a glenoid component that would adhere to the principle of minimal removal of bone stock from

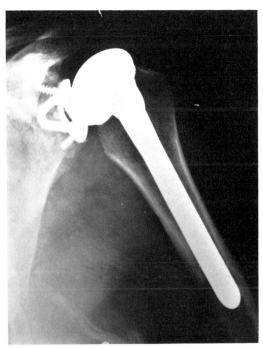

Figure 17–88. There are some situations in which cement fixation may seem somewhat tenuous in spite of seemingly adequate bone stock. In this patient, in spite of excellent bone stock, the texture of the bone within the glenoid neck was extremely firm and sclerotic. Cement interdigitation was compromised because of this. It was elected to use a cemented glenoid component with supplemental screw fixation to enhance glenoid component attachment to the scapula.

the glenoid and yet could be quite accurately fitted to the bone by using a simple but precise instrumentation system. The implant would be stable in the glenoid without the use of methyl methacrylate and could incorporate the potential for bony ingrowth into the component. Such a component became available to the author in 1983, and preliminary results were reported in 1986.[46] Continuing revisions of the system have been undertaken with a number of engineers, so that currently the author has come to use this implant system for the majority of patients requiring total shoulder arthroplasty. The surgical exposure is the same. The preparation of the humerus is the same except for the availability of a highly precise humeral cutting guide. The glenoid placement, however, is significantly different and will be described here briefly.

The glenoid is exposed, and the margins of the glenoid are carefully defined. A centering hole is started with an awl or a small burr. A long quarter-inch drill is then held perpendicular to the planned surface for the prosthetic glenoid component, and a central one-quarter-inch drill hole is made (Fig. 17–89). This then allows positioning of a bullet-tipped facing reamer. This reamer is very carefully used to remove 1 to 2 mm of subchondral bone (Fig. 17–90). In most patients, this will allow a slight admixture of cancellous bleeding bone among the harder surface areas of the subchondral plate. A template of appropriate size is then positioned over the glenoid face. A second quarter-inch drill with a stop is then introduced into the central drill hole and drilled to the appropriate

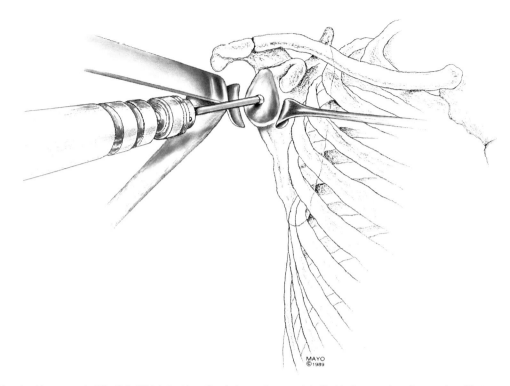

Figure 17–89. The glenoid component of the Cofield total shoulder arthroplasty may be accurately fitted to the scapula, using a series of instruments. The first step is selecting a centering hole, using a bone awl, and then preparing this hole with a one-quarter-inch drill. (By permission of Mayo Foundation.)

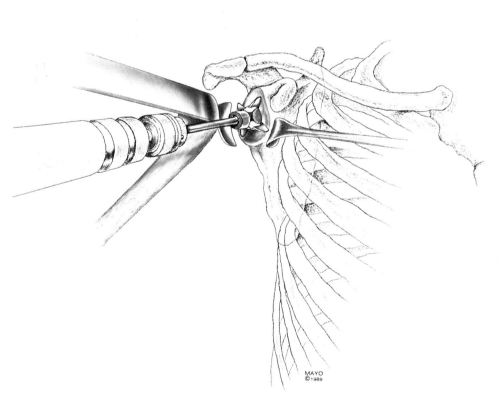

Figure 17–90. After the centering hole is prepared (see Fig. 17–89), a glenoid facing reamer is positioned in the hole, and approximately 1 to 1.5 mm of bone is removed to recontour the glenoid surface and obtain a mixture of cortical and cancellous bone on the glenoid surface. One must be extremely cautious not to ream away the entire subchondral plate. (By permission of Mayo Foundation.)

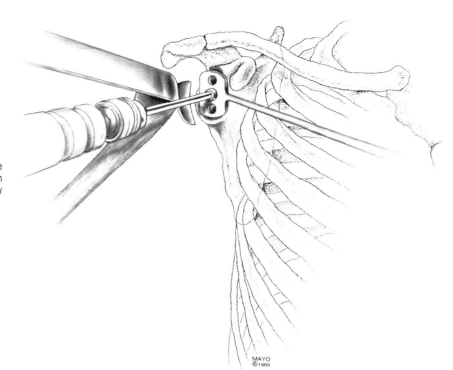

Figure 17–91. After preparing the glenoid surface, the first template is positioned and a quarter-inch drill with a stop is reintroduced into the centering hole. (By permission of Mayo Foundation.)

depth (Fig. 17–91). This drill is left in place. Two other quarter-inch holes are made in the superior and inferior aspects of the glenoid to the correct depth using the alternate quarter-inch drill with drill stop (Fig. 17–92). These drills and the template are removed, a second template is applied, and two eighth-inch drill holes are constructed through the superior and inferior one-quarter-inch drill holes (Fig. 17–93). A trial component is fitted, and a trial reduction of the shoulder may also be done to assess tension and stability.

The trial component is removed, and the real component is impacted into position. Ordinarily, the component is quite stable at this point and can be removed only with difficulty. Should the patient be a candidate for an ingrowth type of prosthesis, the screws are then placed through the upper and lower columns of the

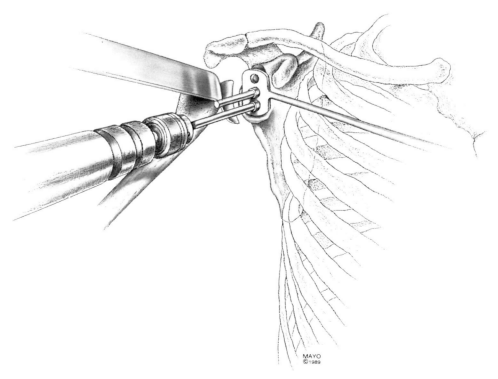

Figure 17–92. Quarter-inch drills with shorter stops are then introduced into superior and inferior holes in the first glenoid template. The template is rotated so that these holes rest in the superior to inferior axis of the glenoid surface. (By permission of Mayo Foundation.)

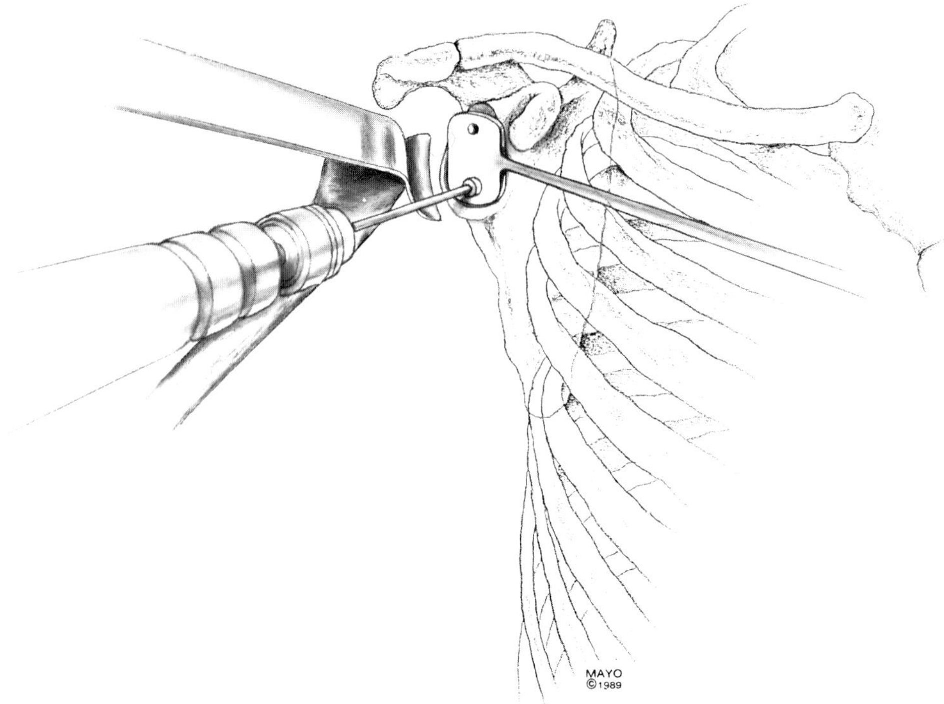

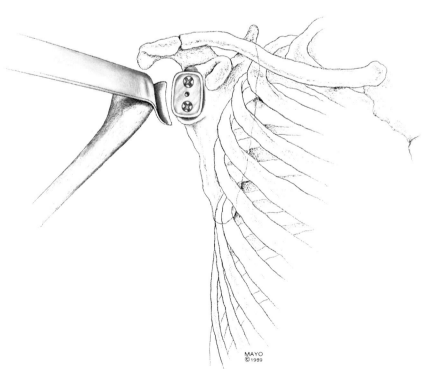

Figure 17–93. The second template is positioned, and one-eighth-inch drills with stops are placed in superior and inferior holes in this template. The smaller drills deepen the holes prepared by the larger one-quarter-inch drills. (By permission of Mayo Foundation.)

implant and tightened, holding the porous surface of the undersurface of the tray firmly against the glenoid articular face (Fig. 17–94). The polyethylene component is then impacted into position in its metal tray (Fig. 17–95).

If cement is used to fix the component, the cement may be introduced into the three column holes before placing the metal tray, and screws are then placed through the tray into the scapula and the cement. Alternatively, the tray can be impacted into position without prior placement of the cement. Cement can then be injected through the column holes to stabilize the columns and the screws introduced into the bone and cement. This second technique will use methyl methacrylate for fixation of the screws and columns of the implant system but will also allow for the possibility of long-term stabilization of the implant by bone ingrowth between the undersurface of the glenoid component tray and the glenoid articular surface.

Following placement of the glenoid component, the

Figure 17–94. The drills and templates are removed, and the component with its three columns is impacted into position. Typically, the component is quite secure at this point. Screws are then placed through the superior and inferior columns to further supplement fixation. If fixation is not absolutely secure at this point, the fixation is supplemented with methyl methacrylate. (By permission of Mayo Foundation.)

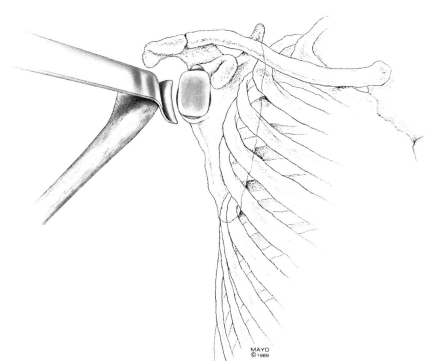

Figure 17–95. Following seating of the screws, the high-density polyethylene portion of the glenoid component is impacted into position within the metal tray. (By permission of Mayo Foundation.)

arm is externally rotated, pulled forward, slightly extended, and adducted. The humeral component is impacted into position if the bone quality is good and the fit in both the metaphyseal and diaphyseal areas is tight. The press-fitted component is tested for security, and, if secure, it is elected not to augment the fixation with polymethyl methacrylate. Should the fit in the diaphysis not be tight or should there be deficient metaphyseal bone, a plug is placed in the humeral canal, the canal is cleansed with pulsatile lavage, and, using a syringe, methacrylate is injected into the upper humerus. The humeral component is then positioned, and excess cement is trimmed.

The shoulder is reduced and again assessed for range of motion and stability. The arthrotomy incision is closed and sutures that have been placed in the proximal humerus for tuberosity repositioning or rotator cuff repair are tied, correcting tuberosity position or closing rotator cuff tears. Range of motion of the shoulder is again tested, the wound is irrigated, a suction drain is placed, and standard closure is done.

Most patients are then positioned in a shoulder immobilizer. A few patients who have a tendency for posterior humeral instability, who have a posterior-superior rotator cuff repair, who were stiff prior to surgery, or who for one reason or another may be poor candidates for rehabilitation are then positioned in a humeral abduction splint. If the rotator cuff repair is quite tenuous, a splint may be used temporarily, and a light plastic shoulder spica cast may be applied when wound healing has occurred.

Postoperative Rehabilitation

Many different rehabilitation regimens have been described for the care of patients following prosthetic shoulder arthroplasty. All of these will depend on the underlying condition being treated and the surgeon's interpretation of the stability of the implants and the quality of the soft tissue or bone repair following the surgical procedure. The variation in the regimens will also be determined by the surgeon's beliefs concerning the advisability or lack of advisability of early movement programs.

The most complete rehabilitation program has been described by Hughes and Neer[106] and has been modified over time.[155, 157] Most recently, the possibility of continuous passive motion machines as an adjunct to rehabilitation has been considered.[51] The rehabilitation program will, of course, be individualized according to specific patient needs; however, Neer has suggested dividing the patients into two groups. The first group consists of those patients who could undergo a reasonably normal rehabilitation program, and the second is a group of patients with tissue deficiencies, usually involving the muscles, bone, or both, who must be placed in a limited-goals category of rehabilitation. For this latter group of patients, rehabilitation is aimed at maintaining joint stability and achieving a lesser range of motion with reasonable muscle control through this more limited range. This concept can seem quite foreign to reconstructive surgeons dealing mainly with hip and knee prostheses; however, it is eminently reasonable when considering shoulder joint arthroplasty, with its reliance for stability upon soft tissue healing and the limited amount of stability supplied by the resurfacing or unconstrained types of implants.

Hughes and Neer have divided the typical physical therapy program into three phases.[106] The first phase initially began at four to five days postoperatively. Subsequent experience indicated that with careful surgery it was possible to begin the initial phase of rehabilitation at approximately two days following the surgical procedure.[157] This phase includes early passive or gentle active assisted motion, which helps to prevent adhesions or retard their maturation. These early movements are often accomplished in the supine position and include assisted forward elevation and assisted external rotation with the arm at the side, and then, in a progressive fashion over the first six weeks, pendulum exercises, assisted extension, pulley exercises, assisted internal rotation posterior to the trunk, and assisted external rotation with the arms clasped behind the neck. During the third postoperative week, isometric exercises are initiated for the external rotators, internal rotators, extensors, flexors, and abductors. It is important that these early exercises be guided by the surgeon, often in an in-patient setting, and carried out by the surgeon or by a physical therapist very familiar with the specific needs of the patient and the limitations described by the operating surgeon. Although hospital stays for many upper extremity procedures are quite brief, hospitalization for this procedure may extend into the second, third, or fourth week to allow this early rehabilitation regimen to be accomplished safely and effectively.

The second phase is a more active exercise program and is commenced at four to six weeks postoperatively. The program includes supine forward elevation, forward elevation in the standing position assisted by the other extremity, and continuation of rotational exercises with some element of controlled self-stretching added. Strengthening exercises may be converted from isometrics to resistance exercises using various grades of elastic tubing, with strengthening continuing in each of the five directions mentioned earlier.

After three months, residual deficiencies in range of movement and strength can be addressed by stretching and by continued strengthening. The latter can include continuation of the use of elastic tubing or other strengthening modalities such as light weights.

Neer has recently documented the safety and effectiveness of this early passive motion program done under the guidance of the surgeon or a carefully instructed physical therapist.[157] Continuous passive motion machines may be an adjunct to this rehabilitation protocol, but he feels they are mainly of use in patients who have involvement of both shoulders, which precludes the use of the assistive exercise program using the opposite upper extremity. Craig has recently demonstrated that continuous passive motion used as an adjunct to the physical therapy program can be effective in the rehabilitation of the surgically reconstructed shoulder.[51] He feels that it allows patients to achieve satisfactory range of motion slightly earlier than those who do not have the benefit of the use of a machine. Continuous passive motion did allow somewhat earlier hospital discharge, and postoperative pain seemed to be lessened. Craig could not identify any adverse effects of the use of continuous passive motion, but it is important to recognize that this program was also carried out in a controlled environment with very careful in-patient physician supervision.

In patients with muscle or bone deficiencies where it is necessary to alter rehabilitation goals to maintain stability and prevent muscle, tendon, or bone disruption, a limited-goals category of rehabilitation has been suggested.[155] In this setting, the initiation of exercises may be delayed somewhat, and the extent of passive or assisted early motion is reduced. Typically, elevation may be limited to 90 degrees and external rotation to 20 degrees. These limited arcs of movement allow the possibility of more scar formation, fibrous tissue maturation, and maintenance of joint stability to a greater degree than in a fuller rehabilitation program.

As mentioned above, there are many variations in rehabilitation programs. The most cautiously aggressive program has been described here. There are certainly patients with conditions that will suggest the need for more limitations on the timing of physical therapy, the extent of motion, and the extent of strengthening activities included within their rehabilitation plans.

Results

HEMIARTHROPLASTY

The results for the Neer design of hemiarthroplasty, or proximal humeral prosthetic replacement, are reported in Table 17–15. The results have been reported for osteonecrosis, osteoarthritis, rheumatoid arthritis, and the residuals of trauma. When this procedure is applied to the treatment of proximal humeral osteonecrosis, the pain relief has been quite good, ranging from 91 to 100 per cent, and the range of motion of the shoulder approaches normal. When this operation is applied to patients with rheumatoid arthritis, osteoarthritis, or the residuals of trauma, satisfactory pain relief is less consistently achieved but, with the exception of 3 of the 11 reported series, is still quite acceptable in the 80 to 100 per cent range. Range of motion in these latter patients tends to be less and is variable from series to series. In the series reported in this chapter, the average active abduction ranged from one-third to three-quarters normal.

The results for various other designs of hemiarthroplasty in the forms of either proximal humeral prosthetic replacement or interpositional arthroplasty are reported in Table 17–16. In 1951, Krueger reported

Table 17-15. RESULTS OF SHOULDER HEMIARTHROPLASTY—NEER DESIGN

Author, Year	Diagnosis	No. Shoulders	No or Slight Pain (%)	Average Active Abduction (°) or Overall Rating
Neer, 1955[148]	Osteonecrosis	3	100	Excellent, good, good
Neer, 1974[151]	Osteoarthritis	47		20 excellent
				20 satisfactory
				6 unsatisfactory
Cruess, 1976[53]	Osteonecrosis	5	100	Approached normal
Bodey and Yeoman, 1983[23]	Osteoarthritis Rheumatoid arthritis	8	88	63°
Tanner and Cofield, 1983[209]	Old trauma	28	89	112°
Bell and Gschwend, 1986[17]	Mixed	17	59	91°
Petersson, 1986[167]	Rheumatoid arthritis	11	36	74°
Zuckerman and Cofield, 1986[228]	Osteoarthritis	39	82	134°
	Rheumatoid arthritis	44	91	112°
Hawkins et al, 1987[102]	Chronic dislocation	9	67	140°
Pritchett and Clark, 1987[174]	Chronic dislocation	7	100	5 good, 2 fair
Rutherford and Cofield, 1987[189]	Osteonecrosis	11	91	161°
Total		229	Weighted mean, 82%; median, 89%	Weighted mean of 8 series, 115°; median, 112°

on a chrome-cobalt custom design not unlike the Neer proximal humeral prosthesis.[128] This very early report was quite encouraging in that the patient so treated had an excellent result. Plastic implants have been used to a much greater degree in Europe and Great Britain than they have been in North America. The isoelastic prosthesis was designed so that the implant would have a flexibility approximating that of bone. In the patients treated with this device, pain relief is usually achieved; return of active movement is moderate at best. A Silastic interpositional cup was first applied by Varian and then also reported on in a series by Spencer and Skirving.[200, 215] Pain relief was not consistently achieved in these patients, and often the improvment in movement was modest or no gains occurred.

Jónsson and co-workers and Steffee and Moore have reported on the use of a metal cup for patients with rheumatoid arthritis or other mixed diagnostic groups.[113, 114, 201] Pain relief seems to be quite acceptable after insertion of this implant. Return of movement varies greatly among the series reported, ranging from a mean active abduction of 57 degrees to a mean active abduction of 147 degrees.

Swanson has developed and described the use of a bipolar type of proximal humeral prosthetic replacement in 15 shoulders.[206] Pain relief was uniformly achieved. Return of active abduction was disappointing, averaging 78 degrees.

Various types of unconstrained shoulder prostheses can also be used as hemiarthroplasties in certain situations. Kay and Amstutz have reported on the use of the Dana implant for the treatment of osteonecrosis and osteoarthritis.[117] The results seem similar to those

Table 17-16. RESULTS OF SHOULDER HEMIARTHROPLASTY—VARIOUS IMPLANT DESIGNS

Author, Year	Design	Diagnosis	No. Shoulders	No or Slight Pain (%)	Average Active Abduction (°)
Krueger, 1951[128]	Custom	Osteonecrosis	1	100	Full overhead motion
Varian, 1980[215]	Silastic cup	Rheumatoid arthritis, 28 Osteoarthritis, 2	32	94	Improved in 21 cases
Cockx et al, 1983[36]	Isoelastic	Mixed	25	72	Acute injuries, 73° Old injuries, 45°
Steffee and Moore, 1984[201]	Metal cup	Mixed	51	82	147°
Swanson, 1984[206]	Bipolar	Rheumatoid arthritis, 9 Osteoarthritis, 5	15	100	78°
Tonino and van de Werf, 1985[211]	Isoelastic	Mixed	14	100	Moderate improvement
Jónsson et al, 1986[113]	Metal cup	Rheumatoid arthritis	26	100	57°
Spencer and Skirving, 1986[200]	Silastic cup	Rheumatoid arthritis, 9 Osteoarthritis, 3	12	42	Little change
Jónsson et al, 1988[115]	Metal cup	Rheumatoid arthritis	5	100	73°
Kay and Amstutz, 1988[117]	2 Dana/2 Neer	Osteonecrosis, 3 Osteoarthritis, 1	4	100	Osteonecrosis, 140–150° Osteoarthritis, 99°
Total			185	Weighted mean 86%; median, 100%	Weighted mean of 6 series, 109°; median, between 78° and 99°

reported for the implant of the Neer design, and this is not unexpected.

TOTAL SHOULDER ARTHROPLASTY

As with hemiarthroplasty, it is more difficult to tabulate and report results than one might initially perceive. Many of the series report their findings using different evaluative guidelines, and, on a number of occasions, a rating system is applied in lieu of reporting actual data. By far the most commonly used total shoulder arthroplasty has been the Neer design. The results for this system are tabulated in Table 17–14. Most patient series contain a mixed diagnostic grouping, including patients with rheumatoid arthritis, osteoarthritis, old trauma, and a variety of less common diagnostic categories. As can be seen from the table, the percentage of patients achieving satisfactory pain relief is quite high, and, quite typically, slightly greater than 90 per cent of patients report no or only slight pain following surgery. Motion data following surgery have not been as consistently reported as one might desire, but the amount of motion regained seems variable and dependent on diagnostic category. For example, in the series reported by Cofield, the mean active abduction following surgery for the entire group of patients reported was 120 degrees.[43] The average return of active abduction varied greatly according to diagnosis: 141 degrees for osteoarthritis, 109 degrees for those with post-traumatic arthritis, and 103 degrees for patients with rheumatoid arthritis. The return of movement in Cofield's series was not only dependent on diagnosis but was also highly dependent on the condition of the rotator cuff and shoulder capsule and on the avoidance of complications.[43]

The largest series of total shoulder arthroplasties of this category has been reported by Neer.[155] He has suggested two systems for grading results. Patients who received a full rehabilitation program were graded as excellent, satisfactory, or unsatisfactory. To achieve an excellent result, the patient was enthusiastic about the operation, had no significant pain, could use the arm without limitations, strength approached normal, and active elevation of the arm was within 35 degrees of the opposite normal side. In these patients, external rotation was 90 per cent of the normal side. In patients with a satisfactory result, there was no more than occasional pain or aching with weather changes, good use of the shoulder for daily activities, movement in elevation from 90 to 135 degrees, and rotation to 50 per cent of the normal side. Muscle strength was 30 per cent of the normal side or greater, and the patients expressed satisfaction with the operation. In an unsatisfactory result, the above criteria were not achieved. Neer has suggested a separate evaluation category for patients who have total shoulder replacement but whose muscles could be classified as detached and not capable of recovering function after repair because of fixed contracture or denervation. Patients with substantial bone loss, particularly bone loss in the proximal humerus, might also be included within this evaluative category. In this setting, rehabilitation is aimed at achieving limited goals, the purpose being to gain a lesser range of motion but maintain stability. Neer has suggested that this limited-goals rehabilitation is successful when patients with these muscle or bone deficiencies achieve 90 degrees of elevation and 20 degrees of external rotation, maintain reasonable stability, and achieve satisfactory pain relief. The results achieved for Neer's large series of patients, including the many diagnostic categories, are displayed in Table 17–17.

Roentgenographic assessment of component position and the security of the attachment of the components to their respective bones can be quite difficult following total shoulder replacement. There is no standard system for describing the radiographic appearance of total shoulder components. Franklin and co-authors have suggested a classification system for describing the radiographic appearance of the glenoid component.[82] In Class 0, there is no lucency. In Class 1, there is lucency at the superior or inferior flange only. In Class 2, there is incomplete lucency at the keel. In Class 3, there is complete lucency up to 2 mm around the component. In Class 4, there is complete lucency greater than 2 mm around the component. In Class 5A, the component has translated, tipped, or shifted in position. And in Class 5B, the component has become dislocated from the bone. A number of investigators might disagree with this system of analysis, but

Table 17–17. FOLLOW-UP ON 194 TOTAL SHOULDER ARTHROPLASTIES* (CLINICAL RATINGS)

Diagnosis	No. Shoulders	Excellent	Full Exercise Program		Limited Goals Rehabilitation	
			Satisfactory	Unsatisfactory	Successful	Unsuccessful
Osteoarthritis (primary and secondary)	40	36	3	0	1	0
Arthritis of recurrent dislocation	18	13	3	1	1	0
Rheumatoid arthritis	50	28	12	3	7	0
Old trauma	41	16	7	12	6	0
Prosthetic revision	26	7	3	5	11	0
Cuff-tear arthropathy	11	—	—	—	10	1
Miscellaneous (tumor, glenoid dysplasia, failed arthrodesis)	8	1	—	—	6	1
Total	194	101	28	21	42	4

*Adapted from Neer CS, Watson KC, and Stanton FJ: Recent experience in total shoulder arthroplasty. J Bone Joint Surg 64A:319–337, 1982.

Table 17–18. RESULTS OF ROENTGENOGRAPHIC ANALYSIS OF NEER TOTAL SHOULDER ARTHROPLASTY

| Author, Year | No. Shoulders | Glenoid Bone-Cement Junction Lucent Zones (%) | | | Shift in Position |
		None	*Any Area*	*Keel*	
Neer et al, 1982[155]	194	70	30	12	
Bade et al, 1984[7]	38	33	67		
Cofield, 1984[43]	73	29	71	33	11
Wilde et al, 1984[222]	38	7	93	68	
Adams et al, 1986[1]	33			36	
Brems et al, 1986[25]	69	31	69		
Barrett et al, 1987[12]	50	26	74	36	10
Kelly et al, 1987[118]	40	17	83	63	

really the major point of disagreement can be related to the clinical relevance of the lucent zone. The area of attachment of a glenoid implant to the scapula is certainly much less than the area of attachment of an acetabular component to the pelvis. A lucent zone of 2 mm at the glenoid may be too wide to serve as a distinguishing point between a prosthesis that is securely affixed to the bone and one that has an interposing fibrous or fibrous and histiocytic membrane.

Roentgenographic analyses for a number of series of total shoulder arthroplasties using the Neer design are displayed in Table 17–18. Note that all series report lucent lines or lucent zones at the glenoid-bone cement junction. These vary considerably in frequency among the different series, ranging from 30 to 93 per cent of shoulders reported. The keel portion of this implant serves as the significant means of attachment to the scapula, and the lucent zones seen at the cement-bone junction surrounding the keel are of great concern. The median percentage of the number of shoulders analyzed in which a lucent line was identified at the bone-cement junction of the keel part of the component is 36. The argument has been presented that when these lucent lines or zones are seen in patients they are almost always present immediately postoperatively and clearly represent an error in surgical technique.[155] This may be the most common sequence of events associated with roentgenographic lucent zones at the glenoid bone-cement junction and speaks for the need

for meticulous preparation of the bony bed and cementing at the time of surgery. However, it has also been reported that these lucent zones have not been present immediately after surgery but rather have developed over time.[43]

In the series by Barrett[12] and Cofield,[13] analyses have also included a shift in glenoid component position relative to the position achieved immediately following surgery. Analysis of component movement relative to the bone requires the viewing of sequential x-rays over time because often a lucent zone is not seen. This finding implies component loosening, but it can easily be overlooked if serial x-rays are not studied. In summary, the roentgenographic analysis of patient series provokes some concern, but, as will be seen in the section on complications, the frequency of clinically significant glenoid loosening has been quite small to date.

Table 17–19 displays the results for other designs of total shoulder arthroplasty. In the series reported by Engelbrecht and Heinert,[71] Gristina and co-workers,[92, 93] and Amstutz,[5] the prosthetic design does not differ greatly from that of the Neer prosthesis. The designs used in the series are resurfacing implants with little additional constraint built into the articulation. The results reported by Gristina and Amstutz parallel those reported in the series of total shoulder replacements using the Neer design. The same is true for the series reported by Engelbrecht, but, unfortunately, as

Table 17–19. RESULTS OF TOTAL SHOULDER ARTHROPLASTY—VARIOUS IMPLANT DESIGNS

Author, Year	Mean Follow-up (Yr)	Prosthetic Design	No. Shoulders	No or Slight Pain (%)	Average Active Abduction (°)
Coughlin et al, 1979[50]	2.0	Stanmore	16	100 (?)	104
Post et al, 1980[171]	1.3–6.0	Michael Reese	28	96	
Beddow and Elloy, 1982[16]	2.5	Liverpool	13	85	
Gristina and Webb, 1982[91]	1.0–3.5	Trispherical	20	100	58
Kessel and Bayley, 1982[122]	3.5	Kessel	33	85	
Lettin et al, 1982[131]		Stanmore	40	90	70
Mazas and de la Caffinière, 1982[139]	(range, 1.0–6.0)	Nonretentive	32	91	
Faludi and Weiland, 1982[76]	3.7	English-Macnab	13		75
Swanson, 1984[206]	3.4	Bipolar	15	100	70
Engelbrecht and Heinert, 1987[71]	4.0	St. Georg (most of series)	51	88	
Gristina et al, 1987[93]	3.2	Monospherical	100	90	115
McElwain and English, 1987[142]	3.1	English-Macnab	13	85	56
Amstutz et al, 1988[5]	3.5	Dana (regular)	46	91	120
		Dana (hooded)	10	100 (85–100)	85

will be seen in the complications section, glenoid loosening was quite frequent in this series.

The two series reported by Faludi and Weiland[76] and McElwain and English[142] describe the results with the English-Macnab type of prosthesis. This implant system is slightly more constrained than the earlier-mentioned series, but, perhaps more important, this implant also incorporates the potential for bone ingrowth for both glenoid and humeral components. Pain relief has been quite satisfactory with this implant system. Unfortunately, the return of active movement has been less than one might wish.

Mazas and de la Caffinière[139] and Amstutz and co-workers[5] reported results on the use of a hooded glenoid component, designed to replace the stabilizing functions of the superior aspect of the rotator cuff and capsule. Again, pain relief has been satisfactory in these patients, and return of motion has been less than for the minimally constrained implants. As will be seen in the following section, complications with these implants have been more frequent than with those of the unconstrained design.

Ball-in-socket or constrained-type implants have been made in a variety of configurations. Results are available for implants of the Stanmore,[50, 131] Michael Reese,[171, 172] Liverpool,[16] Kessel,[122] and trispherical designs.[91] In implants of this category, pain relief is satisfactory unless a complication develops. Typically, return of active abduction ranges between one-third and one-half normal.

Complications

The complications for shoulder hemiarthroplasty of the Neer design are presented in Table 17–20. Of the 11 reported series, 5 record no complications. Of the 229 shoulders analyzed, 18 complications (8 per cent) have been described and are displayed in the table. Of these 18 complications, 2 included late infections, 3 were subluxations that resolved, 2 were nerve injuries that resolved, and 1 was an intraoperative fracture treated with internal fixation and no subsequent sequelae. Thus, 10 of the complications were directly related to the initial surgical event and continued to have significance. This represents a complication rate of 5 per cent for the entire series of patients reported. It should be noted that 7 of these 10 significant complications occurred in the placement of a prosthesis for the care of old trauma. The difficulties encountered in the care of these patients with complications of trauma are discussed in the article by Tanner and Cofield.[209] The complications relate both to the increasing difficulty of the surgical procedure and to the alteration of tissue quality, stiffness of the rotator cuff and capsule, and often osteopenia rendering reconstructive bony work at the time of surgery difficult and bone fixation tenuous.

The complications of shoulder hemiarthroplasty of other various implant designs are presented in Table 17–21. Thirty-two complications occurred following the care of 185 shoulders, a frequency of 17 per cent. This figure is more than twice as high as the number of complications reported for the Neer type of prosthetic design. Of the 32 complications, 2 included mechanical failure that was not clinically significant, one represented an impingement syndrome, and one was transient postoperative instability. Thus, 28 significant complications occurred. It should be noted that 25 of these 28 occurred with the use of nonmetallic or plastic implants—an experience that has developed in Europe and the British Isles. To date, the metallic cup arthroplasties have had very few complications.

There are a greater variety and number of compli-

Table 17–20. COMPLICATIONS OF SHOULDER HEMIARTHROPLASTY—NEER DESIGN

Author, Year	Diagnosis	No. Shoulders	None	Infection	Intraoperative Fracture	Nerve Injury	Ectopic Ossification	Instability	Rotator cuff tear, Tuberosity nonunion or malunion
Neer, 1955[148]	Osteonecrosis	3	—						
Neer, 1974[151]	Osteoarthritis	47						2	
Cruess, 1976[53]	Osteonecrosis	5		1			1		
Bodey and Yeoman, 1983[23]	Rheumatoid arthritis Osteoarthritis	8						2	
Tanner and Cofield, 1983[209]	Old trauma	28				1	1	1	4
Bell and Gschwend, 1986[17]	Mixed	17						1	
Petersson, 1986[167]	Rheumatoid arthritis	11	—						
Zuckerman and Cofield, 1986[228]	Osteoarthritis	39	—						
	Rheumatoid arthritis	44		1	1	1			
Hawkins et al, 1987[102]	Chronic dislocation	9	—						
Pritchett and Clark, 1987[174]	Chronic dislocation	7				1			
Rutherford and Cofield, 1987[189]	Osteonecrosis	11	—						
Total		229		2	1	3	2	6	4

Table 17–21. COMPLICATIONS OF SHOULDER HEMIARTHROPLASTY—VARIOUS IMPLANT DESIGNS

Author, Year	Implant Design	Diagnosis	No. Shoulders	Complication						
				None	Infection	Nerve Injury	Instability	Impingement	Mechanical Failure	Loosening
Krueger, 1951[128]	Custom	Osteonecrosis	1	—						
Varian, 1980[215]	Silastic cup	Rheumatoid arthritis, 28 Osteoarthritis, 2	32				5		4	
Cockx et al, 1983[36]	Isoelastic	Mixed	25		2	2	5			3
Steffee and Moore, 1984[201]	Metal cup	Mixed	51		1					
Swanson, 1984[206]	Bipolar		15				1			
Tonino and van der Werf, 1985[211]	Isoelastic	Mixed	14	—						
Jónsson et al, 1986[113]	Metal cup	Rheumatoid arthritis	26					1		
Spencer and Skirving, 1986[200]	Silastic cup	Rheumatoid arthritis, 9 Osteoarthritis, 3	12				4		2	
Kay and Amstutz, 1988[117]	2 Danna 2 Neer		4				1	1		
Jónsson et al, 1988[115]	Metal cup		5							
Total			185		3	2	16	2	6	3

cations following total shoulder arthroplasty than have arisen following hemiarthroplasty. The complications of the Neer design of total shoulder arthroplasty are presented in Table 17–22. The most common complication following this type of surgery is difficulty with the rotator cuff or with tuberosity healing. This is followed in frequency by glenoid loosening and instability. A few intraoperative and postoperative fractures have occurred, and subacromial impingement has been identified in a few patients following this surgery. Nerve injury, although uncommon, does occur but fortunately tends to resolve. Infection has been quite uncommon and perhaps is less frequent in this type of surgery than in any other major total joint replacement. Three infections were identified in 586 operative procedures (0.51 per cent). Also quite fortunately, ectopic bone formation following this procedure is quite rare.

Reported series of other relatively unconstrained total shoulder arthroplasties have revealed complications mimicking those seen in the Neer design. Gristina and co-workers have reported on a series of 100 monospherical total shoulder arthroplasties,[92, 93] in which there were four clinically loosened glenoid components, two dislocations, one loosened humeral component, one axillary nerve injury, and one late infection metastatic from another site. Amstutz and associates have reported on 46 Dana total shoulder arthroplasties using the standard glenoid component.[5] Complications included two subluxations and one dislocation following surgery. Also, one infection, one rotator cuff tear, and one loosened glenoid were reported.

Engelbrecht and co-workers reported on a variety of rather unconstrained total shoulder devices, many of which were the St. Georg design.[70–72] Their experi-

Table 17–22. COMPLICATIONS OF TOTAL SHOULDER ARTHROPLASTY—NEER DESIGN

Author, Year	No. Shoulders	Complication									
		None	Infection	Intra-operative Fracture	Nerve Injury	Ectopic Ossification	Instability	Impinge-ment	Rotator Cuff Tear, Tuberosity Nonunion or Malunion	Loosening	
										Glenoid	Humerus
Neer et al, 1982[155]	194		1	1			6	1	6		
Bade et al, 1984[7]	38			1				2	5	1	2
Cofield, 1984[43]	73			1					6	3	
Wilde et al, 1984[222]	38		1			1	2	2		1	
Adams et al, 1986[1]	33		1				1				
Hawkins et al, 1986[101]	70			2						3	
Barrett et al, 1987[12]	50			3	1		1	1	1	4	
Kelly et al, 1987[118]	40			2					2		
Frich et al, 1988[83]	50				1		1			3	
Total	586		3 (.51)*	8 (1.4)	4 (.68)	1 (.17)	11 (1.9)	6 (1.0)	20 (3.4)	15 (2.6)	2 (.34)

*Percentages in parentheses

ence was much different from that occurring in the other unconstrained prosthetic designs. Glenoid loosening was recognized in 32 shoulders (51 per cent), dislocation occurred in 17, subluxation in 7, ectopic ossification in 4, infection in 2, and humeral loosening in 1. This experience has suggested to these authors that hemiarthroplasty without placement of a glenoid component may offer a more consistently satisfactory result, avoiding many of the complications reported above.

Only a few series have been reported analyzing the results and complications of total shoulder arthroplasties with hooded glenoid components. The largest series is by Mazas and de la Caffinière.[139] In 1982, they reported on 32 nonretentive total shoulder arthroplasties. Complications included subluxation or dislocation in nine shoulders, infections in three, component loosening in two, axillary nerve paralysis in one, and pulmonary embolus in one. The English-Macnab prosthesis may include a hooded glenoid component. The standard glenoid component also incorporates more concavity than other nonconstrained designs. In the series using the English-Macnab prosthesis reported by Faludi and Weiland,[76] there were 2 intraoperative humeral fractures, 1 intraoperative perforation of the humeral shaft, 1 postoperative dislocation, and 1 late infection in 13 shoulders analyzed. McElwain and English also analyzed 13 arthroplasties with this design.[142] Complications included two screw fractures, one humeral shaft fracture, one dislocation, one loosened plastic insert, one loosened glenoid component, and one loosened humeral component. Most recently, Amstutz and co-workers and Ellman and Jinnah have reported on the placement of 10 hooded components as a part of Dana total shoulder arthroplasty.[5, 68] In these patients, one experienced an acromial fracture, and the glenoid loosened in another. Thus, one can recognize an increased frequency of complications in patients having this variety of total shoulder arthroplasty. In spite of the hooded component supposedly offering greater stability, subluxation or dislocation is more commonly reported than with the unconstrained design, glenoid component loosening is slightly more common, and apparently the humeral component of the English-Macnab prosthesis is quite difficult to place with safety, avoiding humeral fracturing or perforation.

Various authors have presented series of patients using ball-in-socket designs of total shoulder arthroplasties and, as a part of their report, have detailed the complications. Gristina and co-workers, reporting on 20 Trispherical total shoulder arthroplasties, recognized two component disruptions with subluxation.[91, 93] Kessel and Bayley, reporting on 33 shoulder arthroplasties of Kessel's design, reported on three dislocations and two brachial plexus traction injuries.[122] Beddow and Elloy, analyzing 13 Liverpool shoulder arthropasties, reported four loose scapular components, one clavicle fracture, and one instance of heterotopic ossification.[15, 16]

Lettin and colleagues described a large series of Stanmore total shoulder arthroplasties.[131] Fifty shoulders were followed. In ten, glenoid loosening occurred, three dislocated, and one became infected as a result of seeding from a distant site. Coughlin and associates also reported on this prosthetic design.[50] Sixteen shoulders were analyzed. Post and co-workers presented the results obtained using the Michael Reese prosthesis in 1980 and offered an update on the results and complications in 1987.[171, 172] At the time of the more recent report, an alarming number of complications were described. In the first design of this type of arthroplasty, the humeral neck became bent or broken in 13; there were dislocations in six shoulders; three shoulders experienced humeral loosening; and three developed loosened glenoids. The prosthesis was modified (Series II), eliminating the bending and fracturing of the prosthetic humeral neck. Unfortunately, other complications became more frequent. There were dislocations in 13 shoulders, five loose humeral components, and four loose glenoid components. It is not difficult to recognize that the complications that have occurred following the use of the constrained ball-in-socket types of total shoulder arthroplasty units have been quite frequent and serious, usually requiring revision surgery.

Revision Surgery

Neer and Kirby have published the only article directed specifically toward revision surgery for humeral head and total shoulder arthroplasties.[154] The contents of this article were based on experience with 40 hemi/total shoulder arthroplasties requiring revision. The authors identified many potential causes of failures and suggested a broad approach to analysis of problems with this type of shoulder surgery. As such, they recommended analysis of preoperative, surgical, and postoperative considerations (Table 17–23) with the thought that each of these areas could contribute to the cause of failure and also preclude successful revision surgery.

In this same article, selected causes of failure were discussed.[154] For the fixed fulcrum or constrained arthroplasty, the two outstanding problems identified were loss of the external rotators and mechanical failure of the implant device. For the unconstrained or resurfacing arthroplasties, prominent problems included deltoid detachment and fibrosis, tightening of the subscapularis and anterior shoulder capsule, adhesions about the rotator cuff possibly in association with subacromial impingement, the presence of a prominent or retracted tuberosity, loss of humeral length, uneven or central glenoid wear, and lack of a supervised postoperative rehabilitation program. Treatment recommendations included "clean-out" and fusion when there was infection or extensive loss or paralysis of

Table 17–23. EVALUATION OF FAILED HUMERAL HEAD AND TOTAL SHOULDER ARTHROPLASTIES

I. Preoperative (general) considerations
    Psychological
    Neuromuscular
    Adjacent joints
    Infection
II. Surgical considerations
    Soft tissue
        Deltoid
        Rotator cuff
        Heterotopic ossification
    Bone
        Coracoid
        Acromion
        Acromioclavicular joint
        Tuberosities
        Retained humeral head or osteophytes
        Loss of humeral length
        Glenoid
    Prosthesis
        Humeral component
            Version
            Height
            Head length
            Stem size
            Stability
            Loosening or breakage
        Glenoid component
            Version
            Height
            Loosening or breakage
        Cement
III. Postoperative considerations
    Residual instability
    Capability of remaining muscles

(Adapted from Neer CS II, and Kirby RM: Revision of humeral head and total shoulder arthroplasties. Clin Orthop *170*:189–195, 1982.)

both the deltoid and rotator cuff muscles. Fusions, when required, were often done using autogenous iliac grafts, internal fixation, and external cast support. The other major treatment option was total shoulder arthroplasty. In this series of patients, 34 were revised in this manner. The authors considered this the most technically difficult of any category of prosthetic shoulder surgery. They commented that satisfactory pain relief and function for daily living were obtained in all but five patients; however, the results in the majority of patients were not as good as the unconstrained arthroplasties done for other diagnostic categories.

Review of the literature since the early 1970s allows the collection of sufficient data to identify the compli-

cations that have occurred in total shoulder arthroplasties. These have been defined in the previous section. Information on the reoperations done for these complications is less ample, and the results of revision surgery are somewhat uncertain.

As mentioned earlier, the infection rate following total shoulder arthroplasty is less than 1 per cent. The majority of infections occur late, and many are related to hematogenous spread from other infected sites. *Staphylococcus aureus* is the most commonly isolated organism. Amstutz and colleagues reported on exchanging an unconstrained for a constrained glenoid in one patient with septic loosening of the glenoid.[5] However, in all other situations, resection arthroplasty with removal of the prosthetic components and cement has been necessary.

Nerve injuries are uncommon but do occur. Almost all have resolved spontaneously with time. Thus, it would seem that treatment for this problem following surgery should be expectant, with repeated examinations and electromyography when necessary. If there is no evidence of recovery after a period of time, perhaps three to six months, and there is concern that local injury to the nerve may have occurred, there is indication for exploration of the area.

Should a fracture occur adjacent to prosthetic components at some time during the postoperative period, there is little guidance that one can obtain from reading the literature. It is suggested that the fractures can be treated on their own merit. However, if they are associated with component loosening, revision will probably be necessary. In patients with certain fractures or with lack of prompt healing, internal fixation with or without bone grafting may be required.

In unconstrained shoulder arthroplasty, postoperative rotator cuff tearing is one of the more common complications encountered (Table 17–24). Of those that have occurred in the reported series, approximately one-quarter of the patients have undergone further surgery for repair of their torn tendons. The apparent reason for the conservative attitude toward this complication is that most of the patients seemingly continued to have satisfactory relief of pain, and, although they had functional limitations, were not impaired to the extent that revision surgery was thought necessary. Figgie and associates have noted a significant correlation between an intact rotator cuff and the successful outcome from arthroplasty.[79] This

Table 17–24. REVISION SURGERY FOR UNCONSTRAINED TOTAL SHOULDER ARTHROPLASTY—NEER DESIGN

Complication	Treatment at Revision Surgery				
	Replace Component	Remove Component(s)	Rotator Cuff Repair	Open Reduction and Internal Fixation	Acromioplasty
Glenoid loosening	4[43, 101]	4[9, 222]			
Rotator cuff tear			4[9, 118, 155]		
Fracture	1[155]			1[9]	
Impingement					2[222]
Infection		1[155]			

has also been reported by Cofield.[43] Franklin and co-authors studied seven total shoulder arthroplasty procedures that exhibited objective radiographic signs of loosening.[82] Six of these shoulders had massive rotator cuff tearing that was incompletely repaired at the time of arthroplasty and redeveloped more extensive tearing following surgery. These authors felt that superior subluxation of the humeral head component associated with rotator cuff tearing contributed to glenoid loosening by creating eccentric loads across the glenoid. Thus, although the literature seems to support repair of rotator cuff tearing based solely on symptomatology, there may be some rationale for performing rerepair of rotator cuff tears more frequently in this setting with the hopes of increasing the longevity of the arthroplasty.

All large series of unconstrained shoulder replacements contain reports of joint instability with subluxation or occasional dislocations. The instability has been reported for all directions: anterior, posterior, inferior, and, most comonly, superior. It is thought that superior subluxation is associated with rotator cuff pathology and should be treated as such. Statements are made that inferior subluxation is usually benign and resolves with time and rehabilitative care. Neer and co-workers have noted, however, that if humeral length is not restored, the prosthesis may subluxate inferiorly and remain in that position.[155] Of the cases with anterior instability, approximately one-third were treated by closed reduction and support, and surgical treatment was undertaken in the remaining two-thirds. Occasionally, capsule and rotator cuff repair was all that was necessary, but, most commonly, component revision was also needed.

Posterior instability has been successfully treated with exercises and support, but, as with anterior instability, it has also been treated with open revision surgery repairing the posterior capsule and muscle structures or repairing these plus revising components to effect a more stable articulation. Posterior instability may be most common in osteoarthritis, as there is often a tendency for posterior glenoid wear and posterior humeral subluxation to occur in this condition in the preoperative state. It has been suggested that it may be necessary to bone graft symmetrical posterior deficiencies of the glenoid to eliminate the tendency for posterior subluxation.[158] It may also be necessary to alter humeral component torsion or tighten the posterior capsule. The author has seen several patients whose humeral osteotomy has resulted in incision of the external rotators and posterior capsule and has fostered postoperative posterior instability. This may occur when the osteotomy is slightly too inferior or when slightly more than normal retrotorsion is incorporated into the bone cut.

Somewhat surprisingly, dislocation is more common following placement of a constrained implant system than if an unconstrained design is used. Only a few of the constrained designs (Stanmore) will allow closed treatment of a dislocation, and 16 out of the 21 reported dislocations were, in fact, treated surgically.

Thirteen had successful revision surgery. In the remaining patients, further treatment often included removal of the implant system.

Mechanical failure of the components of a shoulder arthroplasty has been a substantial problem only in those of constrained design. Post and co-workers reported successful revisions of Series I Michael Reese total shoulder arthroplasties with broken or bent humeral necks to Series II designs using components with stronger humeral necks.[171, 172] Modular components may become disassembled and require revision surgery. This has occurred in the English-Macnab prosthesis and in the Trispherical design may become disassembled and require revision surgery.[94, 142]

As with many other joint replacements, the most frequent problem associated with total shoulder arthroplasty over the long term may be component loosening. To date, however, the need for revision of surgery for component loosening in unconstrained systems has been quite uncommon. Of slightly more than one dozen patients with glenoid loosening reported who underwent revision surgery, approximately three-quarters had reinsertion of a glenoid implant, and in one-quarter of patients, the component was removed, presumably because of insufficient bone stock remaining at the time of revision surgery. The results of these revisions are not reported to any extent. As can be seen from the data in the complications sections of this chapter, the frequency of humeral loosening is quite low in the unconstrained systems. Should humeral loosening occur, it should be possible to reinsert a new component with or without methyl methacrylate as a supplement to the fixation.

Total shoulder arthroplasties of the constrained type have a higher frequency of component loosening than has occurred in the unconstrained design. Of the reported series of constrained implants, 23 cases of component loosening have been reported for an incidence of 9.9 per cent. In these systems, the glenoid component was revised in 18 shoulders, reinsertion of a new component was possible in 12, and resection arthroplasty was necssary in six. Unfortunately, Lettin and co-workers reported failure in six of eight Stanmore prostheses reimplanted, and later it was necessary to perform resection arthroplasty on these.[131] Because of the high failure rate associated with constrained implants, revision of failed constrained implants to unconstrained total shoulder arthroplasties has been considered. Amstutz and colleagues revised two loosened hooded glenoid components to the unconstrained regular glenoid component in the Dana system.[5] This approach has also been suggested by Neer and Kirby.[154]

Thus, in summarizing failures of total shoulder arthroplasty and the need for revision surgery, it is important to define quite specifically the problem or problems involved. When infection arises, removal of the components and cement will almost always be necessary. When nerve injuries occur, observation will usually suffice, as spontaneous recovery is common. Unless component loosening has occurred, fractures surrounding total shoulder arthroplasty components can usually be treated on their own merit. Rotator cuff tearing following shoulder arthroplasty is usually treated symptomatically, but, even if there is absence of substantial pain, shoulder function and component longevity may be improved by repeat rotator cuff repair. When inferior instability develops following surgery, exercises and time may be sufficient to allow this to resolve. Superior subluxation is often associated with rotator cuff disease. Anterior or posterior instability may be treated with closed reduction but may also require capsular repair with or without revision of the prosthetic components. Mechanical failure of constrained arthroplasty components will almost always require revision surgery, reinserting a component of the same system or components of a less constrained design. Loosening of constrained components may require removal of the components, or revision to a less constrained system might be considered. For glenoid loosening in the unconstrained designs of implants, revision surgery is considered for symptomatic patients. It will often include placement of a new, securely fixated glenoid component; however, the lack of bone remaining in the scapula may require component removal without replacement of a new glenoid part.

As can be appreciated from this discussion, the complications of shoulder arthroplasty are quite varied, as are their proposed solutions. There is not enough experience with each of these complications and their treatment alternatives for the literature to offer concrete suggestions about care for these problems. However, a number of the complications seen in the shoulder have been recognized in other anatomical regions, and treatment guidelines may be extrapolated from these other areas to the shoulder. Revision surgery in the shoulder does present some unique features. Mobility is a primary requisite of a satisfactorily functioning shoulder. The scar that has developed as a result of the disease process and the initial surgery may preclude an excellent result at the time of revision. Repeat rotator cuff surgery may be exceedingly difficult and require limited-goal rehabilitation following the revision procedure. Instability may be a combination of bone deficiency, component positioning, capsule and rotator cuff deficiency, or muscle weakness. It may be difficult to control all these variables, and instability following total shoulder arthroplasty may be exceedingly resistant to successful treatment.

References

1. Adams MA, Weiland AJ, and Moore JR: Nonconstrained total shoulder arthroplasty: An eight-year experience. Orthop Trans 10:232–233, 1986.
2. Agarwal A, Ferrante J, Schmidt R, and Eisenbeis CH: Bilateral giant cyst of the shoulder. Clin Exp Rheumatol 5:271–273, 1987.
3. Amstutz HC, Sew Hoy AL, and Clarke IC: UCLA anatomic total shoulder. Clin Orthop 155:7–20, 1981.
4. Amstutz HC: The Dana Shoulder Replacement. Howmedica, Inc.: Rutherford, NJ, 1982.
5. Amstutz HC, Thomas BJ, Kabo JM, et al: The Dana total shoulder arthroplasty. J Bone Joint Surg 70A:1174–1182, 1988.
6. Armbuster TG, Slivka J, Resnick D, et al: Extraarticular manifestations of septic arthritis of the glenohumeral joint. J Roentgenol 129:667–672, 1977.
7. Bade HA III, Warren RF, Ranawat C, and Inglis AE: Long term results of Neer total shoulder replacement. In Bateman JE, and Welsh RP (eds): Surgery of the Shoulder. St. Louis: CV Mosby Company, 1984, pp 294–302.
8. Baker GL, Oddis CV, and Medsger TA, Jr: Pasteurella multocida polyarticular septic arthritis. J Rheumatol 14:355–357, 1987.
9. Barton NJ: Arthrodesis of the shoulder for degenerative conditions. J Bone Joint Surg 54A:1759, 1972.
10. Bayley JIL, and Kessel L: The Kessel total shoulder replacement. In Bayley I, and Kessel L (eds): Shoulder Surgery. New York: Springer-Verlag, 1982, pp 160–164.
11. Bateman JE: Arthritis of the glenohumeral joint. In The Shoulder and Neck. Philadelphia: WB Saunders, 1978, pp 343–362.
12. Barrett WP, Franklin JL, Jackins SE, et al: Total shoulder arthroplasty. J Bone Joint Surg 69A:865–872, 1987.
13. Bechtol CO: Bechtol Total Shoulder. Richards Manufacturing Co.: Memphis, TN, 1976.
14. Becker W: Arthrodesis of the shoulder joint (review of 47 cases). In The Arthrodesis in the Restoration of Working Ability. Stuttgart: Georg Thieme, 1975, p 25.
15. Beddow FH, and Elloy MA: The Liverpool total replacement for the gleno-humeral joint. In Joint Replacement in the Upper Limb, I Mech E Conference Publications 1977–5. Conference Sponsored by the Medical Engineering Section of The Institution of Mechanical Engineers and the British Orthopaedic Association, London, 1977, pp 21–25.
16. Beddow FH, and Elloy MA: Clinical experience with the Liverpool shoulder replacement. In Bayley I, and Kessel L (eds): Shoulder Surgery. New York: Springer-Verlag, 1982, pp 164–167.
17. Bell S, and Gschwend N: Clinical experience with total arthroplasty and hemiarthroplasty of the shoulder using the Neer prosthesis. Int Orthop 10:217–222, 1986.
18. Beltran JE, Trilla JC, and Barjau R: A simplified compression arthrodesis of the shoulder. J Bone Joint Surg 57A:538, 1975.
19. Benhamou CL, Tourliere D, Brigant S, et al: Synovial metastasis of an adenocarcinoma presenting as a shoulder monoarthritis. J Rheumatol 15:1031–1033, 1988.
20. Benjamin A, Hirschowitz G, and Arden GP: The treatment of arthritis of the shoulder joint by double osteotomy. Int Orthop 3:211–216, 1979.
21. Benjamin A, Hirschowitz D, Arden GP, and Blackburn N: Double osteotomy of the shoulder. In Bayley I, and Kessel L (eds): Shoulder Surgery. New York: Springer Verlag, 1982, pp 170–175.
22. Blauth W, and Hepp WR: Arthrodesis of the shoulder joint by traction absorbing wiring. In Chapchal G. (ed): The Arthrodesis in the Restoration of Working Ability. Stuttgart: Georg Thieme, 1975, p 30.
23. Bodey WN, and Yeoman PM: Prosthetic arthroplasty of the shoulder. Acta Orthop Scand 54:900–903, 1983.
24. Bradford DS, Szalapski EW Jr, Sutherland DER, et al: Osteonecrosis in the transplant recipient. Surg Gynecol Obstet 159:328–334, 1984.
25. Brems JJ, Wilde AH, Borden LS, and Boumphrey FRS: Glenoid lucent lines. Orthop Trans 10:231, 1986.
26. Brett AL: A new method of arthrodesis of the shoulder joint, incorporating the control of the scapula. J Bone Joint Surg 15:969, 1933.
27. Brittain HA: Architectural Principles in Arthrodesis. Baltimore: Williams & Wilkins, 1942, p 1070.
28. Brownlee RC, and Cofield RH: Shoulder replacement in cuff tear arthropathy. Orthop Trans 10:230, 1986.
29. Buechel FF, Pappas MJ, and DePalma AF: "Floating-socket" total shoulder replacement: Anatomical, biomechanical, and surgical rationale. J Biomed Mater Res 12:89–114, 1978.

30. Burdge DR, Reid GD, Reeve CE, et al: Septic arthritis due to dual infection with Mycoplasma hominis and Ureaplasma urealyticum. J Rheumatol 15:366–368, 1988.

31. Burri C: Indication, technique and results in prosthetic replacement of the shoulder joint. Acta Orthop Belg 51:606–615, 1985.

32. Carroll RE: Wire loop in arthrodesis of the shoulder. Clin Orthop 9:185, 1957.

33. Casagrande PA: Surgical rehabilitation of shoulder and elbow in rheumatoid arthritis. Semin Arthritis Rheum 1:3–6, 1971.

34. Charnley J: Compression arthrodesis of the ankle and shoulder. J Bone Joint Surg 33B:180–191, 1951.

35. Charnley J, and Houston JK: Compression arthrodesis of the shoulder. J Bone Joint Surg 46B:614, 1964.

36. Cockx E, Claes T, Hoogmartens M, and Mulier JC: The isoelastic prosthesis for the shoulder joint. Acta Orthop Belg 49:275–285, 1983.

37. Cofield RH: Status of total shoulder arthroplasty. Arch Surg 112:1088–1091, 1977.

38. Cofield RH, and Stauffer RN: The Bickel glenohumeral arthroplasty. In Joint Replacement in the Upper Limb, I Mech E Conference Publications 1977–5. Mechanical Publications Limited for The Institution of Mechanical Engineers, 1977, London, pp 15–19.

39. Cofield RH, and Briggs BT: Glenohumeral arthritis. J Bone Joint Surg 61A:668–677, 1979.

40. Cofield RH: Unconstrained total shoulder prostheses. Clin Orthop 173:97–108, 1983.

41. Cofield RH: Arthrodesis and resection arthroplasty of the shoulder. In McCollister Evarts C (ed): Surgery of the Musculoskeletal System. New York: Churchill Livingstone, 1983, pp 109–124.

42. Cofield RH: Total shoulder arthroplasty: Associated disease of the rotator cuff, results, and complications. In Bateman JE, and Welsh RP (eds): Surgery of the Shoulder. St. Louis: CV Mosby, 1984, pp 229–233.

43. Cofield RH: Total shoulder arthroplasty with the Neer prosthesis. J Bone Joint Surg 66A:899–906, 1984.

44. Cofield RH: Shoulder arthrodesis and resection arthroplasty. AAOS Instruct Course Lect 34:268–277, 1985.

45. Cofield RH, and Berquist TH: The shoulder. In Berquist TH (ed): Imaging of Orthopaedic Trauma and Surgery. Philadelphia: WB Saunders, 1986, pp 499–566.

46. Cofield RH: Preliminary experience with bone ingrowth total shoulder arthroplasty. Orthop Trans 10:217, 1986.

47. Cofield RH: Total shoulder arthroplasty with bone ingrowth fixation. In Kölbel R, Helbig B, and Blauth W (eds): Shoulder Replacement. Berlin: Springer-Verlag, 1987, pp 209–212.

48. Cofield RH: Subscapularis tendon transposition for large rotator cuff tears. Techniques Orthop 3:58, 1989.

49. Cosendai A, Gerster JC, Vischer TL, et al: Destructive arthropathies associated with articular chondrocalcinosis. Clinical and metabolic study of 16 cases. Schweiz Med Wochenschr 106:8–14, 1976.

50. Coughlin MJ, Morris JM, and West WF: The semiconstrained total shoulder arthroplasty. J Bone Joint Surg 61A:574–581, 1979.

51. Craig EV: Continuous passive motion in the rehabilitation of the surgically reconstructed shoulder. Orthop Trans 10:233, 1986.

52. Crossan JF, and Vallance R: The shoulder joint in rheumatoid arthritis. In Bayley I, and Kessel L (eds): Shoulder Surgery. New York: Springer-Verlag, 1982, pp 131–143.

53. Cruess RL: Steroid-induced avascular necrosis of the head of the humerus. J Bone Joint Surg 58B:313–317, 1976.

54. Cruess RL: Corticosteroid-induced osteonecrosis of the humeral head. Orthop Clin North Am 16:789–796, 1985.

55. Cruess RL: Osteonecrosis of bone. Current concepts as to etiology and pathogenesis. Clin Orthop 208:30–39, 1986.

56. Curran JF, Ellman MH, and Brown NL: Rheumatologic aspects of painful conditions affecting the shoulder. Clin Orthop 173:27–37, 1983.

57. Davis JB, and Cottrell GW: A technique for shoulder arthrodesis. J Bone Joint Surg 44A:657, 1962.

58. Debrunner AM, and Cech O: Primär Stabile Schulterarthrodese. Z Orthop 13:82, 1975.

59. DeJager JP, and Fleming A: Shoulder joint rupture and pseudothrombosis in rheumatoid arthritis. Am Rheum Dis 43:503–504, 1984.

60. DeSmet AA, Ting YM, and Weiss JJ: Shoulder arthrography in rheumatoid arthritis. Diag Radiol 116:601–605, 1975.

61. De Velasco Polo G, and Cardoso Monterrubio A: Arthrodesis of the shoulder. Clin Orthop 90:178, 1973.

62. Dijkstra J, Dijkstra PF, and Klundert Wvd: Rheumatoid arthritis of the shoulder. Fortschr Röntgenstr 142:179–185, 1985.

63. Dorwart RH, Genant HK, Johnston WH, and Morris JM: Pigmented villonodular synovitis of synovial joints: clinical, pathologic, and radiologic features. AJR 143:87–885, 1984.

64. Dorwart RH, Genant HK, Johnston WH, and Morris JM: Pigmented villonodular synovitis of the shoulder: radiologic-pathologic assessment. AJR 143:886–888, 1984.

65. Doube A, and Calin A: Bacterial endocarditis presenting as acute monoarthritis. Ann Rheum Dis 47:598–599, 1988.

66. Drvaric DM, Rooks MD, Bishop A, and Jacobs LH: Neuropathic arthropathy of the shoulder. A case report. Orthopedics 11:301–304, 1988.

67. Egund N, Jonsson E, Lidgren L, et al: Computed tomography of humeral head cup arthroplasties. A preliminary report. Acta Radiol 28:71–73, 1987.

68. Ellman H, and Jinnah R: Experience with the Dana hooded component for cuff deficient shoulder arthroplasty. Orthop Trans 10:217, 1986.

69. Ellman MH, and Curran JJ: Causes and management of shoulder arthritis. Compr Ther 14:29–35, 1988.

70. Engelbrecht E, and Stellbrink G: Total Schulterendoprothese Modell "St. Georg." Chirurg 47:525–530, 1976.

71. Engelbrecht E, and Heinert K: More than ten years' experience with unconstrained shoulder replacement. In Kölbel R, Helbig B, and Blauth W (eds): Shoulder Replacement. Berlin: Springer-Verlag, 1987, pp 85–91.

72. Engelbrecht E: Ten years of experience with unconstrained shoulder replacement. In Bateman JE, and Welsh RP (eds): Surgery of the Shoulder. St. Louis: CV Mosby, 1984, pp 234–239.

73. Engelhardt P: 10-Jahres-Resultate bei Schulterarthrodese. Orthopäde 8:218–222, 1979.

74. Ennevaara K: Painful shoulder joint in rheumatoid arthritis: a clinical and radiological study of 200 cases with special reference to arthrography of the glenohumeral joint. Acta Rheum Scand [Suppl 11] pp 1–108, 1967.

75. Epps CH Jr: Painful hematologic conditions affecting the shoulder. Clin Orthop 173:38–43, 1983.

76. Faludi DD, and Weiland AJ: Cementless total shoulder arthroplasty: preliminary experience with thirteen cases. Orthopedics 6:431–437, 1982.

77. Fenlin JM, Jr: Total glenohumeral joint replacement. Orthop Clin North Am 6:565–583, 1975.

78. Fenlin JM: Semi-constrained prosthesis for the rotator cuff deficient patient. Orthop Trans 9:55, 1985.

79. Figgie HE III, Inglis AE, Goldberg VM, et al: An analysis of factors affecting the long-term results of total shoulder arthroplasty in inflammatory arthritis. J Arthroplasty 3:123–130, 1988.

80. Fishel B, Weiss S, Eventov E, et al: Chylous cyst of shoulder joint in a patient with rheumatoid arthritis. Clin Exp Rheumatol 6:79–80, 1988.

81. Fournie B, Railhac J-J, Monod P, et al: The enthesopathic shoulder. Rev Rhum Mal Osteoartic 54:447–451, 1987.

82. Franklin JL, Barrett WP, Jackins SE, and Matsen FA III: Glenoid loosening in total shoulder arthroplasty. J Arthroplasty 3:39–46, 1988.

83. Frich LH, Møller BN, and Sneppen O: Shoulder arthroplasty with the Neer Mark-II prosthesis. Arch Orthop Trauma Surg 107:110–113, 1988.

84. Friedman RJ, and Ewald FC: Arthroplasty of the ipsilateral shoulder and elbow in patients who have rheumatoid arthritis. J Bone Joint Surg 69A:661–666, 1987.

85. Fukuda K, Chen C-M, Cofield RH, and Chao EYS: Biomechanical analysis of stability and fixation strength of total shoulder prostheses. Orthopedics 11:141–149, 1988.

86. Garancis JC, Cheung HS, Halverson PB, and McCarty DJ: "Milwaukee shoulder"—association of microspheroids containing hydroxyapatite crystals, active collagenase, and neutral protease with rotator cuff defects. Arthritis Rheum 24:484–491, 1981.

87. Gariépy R: Glenoidectomy in the repair of the rheumatoid shoulder. J Bone Joint Surg 59B:122, 1977.

88. Gerard PrY, Leblanc J-P, and Rousseau B: Une prothèse totale d'épaule. Chirurgie 99:655–663, 1973.

89. Gill AB: A new operation for arthrodesis of the shoulder. J Bone Joint Surg 13:287, 1931.

90. Gompels BM, and Darlington LG: Septic arthritis in rheumatoid disease causing bilateral shoulder dislocation: Diagnosis and treatment assisted by grey scale ultrasonography. Ann Rheum Dis 40:609–611, 1981.

91. Gristina AG, and Webb LX: The trispherical total shoulder replacement. In Bayley I, and Kessel L (eds): Shoulder Surgery. New York: Springer-Verlag, 1982, pp 153–157.

92. Gristina AG, Webb LX, and Carter RE: The monospherical total shoulder. Orthop Trans 9:54, 1985.

93. Gristina AG, Romano RL, Kammire GC, and Webb LX: Total shoulder replacement. Orthop Clin North Am 18:445–453, 1987.

94. Gschwend N, and Kentsch A: Arthritic disorders. Surgery of the rheumatoid shoulder. In Bateman JE, and Welsh RP (eds): Surgery of the Shoulder. St. Louis: CV Mosby, 1984, pp 269–280.

95. Halverson PB, Cheung HS, McCarty DJ, et al: "Milwaukee shoulder"—association of microspheroids containing hydroxyapatite crystals, active collagenase, and neutral protease with rotator cuff defects. II. Synovial fluid studies. Arthritis Rheum 24:474–483, 1981.

96. Halverson PB, Cheung HS, and McCarty DJ: Enzymatic release of microspheroids containing hydroxyapatite crystals from synovium and of calcium pyrophosphate dihydrate crystals from cartilage. Ann Rheum Dis 41:527–531, 1982.

97. Halverson PB, Garancis JC, and McCarty DJ: Histopathological and ultrastructural studies of synovium in Milwaukee shoulder syndrome—a basic calcium phosphate crystal arthropathy. Ann Rheum Dis 43:734–741, 1984.

98. Halverson PB, McCarty DJ, Cheung HS, and Ryan LM: Milwaukee shoulder syndrome: eleven additional cases with involvement of the knee in seven (basic calcium phosphate crystal deposition disease). Semin Arthritis Rheum 14:36–44, 1984.

99. Hardin CW, and Manaster BJ: Rheumatoid arthritis with massive osteolysis and deformity of cervical spine; consequent neuropathic arthropathy of the shoulders. Skeletal Radiol 16:232–235, 1987.

100. Hauge MF: Arthrodesis of the shoulder: A simple elastic band appliance utilizing the compression principle. Acta Orthop Scand 31:272, 1961.

101. Hawkins RJ, Bell RH, and Jallay B: Experience with the Neer total shoulder arthroplasty: a review of 70 cases. Orthop Trans 10:232, 1986.

102. Hawkins RJ, Neer CS II, Pianta RM, and Mendoza FX: Locked posterior dislocation of the shoulder. J Bone Joint Surg 69A:9–18, 1987.

103. Hawkins RJ, and Neer CS II: A functional analysis of shoulder fusions. Clin Orthop 223:65–76, 1987.

104. Hjelkrem M, and Stanish WD: Synovial chondrometaplasia of the shoulder. A case report of a young athlete presenting with shoulder pain. Am J Sports Med 16:84–86, 1988.

105. Hucherson DC: Arthrodesis of the paralytic shoulder. Am Surg 25:430, 1959.

106. Hughes M, and Neer CS II: Glenohumeral joint replacement and postoperative rehabilitation. Physical Med 55:850–858, 1975.

107. Huston KA, Nelson AM, and Hunder GG: Shoulder swelling in rheumatoid arthritis secondary to subacromial bursitis. Arthritis Rheum 21:145–147, 1978.

108. Huten D, and Duparc J: L'arthroplastie prothétique dans les traumatismes complexes récents et anciens de l'épaule. Revue de Chir Orthop 72:517–529, 1986.

109. Huten D, Duparc J, Lajoie D, and Garcon P: Arthroplasty for shoulder injuries. Orthop Trans 12:206, 1988.

110. Johnson CA, Healy WL, Brooker AF Jr, and Krackow KA: External fixation shoulder arthrodesis. Clin Orthop 211:219–223, 1986.

111. Jones L: Reconstructive operation for nonreducible fractures of the head of the humerus. Ann Surg 97:217, 1933.

112. Jones L: The shoulder joint—observations on the anatomy and physiology: with an analysis of a reconstructive operation following extensive injury. Surg Gynecol Obstet 75:433, 1942.

113. Jónsson E, Egund N, Kelly I, et al: Cup arthroplasty of the rheumatoid shoulder. Acta Orthop Scand 57:542–546, 1986.

114. Jónsson E: Surgery of the Rheumatoid Shoulder with Special Reference to Cup Hemiarthroplasty and Arthrodesis. The University Department of Orthopaedics, Lund, Sweden. Malmo, Sweden: Infotryck, 1988.

115. Jónsson E, Brattström M, and Lidgren L: Evaluation of the rheumatoid shoulder function after hemiarthroplasty and arthrodesis. Scand J Rheumatol 17:17–26, 1988.

116. Kalamchi A: Arthrodesis for paralytic shoulder: review of ten patients. Orthopedics 1:204–208, 1978.

117. Kay SP, and Amstutz HC: Shoulder arthroplasty at UCLA. Clin Orthop 228:42–48, 1988.

118. Kelly IG, Foster RS, and Fisher WD: Neer total shoulder replacement in rheumatoid arthritis. J Bone Joint Surg 69B:723–726, 1987.

119. Kenmore PI, MacCartee C, and Vitek B: A simple shoulder replacement. J Biomed Mater Res 5:329–330, 1974.

120. Kenzora JE, and Glimcher MJ: Pathogenesis of idiopathic osteonecrosis: the ubiquitous crescent sign. Orthop Clin North Am 16:681–696, 1985.

121. Kerr R, Resnick D, Pineda C, and Haghigli P: Osteoarthritis of the glenohumeral joint: a radiologic-pathologic study. AJR 144:967–972, 1985.

122. Kessel L, and Bayley JL: The Kessel total shoulder replacement. In Shoulder Surgery. New York: Springer-Verlag, 1982, pp 160–164.

123. Kirschner Medical Corporation: The New Neer II-C and the Neer II. Fairlawn, NJ.

124. Knight RA, and Mayne JA: Comminuted fractures and fracture-dislocations involving the articular surface of the humeral head. J Bone Joint Surg 39A:1343, 1957.

125. Kölbel R, and Friedebold G: Schultergelenkersatz. Z Orthop 113:452–454, 1975.

126. Kölbel R, Rohlmann A, and Bergmann G: Biomechanical considerations in the design of a semi-constrained total shoulder replacement. In Bayley I, and Kessel L (eds): Shoulder Surgery. New York: Springer-Verlag, 1982, pp 144–152.

127. Kraft SM, Panush RS, and Longley S: Unrecognized staphylococcal pyarthrosis with rheumatoid arthritis. Semin Arthritis Rheum 14:196–201, 1985.

128. Krueger FJ: A Vitallium replica arthroplasty on the shoulder. A case report of aseptic necrosis of the proximal end of the humerus. Surgery 30:1005–1011, 1951.

129. Laine VAI, Vainio KJ, and Pekanmaki K: Shoulder affections in rheumatoid arthritis. Ann Rheum Dis 13:157–160, 1954.

130. Laumann U, and Schilgen L: Varisierende subkapitale Osteotomie in Verbindung mit Schulterarthrodese und Oberarmamputation bei Plexusparese. Z Orthop 115:787, 1977.

131. Lettin AWF, Copeland SA, and Scales JT: The Stanmore total shoulder replacement. J Bone Joint Surg 64B:47–51, 1982.

132. Levine RB, and Sullivan KL: Rheumatoid arthritis: skeletal manifestations observed on portable chest roentgenograms. Skeletal Radiol 13:295–303, 1985.

133. Lugli T: Artificial shoulder joint by Péan (1893). The facts of an exceptional intervention and the prosthetic method. Clin Orthop 133:215–218, 1978.

134. Marks SH, Barnett M, and Calin A: Ankylosing spondylitis in women and men: a case-control study. J Rheumatol 10:624–628, 1983.

135. Mason JM: The treatment of dislocation of the shoulder-joint complicated by fracture of the upper extremity of the humerus. Ann Surg 47:672, 1908.

136. Matsunaga M: A new method of arthrodesis of the shoulder. Acta Orthop Scand 43:343, 1972.

137. Mau H, and Nebinger G: Arthropathy of the shoulder joint in syringomyelia. Z Orthop 124:157–164, 1986.

138. May VR Jr: Shoulder fusion: a review of 14 cases. J Bone Joint Surg 44A:65, 1962.

139. Mazas F, and de la Caffinière JY: Une prothèse totale d'épaule non rétentive. A propos de 38 cas. Revue Chir Orthop 68:161–170, 1982.

140. McCarty DJ, Halverson PB, Carrera GF, et al: "Milwaukee shoulder"—association of microspheroids containing hydroxyapatite crystals, active collagenase, and neutral protease with rotator cuff defects. I. Clinical aspects. Arthritis Rheum 24:464–473, 1981.

141. McCarty D: Crystals, joints, and consternation. Ann Rheum Dis 42:243–253, 1983.

142. McElwain JP, and English E: The early results of porous-coated total shoulder arthroplasty. Clin Orthop 218:217–224, 1987.

143. Meachim G: Effect of age on the thickness of adult articular cartilage at the shoulder joint. Ann Rheum Dis 30:43–46, 1971.

144. Medsger TA, Dixon JA, and Garwood VF: Palmar fasciitis and polyarthritis associated with ovarian carcinoma. Ann Intern Med 96:424–432, 1982.

145. Meythaler JM, Reddy NM, and Mitz M: Serratus anterior disruption: a complication of rheumatoid arthritis. Arch Phys Med Rehabil 67:770–772, 1986.

146. Mills KL: Severe injuries of the upper end of the humerus. Injury 6:13, 1974.

147. Neer CS, Brown TH Jr, and McLaughlin HL: Fracture of the neck of the humerus with dislocation of the head fragment. Am J Surg 85:252–258, 1953.

148. Neer CS II: Articular replacement for the humeral head. J Bone Joint Surg 37A:215–228, 1955.

149. Neer CS II: Follow-up notes on articles previously published in the journal. Articular replacement for the humeral head. J Bone Joint Surg 46A:1607–1610, 1964.

150. Neer CS II: The rheumatoid shoulder. In Cruess RR, and Mitchell NS (eds): Surgery of Rheumatoid Arthritis. Philadelphia: JB Lippincott, 1971, pp 117–125.

151. Neer CS II: Replacement arthroplasty for glenohumeral osteoarthritis. J Bone Joint Surg 56A:1–13, 1974.

152. Neer CS II: Reconstructive surgery and rehabilitation of the shoulder. In Kelley WN, Harris ED, Jr, Ruddy S, and Sledge CB (eds): Textbook of Rheumatology. Philadelphia: WB Saunders, 1981, pp 1944–1959.

153. Neer CS II: Surgical Protocol. Neer II Proximal Humerus. Arthroplasty of the Shoulder: Neer Technique. St. Paul, MN: Minnesota Mining and Manufacturing Company, 1982.

154. Neer CS II, and Kirby RM: Revision of the humeral head and total shoulder arthroplasties. Clin Orthop 170:189–195, 1982.

155. Neer CS II, Watson KC, and Stanton FJ: Recent experience in total shoulder replacement. J Bone Joint Surg 64A:319–337, 1982.

156. Neer CS II, Craig EV, and Fukuda H: Cuff-tear arthropathy. J Bone Joint Surg 65A:1232–1244, 1983.

157. Neer CS II, McCann PD, Macfarlane EA, and Padilla N: Earlier passive motion following shoulder arthroplasty and rotator cuff repair. A prospective study. Orthop Trans 2:231, 1987.

158. Neer CS, and Morrison DS: Glenoid bone-grafting in total shoulder arthroplasty. J Bone Joint Surg 70A:1154–1162, 1988.

159. Neviaser RJ, and Neviaser TJ: Transfer of subscapularis and teres minor for massive defects of the rotator cuff. In Bayley I, and Kessel L (eds): Shoulder Surgery. New York: Springer-Verlag, 1982, pp 60–63.

160. Nussbaum AJ, and Doppman JL: Shoulder arthropathy in primary hyperparathyroidism. Skeletal Radiol 9:98–102, 1982.

161. Orr TE, and Carter DR: Stress analyses of joint arthroplasty in the proximal humerus. J Orthop Res 3:360–371, 1985.

162. Ovesen J, and Nielsen S: Prosthesis position in shoulder arthroplasty. Acta Orthop Scand 56:330–331, 1985.

163. Ovesen J, Sojbjerg JO, and Sneppen O: A humeral head cutting guide: instrument to secure correct humeral component retroversion in shoulder joint arthroplasty. Clin Orthop 216:193–194, 1987.

164. Pahle JA, and Kvarnes L: Shoulder synovectomy. Ann Chirurg Gynaecol [74 Suppl] 198:37–39, 1985.

165. Petersson CJ: Degeneration of the gleno-humeral joint. Acta Orthop Scand 54:277–283, 1983.

166. Petersson CJ: Painful shoulders in patients with rheumatoid arthritis. Scand J Rheum 15:275–279, 1986.

167. Petersson CJ: Shoulder surgery in rheumatoid arthritis. Acta Orthop Scand 57:222–226, 1986.

168. Podgorski M, Robinson B, Weissberger A, et al: Articular manifestations of acromegaly. Aust NZ J Med 18:28–35, 1988.

169. Post M, and Haskell S: Michael Reese Total Shoulder. Memphis TN: Richards Manufacturing Company, Inc., 1978.

170. Post M, Jablon M, Miller H, and Singh M: Constrained total shoulder joint replacement: a critical review. Clin Orthop 144:135–150, 1979.

171. Post M, Haskell SS, and Jablon M: Total shoulder replacement with a constrained prosthesis. J Bone Joint Surg 62A:327–335, 1980.

172. Post M: Constrained arthroplasty of the shoulder. In Neviaser RJ (ed): Orthopedic Clinics of North America. Philadelphia: WB Saunders, 1987, pp 455–462.

173. Post M: Shoulder arthroplasty and total shoulder replacement. In Post, M (ed): The Shoulder. Philadelphia: Lea & Febiger, 1988, pp 221–278.

174. Pritchett JW, and Clark JM: Prosthetic replacement for chronic unreduced dislocations of the shoulder. Clin Orthop 216:89–93, 1987.

175. Putti V: Artrodesi nella tubercolosi del Ginocchio e della Spalla. Chir Organi Mov 18:217, 1933.

176. Rand JA, and Sim FH: Total shoulder arthroplasty for the arthroplasty of hemochromatosis: a case report. Orthopedics 4:658–660, 1981.

177. Rask MR: Suprascapular axonotmesis and rheumatoid disease: report of a case treated conservatively. Clin Orthop 134:266–267, 1978.

178. Reeves B, Jobbins B, Dowson D, and Wright V: A total shoulder endo-prosthesis. Eng Med 1:64–67, 1974.

179. Rhoades CE, Neff JR, Rengachary SS, et al: Diagnosis of post-traumatic syringohydromyelia presenting as neuropathic joints. Clin Orthop 180:182–187, 1983.

180. Richard A, Judet R, and René L: Acrylic prosthetic reconstruction of the upper end of the humerus for fracture-luxations. J Chir 68:537–547, 1952.

181. Richards RR, Waddell JP, and Hudson AR: Shoulder arthrodesis for the treatment of brachial plexus palsy. Clin Orthop 198:250–258, 1985.

182. Richards RR, Sherman RMP, Hudson AR, and Waddell JP: Shoulder arthrodesis using a pelvic-reconstruction plate. J Bone Joint Surg 70A:416–421, 1988.

183. Riggins RS: Shoulder fusion without external fixation: a preliminary report. J Bone Joint Surg 58A:1007, 1976.

184. Rossleigh MA, Smith J, Straus DJ, and Engel IA: Osteonecrosis in patients with malignant lymphoma. Cancer 58:1112–1116, 1986.

185. Rountree CR, and Rockwood CA Jr: Arthrodesis of the shoulder in children following infantile paralysis. South Med J 58:861, 1959.

186. Rowe CR: Re-evaluation of the position of the arm in arthrodesis of the shoulder in the adult. J Bone Joint Surg 56A:913, 1974.

187. Rowe CR, and Zarins B: Chronic unreduced dislocations of the shoulder. J Bone Joint Surg 64A:494–505, 1982.

188. Russe O: Schulterarthrodese nach der AO-methode. Unfallheilkunde 81:299, 1978.

189. Rutherford CS, and Cofield RH: Osteonecrosis of the shoulder. Orthop Trans 11:239, 1987.

190. Rybka V, Raunio P, and Vainio K: Arthrodesis of the shoulder in rheumatoid arthritis: a review of 41 cases. J Bone Joint Surg 61B:155, 1979.

191. Saha AK, Bhattacharyya D, and Dutta SK: Total Shoulder Replacement. A Preliminary Report. Calcutta: SK Sircar, 1975.

192. Salzer M, Knahr K, Locke H, et al: A bioceramic endoprosthesis for the replacement of the proximal humerus. Arch Orthop Trauma Surg 93:169–184, 1979.

193. Samilson RL, and Prieto V: Dislocation arthropathy of the shoulder. J Bone Joint Surg 65A:456–460, 1983.

194. Sharon E, Vieux U, and Seckler SG: Giant synovial cyst of the shoulder and perforation of the nasal septum in (a patient with) rheumatoid arthritis. Mt Sinai J Med (NY), 45:103–105, 1978.

195. Sillár P, Mészáros T, Horváth F, et al: Gerontological aspects of degenerative changes of the shoulder-joint. Z Alternsforsch 34:411–421, 1979.

196. Silver R, and Post M: Post-traumatic resection of the proximal humerus. Orthopaedic Consultation 4:1–12, 1983.

197. Simon L, Pjol H, Blotman F, and Pelissier J: Aspects of the pathology of the arm after irradiation of breast cancer. Rev Rheum Mal Osteoartic 43:133–140, 1976.

198. Smith-Peterson MN, Aufranc OE, and Larson CB: Useful surgical procedures for rheumatoid arthritis involving joints of the upper extremity. Arch Surg 46:764–770, 1943.

199. Souter WA: The surgical treatment of the rheumatoid shoulder. Ann Acad Med 12:243–255, 1983.

200. Spencer R, and Skirving AP: Silastic interposition arthroplasty of the shoulder. J Bone Joint Surg 68B:375–377, 1986.

201. Steffee AD, and Moore RW: Hemi-resurfacing arthroplasty of the shoulder. Contemp Orthop 9:51–59, 1984.

202. Steindler A: Orthopedic Operations: Indications, Technique, and End Results. Springfield, IL: Charles C Thomas, 1940, p 302.

203. Steindler A: Arthrodesis of the shoulder. AAOS Instruct Course Lect 2:293, 1944.

204. Svend-Hansen H: Displaced proximal humeral fractures: a review of 49 patients. Acta Orthop Scand 45:359, 1974.

205. Swanson AB: Implant resection arthroplasty of shoulder joint. In Swanson AB (ed): Flexible Resection Arthroplasty in the Hand and Extremities. St. Louis: CV Mosby, 1973, pp 287–295.

206. Swanson AB: Bipolar implant shoulder arthroplasty. In Bateman JE, and Welsh RP (eds): Surgery of the Shoulder. St. Louis: CV Mosby, 1984, pp 211–223.

207. Swanson AB, deGroot G, Maupin BK, et al: Bipolar implant shoulder arthroplasty. Orthopedics 9:343–351, 1986.

208. Svend-Hansen H: Displaced proximal humeral fractures: A review of 49 patients. Acta Orthop Scand 45:359, 1974.

209. Tanner MW, and Cofield RH: Prosthetic arthroplasty for fractures and fracture-dislocations of the proximal humerus. Clin Orthop 179:116–128, 1983.

210. Tillmann K, and Braatz D: Results of resection arthroplasty and the Benjamin double osteotomy. In Kölbel R, Helbig B, and Blauth W (eds): Shoulder Replacement. Berlin: Springer-Verlag, 1987, pp 47–50.

211. Tonino AJ, and van de Werf GJIM: Hemi arthroplasty of the shoulder. Acta Orthop Belg 51:625–631, 1985.

212. Tully JG Jr, and Latteri A: Paraplegia, syringomyelia tarda and neuropathic arthrosis of the shoulder: a triad. Clin Orthop 134:244–248, 1978.

213. Uematsu A: Arthrodesis of the shoulder: posterior approach. Clin Orthop 139:169, 1979.

214. Vainio K: Orthopaedic surgery in the treatment of rheumatoid arthritis. Ann Clin Res 7:216–224, 1975.

215. Varian JPW: Interposition Silastic cup arthroplasty of the shoulder. J Bone Joint Surg 62B:116–117, 1980.

216. Wainwright D: Glenoidectomy in the treatment of the painful arthritic shoulder (abstract). J Bone Joint Surg 58B:377, 1976.

217. Watson-Jones RW: Extra-articular arthrodesis of the shoulder. J Bone Joint Surg 15:862, 1933.

218. Weigert M, and Gronert HJ: Zur Technik der Schultergelenk-sarthrodese. Z Orthop 112:1281, 1974.

219. Weiss JJ, Good A, and Schumacher HR: Four cases of "Milwaukee shoulder" with a description of clinical presentation and long-term treatment. J Am Geriatr Soc 33:202–205, 1985.

220. Weiss JJ, Thompson GR, Doust V, and Burgener F: Rotator cuff tears in rheumatoid arthritis. Arch Intern Med 135:521–525, 1975.

221. Wheble VH, and Skorecki J: The design of a metal-to-metal total shoulder joint prosthesis. In Joint Replacement in the Upper Limb. I Mech E Conference Publications 1977–5. Conference sponsored by the Medical Engineering Section of the Institution of Mechanical Engineers and the British Orthopaedic Association, London, 1977, pp 7–13.

222. Wilde AH, Borden LS, and Brems JJ: Experience with the Neer total shoulder replacement. In Bateman JE, and Welsh RP (eds): Surgery of the Shoulder. St. Louis: CV Mosby, 1984, pp 224–228.

223. Wolff R, and Kölbel R: The history of shoulder joint replacement. In Kölbel R, Helbig B, and Blauth W (eds): Shoulder Replacement. Berlin: Springer-Verlag, 1987, pp 3–13.

224. Woolf AD, Cawston TE, and Dieppe PA: Idiopathic haemorrhagic rupture of the shoulder in destructive disease of the elderly. Ann Rheum Dis 45:498–501, 1986.

225. Zimmer Total Shoulder Prostheses, Specialty Product Services, Research and Development Department, Warsaw, IN.

226. Zippel J: Luxationssichere Schulterendoprothese Modell BME. Z Orthop 113:454–457, 1975.

227. Zuckerman JD, and Matsen FA III: Complications about the glenohumeral joint related to the use of screws and staples. J Bone Joint Surg 66A:175–180, 1984.

228. Zuckerman JD, and Cofield RH: Proximal humeral prosthetic replacement in glenohumeral arthritis. Orthop Trans 10:231, 1986.

Neurological Problems

Robert D. Leffert, M.D.

The shoulder girdle and its environs encompass an anatomical area that constitutes a meeting ground for the interests of orthopedics, neurology, neurosurgery, and vascular and thoracic surgery, since all of these specialties are concerned with disorders that are manifested in this same region. Yet it is precisely because of this overlapping of interest that patients with clinical problems in this area may fail to obtain diagnosis and treatment since each specialty may assume that the problem belongs to someone else. This is particularly true for neurological problems, since they tend to be relatively uncommon and symptoms are often vague and difficult to interpret. Differential diagnosis may involve consideration of entities that are rarely encountered or are totally unknown to the orthopedic surgeon.[71]

The understanding of the function of the normal shoulder is totally dependent on anatomical and biomechanical considerations, which are thoroughly covered in other chapters of this book, so that no attempt will be made to recapitulate that material in detail. In addition, there are several useful references to which the reader is directed.[32, 39, 45, 84, 86] However, from the study of abnormal shoulders, and particularly those paralyzed by poliomyelitis, comes much of the information that we have regarding the treatment of neurological problems. This is not surprising since the disease has provided a continuous supply of patients with paralysis of virtually every muscle in the upper limb, and it was only natural that their patterns of motor loss should be studied.

Probably the most intensive work on this subject is that of Duchenne, the 19th century anatomist whose masterful treatise *The Physiology of Motion* was translated by E. B. Kaplan in 1949.[22] It should be consulted by anyone interested in motor loss or who would do tendon transfers about the shoulder (Fig. 18–1). In this century, the curator of this subject was Arthur Steindler, whose book *Kinesiology*[83] and contributions to the armamentarium of surgical procedures have been of enormous value. Among the many who have contributed to our understanding of the surgical reconstruction of the shoulder paralyzed by polio are Schottsteadt, Larsen, and Bost,[72] Ober,[59] Harmon,[28] Saha[70] and others.[51]

After the virtual elimination of poliomyelitis as a serious cause of paralysis in the industrialized world, brachial plexus injuries became the most common cause of shoulder paralysis, and many of the lessons that were learned from the polio experience were applied to plexus injuries. Sir Herbert Seddon and the

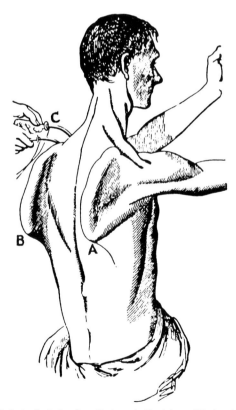

Figure 18–1. An illustration from Duchenne's Physiology of Motion showing the winging of the scapula caused by paralysis of the serratus anterior *(A)*, and a similar deformity elicited experimentally by electrical stimulation of the deltoid *(B)*. (Reproduced with permission from Duchenne GB: The Physiology of Motion (trans. EB Kaplan.) Philadelphia: WB Saunders, 1959.)

group that he inspired at the Royal National Orthopaedic Hospital in London contributed significantly to our knowledge.[6, 10, 43, 72, 74]

It is of interest that the relatively recent advances in nerve repair for the brachial plexus have not proved to be as dramatically beneficial to the restoration of adult shoulder function as those for the elbow or wrist. Finally, as techniques of surgical reconstruction and rehabilitation have become more widespread, they have also been applied to treatment of the paralytic shoulder of muscular dystrophy and the shoulders of stroke patients.[13, 55] Suffice it to say that the need for work in this area continues.

Clinical Presentation

Clearly, when there has been a history of trauma to the shoulder and there is a localized neurological deficit, there should be little diagnostic confusion as to the cause. Nevertheless, when patients who have sustained multisystem trauma are first encountered, either in a life-threatening situation or under anesthesia when they cannot be properly examined by the soon-to-be-treating orthopedist, a potentially difficult situation can arise if a nerve injury is recognized after treatment. Inasmuch as possible, these difficulties can be minimized by careful preoperative evaluation, including a detailed neurological examination, which takes surprisingly little time to accomplish.

The history and presenting complaints generated by a neurological problem about the shoulder may be complicated by the anatomical situation of the shoulder as a "way station" through which the nerves and vessels to the upper limb must pass. Consequently, there may be local shoulder discomfort referred from lesions of the spinal cord or the cervical roots. In brachial plexus injuries or thoracic outlet syndrome, nerves have been affected by pathology in the region of the shoulder, yet the symptoms will appear further distally in the arm or hand.

The anatomy of the brachial plexus is shown in Figure 18–2. In addition, since cervical radiculopathy may be expressed as pain, paresthesias, or motor weakness in the limb, Figures 18–3 and 18–4 summarize the segmental distribution of the motor and sensory components of the nerve supply.

Consideration must also be given to those referred pains that originate in the pleural or abdominal cavities but are interpreted as shoulder pain. One does see the occasional patient whose cholecystitis is manifested as shoulder pain, and there are others whose intrapleural or cardiac problems can be diagnostic challenges. Consider the patient who recently came to my office with the complaint that his frozen shoulders were symptomatic when he was walking against the wind or up stairs.

General medical history and family history are extremely important. When one sees the painless and atraumatic onset of weakness and atrophy about the shoulder girdle of a patient in the first or second decades of life, and especially if the condition is bilateral, one must consider the possibility of an underlying neurological disease, either neurogenic or myopathic. A positive family history may often be obtained.[1, 5, 23]

The physical examination must begin with the head and neck, since it is not at all uncommon for shoulder pain to come from discogenic radiculopathy. Foramenal closure tests, done by gently hyperextending the cervical spine and laterally flexing it to the affected side, may completely reproduce the patient's shoulder pain and exonerate this joint as the culprit. It should be remembered, however, that patients may have pathology and symptoms coming from both areas at the same time, and each area may require treatment.

The entire upper limb must be examined next, and a thorough manual muscle test and sensory examination must be conducted and recorded. The contralateral limb must be similarly examined, and when indicated, particularly if a generalized neurological condition is suspected, the lower extremities must be evaluated. The deep tendon responses are tested, since the finding of hyper-reflexia or pathological plantar responses will indicate the presence of an upper motor neuron lesion. Because it is not unheard of for an intracranial or intraspinal lesion to present as a disability of the upper limb and sometimes of the shoulder girdle, we must not forget this possibility or neglect to examine the patient with this in mind.

I am reminded of a personal case many years ago of a woman who had a particularly intractable case of frozen shoulder with reflex sympathetic dystrophy. Ultimately, a brain tumor was found to be the cause of her inability to move the limb. I have also seen three relatively young women who had been thought to have thoracic outlet syndrome (TOS) and who ultimately proved to have apical lung tumors.

X-ray and Laboratory Evaluation

In all patients in whom there is a neurological disorder about the shoulder or one further distally in the limb that is felt to originate proximally, it is most important to obtain plain radiographs of the shoulder and cervical spine in three planes (Fig. 18–5). This is important even in cases where there is no known bony injury, such as brachial plexus trauma without clinically obvious fractures. In such patients it behooves us to look for displaced fractures of the cervical transverse processes, since they are presumptive evidence of avulsion of cervical nerve roots.[75] Patients with thoracic outlet syndrome may have cervical ribs or long transverse processes at C7 that may materially contribute to the problem of compression, although only about 20 per cent of patients in whom I make the diagnosis of thoracic outlet syndrome do have such bony abnor-

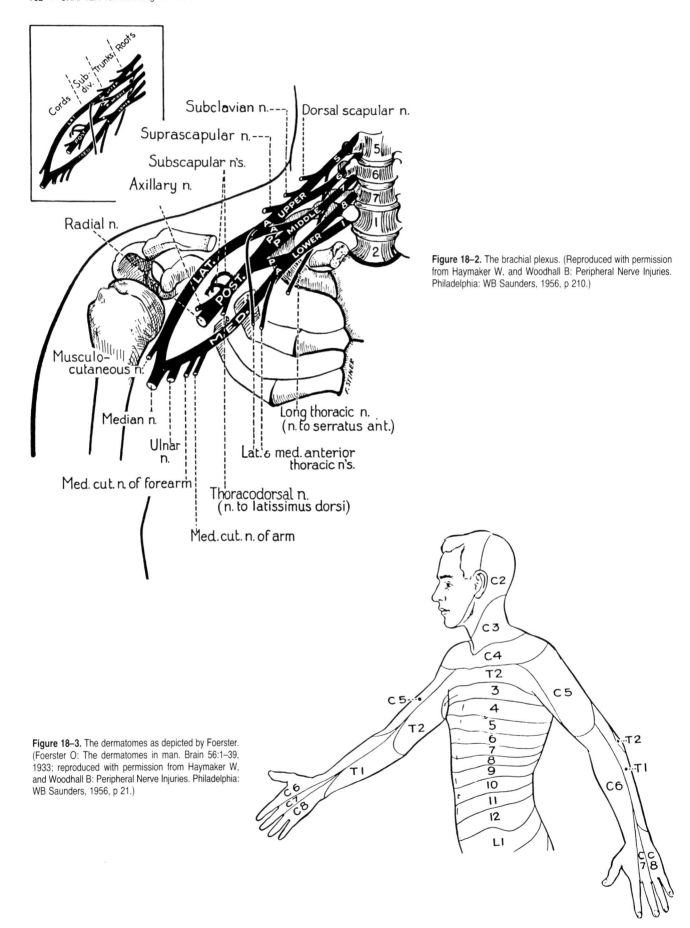

Figure 18–2. The brachial plexus. (Reproduced with permission from Haymaker W, and Woodhall B: Peripheral Nerve Injuries. Philadelphia: WB Saunders, 1956, p 210.)

Figure 18–3. The dermatomes as depicted by Foerster. (Foerster O: The dermatomes in man. Brain 56:1–39, 1933; reproduced with permission from Haymaker W, and Woodhall B: Peripheral Nerve Injuries. Philadelphia: WB Saunders, 1956, p 21.)

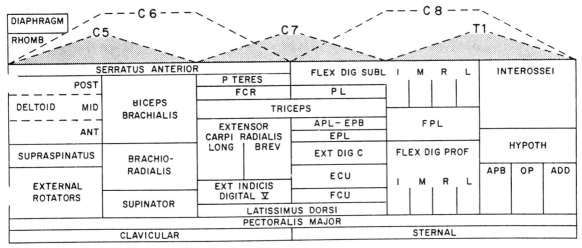

Figure 18–4. The segmental supply of the muscles of the upper limb. (Reproduced with permission from Leffert RD: Brachial Plexus Injuries. New York: Churchill Livingstone, 1985, p 76.)

malities. In some patients with TOS, an ununited or malunited clavicular fracture may be present.[36]

Occasionally one may see a nerve lesion that has occurred as a result of a totally unsuspected bone tumor. In addition, chest x-rays, particularly in patients who smoke, are helpful, since lesions of the apical pleura can be the reason for pain in the shoulder (Fig. 18–6). When there is suspicion of pathology that cannot be clearly demonstrated by plain radiographs, tomography or computer-assisted tomography may be help-

ful. The use of magnetic resonance imaging of the cervical spine has materially advanced the diagnosis of discogenic radiculopathy and many other lesions about the shoulder.

Arthrography of the shoulder joint is particularly useful in differential diagnosis of atrophy and weakness of the supraspinatus and infraspinatus. This finding may be due to a lesion of the suprascapular nerve[62] or a rotator cuff tear, and sometimes, although not commonly, the two may coexist. Ultrasonography and

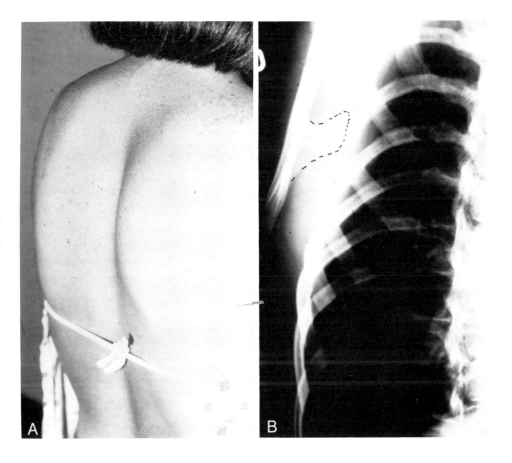

Figure 18–5. *A*, A 24-year-old woman referred with a diagnosis of winged scapula thought to be due to an idiopathic serratus palsy. *B*, Axial view of her scapula showing the large osteochondroma that was the cause of her problem. There was complete relief of the deformity following removal of the lesion.

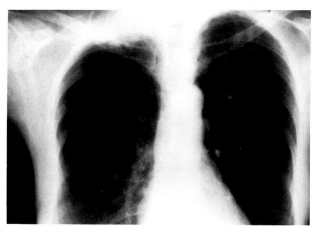

Figure 18–6. Chest radiograph of a 38-year-old woman with undiagnosed pain in the right shoulder. The patient smoked two packs of cigarettes a day.

magnetic resonance imaging can provide alternative means of obtaining much of the same information and may, in specific cases, be preferable. Nevertheless, a patient with severe atrophy thought to be caused by a suprascapular nerve lesion ought to have an arthrogram or equivalent, and one with a cuff tear and an unexpectedly severe degree of atrophy should have an EMG.

Electrodiagnostic testing may be tremendously helpful in refining the clinical diagnosis of a neurological disorder in those situations in which there is a lower

motor neuron lesion.[3, 41, 79, 89] Electromyography may reveal extension of the pathological process beyond the confines of a single peripheral nerve, as in the case of idiopathic brachial neuritis,[92] or may indicate that the observed neuropathy is part of a generalized peripheral neuropathy. Although a detailed consideration of the fine points of electromyographic theory and practice is probably not necessary for most orthopedic surgeons, a basic understanding of its applications and limitations is as necessary as the corresponding considerations of bone radiology. A general discussion of the pathology of nerve injury and electromyographic findings is to be found in the next section of this chapter.

The use of nerve conduction velocity determination, an extension of the EMG, may help to further localize a specific lesion along the length of the motor unit and peripheral nerve. The specific applications will be described within the sections devoted to particular entities.

Electromyography is also very useful in the identification of myopathies of a chronic nature such as muscular dystrophy. It may be difficult to classify precisely myopathies of an acute nature, such as acute polymyositis, on the basis of EMG, but these disorders are not confined to the shoulder girdles, which are more likely to be affected by the localized fascioscapulohumeral (Fig. 18–7) or limb girdle dystrophies. In these cases, diagnosis will have to include further study of muscle biopsies by means of electronmicroscopy and

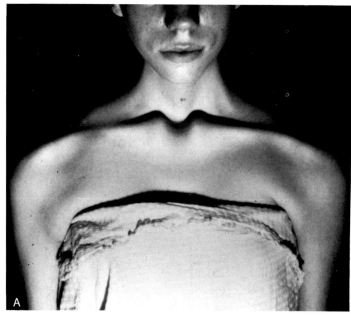

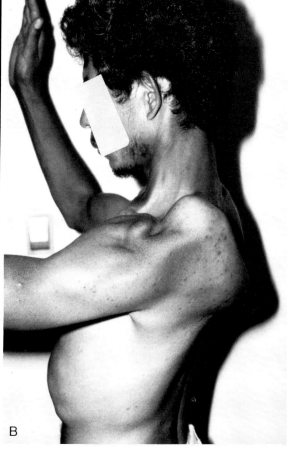

Figure 18–7. *A,* A patient with fascioscapulohumeral muscular dystrophy causing severe atrophy and weakness about the shoulder girdles. *B,* Another patient with fascioscapulohumeral dystrophy. The deltoid has been preserved, but the scapulothoracic muscles are paralyzed.

histochemistry. The study of serum enzymes will also be an important part of the evaluation.[5]

Pathology and Classification

The classification of all disorders of the nervous system that can affect shoulder function or be influenced by pathology in the region of the shoulder joint complex can be approached in several ways. It makes little sense merely to list as many diseases as possible for the sake of being inclusive, since this is not a textbook of neurology. Rather, it would appear appropriate to group these diseases according to the unique functional consequences that will have to be addressed by the shoulder surgeon during the course of treatment. No attempt will be made to be encyclopedic, although the more commonly encountered entities will be included under the category in which the most pronounced manifestation belongs.

In addition, because of the varying pathology inherent in traumatic lesions of the peripheral nerves and their problems of prognostication, it will be necessary to discuss their specific classification.

Finally, we will complete this section of the chapter with a discussion of the differential diagnosis of organic and functional causes of dysfunction of the shoulder complex.

CLASSIFICATION OF NEUROLOGICAL DISEASES PRODUCING SHOULDER DYSFUNCTION

Neurological diseases that produce shoulder dysfunction include:
1. Upper motor neuron diseases
   A. Stroke
   B. Head injury
   C. Tumors of brain and spinal cord
   D. Cerebral palsy
   E. Multiple sclerosis
2. Lower motor neuron diseases
   A. Idiopathic brachial neuritis
   B. Infectious or idiopathic myelopathy or neuropathy
      (1) Poliomyelitis
      (2) Guillain Barré syndrome
      (3) Motor neuron disease (progressive muscular atrophy)
      (4) Herpes zoster
      (5) Mononeuritis multiplex, metabolic or other
      (6) Diffuse peripheral neuropathy
   C. Brachial plexus injuries
      (1) Supraclavicular
      (2) Subclavicular
      (3) Infraclavicular
      (4) Open wounds
      (5) Postanesthetic palsy
      (6) Radiation neuropathy

   D. Cervical radiculopathy, discogenic or due to spondylosis
   E. Spinal cord tumors (intrinsic or extrinsic)
   F. Compression neuropathy
      (1) Suprascapular nerve
      (2) Thoracic outlet syndrome
      (3) Quadrilateral space syndrome
   G. Cranial nerve injury
      (1) Spinal accessory nerve
   H. Peripheral nerve injuries
      (1) Axillary
      (2) Musculocutaneous
      (3) Long thoracic
      (4) Suprascapular
3. Myopathies
   A. Muscular dystrophy
      (1) X-linked
         (a) Duchenne, Becker
      (2) Autosomal recessive
         (a) Limb girdle, scapulohumeral
         (b) Childhood
         (c) Congenital
      (3) Autosomal dominant
         (a) Fascioscapulohumeral
   B. Metabolic myopathies
   C. Inflammatory myopathies
      (1) Polymyositis
      (2) Dermatomyositis
   D. Endocrine myopathies
   E. Toxic and drug-induced myopathies
4. Mixed pathology and miscellaneous
   A. Reflex sympathetic dystrophy
      (1) Shoulder-hand syndrome
   B. Arthrogryposis

CLASSIFICATION OF THE PATHOLOGY OF PERIPHERAL NERVE INJURIES

With the publication in 1934 of his seminal article, "Three Types of Nerve Injury," H. J. Seddon provided clinicians with a common language by which they could not only describe a nerve injury, but also understand the nature of the pathology and the basis for the prognosis, as well as formulate a rational treatment program.[73]

The first grade of nerve injury, neurapraxia (nonaction of nerve) describes the most benign situation. It commonly results from milder degrees of compression or traction and is clinically expressed in motor loss that may be quite profound, yet usually accompanied by a partial sensory deficit and little or no disturbance of the sympathetic innervation. There are no evidences of wallerian degeneration, and the electrical changes are limited to a local conduction block with intact conduction distal to the lesion. Electromyographic examination will fail to demonstrate any spontaneous electrical activity at rest, so there will be no fibrillations or sharp positive waves seen if the patient is still paralyzed at three weeks from onset.

The circumstances under which these lesions occur vary from the "foot falling asleep" to crutch palsy and the milder tourniquet palsies. Many gunshot wounds involve "near-misses" of the nerves by bullets that generate shock-waves in the tissues. In these cases, it is a local stretching of the nerves that is expressed in a local conduction block without degeneration of the axon. Consequently, there is rapid recovery of function. This clinical picture was first described by the American Civil War neurologist Silas Weir Mitchell in 1872,[97] when he noted the speed with which many patients with nerve injuries incurred in this manner recovered. In fact, the duration of the paralysis with neurapraxia may vary from moments to days to weeks, and there is usually complete recovery within 10 weeks, and often in considerably less time. Although the more transient of these palsies may be solely attributed to local vascular compromise, the experiments of Denny-Brown and Brenner in 1944[20] using spring clips to produce nerve compression demonstrated degeneration of the myelin sheaths at the site of the lesion and edema of the axon above and below it. They characterized this lesion as one of ischemic demyelination.

The term *axonotmesis* was used by Seddon to describe the situation in which the damage to the nerve is confined to loss of continuity of the axon and the myelin sheath. Usually this results from a more severe crush or traction injury than that in the former circumstance, but the supporting stromata of the nerve, including Schwann's sheath, the endoneurium, and successively larger subdivisions of the nerve, remain intact. This lesion in continuity results in complete loss of motor and sensory function below the level of the lesion and is indistinguishable from a complete transection of the nerve, and wallerian degeneration does take place. The appropriate electrical changes of denervation are found after three weeks. However, because the Schwann's sheaths and endoneurial tubes are intact, these lesions recover spontaneously at a rate of regeneration of the nerves of approximately an inch a month or a millimeter per day. Because of the persistence of the supporting stromata, which precludes loss of axonal material as well as confused reinnervation, the quality of neurological recovery is excellent. Assuming that the temporarily denervated parts are protected from injury and contractures, functional recovery should follow suit.

For the clinician encountering a complete loss of motor and sensory function following an injury to a peripheral nerve, the dilemma will usually be that of differentiating the more benign lesion of axonotmesis with its excellent prognosis from the situation in which there is complete division of all the structural elements of the nerve, axon, and Schwann's sheath. This was called neurotmesis by Seddon and requires surgical manipulation to re-establish the continuity of the peripheral nerve with the fascicular alignment sufficiently correct to allow for regeneration and functional recovery. The electromyographic findings after the three-week period needed for wallerian degeneration will be the same as the previous case, with fibrillation potentials at rest and, in the case of a complete lesion, no action potentials seen on attempted voluntary contraction.

In most cases, the history of the mode of injury will be of help in making the correct diagnosis. For example, a patient with a nerve injury caused by a knife is far more likely to have sustained a laceration rather than a lesser degree of damage. Closed fractures, unless they involve extremely displaced or very sharp bone fragments, are less prone to cause lacerations of nerves and, since they are usually axonotmeses, have a relatively good prognosis for spontaneous recovery.

At this point it would be well to consider those injuries to the nerves about the shoulder girdle that may occur during the course of surgical operations about the shoulder, particularly anterior repair. Richards, Waddell, and Hudson[64] studied these and concluded that if a brachial plexus deficit is present following anterior shoulder stabilization, there is a high likelihood of structural injury if function does not return rapidly. They found the musculocutaneous nerve to be at greatest risk and recommended early brachial plexus exploration in these situations. It should be noted that with misplacement of the anterior portal for arthroscopy, it is possible to cause plexus injury, and these injuries should be treated similarly, as should those lesions of the axillary nerve that can be incurred during the course of capsular shift procedures. The axillary nerve should be identified and can be palpated during the exposure for the capsular shift. The Bristow procedure puts the musculocutaneous nerve at particular risk, not only at the time of the original surgery but also in cases where reoperation is necessary after this procedure has failed. Further discussion of this topic will continue under the headings of the individual nerves.

Although the classification of Seddon has been very useful, there are some situations in which additional descriptive terms are needed. For this reason, the classification advanced by Sunderland[85] is of use. It has five categories, the first, second, and fifth grades being equivalent to neurapraxia, axonotmesis, and neurotmesis as above. The fourth grade, according to Sunderland, describes the situation wherein all that remains in continuity of the nerve is the external or epifascicular epineurium, giving the false impression that the nerve is intact and will recover with time. This situation may be encountered clinically but can be recognized if the nerve is carefully dissected under magnification; this will reveal that there are really no intact elements beneath the epineurium. In these circumstances, nerve repair will be necessary. Finally, Sunderland's third degree of injury represents the situation wherein the perineurium is intact, but the fascicles themselves have been disrupted. Although some degree of regeneration may occur, its quality is extremely poor, and such lesions usually require formal repair.

Having these considerations of the spectrum of pathology of the peripheral nerves in mind, the surgeon can approach a clinical problem with a better understanding of the diagnostic and prognostic possibilities for a particular case. Knowledge of the mechanism of injury allows for an informed presumption of the state of the nerve.

DIFFERENTIAL DIAGNOSIS OF ORGANIC VERSUS FUNCTIONAL CAUSES OF PROBLEMS OF THE SHOULDER JOINT COMPLEX

This area of evaluation is not only one of the most difficult, it also has the greatest risk in terms of the consequences of misdiagnosis. Yet, clinicians are often called upon to make such distinctions, with the full realization that organic and functional disorders may coexist in the same patient and that there is no organic entity that cannot be mimicked by its counterpart in psychogenic or factitious disease. For this section, as in my clinical practice over the past 22 years, I have relied heavily on and drawn from the excellent chapter in *The Neurological Examination* by DeJong[19] entitled "Examination in Cases of Suspected Hysteria and Malingering."

If we are to differentiate between organic and nonorganic disorders as expressed about the shoulder girdle, a few definitions are essential. First, the term hysteria probably should be replaced by conversion reaction, since it describes the process whereby emotional disturbances are converted into physical symptoms and signs. It is a psychoneurosis in which the patient is unaware that the disability or symptoms are not the result of an alteration of anatomy or physiology so that to him or her, they are real. This condition must be differentiated from malingering, which is a deliberate and willful, fraudulent imitation or exaggeration of illness. It is conscious and involves deception for the purpose of attaining a goal. Unfortunately, it must be stated that these two entities may sometimes overlap, making a clean and precise diagnosis impossible. However, some useful generalizations may be articulated.

In cases of malingering, the symptoms rarely vary from time to time. A malingerer with pain may insist that the quality of the discomfort is always the same (usually excruciating) no matter what the time of day, degree of activity, or modalities used to treat it. The pain and disability will often appear to be greater than one would expect from the situation. It should be noted, however, that this aberration is also to be found in patients with reflex sympathetic dystrophy.

Symptoms may fail to fit a pattern consistent with an anatomical lesion and may seem completely bizarre. Often the patient may not be able to give an exact description of just what the complaint is and may be evasive in answering questions directed at clarification. In addition, he or she may be sullen and uncooperative in the process.

By contrast, the patient with a conversion reaction may appear honest, sincere, and cooperative in all aspects of treatment, including submitting to surgery.

Unfortunately, either conversion reactions or malingering may follow trauma, including industrial situations, although in the latter case, if there are persistent symptoms associated with the process of attempting to secure compensation, appropriate inferences may usually be made. Taking a history of activities of daily living, including questions regarding ability to sleep or engage in recreational activities in addition to employment, may be extremely enlightening. The patient with organic pathology who is disabled is generally globally impaired.

Although there really is no foolproof process that one may use to detect nonorganic disease, there are observations within a routine, carefully detailed neurological examination that can be extremely helpful. Specifically, in the history taking, it is important to search for prior episodes similar to the present one or evidence of adjustment problems. The patient can be asked to reenact the accident if there was one, and occasionally a very naive malingerer may move the allegedly weak or paralyzed limb to demonstrate its former utility. The patient should be surreptitiously observed in the process of entering the room and disrobing as well as gesturing. Facial expression and vital signs must be assessed, particularly when the examination is likely to produce discomfort. A departure from what would be expected should be noted, particularly theatrical or dramatic gesturing in response to the physical examination. The examiner should be sympathetic and nonjudgmental in approach but consciously testing the patient at all times. It is useful to exclude family, friends, lawyers, or rehabilitation counselors from the examination room, although they may return for any discussion that takes place at the end of the session.

Hyperesthesia and tenderness may be found in both organic and functional disorders. In the latter, however, patients may exhibit an inconstant response to stimulation in that they may wince and cry out when barely touched, only to hardly react to deep pressure over the same area when distracted. Mankoff's sign may be useful in differentiating between organic and malingering pain; in organic pain, pressure over a painful area usually causes an increase in pulse of from 20 to 30 beats per minute, while the malingerer's pulse will remain unchanged.

Disturbances of sensibility are commonly found in nonorganic as well as organic neurological disorders. Unfortunately, it is the rare patient who will succumb to the old "say yes when you feel my touch, and no when you don't" routine. Nevertheless, those patients with sensory deficits that do not conform to known anatomical distributions are suspect. The glove or stocking sensory loss found in peripheral neuropathies differs from that which is feigned or is a manifestation of a conversion reaction in that it does not have a sharply defined margin. Hemisensory loss involving the head, neck, and trunk, changing at the midline, should be evaluated by proceeding from the anesthetic side to the side with sensibility. Using this approach, in organic lesions, sensation begins to return slightly before the midline is reached. All sensory modalities may be lost with nonorganic disorders, and these may include vibration sense over the skull or sternum. However, since vibration is partially conducted through bone, such sharp midline changes cannot be attributed to organic lesions. In situations where there is a hemisensory defect, the cutaneous reflexes may be compared on both sides. If they are retained on the anesthetic side, it cannot be truly anesthetic. Furthermore, an anesthetic area with a preserved psychogalvanic response (mediated by sweating) is inconsistent, since in organic anesthesia caused by a nerve lesion, this response would be abolished.

The motor system must be carefully evaluated in all patients with reference to muscle bulk, tone, volume, strength, and coordination. The presumptive diagnostic impression can then be further clarified by means of electrodiagnostic testing. It would be rare to see changes of volume or contour in muscles apparently paralyzed or weakened by nonorganic disease, except in long-term situations where disuse atrophy may supervene. However, it should be noted that significant psychopathology or factitious disorders may result in contractures and deformities if they are allowed to persist long enough.

The examiner should be aware of the variety of tricks that may be encountered during the course of detailed manual muscle testing. Patients may make little effort to contract muscles when asked to do so. The antagonist of the muscle or group under consideration should be observed and palpated, since it may be contracted in an effort to simulate weakness of the agonist. On passive movement there may be evidence of contraction of the agonists when the antagonists are moved.

The muscle contractions in nonorganic weakness may be poorly sustained or of the "give-way" variety. There may be absence of follow-through when the examiner withdraws his pressure.

If the examiner drops the flail upper limb, particularly when the patient is lying supine on the examining table and the hand is above the face, it will gracefully and slowly glide away from the patient so that it will not strike him. A truly paralyzed limb will lack the motor control needed to avoid having the patient hit himself in the face. Of course, one must be very confident before trying this particular maneuver.

Muscle testing should be done with the patient and the limb in different positions. For example, testing the power of forward flexion of the humerus with the patient supine and then prone may confuse the unsophisticated malingerer if the test is done in the context of asking the patient to first push up and then push down, implying that these are really two different functions that employ different muscle groups. However, I would hasten to add that for the patient with the residua of stroke, there will often be a bona fide difference in the responses elicited when the patient is sitting up or lying down.

Finally, one may ask the patient to exert maximal effort on one side, such as that involved in adducting the humerus tightly against the body. The examiner feels the contralateral adductors, and unless these muscles are truly paralyzed, they will be felt to contract, since it is extremely difficult to suppress this phenomenon.

Stereotyped tests of coordination may convey the impression of significant ataxia or clumsiness of the upper limb, which may be totally abolished when at the end of the examination the patient is putting on his shirt. It is useful to have a mirror on the wall near the door to the examining room as the doctor exits.

As one becomes more experienced in the art of examination, these techniques and others can be smoothly integrated into the process of evaluation and should not be treated any differently from the standard neurological examination. Remember, however, that symptoms often are not totally clearly defined, and the last thing a responsible examiner would want to do would be to dismiss a patient's complaints as nonorganic without having employed every possible technique to make that diagnosis on as firm a basis as possible. When that has been done, however, there is the problem of what one writes in a report and what one tells the patient. No report should ever be written that cannot be read in open court or to the patient and his lawyer, since this will invariably come to pass if the opinion is not founded on solid grounds. When there are inconsistencies in the examination or bizarre responses, I describe them as such and then comment that they do not, in my opinion, conform to known organic neurological deficits. When patients complain of pain, I do not presume to say that they don't feel it, only that I can find no evidence of organic pathology with which to diagnose their subjective complaint. Although there are numerous psychological tests and personality indices that have been used to differentiate the malingerer from the psychoneurotic, I resist the temptation to enter this minefield, for little good can come to an orthopedic surgeon from such excursions.

Methods of Treatment of Kinesiological Abnormalities of the Shoulder

Because normal function of the shoulder joint complex depends on the smooth integration of nerve, muscle, bone, and joint, the treatment of its kinesiological abnormalities must be based on knowledge of the functional status of each of these interrelated components. Only in this way can the varied pathological entities be approached in a logical fashion, using available techniques of medical or surgical therapy as required. When, for example, there is muscle weakness about the shoulder caused by a generalized myopathy that can be treated or that will recover spontaneously, one must await the limit of improvement before proceeding to considerations of surgical therapy. However, it is important that the orthopedic surgeon be included in the assessment of such patients early in the course of the disease so that reasoned decisions can be made regarding the rehabilitation process. In this way, patients will benefit from the combined knowledge and differing points of view of the various medical and surgical specialists who care for them.

A thorough and complete consideration of the surgical treatment of all the neuropathological entities that can disturb the function of the shoulder girdle complex or impair the limb distally would require an encyclopedic presentation beyond the scope of this chapter. Instead, by describing the management of the more common entities, an attempt will be made to provide a framework from which treatment plans can be established for the less common disorders that must be omitted owing to limitations of space and time.

No matter what the original etiology of the motor deficit about the shoulder, the ultimate result will be a disturbance in the smooth and exquisitely balanced interaction of the force couples that provide a stable yet globally mobile base for the function of the upper limb.[34, 70, 83] Certain basic principles can be enumerated as common to the approach of any of the resulting kinesiological disturbances. Nerves may require decompression and neurolysis when compressed or, with more severe degrees of injury, either direct repair or grafting. The classification of pathology of traumatic neuropathy and the manner in which it leads to therapeutic decisions have already been presented in the previous section on classification.

When muscle power is permanently lost, whether from nerve injury, neuropathy, direct trauma, or myopathy, tendon transfer is an option. This technique preserves mobility more than any other, and most closely simulates normal function. However, since no muscle is added to the limb by the operation, its total strength will remain less than normal. For the paralyzed glenohumeral joint when there are no available motors for transfer, arthrodesis provides useful and reasonably strong function within a limited range of motion, provided the serratus and trapezius are intact.[18, 69, 83] In situations where the scapular motors are deficient and the glenohumeral musculature is intact, an entirely different set of problems exists.

It should be apparent that different avenues of therapeutic approach may be required for management of a single entity, depending on the stage or severity of the lesion. Finally, there are complex interrelations between the components of the shoulder girdle and neurological dysfunction that may be expressed as secondary thoracic outlet syndrome or lesions of the brachial plexus which will require correction before the neurovascular dysfunction can be alleviated.[44, 46] An example of this situation is a fracture of the clavicle with malunion or nonunion that compromises the depth of the costoclavicular space available to the neurovascular structures and thereby creates a thoracic outlet syndrome. In addition, the patient may have superimposed disuse atrophy of the trapezius muscle because

of pain, and this will result in postural ptosis of the scapula, thus aggravating the compression. In a number of patients I have observed with anterior instability of the glenohumeral joint, the symptoms of "dead arm syndrome" have been accompanied by physical findings consistent with the diagnosis of thoracic outlet syndrome. I believe that this association is more than coincidence and that many of the symptoms of what has been labeled "dead arm syndrome" are actually due to thoracic outlet syndrome.[46] The subject will be further discussed later.

Specific neurological disorders for which functional restoration or significant improvement of shoulder dysfunction may be obtained by surgical treatment are as follows:
1. Spinal accessory nerve palsy
2. Muscular dystrophy
3. Serratus anterior palsy
4. Brachial plexus injuries
   A. supraclavicular
   B. infraclavicular
   C. subclavicular
5. Suprascapular nerve compression
6. Axillary nerve injury
7. Musculocutaneous nerve injury
8. Thoracic outlet syndrome
9. Stroke shoulder

Spinal Accessory Nerve Palsy

The spinal accessory nerve, which leaves the jugular foramen at the base of the skull, passes obliquely through the sternomastoid muscle in its upper third and then crosses the posterior triangle of the neck to end in the trapezius. It is the major nerve supply to that muscle, and because it is quite superficially located, the nerve is vulnerable to injury. Unfortunately, this occurs not uncommonly as a result of surgical operations in the neck. It may be damaged by traction with injury to the shoulder girdle (Fig. 18–8).

The nerve may be sacrificed intentionally during the course of radical neck dissection for cancer (Fig. 18–9), although recent appreciation of the disability that this can cause has prompted its preservation whenever possible. Inadvertent spinal accessory nerve lesions may also occur during the course of "minor surgical procedures" in the area, such as lymph node biopsy.[99] Often, the patient does not realize that anything is wrong until days after the biopsy, when the pain from the surgery should have gone away, but there is an inability to abduct the arm without pain. As one might imagine, the actual incidence of this complication is difficult to establish with certainty. Nevertheless, it is not rare, and often the diagnosis takes considerable time to establish. If by three months there is persistent and complete paralysis of the trapezius both clinically and electromyographically, the nerve should be surgically explored. If it appears to be caught in scar, neurolysis should be done. An obvious discontinuity requires a suture or graft if the gap cannot be closed without tension.[29]

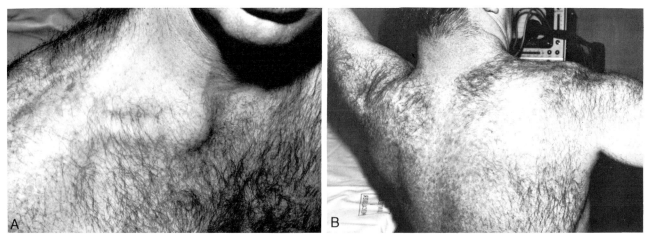

Figure 18–8. *A,* This patient had a 10-year history of pain in the sternoclavicular joint and weakness of abduction of the shoulder following a blow to the posterior aspect of the shoulder from a 5-inch gun aboard ship. He has a complete loss of trapezius muscle function due to a spinal accessory nerve traction injury incurred at the time of sternoclavicular joint dislocation. *B,* Weakness of abduction due to trapezius palsy.

For those patients in whom the trapezius palsy is judged to be permanent, usually six months after attempted repair or injury without electromyographic evidence of recovery, the options for reconstruction are tendon transfer, scapular suspension, or fusion to the ribcage.

The tendon transfer of levator scapulae and rhomboids, the Eden-Lange procedure, has recently received a favorable report from Bigliani.[9] A vertical incision is made halfway between the scapula and the vertebral spines along the length of the scapula so that the levator scapulae and the rhomboids may be detached. The levator is then reattached as far laterally

on the spine of the scapula as it will reach. The infraspinatus is gently elevated from the posterior aspect of the body of the scapula and the rhomboids are brought laterally to be attached to the bone about five cm from their original insertion on the medial border of the scapula. The limb is immobilized in a splint or sling for six weeks, following which gentle mobilization and strengthening exercises are begun. This operation has the greatest potential for maintaining mobility and providing near-normal function. It is particularly useful for elimination of the pain that these patients usually have in their shoulders with any type of activity that requires lifting. The four patients on whom I have done the operation recently have been very enthusiastic about their increased function as a result of surgery. In consideration of the alternatives and their disadvantages, I would judge this to be my first choice in management of this entity, assuming the anatomical prerequisites are present. Biglianai's paper should be consulted for the specifics of techniques and results.[9]

The operation of scapular suspension has been adapted from the polio era, when the Whitman procedure used fascial grafts from the vertebral spines to the medial aspect of the scapula. Dewar and Harris[21] transferred the levator scapulae insertion laterally to substitute for the upper trapezius and used fascial strips in place of the middle and lower parts of the muscle, as was done in the Whitman operation. Because it has been my experience that static procedures subjected to heavy or even everyday loading over a long period of time have a high failure rate, I have not used this one despite the fact that part of it is dynamic since it does use the levator to substitute for the upper trapezius. I do have the experience of a patient of Dr. Mankin's in whom the upper trapezius had to be sacrificed because of a local malignancy, yet the spinal accessory nerve and the lower two-thirds of the muscle were preserved. The result of the levator transfer has been functionally superb.

Another variant of scapulopexy was described by

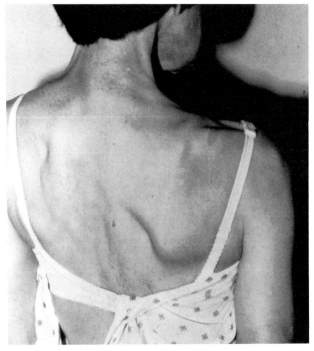

Figure 18–9. Complete loss of the trapezius muscle following radical neck dissection.

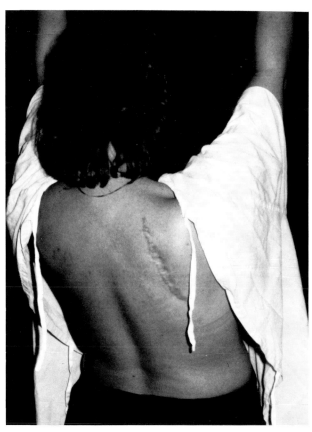

Figure 18–10. Postoperative appearance of a patient whose spinal accessory nerve was severed during a lymph node biopsy and who underwent scapular stabilization.

Ketenjian.[40] The procedure is done using the same vertical incision between the vertebrae and the medial border of the scapula, but in this case, the scapula is positioned in 30 degrees of abduction, which appears to be the optimal one for function of the arms in abduction. Four or five drill-holes are made in the vertebral border of the scapula, through which either fascia lata or mersaline tape may be passed to encircle the subjacent ribs subperiosteally. Although at one time I was enthusiastic about the use of Dacron artificial ligament for this purpose, in four cases it stretched after two to three years. I have, therefore, discontinued its use. The operation is contraindicated in patients with osteoporotic bone or those whose rib cages show the effects of heavy radiation, since the ribs are likely to fracture in these situations. When fascia lata is used, it is usually possible to begin gentle mobilization exercises at six weeks. The degree of motion that may be obtained with a solid suspension is surprisingly good, with forward elevation of 140 degrees being common in the postoperative patients (Fig. 18–10). Rotation and strength are adequate for most activities. However, the success of the Eden-Lange tendon transfer has considerably diminished my enthusiasm for static suspension procedures, unless, as sometimes happens, there is a deficit of available muscles for transfer.

For those patients in whom the above procedures have failed to provide adequate stability or range of motion, the salvage procedure that is most effective is scapulothoracic fusion. Patients who have heavy demands on their shoulders may be best treated with it as the primary procedure. The same longitudinal incision is used and the undersurface of the scapula, as well as the underlying ribcage (usually four or five ribs), is decorticated. A generous amount of iliac crest graft is then placed between the scapula and the ribcage, and the fusion is secured by wires through drill-holes in the scapula and around the ribs. A compression plate may be used on the posterior surface of the scapula to act as a retention device when the wires are passed through its holes before they are tightened. This protects the bone from splintering and distributes the stress over a greater area than that of the drill-holes themselves. I have found that the combination of Lucque wires and a pelvic reconstruction plate works very nicely. The fusion must be protected for 10 to 12 weeks with a shoulder spica, following which graduated exercises are begun. In a few very reliable patients, I have substituted a pelvic support brace for the plaster cast.

A less extensive method of achieving scapular fixation to the ribcage has been described by Spira.[81]

Muscular Dystrophy

Muscular dystrophy, particularly of the fascioscapulohumeral variety, will often cause weakness about the shoulder girdle in a patient who is otherwise unimpaired.[1, 56] Although the affliction may be asymmetrical, leaving one shoulder in comparatively good condition, the disease often progresses so that both shoulders are paralyzed and the patient is significantly handicapped. The deltoids and lateral rotators are less severely involved than the scapular motors in some cases. Consequently, these patients may be approached in the same manner as those with irrevocably damaged spinal accessory nerves, and the same reconstructive techniques may be employed. It is most important in the care of patients with muscular dystrophy that they be mobilized and out of bed as quickly as possible, lest their general condition deteriorate.

Brachial Plexus Injuries

The subject of injuries to the brachial plexus is an extremely complex one that will not be covered in its entirety in this chapter, although it is extremely important when considering the neurological lesions about the shoulder. Not only may shoulder function be severely compromised by the nerve injuries, but the nerves themselves may be injured by fractures and dislocations within the shoulder joint complex.[43]

Most closed brachial plexus injuries result from traction on the nerves that occurs when a motorcyclist falls and lands on his helmet and shoulder.[6] The forces that can be brought to bear on the soft tissues between these two points may be sufficient either to avulse individual nerve roots from the spinal cord or to rupture the nerves distally in the supraclavicular fossa. The former situation is one for which there is as yet no surgical remedy, since the nerves cannot be reimplanted into the spinal cord. In the case of distal rupture, however, some function may be regained by nerve grafting, particularly in the upper and intermediate trunk outflow.[53, 58]

If confronted by a traction injury of the plexus with paralysis of the shoulder, the surgeon must ascertain whether there is a possibility of spontaneous recovery before considering the surgical options.[10] The clinical appearance of the shoulder may provide important insights into the localization and severity of the lesion. If, for example, the patient with a traction lesion and a flail shoulder has lost the function of the serratus anterior and rhomboids as well as the deltoid and rotator cuff, it is highly likely that root avulsion has occurred, since these two muscles are innervated by root collaterals, which originate where the spinal nerve exits from the intervertebral foramen. Preservation of these two muscles with loss of glenohumeral control would imply that the lesion is beyond the branches that supply them so that distal rupture is probably present. An electromyographic examination which includes the cervical paravertebral muscles would be extremely useful in defining the two types of injury, and it should be done at about one month from the time of injury.[11] Particularly if the patient has a flail and anesthetic arm, a myelogram using water-soluble contrast material and CT follow-up will help to clarify the issue, and this can be done in conjunction with the electrodiagnostic studies.[45, 100]

The questions that must be addressed about the shoulder are as follows:

1. What is the prognosis for spontaneous reinnervation of the paralyzed muscles and what is the time frame?

2. Can the outlook for recovery of the muscles be significantly enhanced by surgical manipulation of the nerves, and what are the time limits for neurological reconstruction?

3. Would tendon transfer or arthrodesis be applicable in this situation? If so, how would these procedures affect the timetable or sequence of any other reconstructive procedures in the distal parts of the limb?

In general, these issues may be summarized as follows: For lesions of the upper trunk of the plexus that are determined to be root avulsions, the prognosis for spontaneous recovery of function is virtually nil, not only for the glenohumeral joint but also for the possibility of reconstruction by means of shoulder fusion, since the all-important serratus anterior will have been paralyzed, and no forward flexion of the fusion would be possible. Fortunately, the incidence of root avulsions at these levels is considerably less than that for the lower roots of the plexus. Although the trapezius would be intact unless the spinal accessory nerve has been injured as well, its function as a transfer will simply not duplicate all of the force couples about the shoulder to the point that will provide satisfactory function.

When the weakness is a result of distal rupture of the upper trunk, it usually occurs proximal to the origin of the suprascapular nerve, with the result that the power of lateral rotation is lost as well. Although that would seem relatively unimportant with the arm at the side, when the arm is brought into forward flexion, as it is for most functional activities, unless there is the stabilization conveyed by active lateral rotators, the arm will medially rotate and the hand will drop below the functional plane. In the absence of active control of the lateral rotatory components of the cuff, forward flexion and abduction will be severely compromised and reduced to shrugging of the shoulder or the ability to overcome the downward subluxation of the glenohumeral joint.

In evaluation of an individual patient with a plexus injury involving the shoulder, if the loss of motor power is incomplete, the outlook is relatively good, particularly if there is no muscle that is totally paralyzed. However, it is mandatory that the passive range of motion be preserved by means of daily exercise, active when possible, and gentle, passive exercise by the patient when it is not, or else the joint will stiffen while awaiting full recovery. The prognosis for recovery of the shoulder is considerably better for the patient in whom the injury is confined to upper trunk as opposed to one in whom more roots, or the entire plexus is involved, since the incidence of nondegenerative or neu.practic lesions is much higher in the more restricted lesions.[6] In general, if there has been no evidence of either electromyographic or clinical recovery of the muscles by nine months following injury, the outlook for meaningful recovery is poor.

The next question that must be addressed is whether the outlook for the nerves can be substantially improved by surgical manipulation of any type. Here it is most important to be critical in evaluation of the published reports of brachial plexus neural reconstructions. Function must be considered as the measure of success rather than an ability to shrug the shoulder or to overcome the inferior subluxation of the glenohumeral joint.[76] Although there have been some documented cases of significant functional improvement following surgery compared with the results of observation of the paralyzed shoulder in infants with obstetrical paralysis,[26] the prognosis in the adult brachial plexus injury is considerably less favorable,[58] and most patients will not be able to raise their arms overhead as a result of surgical reinnervation of their shoulder musculature. In fact, in all cases, it is absolutely vital that the suprascapular nerve be repaired, or else the all-important lateral rotatory stability will be lacking. It should be stated that the results of repair of the upper trunk for the restitution of elbow flexion are significantly better than those for shoulder function, and about 75 per cent of these patients will achieve the ability to flex the elbow against gravity and resistance. The general consensus regarding the time frame in which surgery holds promise for reinnervation is that the operation should be done within the first six months postinjury if at all possible, and a lapse of more than a year and a half makes it hardly worthwhile. Since most of the lesions are the result of traction

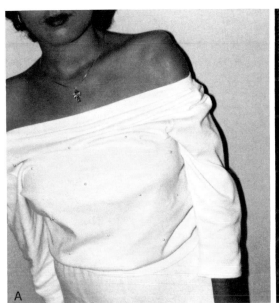 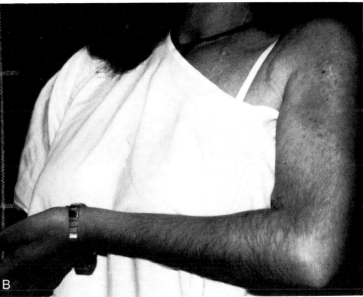

Figure 18–11. *A,* A 26-year-old woman with a flail, anesthetic arm following a motorcycle accident causing traction injury to the left brachial plexus. *B,* Eighteen months after an 11-cm sural nerve graft from the upper trunk to the musculocutaneous nerve and neurolysis of the remainder of the plexus, she regained finger flexion but no intrinsic function.

injuries, direct repair of these distal ruptures will not be possible, and an autograft is usually required. The sural nerve is the most often used donor nerve, and the interval between surgical repair and the onset of observable recovery of elbow flexion is between a year and 18 months in successful cases (Fig. 18–11).

It is because of the poor functional results of neural recontructions in adult traumatic injury that peripheral reconstruction is, in my opinion, the mainstay of surgical therapy of these shoulders.[45] Despite the fact that within the first two decades of this century there were reports of repair of brachial plexus injuries, particularly in the neonatal population,[16, 27, 38, 77] the majority of paralyzed shoulders were a result of poliomyelitis. For these patients, there have been numerous attempts to use the trapezius as a substitute for the multiple force couples that are necessary to control the glenohumeral joint,[8, 52] with some encouraging results, including a recent report by Karev.[37] For the most part, the transfer has not enjoyed wide popularity because of its biomechanical shortcomings. In 1906 Hildebrand[30] used the pectoralis major, elevated and attached to the lateral third of the clavicle and acromion. Others such as Spitzy,[82] Mau,[51] and Ansart[4] used multiple transfers about the shoulder. Ober[59] in 1932 brought the long head of the triceps and the short head of the biceps to the acromion, and in 1950 Harmon[28] described multiple transfers for the combination of deltoid and lateral rotator paralysis. The latissimus dorsi and teres major were transferred for lateral rotation, as in the L'Episcopo[48] procedure for obstetrical palsy, and the posterior deltoid was shifted anteriorly if this was available. The clavicular pectoralis major could be brought laterally to the acromion and then the short head of the biceps and long head of the triceps moved to the acromion. The long head of the biceps can similarly be shifted to the acromion as an aid to forward flexion of the humerus.

The work of Saha[70] in 1967 is particularly notable in terms of its analysis of the mechanics of tendon transfers for the shoulder paralyzed by polio. He argued that these methods are equally applicable to the patient with brachial plexus injury and that arthrodesis of the shoulder is, therefore, no longer required. I have not used the transfer that he had advocated for the totally flail shoulder, which includes the upper two digitations of the serratus anterior, the levator scapulae, and a modification of the trapezius transfer. However, I would comment that since the serratus and trapezius are both essential to the success of a shoulder fusion, if the transfer were to fail, the only bridge to a salvage procedure would have been burned.

In my experience, arthrodesis of the flail glenohumeral joint owing to brachial plexus injury can provide the patient with function that allows use of the limb as an assistive member and overcomes the often painful subluxation of the joint. It is an operative procedure that is well within the technical abilities of the average orthopedic surgeon, whereas most of the complex tendon transfers are best done by those who do them frequently, although obviously even they are not so technically demanding that they cannot be attempted. As was previously stated, it is imperative that the trapezius and the serratus function normally, since this is the minimal muscle pattern that will allow good function postoperatively. If the lesions of C5 and C6 are root avulsions, the upper serratus will have been denervated, thus compromising control.

Assuming that the muscles are intact, the remaining considerations are of operative approach, choice of position for the fusion, and method of fixation.

Although I have, in the past, used anterior, lateral, or posterior approaches for fusion, the last of these has been my preference for the past 15 years because of the ease of dissection, free of vital structures; less vascularity; and general lack of wound problems.

The patient is anesthetized in the lateral decubitus position, and the arm is supported on a sterile Mayo stand so that an assistant will not have to support it during the course of a two-hour procedure. The incision is made just caudad to and parallel to the spine of the scapula then continues across the midacromial point and down the lateral aspect of the proximal third of the arm. Hemostasis is assisted by the use of self-retaining retractors and the cutting cautery, and dissection is carried sharply down in the plane of the incision to the level of the rotator cuff muscles. These are then sectioned transversely in line with the joint, which is then opened so that the humeral head can be dislocated. A Fukuda retractor is extremely helpful in holding the head out of the way so that the cartilage of the glenoid can be cleared of all soft tissue attachments. Then, a three- to four-cm osteotome is used to remove the glenoidal joint surface perpendicular to the neck of the scapula down to the level of bleeding bone. At this point, the position for fusion must be verified by palpation of the shaft of the humerus and the vertebral border of the scapula as well as its posterior surface. I generally aim for about 20 degrees of abduction, just enough to permit access to the axilla, 30 degrees of forward flexion, and 30 to 40 degrees of medial rotation. This combination should allow the patient to reach the opposite axilla, the midline, and both front and rear pants pockets on the ipsilateral side as well as to get the arm to the horizontal and the hand to the mouth. These recommendations are according to Rowe.[69]

Fixation of the fusion site is usually by means of a 10-hole dynamic compression plate that is contoured to fit along the spine of the scapula, over the midline of the acromion, and laterally down the proximal shaft of the humerus. It is of advantage to translocate the humerus cephalad and to decorticate both the undersurface of the acromion and the upper surface of the humerus and greater tuberosity so that a secondary site for fusion can be obtained. Some of the cancellous screws can transfix the joint through the plate, while others may be introduced down the body of the scapula; the remaining ones will be cortical screws to the shaft of the humerus, for which one would hope to have at least two. Additional fixation with cancellous screws can be obtained on either side of the plate at the level of the joint.

Postoperative immobilization of the patient who is cooperative and reliable can be a light orthoplast pelvic-support brace for six weeks, although I do not hesitate to use a shoulder spica in those cases where I have reason to doubt the ability of the patient to protect the fusion. It should be noted that, as in all things, there are definite advantages and disadvantages, and fusion of the shoulder is no exception. Some patients will continue to have pain in the shoulder despite a solid fusion; in my experience, this is more likely if there is neurogenic pain rather than that which comes from the traction of the inferiorly subluxating joint. Sleeping on the fused shoulder may be uncomfortable for some patients, and others may have an increased tendency to fracture of the humerus if the arm is subjected to unusually violent stress. I have seen four such fractures in the last 20 years, and all of them healed with further immobilization.

Infraclavicular Brachial Plexus Injuries

Fractures and fracture dislocations in the region of the shoulder joint complex can produce injuries to the nerves and vessels that have a mechanism different from that described above. Rather than the indirect traction produced as the head and shoulder are forced apart, the plexus is compressed or locally injured in its infraclavicular portion as a result of pressure from the displaced bones or joints. Assuming that there are no sharp fracture fragments that lacerate the nerves, the amount of damage that can be inflicted is of a different order of magnitude compared with the supraclavicular injuries. The mode of injury is usually different as well, with fewer high velocity situations. More of these patients are hurt in falls or low velocity vehicular accidents. As reported by Leffert and Seddon[43] in 1965, their prognosis for recovery is usually very good. It is important to differentiate this group of patients from the larger group of patients with supraclavicular injuries and their worse prognosis. However, it is important to realize that if there is evidence of injury to supraclavicular branches of the plexus such as the suprascapular nerve or evidence of root avulsion such as Horner's syndrome, the prognosis is the same as that for the supraclavicular injury, even if it has been accompanied by a dislocated shoulder. For the most part, patients with infraclavicular injuries will not require surgery on their nerves, although occasionally one will see a patient with direct blunt injury to the infraclavicular plexus that will benefit from local neurolysis. As in other injuries where recovery is anticipated, it is most important to maintain, by daily exercise and stretching, the range of motion of those joints that lack normal voluntary control.

Subclavicular Brachial Plexus Injuries

Direct injury to the subjacent nerves of the plexus by bone fragments resulting from a closed fracture of the clavicle is unusual on an acute basis, and when it does occur, it is usually the upper trunk and suprascapular nerve that are involved. However, when the clavicle fails to heal or does so with hypertrophic callus posteriorly, there is danger that the underlying nerves and vessels will be compressed.[36] The subclavian vein is also at risk and is a major consideration for the surgeon who must decompress the nerves, since it may become adherent to the callus. The onset of the neurological deficit may be insidious, with weakness of the shoulder abductors, lateral rotators, and elbow flexors developing gradually. In most cases the clavicle has ceased to be painful and is presumed to have healed, yet the buildup of callus continues. Operative intervention should be preceded by CT scanning, angiography, and venography, and the surgeon should be prepared for the eventuality of a major vascular complication, since it is certainly within the realm of possibility. A high-speed air drill and bur facilitate the removal of the compressing bone, and the nerves and vessels may be shielded by malleable retractors. Attention may then be directed to the state of union of the clavicular fracture, which may require plating and bone grafting.[36] Of course, one would be well advised to avoid placing the grafts posteriorly so as to avoid a recurrence.

Suprascapular Nerve Compression

As indicated above, the suprascapular nerve is not often injured acutely as an isolated lesion owing to a closed fracture of the clavicle. However, its path from the upper trunk of the plexus to its eventual termination in the supraspinatus and infraspinatus leads through the unyielding confines of the notch in the scapula adjacent to the base of the coracoid process. Here it is separated from its accompanying artery by the transverse suprascapular ligament, which can cause compression resulting in pain and motor weakness (Fig. 18–12).[62] Clearly there is little problem in making the diagnosis when there has been a fracture that has distorted the bony confines of the notch and the patient

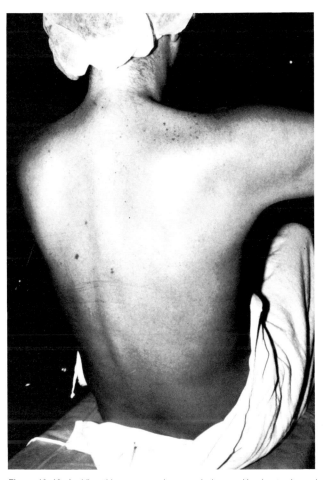

Figure 18–12. An idiopathic suprascapular nerve lesion resulting in atrophy and weakness of the supraspinatus and infraspinatus muscles.

subsequently has weakness and atrophy of the supraspinatus and infraspinatus.[80] It is in the chronic situation, particularly when there is no history of trauma and the patient complains of loss of power and vague pain in the posterior aspect of the shoulder and has only slight atrophy of the lateral rotators on physical examination, that the diagnosis must be entertained. It is of value to obtain electromyographic examination and to measure the velocity of nerve conduction (actually latency from stimulus at Erb's point to response in the supraspinatus: normal range 1.7 to 3.7 msec) to confirm the clinical diagnosis.[62]

In some cases there can be atrophy and weakness of the infraspinatus without involvement of the supraspinatus, and the electromyogram will confirm the clinical impression of the sparing of the supraspinatus. These have been explained by compression of the nerve by a ganglion as it crosses the root of the spine of the scapula and before the innervation to the infraspinatus is given off.[90] Where there is significant atrophy of the lateral rotators and weakness of abduction of the arm, the differential diagnosis of the rotator cuff tear may make arthrography necessary as well.

The surgery of compression lesions of the suprascapular nerve in the notch is deceptively simple in description.[57] The approach is a transverse incision parallel to the spine of the scapula, splitting the fibers of the trapezius short of the medial border of the scapula to avoid injury to the spinal accessory nerve. The superior surface of the supraspinatus is then identified and retracted posteriorly so that the notch may be uncovered. This is actually a very deep wound in which vision is difficult. It is helpful to palpate along the superior surface of the scapula to feel the notch before proceeding further. The suprascapular artery crosses above the ligament and must be gently retracted and either preserved or ligated, or else troublesome bleeding will obscure the field and make safe dissection impossible. The ligament is a very thick and unyielding structure, and the nerve should be protected by a probe between it and the ligament when it is divided. The configuration of the notch has been the subject of considerable interest from an anatomical point of view.[63] If it is apparent that the bone itself is continuing to contribute to the compression, the notch can be enlarged with a rongeur. The results of the surgery are generally good with reference to pain relief, although severe atrophy of the muscles may not be reversed by surgery if the atrophy is of long duration.

Axillary Nerve Injury

The axillary nerve, derived from the posterior cord, is a terminal branch representing C5 and C6. In its course behind the axillary artery, it lies on the subscapularis muscle and then proceeds posteriorly in intimate relationship to the inferior aspect of the glenohumeral joint to emerge from the quadrangular space where it supplies the teres minor and the deltoid muscles. The anterior and middle deltoids are supplied by the anterior division of the nerve, which is subfas-

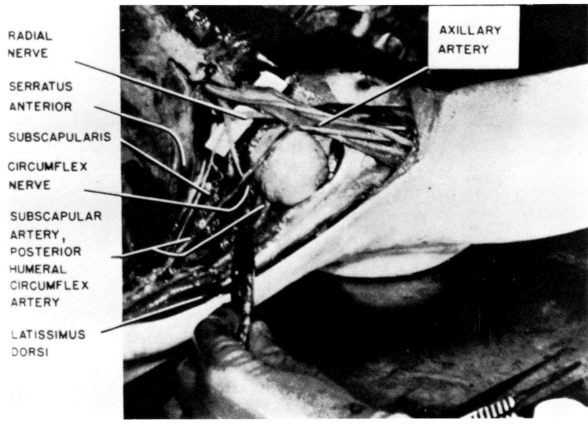

RADIAL
NERVE

SERRATUS
ANTERIOR

SUBSCAPULARIS

CIRCUMFLEX
NERVE

SUBSCAPULAR
ARTERY,
POSTERIOR
HUMERAL
CIRCUMFLEX
ARTERY

LATISSIMUS
DORSI

AXILLARY
ARTERY

Figure 18–13. The axillary (circumflex) nerve stretched over the humeral head during experimental dislocation of the shoulder in a cadaver dissection. (Reproduced with permission from Milton GW: The mechanism of circumflex and other nerve injuries in dislocation of the shoulder and the possible mechanism of nerve injury during reduction of dislocation. Aust NZ J Surg 23:4, 1953.)

cially applied to the muscle, while the posterior division supplies the posterior third of the muscle and ultimately becomes cutaneous to supply the skin on the lateral aspect of the arm over the deltoid. The relationships to the joint are most important with reference to the liability to injury. Fractures and fracture dislocations are very likely to directly traumatize the nerve, since it becomes stretched across the humerus as it dislocates anteriorly and inferiorly. This mechanism was well described and illustrated by the work of Milton (Fig. 18–13).[54] In fact, examination of the anatomical relationships of the nerve to the joint leaves one wondering why the nerve isn't injured whenever the joint dislocates. It is for this reason that the findings that Sir Herbert Seddon and I published in 1965[43] were troublesome. Specifically, we found little or no recovery in six cases of isolated axillary nerve lesions accompanying dislocations and fractures in this region and stated that the prognosis for such lesions was poor. I now believe that the incidence of axillary nerve lesions with such skeletal injuries is not only considerably more common but also the prognosis for recovery is much better than we had stated. The reason for this change of opinion is not only the anatomical consideration but also the experience of specifically looking for evidence of nerve lesions in such patients seen fresh after their injuries, finding them, and then watching them go on to recovery, usually complete. Probably our spurious conclusion stemmed from the population selected for

our study—patients from two peripheral nerve injury centers at the Royal National Orthopaedic Hospital in London and the Oxford Nerve Injury Center. There were doubtless many patients whose lesions were never picked up at the time of injury, or they spontaneously recovered and were therefore never referred to the Nerve Injury Center.

In addition to the possibility of axillary nerve injury accompanying closed injury to the glenohumeral joint, the nerve is extremely vulnerable in any operative procedure at the inferior aspect of the shoulder, such as one for capsular shift. One must also remember that the nerve runs horizontally 5 cm inferior to the acromion so that deltoid-splitting incisions must not be prolonged distally, lest they divide the nerve and denervate all of the deltoid muscle anterior to the incision (Fig. 18–14). Finally, blunt injury to the deltoid from heavy falls on the shoulder or blows can injure the nerve in its course through the muscle.

Watson-Jones[95, 96] described 15 cases of dislocation of the shoulder with axillary palsy and reported a considerably brighter picture for recovery. Of these patients, 10 recovered spontaneously over 6 months, 3 between 6 and 12 months, and 2 remained permanently paralyzed.

The problem of when and how to explore the nerve following closed injury has been addressed by several authors, including Coene[17] from Narakas' clinic in Lausanne and Petrucci, Morelli, and Raimondi[61] from

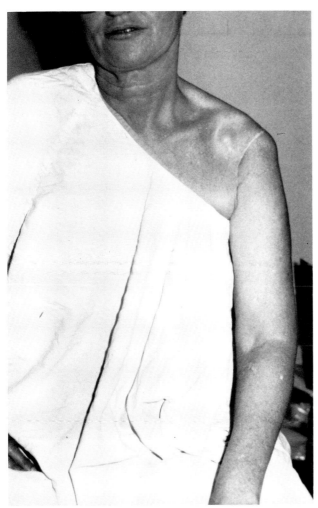

Figure 18–14. This patient had a misplaced deltoid-splitting incision that transected her axillary nerve and denervated the entire anterior deltoid muscle. The disability was severe, and forward flexion of the humerus was lost.

Legano, Italy. There is agreement that if there is no sign of recovery three to four months after injury, the nerve should be explored. Coene described the results of 54 operations, with recovery to at least grade 4 in 60 per cent and at least grade 3 in over 70 per cent at one year following surgery. The Legano group reported on 21 patients and also had extremely favorable results. The reader is referred to their papers for the specifics of the anatomical and technical details.[17, 61]

It is well known that patients with complete paralysis of the deltoid may still, by trick and supplementary motions, be able to elevate their arms quite well. However, not all patients are able to use these mechanisms, and so loss of the deltoid can be, as expected, quite disabling. For these patients, the reconstructions are similar to those that have already been described for brachial plexus injuries, with the same considerations of arthrodesis if nothing else is possible. For the patient with denervation of the anterior deltoid owing to a misplaced deltoid-splitting incision, a rotational transfer of the entire deltoid with excision of the denervated portion has been of value on several occasions in my practice.

Musculocutaneous Nerve Injury

The musculocutaneous nerve is rarely injured in the absence of an open wound to the area. Nevertheless, it is at risk during surgery about the shoulder, particularly during procedures done for anterior instability of the glenohumeral joint.[64] Although it is stated that the nerve crosses obliquely to enter the coracobrachialis muscle 5 cm below the coracoid process, this safe interval may diminish because of the abducted position of the arm or because of anatomical variations, which are not rare. The result is that unless the surgeon keeps the nerve in mind, there is the possibility of the patient's awakening with paralysis of the biceps and brachialis and numbness along the radial aspect of the forearm.

There are two alternative techniques for anatomical approach to the area and protection of the nerve during surgery. The first is not to take the conjoined tendon down from the coracoid but to incise part of its origin just below the bone and then gently retract the tendon. The other, which I favor, is to do an osteotomy of the tip of the coracoid to allow the muscle to retract medially so that tension on the nerve is lessened. At the end of the procedure, the osteotomy may be fixed by means of two nonabsorbable sutures, a method that has proved quite dependable.

The question that usually comes up with reference to the musculocutaneous nerve is what to do if the patient awakens from anesthesia with total inability to flex the elbow following an operation in the region of the shoulder joint. He or she may be able to flex the elbow by means of the brachioradialis muscle even with profound weakness or complete paralysis of the biceps and brachioradialis (Fig. 18–15). The first thing that must be established is that there is a true lesion of the musculocutaneous nerve rather than a brachial plexus lesion owing to plexus traction on the operating table, since the two entities can present in very similar fashion. Obviously, if the shoulder is weak in abduction and lateral rotation, elbow flexion is deficient, and there is sensory loss over the lateral aspect of the arm,

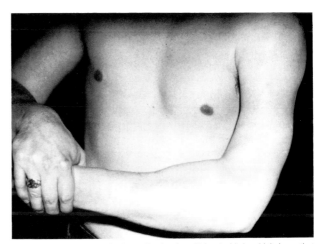

Figure 18–15. This patient had sustained a closed injury to his brachial plexus that completely denervated his biceps and brachialis. Nevertheless, he had powerful elbow flexion by his brachioradialis.

this would correspond more with a lesion of the upper trunk of the plexus than with a localized lesion of the musculocutaneous nerve caused by injury in the operative field. The prognosis for anesthetic palsies is extremely favorable, and such patients usually recover within six weeks of their surgery, although some may take longer.[42] For the patient who appears to have a lesion of the musculocutaneous nerve following shoulder surgery, there is little indication for immediate reoperation unless it is known with certainty that the nerve has been divided, in which case every effort should have been made to find and repair the nerve before the wound was closed. Otherwise, a short-term conservative approach, with maintenance of range of motion for the elbow, is taken for the first three weeks. At that time, unless there is definite evidence of beginning recovery, an electromyographic examination of the paralyzed muscles should be done. Failure to demonstrate the presence of voluntary action potentials and the finding of fibrillations at rest indicate a degenerative lesion of the nerve but do not give any information as to whether this represents a neurotmesis or an axonotmesis. That will become evident within three months of the injury, since at the rate of regeneration of an inch per month, one would expect a local traction lesion to have shown evidence of recovery by this time. If it hasn't, I believe that surgical exploration of the nerve should be done without delay, since the likelihood of an anatomical lesion requiring repair is extremely high.

Long Thoracic Nerve Palsy

The nerve to the serratus anterior is derived from the C5, C6, and C7 nerve roots immediately after their exit from the intervertebral foramina. As root collaterals, they are often spared the effects of traction injury when the entire plexus is affected, since root avulsions are less common at the upper parts of the plexus than at the lower roots. However, the nerve is heir to a number of poorly understood lesions that result in paralysis of the serratus anterior. Isolated serratus palsy may follow viral illnesses, immunizations, recumbency for a prolonged period of time and, unfortunately, lying on an operating table during the course of general anesthesia.[25] For those cases in which there has been a viral illness, Horowitz[31] has proposed an intriguing explanation of the pathomechanics that hinges on the anatomical location of the multiple bursae that he has described along the course of the nerve.

Open injury to the nerve is unusual, except as a complication of surgical procedures done in the area of the axilla, and both breast surgery for cancer and that done to relieve thoracic outlet compression can produce paralysis. In the latter case, although minor degrees of weakness following transaxillary first rib resection are not uncommon and have a good prognosis,[47] a complete paralysis has a poor outlook. I do not believe that a surgical repair is practical, and I have no personal experience with trying to repair the

nerve in this situation. I have done tendon transfers for several of these patients with gratifying results.

Closed trauma to the shoulder girdle or upper limb may cause a traction lesion of the long thoracic nerve, and when this is an isolated lesion, the prognosis is usually favorable. Some patients will become aware of the problem either because of significant pain in the shoulder and difficulty raising the arm, or they may suddenly realize that the scapula is winging because they are uncomfortable when sitting in a chair with a high back. In any case, the loss of the stabilization that the serratus conveys to the scapula in forward elevation of the arm becomes a functional problem in many activities, since lifting weights is difficult, and the shoulder may become quite painful as a result.

In my experience, if a patient has either a closed injury or an atraumatic and essentially idiopathic one, the paralysis usually recovers. However, if it persists for a year without any clinical or electromyographic evidence of recovery, the prognosis is poor. A recent paper expressed the opinion that recovery may occur after as long as two to three years.[25] During the period of waiting for recovery, there is little in the way of therapy that is effective, although some patients will get relief from the dragging, painful feeling in the shoulder by the use of a pelvic-support orthotic. Braces that try to hold the scapula to the ribcage are usually ineffective and very uncomfortable.

Some patients with permanent serratus palsies learn to live with their disability by altering their functional activities and do not consider the possibility of reconstructive surgery to alleviate the weakness. Some of these people have been told that there is nothing that can be done for them, and others are simply frightened of surgery. There are a number of surgical options that are available, but I do not consider scapulopexy or scapulothoracic fusion among them, since it is possible to maintain the mobility of the scapula by means of tendon transfers. The pectoralis minor can be detached from the coracoid and prolonged with a fascial graft to reach to the vertebral border of the scapula with good resulting function.[14] Recently I have preferred the pectoralis major extended in the same way, since the mass of the muscle is greater and the strength is correspondingly increased.[50] Four patients whom we have followed for two years after this transfer have had good results in terms of pain relief and loss of the winging as well as return of function (Fig. 18–16).

Thoracic Outlet Syndrome

Thoracic outlet syndrome (TOS) is a complex of signs and symptoms caused by compression of the nerves and vessels to the upper limb where they pass through the interval between the scalene muscles, over the first rib, and down into the axilla. There is a very significant relationship between the posture of the shoulder girdle and the production of symptoms that was well described by Todd[91] in 1912. He measured the inclination of the clavicle and the first rib in different age groups and both sexes and related the

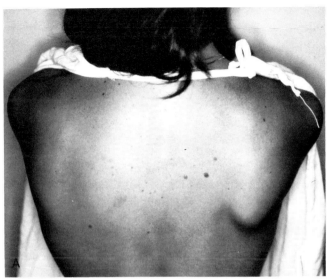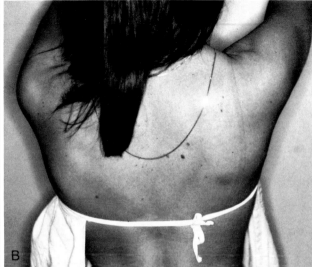

Figure 18–16. *A*, Serratus palsy following injury to the long thoracic nerve during transaxillary first rib resection. *B*, Six months after a pectoralis major transfer.

descent of the scapula to several factors, both normal and abnormal. He reasoned that the inverted U-shaped course of the first thoracic nerve root from the intervertebral foramen over the first rib results in traction on the nerve when, for any reason, the descent of the scapula is greater than normal. Scapular ptosis was therefore identified as a significant factor in the production of the symptoms of thoracic outlet syndrome. This theory predated the indictment of the anterior scalene muscle as the major etiological factor. It has since been significantly neglected because concern then shifted to readily identifiable abnormalities such as cervical ribs. In my own experience, about 20 per cent of the patients in whom I make the diagnosis of TOS have cervical ribs or abnormally long transverse processes at C7. Thus, any pathology in the region of the shoulder girdle, whether traumatic or atraumatic, that alters the posture of the scapula, can cause symptoms of TOS. In cases where there has been a fracture of the clavicle, the space between the clavicle and the first rib may be significantly diminished, leading to compression, or the disuse of the shoulder owing to

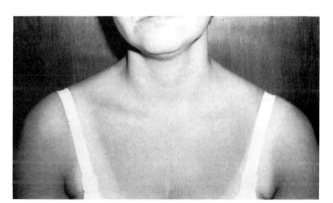

Figure 18–17. This patient had severe symptoms of thoracic outlet syndrome following blunt trauma to the left shoulder. Note the scapular ptosis. She was ultimately cured by transaxillary first rib resection after conservative therapy had failed.

pain or immobilization from any cause may result in atrophy of the trapezius, levator scapulae, and rhomboids. This, in turn, will result in ptosis of the scapula (Fig. 18–17).

There is an interesting relationship between anterior glenohumeral instability and the feeling of fatigue and aching in the arm that has been called "dead arm syndrome." As stated above, I believe that the symptoms in many of these patients are explainable on the basis of thoracic outlet compression.[46]

Because the symptoms are often vague and the signs are subtle to the inexperienced examiner, there is a need for diagnostic criteria for TOS.

The history is often that of pain and paresthesias that extend from the lateral aspect of the neck into the shoulder, down the arm, and into the medial aspect of the forearm and hand to end in the little and ring fingers. Positional changes, particularly raising the hand above the head, tend to bring on symptoms which may be experienced at night and disturb sleep or during the day with such activities as holding a blowdryer to the hair. Carrying heavy loads can provoke symptoms, and sometimes the pain will be felt in the chest. Some patients will complain of headaches.

The most important sign, in my experience, is the ability to reproduce the patient's symptoms by abducting and laterally rotating the arm at the shoulder while palpating the pulses at the wrist (Fig. 18–18). Although many patients will lose the palpable pulse with this maneuver, it is a normal finding that should not be considered as pathological unless there is a concomitant reproduction of symptoms. The overhead exercise test, done by rapidly flexing and extending the fingers as the arms are held overhead, will cause aching and fatigue in the forearm and hand of patients with TOS within 20 to 30 seconds in a high percentage of cases. The classic Adson's maneuver, the arm dependent while the patient turns the head to the affected side and hyperextends the neck, has a low yield in my experience. The neurological findings are usually sub-

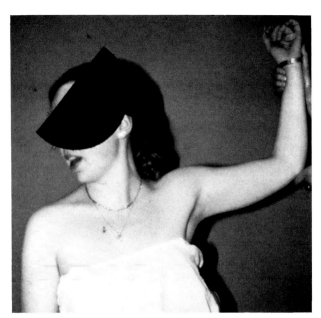

Figure 18–18. Wright's maneuver to elicit symptoms of thoracic outlet compression.

tle, and motor loss, if present, tends to slight wasting and weakness of the interossei and hypothenar muscles as well as the profundi of the little and ring fingers. Sensory deficit, when present, is usually over the little and ring fingers and medial side of the forearm.

Although electrodiagnositic testing, particularly nerve conduction velocity determination, has been thought to be a reliable indicator of TOS,[93, 94] this has not stood the test of time. Noninvasive vascular studies have not been of great value in making the diagnosis in my patients. Invasive studies such as arteriography and venography are rarely indicated unless there has been previous surgery in the area or there is a large cervical rib present.[35, 88] The diagnosis remains a clinical one, but it is most important that other conditions that can cause paresthesias, weakness, and numbness in the limb be sought and ruled out as well. Primary among these are cervical radiculopathies and peripheral compression lesions of the median and ulnar nerves. It cannot be overemphasized that patients with apical lung tumors may present with very similar complaints.

Treatment of the TOS patient should be directed towards reversing the pathological condition that appears responsible for the compression. For example, when patients with ununited clavicular fractures have TOS symptoms, they must undergo osteosynthesis before they will get relief.[36] Those who have had technically successful surgery but persistent scapular ptosis owing to muscle atrophy and who have arm paresthesias will usually respond positively to intelligently directed muscle strengthening exercises and postural re-education. When the patient is obese, weight reduction is indicated along with the muscle exercises. Emotional depression can negatively affect TOS because it can be expressed physically in scapular ptosis. It should be dealt with appropriately with either psychotherapy or antidepressants. A program of muscle strengthening and postural re-education is the major facet of the

conservative management of this complex problem. Because patients may have compression caused by different anatomical and physiological factors, the rehabilitation program must be adjusted to consider these individual needs. The exercise program[60] must be introduced gently so as to avoid provocation of symptoms, and the therapist must be in contact with the patient so that the program can be monitored closely. If a particular exercise causes significant pain, it must be modified or eliminated. Simply admonishing the patient to "stand up like a West Pointer, and get the shoulders back" is likely to result in frustration rather than relief. Sometimes the patient's activities of daily living or conditions of employment are causing exacerbation of the condition, and these should be scrutinized so that appropriate adjustments may be made. In all, such a program should have a time limit, which in my patients is usually three or four months.

The indications for surgical intervention in TOS are as follows:

1. Failure to respond to a carefully supervised conservative program of muscle strengthening and postural re-education exercises.

2. Functionally significant muscle weakness or sensory loss in the hand.

3. Intractable pain.

4. Impending vascular catastrophe.

The purpose of surgery for TOS is to relieve the compression of the neurovascular structures. A detailed description of all the techniques that can be used to accomplish this end is beyond the scope of this chapter, since most shoulder surgeons do not usually do this type of surgery. For those who are interested, there are a number of very informative references[2, 15, 24, 66–68] The procedures include scalenotomy, scalenectomy, first rib resection, and cervical rib resection. In addition, the anatomical approaches that have been used for these operations are posterior, supraclavicular, subclavicular, and axillary.

The transaxillary approach to and resection of the first rib, along with the cervical rib if it is present or any congenital bands that are found to be causing compression, is, in my experience, the most physiological in that it does not cause significant damage to the important suspensory musculature of the scapula, the trapezius, and rhomboids.[66–68] In addition, assuming all goes well with the surgery and there are no complications, the blood loss is trivial, since no important muscles are divided. It is, however, a technically demanding procedure with little margin of error, so it should not be done by the occasional operator. The results in patients who are carefully selected on the basis of the above criteria have, in my experience, been very favorable.

Stroke Shoulder

The so-called "stroke shoulder" can be characterized as a painful and stiff shoulder in a patient who has had a cerebrovascular accident affecting the same side. It can be responsible for the inability of the patient to progress in a rehabilitation program and may be the major factor that prevents independence.[13, 55] Although it is a common occurrence, there are still a number of unanswered questions regarding the pathogenesis and treatment. Some of the patients have pre-existing disease of the shoulder involving either the articular surfaces or the soft tissues such as the rotator cuff, but the majority of them do not. The incidence of true thalamic pain syndrome in the general stroke population is not high enough to be responsible for the stroke shoulder nor is reflex sympathetic dystrophy, and these two entities are sufficiently distinct to be ruled out on the basis of clinical findings.

Quite commonly, patients exhibit downward subluxation of the glenohumeral joint that comes on in the initial flaccid period following the vascular accident, and it becomes manifest when the patient assumes the vertical position. The mechanism of the downward subluxation is debated. Basmajian and Bazart[7] theorized that in the normal shoulder, the obliquity of the glenoid and tightening of the upper capsule and coracohumeral ligament and the activity of the supraspinatus muscle combined to prevent downward drift. Poststroke, with flaccidity of the muscles, the obliquity of the scapula would be lost, and the scapula would rotate to allow the subluxation. Caillet[12] said that loss of the trapezius and serratus allowed this rotation. The depressors of the humeral head may be spastic and contribute to the forces encouraging subluxation. A prospective study of stroke patients by Smith and Cruikshank and colleagues[78] demonstrated that the subluxation occurred during the initial period of flaccidity, but found no correlation with the degree of spasticity.

With time, the adductors and medial rotators of the glenohumeral joint become tight, the joint capsule contracts, and if an arthrogram is done, the capsule appears contracted like that of the typical frozen shoulder in a high percentage of patients.[65]

Although the problem of flaccidity of muscles would appear to allow analogies with polio, brachial plexus injuries, or specific peripheral nerve injuries to formulate treatment plans, it is most important to consider the problem of the stroke shoulder as distinct from these lower motor neuron lesions. In addition to the paralysis, the stroke patient may have to contend with spasticity, proprioceptive defects, and severe distortion of body image. The last of these problems may result in the hemiplegic patient's no longer recognizing the affected side as belonging to him or her. Clearly any of these factors may complicate treatment and seriously prejudice the ultimate functional result. Nevertheless, the stroke shoulder can serve as the prototype for treatment of the shoulder of patients with other upper motor neuron lesions such as head injuries, degenerative lesions, and tumors since they have received the most study.

The overall objective of treatment is to maintain a functional range of motion that will, at minimum, allow for self-care. As soon as the stroke patient can cooperate, he may be taught self-ranging of the affected arm with the assistance of the unaffected limb. Nurses and even the family can assist in this passive exercise, but it is most important that vigorous or forceful stretching be avoided, lest soft tissues be injured. The physical therapist must be brought in as soon as the patient is medically stable. When the patient is in bed, pillows can support the arm to avoid contractures, and turning the patient to the prone position with the arm abducted and laterally rotated can be of benefit as well. Since the emphasis of the rehabilitation program is to attain the vertical position as soon as possible, the shoulder will require support when the patient is sitting up in a chair and, eventually, standing and walking. The use of a sling is controversial.[33] Although it can help to prevent downward subluxation, its uninterrupted use can result in the development of internal rotation and adduction contractures. Thus, it must be used judiciously and with exercises as described. These can be begun with the patient in the supine position and in diagonal patterns, which are usually well tolerated if done gently.

Because of education about stroke rehabilitation, the number of stiff and painful stroke shoulders that are seen has diminished considerably, although they are still often seen in patients who have left the hospital to go to nursing homes or their own homes and who have not regained voluntary control. Because the limb is considered to be "useless," it is neglected, and contractures quickly develop. These patients often have so much pain that it is not possible to treat them with even the most gentle manipulations by the therapist, and the only successful therapy will involve surgical release. This procedure and its subsequent program of exercises were described at Rancho Los Amigos Hospital.[13, 55] An anterior axillary incision is used, and the pectoralis major and subscapularis are released, while the capsule is left intact. At two days postoperatively the exercise program is begun and must be continued indefinitely to prevent recurrence. A light plastic brace may be used to maintain the gains in passive motions. The results have been most satisfactory with reference to relief of pain.

Brachial Plexus Neuropathy

Finally, although the entity of idiopathic brachial neuropathy is not one that can be treated surgically or in any meaningful manner other than by observation, it is most important that the physician who is responsible for care of patients with shoulder disorders be conversant with its clinical manifestations because of the great importance in differential diagnosis.[92] The disorder occurs about twice as frequently in males as in females, particularly those in their 20s and 30s, although it may be seen in other age groups. The most common presenting symptom is severe pain that comes on with no apparent reason. The location of the pain can vary but usually involves the shoulder. It may extend over the scapula and down the arm to the hand, and it may be bilateral, although this is not common. The pain is followed in days or weeks by loss of motor and sensory function in the limb. Rarely is the entire limb involved, and the distribution depends on which part of the plexus is involved, but the roots themselves are usually spared, as is the spinal cord. Most commonly it is the shoulder that is affected, particularly the long thoracic, axillary, and suprascapular nerves, and they may appear to be involved singly or in combinations. The remainder of the plexus may also be involved, but it is unusual in the absence of shoulder dysfunction. The prognosis for recovery in this entity is good in that about 80 per cent of patients experience complete recovery by two years and 90 per cent by three years, although some patients may be left with residual weakness. Recurrences do happen, but they are unusual.[92]

The pathology is unclear, and although it has been characterized as an autoimmune disease, particularly in conjunction with immunizations with various scra and vaccincs, it may occur following viral illncsscs and in the absence of any of these factors. The treatment is supportive, avoiding the use of narcotics for the pain whenever possible. Steroids have been used empirically in treatment, although they have not been shown conclusively to alter the course of the disease, even though they are thought to help diminish the pain. Tegretol may be of use in pain control, but it must be carefully monitored. When the discomfort is most severe, treatment is symptomatic, but range of motion exercises and orthotic devices as needed may be introduced as soon as the patient can tolerate them.

References

1. Adams RD, Denny-Brown D, and Pearson CM: Diseases of Muscle, 2nd ed. New York: Harper & Row, 1962.
2. Adson AW, and Caffey JF: Cervical rib. A method of anterior approach for relief of symptoms by section of the scalenus anterior. Ann Surg 85:839, 1927.
3. Aminoff MJ: Electromyography in Clinical Practice. Menlo Park, CA: Addison-Wesley Publishing Co., 1978.
4. Ansart B: Die Myoplastik bei der Paralyse des Deltoideus. Z Orthop Chir 48:57, 1927.
5. Asbury AK, McKhann GM, and McDonald WI (eds): Diseases of the Nervous System. Philadelphia: WB Saunders, 1986.
6. Barnes R: Traction injuries to the brachial plexus in adults. J Bone Joint Surg 31B:10, 1949.
7. Basmajian JV, and Bazant FJ: Factors preventing downward dislocation of the adducted shoulder joint. J Bone Joint Surg 41A(7):1182, 1959.
8. Bateman JE: The Shoulder and Environs. St. Louis: CV Mosby, 1954.
9. Bigliani L, Perez-Sanz JR, and Wolfe IN: Treatment of trapezius paralysis. J Bone Joint Surg 67A(6):871–877, 1985.
10. Bonney G: Prognosis in traction lesions of the brachial plexus. J Bone Joint Surg 41B:4, 1959.
11. Bufalini C, and Pescatori G: Posterior cervical electromyography in the diagnosis and prognosis of brachial plexus injuries. J Bone Joint Surg 51B:627, 1969.
12. Caillet R: Shoulder in Hemiplegia. Philadelphia: FA Davis, 1980.
13. Caldwell CR, Wilson DJ, and Braun RM: Evaluation and treatment of the upper extremity in the hemiplegic stroke patient. Clin Orthop Rel Res 63:69, 1969.
14. Chavez JP: Pectoralis minor transplanted for paralysis of the serratus anterior. J Bone Joint Surg 33B(2):2128, 1951.
15. Claggett OT: Presidential address: research and prosearch. J Thorac Cardiovasc Surg 44:153–166, 1962.
16. Clark LP, Taylor AS, and Prout TP: Study on brachial birth palsy. Am J Med Sci 130:670, 1905.
17. Coene LNJEM: Axillary nerve lesions and associated injuries. Oegstgeest, Holland: de Kempenaer, 1985 (privately printed).
18. Cofield RH, and Briggs BT: Glenohumeral arthrodesis, operative and long-term functional results. J Bone Joint Surg 61A:668, 1979.
19. DeJong RN: The Neurological Examination, 3rd ed. New York: Hoeber, 1967.
20. Denny-Brown D, and Brenner C: Lesions in peripheral nerve resulting from compression by spring clip. Arch Neurol Psychiatr 52:1, 1944.
21. Dewar FP, and Harris RI: Restoration of the function of the shoulder following paralysis of the trapezius by fascial sling and transplantation of the levator scapulae. Ann Surg 132:1111, 1950.
22. Duchenne GB: The Physiology of Motion. Kaplan, EB (trans.). Philadelphia: JB Lippincott, 1949.
23. Dyck PJ, Thomas PK, and Lambert EH: Peripheral Neuropathy. Philadelphia: WB Saunders, 1975.
24. Falconer MA, and Li FWP: Resection of the first rib in costoclavicular compression of the brachial plexus. Lancet 1:59, 1962.
25. Foo CL, and Swann M: Isolated paralysis of the serratus anterior. A report of 20 cases. J Bone Joint Surg 65B:552–556, 1983.
26. Gilbert A, and Tassin JL: Obstetrical palsy: a clinical, pathologic, and surgical review. In Terzis J (ed): Microreconstruction of Nerve Injuries. Philadelphia: WB Saunders, 1987.
27. Gilmour J: Notes on the surgical treatment of brachial birth palsy. Lancet 2:696–699, 1925.
28. Harmon PH: Surgical reconstruction of the paralytic shoulder by multiple muscle transplantation. J Bone Joint Surg 32A(3):583, 1950.
29. Harris HH, and Dickey JR: Nerve grafting to restore function of the trapezius muscle after radical neck dissection. Ann Otolaryngol 74:880, 1965.
30. Hildebrand A: Uber eine neue Methode der Muskletransplantation. Arch Klin Chir 78:75, 1906.
31. Horowitz MT, and Tocantins LM: An anatomic study of the role of the long thoracic nerve and the related scapular bursae in the pathogenesis of local paralysis of the serratus anterior muscle. Anat Rec 71:375, 1938.
32. Hovelacque A: Anatomie des nerfs craniens et rachidiens et du systeme grand sympathique. Paris: Doin, 1927.
33. Hurd MM, Farrell KH, and Waylonis GW: Shoulder sling for hemiplegia: friend or foe? Arch Phys Med Rehabil 55:519–522, 1974.
34. Inman VT, Saunders JB de CM, and Abbott LC: Observations on the function of the shoulder. J Bone Joint Surg 26(1):1, 1944.
35. Judy KL, and Heyman RL: Vascular complications of thoracic outlet syndrome. Am J Surg 123:521–531, 1972.
36. Jupiter J, and Leffert RD: Non-union of the clavicle: associated complications and surgical management. J Bone Joint Surg 69A(5):753–760, 1987.
37. Karev A: Trapezius transfer for paralysis of the deltoid. J Hand Surg 11B:81–83, 1986.
38. Kennedy R: Suture of the brachial plexus in birth paralysis of the upper extremity. Br Med J 1:298, 1903.
39. Kerr AT: The brachial plexus of nerves in man, the variations in its formation, and its branches. Am J Anat 2:285, 1918.
40. Ketenjian AV: Scapulocostal stabilization for scapular winging in fascioscapulohumeral muscular dystrophy. J Bone Joint Surg 60A:476, 1978.
41. Kimura J: Electrodiagnosis in Diseases of Nerve and Muscle. Philadelphia: FA Davis, 1983.
42. Kwaan JHM, and Rappaport I: Postoperative brachial plexus palsy. Arch Surg 101:612, 1970.
43. Leffert RD, and Seddon, HJ: Infraclavicular brachial plexus injuries. J Bone Joint Surg 47B:9, 1965.
44. Leffert RD: Thoracic outlet and the shoulder. In Jobe F (ed): Clinics in Sports Medicine. Symposium on Injuries to the Shoulder in the Athlete. Philadelphia: WB Saunders, 1983.

45. Leffert RD: Brachial Plexus Injuries. New York: Churchill Livingstone, 1985.

46. Leffert RD, and Gumley G: The relationship between dead arm syndrome and thoracic outlet syndrome. Clin Orthop Rel Res 223:20–31, 1987.

47. Leffert RD: Thoracic outlet syndrome. (In manuscript.)

48. L'Episcopo JB: Restoration of muscle balance in the treatment of obstetrical paralysis. NY State J Med 39:357, 1939.

49. Marinacci AA: Applied Electromyography. Philadelphia: Lea & Febiger, 1968.

50. Marmor L, and Bechtal CO: Paralysis of the serratus anterior due to electric shock relieved by transplantation of the pectoralis major muscle. A case report. J Bone Joint Surg 45A:156–160, 1983.

51. Mau C: Kombinierte Muskelplastik bei Deltoideus Lahmung. Verh Dtsch Ges Orth 22:236, 1927.

52. Mayer L: Transplantation of the trapezius for paralysis of the abductors of the arm. J Bone Joint Surg 36A:775, 1954.

53. Millesi H: Surgical treatment of brachial plexus injuries. J Hand Surg 2(5):367, 1977.

54. Milton GW: Mechanism of circumflex and other nerve injuries in dislocations of the shoulder and the possible mechanisms of nerve injuries during reduction of dislocations. Aust NZ Surg 23:25, 1953.

55. Mooney V, Perry J, and Nickel V: Surgical and non-surgical orthopaedic care of stroke. J Bone Joint Surg 49A:989–1000, 1967.

56. Morgan-Hughes JA: Diseases of striated muscle. In Asbury AK, McKhann GM, and McDonald WI (eds): Diseases of the Nervous System. Philadelphia: WB Saunders, 1986.

57. Murray JWG: A surgical approach for entrapment neuropathy of the suprascapular nerve. Orthop Rev 3:33, 1975.

58. Narakas A: Brachial plexus injury. Orthop Clin N Am 12(2):303, 1981.

59. Ober F: An operation to relieve paralysis of the deltoid. JAMA 99:2182, 1932.

60. Peet RM, Hendricksen JD, Guderson TP, and Martin GM: Thoracic outlet syndrome: evaluation of a therapeutic exercise program. Proc Mayo Clin 31:281, 1956.

61. Petrucci FS, Morelli A, and Raimondi PL: Axillary nerve injuries—21 cases treated by nerve graft and neurolysis. J Hand Surg 7(3):271, 1982.

62. Post M, and Mayer J: Suprascapular nerve entrapment: diagnosis and treatment. Clin Orthop Rel Res 223:126, 1987.

63. Rengachary SS, Burr D, et al.: Suprascapular entrapment neuropathy: a clinical, anatomical and comparative study. Parts 1 & 2. 5:441, 1979.

64. Richards RR, Waddell JP, and Hudson AR: Shoulder arthrodesis for the treatment of brachial plexus palsy: a review of twenty-two patients. Orthop Trans 11(2):240, 1987.

65. Rizk TEW, Christopher RP, Pinals RS, and Salazar JE: Arthrographic studies in painful hemiplegic shoulders. Arch Phys Med 65:254, 1984.

66. Roos DB: Transaxillary approach to the first rib to relieve thoracic outlet syndrome. Ann Surg 163:354, 1966.

67. Roos DB, and Owens JC: Thoracic outlet syndrome. Arch Surg 93:71–74, 1966.

68. Roos DB: Congenital anomalies associated with thoracic outlet syndrome. Anatomy, symptoms, diagnosis and treatment. Am J Surg 132:771–778, 1976.

69. Rowe CR: Re-evaluation of the position of the arm in arthrodesis of the shoulder in the adult. J Bone Joint Surg 56A:913, 1974.

70. Saha AK: Surgery of the paralyzed and flail shoulder. Acta Orthop Scand [Suppl] 97:5–90, 1967.

71. Sandifer P: Neurology in Orthopaedics. London: Butterworths, 1967.

72. Schottsteadt ER, Larsen LJ, and Bost FG: Complete muscle transposition. J Bone Joint Surg 37A:897, 1955.

73. Seddon HJ: Three types of nerve injury. Brain 66:237, 1943.

74. Seddon HJ: Reconstructive surgery of the upper extremity. In Poliomyelitis, Second International Poliomyelitis Congress. Philadelphia: JB Lippincott, 1952.

75. Seddon HJ: Surgical Disorders of the Peripheral Nerves. Baltimore: Williams & Wilkins, 1972.

76. Sedel L: Results of surgical repair of brachial plexus injuries. J Bone Joint Surg 64B:54, 1982.

77. Sharpe W: The operative treatment of brachial plexus paralysis. JAMA 876, 1916.

78. Smith RG, Cruikshank JG, Dunbar S, and Akhtar AJ: Malalignment of shoulder after stroke. Br Med J 284:1224–1226, 1982.

79. Smorto MP, and Basmajian JV: Clinical Electroneuromyography, 2nd ed. Baltimore: Williams & Wilkins, 1979.

80. Solheim LF, and Roaas A: Compression of the suprascapular nerve after fracture of the scapular notch. Acta Orthop Scand 49:338, 1978.

81. Spira E: The treatment of dropped shoulder—a new operative technique. J Bone Joint Surg 30A(1):229, 1948.

82. Spitzy H: Aussprache zur Deltoideuslahmung, Muskleplastik. Verh Dtsch Ges Orthp 22:236, 1927.

83. Steindler A: Kinesiology. Springfield, IL: Charles C Thomas, 1955.

84. Stevens JH: Brachial plexus injuries. In Codman EA (ed): The Shoulder. Brooklyn: G. Miller Medical Publishers, 1934.

85. Sunderland S: A classification of peripheral nerve injuries producing loss of function. Brain 74:491, 1951.

86. Sunderland S: Nerves and Nerve Injuries, 2nd ed. New York: Churchill Livingstone, 1978.

87. Tassin JL: Paralysies obstetricales du plexus brachial: evolution spontanee, resultates des interventions reparatrices precoses. Thesis, Universite Paris VII, 1983.

88. Telford ED, and Stopford JSB: The vascular complications of cervical rib. Br J Surg 18:557, 1931.

89. Thompson LL: The Electromyographer's Handbook. Boston: Little, Brown & Co., 1981.

90. Thompson RC, Schneider W, and Kennedy T: Entrapment neuropathy of the inferior branch of the suprascapular nerve by ganglia. Clin Orthop 166:185, 1982.

91. Todd TW: The descent of the shoulder after birth. Anat Anz 14:41, 1912.

92. Tsairis P, Dyck PJ, and Mulder DW: Natural history of brachial plexus neuropathy; report on 99 patients. Arch Neurol 27:109, 1972.

93. Urschel HC, Paulson DL, and MacNamara JJ: Thoracic outlet syndrome. Ann Thorac Surg 6:1, 1968.

94. Urschel HC, and Rossuk M: Management of thoracic outlet syndrome. N Engl J Med 286:1140, 1972.

95. Watson-Jones R: Fracture in the region of the shoulder joint. Proc R Soc Med 29:1058, 1930.

96. Watson-Jones R: Fractures and Joint Injuries, Wilson JN (ed). Edinburgh: Churchill Livingstone, 1976.

97. Weir Mitchell S: Injuries of Nerves and Their Consequences. London: Smith, Edler, 1872.

98. Wilbourn AJ, and Lederman RJ: Evidence for conduction delay in thoracic outlet syndrome is challenged. N Engl J Med 310:1052–1053, 1984.

99. Woodhall B: Trapezius paralysis following minor surgical procedures in the posterior cervical triangle. Ann Surg 136:375, 1952.

100. Yeoman PM: Brachial plexus injuries. J Bone Joint Surg 47B:187, 1965.

101. Yeoman PM: Cervical myelography in traction injuries of the brachial plexus. J Bone Joint Surg 50B:25, 1968.

Calcifying Tendinitis

Hans K. Uhthoff, M.D.
Kiriti Sarkar, M.D.

Calcifying tendinitis of the rotator cuff is a common disorder of unknown etiology in which reactive calcification undergoes spontaneous resorption in the course of time with subsequent healing of the tendon. During the deposition of calcium, the patient may be either free of pain or suffer only a mild to moderate degree of discomfort, but the disease becomes acutely painful when the calcium is being resorbed.

Historical Review

The subacromial-subdeltoid bursa as a source of painful shoulders was recognized by Duplay[27] as early as 1872, and he described the condition as scapulohumeral periarthritis. Numerous other nomenclatures have since been used. The bursal localization of calcific deposits was first described by Painter,[69] who was also the first to demonstrate the radiological appearance of the disease, and by Stieda and his colleagues.[8, 93] However, surgical explorations soon established that the calcification was primarily in the rotator cuff tendons.[19, 107] In his classic textbook on the shoulder, Codman[20] stated definitively: "The deposits do not arise in the bursa itself, but in the tendons beneath it." Wrede[107] gave a masterly description of the disease, including the pathological changes of the tendon.

The intratendinous localization of calcification has been repeatedly confirmed by later authors.[82, 83, 87] But this did not stop the proliferation of newer nomenclatures, and terms such as peritendinitis calcarea[83] or calcified peritendinitis[26] are well known. In the English literature, calcific or calcified tendinitis is more generally accepted. We, however, prefer calcifying tendinitis following the term "tendinite calcifiante" used by de Sèze and Welfling[24] because it denotes an evolutionary process that is directed to spontaneous healing, whereas other terms imply a progressive deterioration.

Anatomy

The anatomy of the shoulder has been dealt with in earlier chapters. A few aspects of the rotator cuff tendons relevant to calcifying tendinitis will be briefly discussed in this section. The cuff tendons that blend with the capsule of the glenohumeral joint before insertion consist of the supraspinatus in its most superior portion, the infraspinatus and teres minor posteriorly and inferiorly, and the subscapularis anterior to the supraspinatus. The first three tendons insert into the greater tuberosity, whereas the subscapularis attaches to the lesser tuberosity. At the zone of the tendon where calcification takes place, we were unable to distinguish histologically between the deeper, more collagenous tendon and the joint capsule. Cells of the synovial layer were often inconspicuous.

The supraspinatus has the largest bulk among all rotator cuff tendons and is the most frequent site of cuff tendinopathies. It is 2 to 3 cm long, and it traverses the subacromial compartment that is rigidly limited by the coracoacromial arch above and the humeral head below. Codman[20] pointed out that the diseases in the supraspinatus tendon tend to occur in a specific area of the tendon: "about half an inch proximal to the insertion." He called this area the "critical portion," which was later renamed by Moseley and Goldie[62] as the "critical zone." The vascularity of this area has been repeatedly investigated because a possible hypoperfusion is believed to initiate degenerative changes that subsequently result in calcification or tear.

The rotator cuff tendons are regularly supplied by the suprascapular, anterior circumflex humeral, and posterior circumflex humeral arteries. In addition, contributions are received from the thoracoacromial, suprahumeral, and subscapular arteries in a descending order of frequency.[79] The vascularity of the cuff tendons, especially that of the supraspinatus, has been studied in many cadaver shoulders by microangiography simultaneously with histology. Moseley and Goldie[62] found that the supraspinatus was well supplied by a network of vessels coming from both the muscular and the osseous ends of the tendon that anastomosed in the area of the "critical zone." On the other hand, microangiographic studies by Rothman and Parke[80] showed that the "critical zone" was markedly "undervascularized," and their histological examinations corroborated this view. Although the supraspinatus tendon was most frequently involved, the infraspinatus and subscapularis tendons showed zones of hypovascularity as well.

Rathbun and Macnab[77] proposed from their cadaver study that the zone of avascularity in the supraspinatus was dependent on the position of the arm. They showed that when Micropaque (barium sulfate) was injected into the vessels with the arm of the cadaver in the position of adduction, the "critical zone" did not fill. The nonfilling area sometimes extended up to the point of insertion. If the vessels of the contralateral shoulder of the same cadaver were injected after passive abduction, they filled completely throughout the tendon. Therefore, the authors postulated that the zone of avascularity was a "wring-out" effect resulting from pressure of the head of the humerus on the tendon.

Our histological findings have been similar to those of previous authors: There is hardly an area in the supraspinatus tendon that is conspicuously devoid of vascular channels. However, we have observed that vascular channels, especially the larger ones, are abundant in the loose connective tissue underneath the bursa but relatively scarce in the dense collagenous part close to the joint. Interestingly, this is already evident in the supraspinatus tendon of the fetus (Fig. 19–1), even before the fascicular arrangement of the tendon fibers has occurred.

Our histological studies of cadaver tendons were supplemented by microangiographic studies which con-

sistently showed an area of underfilling at the articular aspect of the tendon near its insertion, regardless of the position of the arm.

It is obvious, then, that the question of reduced or lack of vascular perfusion in certain areas of cuff tendons is not entirely settled. Maneuvering the cadaveric arm to obtain optimal results through microangiography is not easy. Furthermore, it is doubtful that microangiography can reveal the entire vasculature up to capillary levels. However, it appears to be a common assumption that anatomical as well as transient hypoperfusion may exist in cuff tendons, particularly in the supraspinatus.

Incidence

Reports on the overall incidence of tendon calcification vary tremendously. The variation depends not only on the clinical material used but also on the radiographic technique. Bosworth[11, 12] examined both shoulders of 6061 office workers and found an incidence of calcification of 2.7 per cent. Welfling and colleagues[104] radiographed 200 shoulders of persons without any complaints and found calcifications in 15 (7.5 per cent). Rüttimann[81] radiographed 100 individuals without symptoms and found an incidence of calcification of 20 per cent.

The incidence of calcification in painful shoulders in Welfling's[104] series of 925 shoulders was 6.8 per cent. When broken down to age groups, patients between 31 and 40 years had a 19.5 per cent incidence of calcification. Evidently the peak at this age did not correspond with the peak seen in patients with painful shoulders. They therefore concluded that both diseases represent different entities. Moreover, no calcification was seen in patients over 71 years. Bosworth[11, 12] estimated that 35 to 45 per cent of patients with calcareous deposits will eventually become symptomatic.

Plenk[76] found that 82 per cent of the calcifications were located in the supraspinatus tendon. Bosworth[11, 12] found 90 per cent in the supraspinatus and infraspinatus. DePalma and Kruper[22] reported an incidence of 74 per cent when assessing the supraspinatus alone, whereas the incidence of simultaneous calcific deposits in the supraspinatus and other short rotators was 90 per cent. In Bosworth's series[11, 12] calcifications in the supraspinatus occurred in 51 per cent, in the infraspinatus in 44.5 per cent, in the teres minor in 23.3 per cent, and in the subscapularis in 3 per cent. Obviously, deposits were sometimes seen in more than one tendon.

In general, authors agree that females are affected more often than males. Bosworth[11, 12] reported an incidence of 76.7 per cent in females, DePalma and Kruper[22] of 60.3 per cent, Welfling[104] of 62 per cent, Lippmann[48] of 64 per cent, and, in our series of 127 patients, it was 57 per cent.

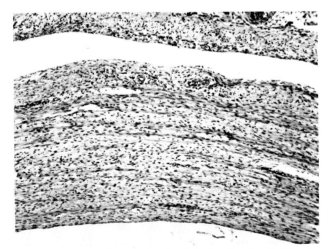

Figure 19–1. The supraspinatus tendon, close to the bony insertion, of a 20-week-old human fetus. Note the rather rich vascular supply in the part of the tendon close to the bursa. On the other hand, vessels are scarce in the articular part. (Goldner, original magnification × 100.)

The age distribution varies slightly among authors. Welfling[104] found the highest incidence between 31 and 40 years, whereas DePalma and Kruper[22] found 36 per cent of patients in the 40 to 50 year group. In our series, 53 patients (42 per cent) were seen in the 40 to 49 year old group. Welfling[104] states that no calcification was seen in patients older than 71 years, and McLaughlin[54] reported that no calcification was discovered in about 1000 older cadavers in an anatomy laboratory. It seems that males peak a bit later than females. Lippmann[48] arrived at similar results: the average age of females was 47 years and of males 51 years.

Occupation seems to play a role in calcifying tendinitis. In DePalma and Kruper's group[22] 41 per cent were housewives and 27 per cent professionals, executives, and salespersons. In our series, 43 per cent were housewives, and 44 per cent were persons having a clerical job.

The right shoulder is usually affected more often than the left shoulder. It amounted to 57 per cent in DePalma and Kruper's series[22] and in ours, 51 per cent. Bilateral involvement was found in 24.3 per cent by Welfling and coworkers.[104] In DePalma and Kruper's series[22] it was 13 per cent. Of our patients, 17 per cent came back with calcification of the opposite shoulder; this incidence increases with increasing length of the follow-up period.

The incidence of simultaneous calcifications around the hip in 23 patients radiographed in Welfling and associates'[104] series amounted to 62.5 per cent, whereas it was only 4 per cent in control subjects.

All authors agree that calcifying tendinitis is not related to any generalized disease process and Welfling and colleagues[104] rightly conclude that tendon calcification constitutes a disease entity on its own. Neither McLaughlin[54] nor Rüttimann[81] could find a correlation between tendon tear and calcific tendinitis. Partial tears occur mostly on the bursal side when the deposit ruptures into the bursa. Ruptures into the glenohumeral joint are said to occur extremely seldom.[36] Patte and Goutallier[70] observed two cases. We did not record a single instance.

The vast majority of authors agree that no relationship exists between calcifying tendinitis and trauma.

Classification

Several classifications of calcifying tendinitis have been proposed. Bosworth[11, 12] divided the deposits into three categories according to their size and corresponding clinical significance: small (up to 0.5 mm), medium (0.5 to 1.5 mm), and large (>1.5 mm). He felt that small deposits are of little clinical significance, while those larger than 1.5 mm are likely to give rise to symptoms. DePalma[23] classified calcifying tendinitis into acute, subacute, and chronic, according to the degree and duration of symptoms. It has been suggested that some patients with the chronic form who suffer from acute exacerbations should be classified in a separate category because they have a better prognosis. Patte and Goutallier[70] classified the deposits into localized and diffuse forms. Radiologically, the localized form is round or oval, dense, and homogeneous and lies close to the bursal wall; it tends to heal spontaneously. In contrast, the diffuse form is situated much deeper in the tendon, close to the bony insertion, and has radiologically a heterogeneous appearance. It produces more symptoms and takes longer to disappear.

We have not used these classifications in the clinical management of our patients with calcifying tendinitis because they do not take into account the cyclic nature of the disease. It is, however, important to remember that radiologically visible calcifications in the cuff tendons may occur with diseases other than calcifying tendinitis. Dystrophic calcifications can be seen around the torn edges of the tendon after complete tear.[106] Massive calcification as seen in the Milwaukee shoulder with complete tear is associated with severe osteoarthritic changes in the glenohumeral joint and, to some extent, in the acromioclavicular joint.[1, 37, 52] Dystrophic calcification associated with tear indicates poor prognosis and progressive degenerative changes and is not comparable to the spontaneous healing of the tendon in calcifying tendinitis.

Pathology

As the etiology of calcifying tendinitis is still a matter of speculation, we believe that a careful study of its pathology is necessary before some logical assumptions about the pathogenetic mechanism can be made.

Under the light microscope, the calcific deposits appear multifocal, separated by fibrocollagenous tissue or fibrocartilage. The latter consists of easily distinguishable chondrocytes within a matrix showing varying degrees of metachromasia (Fig. 19–2). The appearance of chondrocytes within the tendon substance

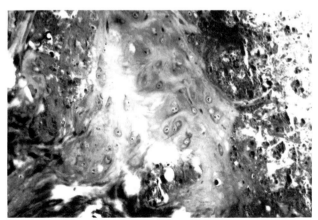

Figure 19–2. A fibrocartilaginous area between calcific deposits (C) shows typical chondrocytes. The appearance characterizes the formative phase. The deposits are partly in clumps and partly granular. (Toluidine blue, × 100.)

near calcification was noted by Wrede[107] in 1912 and illustrated by Pederson and Key in 1951.[72] The ultrastructure of these chondrocytes shows that the cells often have a fair amount of cytoplasm containing a well-developed endoplasmic reticulum, a moderate number of mitochondria, and one or more vacuoles (Fig. 19–3). The margin of the nucleus is indented. The cells are surrounded by a distinct band of pericellular matrix with or without an intervening lacuna. The fibrocartilaginous areas are generally avascular. In contrast to the fibrocartilage, the fibrocollagenous tissue abutting against the calcification may appear compressed, forming a pseudocapsule around the deposits. The neighboring tendon fibers may show thinning and fibrillation.

The calcium deposits may be loosely granular or appear in clumps. With the transmission electron microscope, aggregates of rounded structures containing crystalline material are found in a matrix of amorphous debris or irregularly fragmented collagen fibers (Fig. 19–4). When examined by scanning electron microscope, calcific deposits appear as rocky bulks engulfed in mortar.[30] The irregularly rectangular crystals are sometimes found within membrane-bound structures resembling matrix vesicles. Infrequently, crystalline densities seem to be embedded in collagen fibers.

Examination by chemical methods, x-ray diffraction, and infrared spectrometry as well as thermogravimetry has shown that the crystals are carbonated apatite.[29] However, high-resolution transmission electronmicroscopy revealed that the crystals are much larger than the classic apatite crystals and have a different configuration.

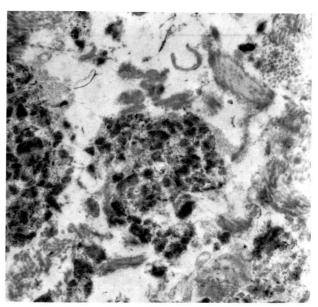

Figure 19–4. Rounded structures resembling matrix vesicles contain electron-dense crystalline structures. (Uranyl acetate and lead citrate, × 23,200.)

Moschkowitz[58] in 1915 identified the deposits within the tendon but stated that the deposits failed to evoke a cellular reaction. A few years before, however, Wrede[107] had already written that, although inflammation or vessels were notably absent around some deposits, "young mesenchymal cells, epithelioid cells, leukocytes, a certain number of lymphocytes and occasionally giant cells" were present at other sites of calcification. Presence of these cells is compatible with a resorptive activity at that stage. Indeed, the marked cellular reaction around calcific deposits—the "calcium granuloma"—was considered by Pederson and Key[72] as the characteristic lesion of calcifying tendinitis. The granulomatous appearance is imparted by the presence of multinucleated giant cells (Fig. 19–5). The cellular reaction is often accompanied by capillary or thin-walled vascular channels around the deposits (Fig. 19–6). The margin and the interior of the deposits are infiltrated by macrophages, a moderate number of

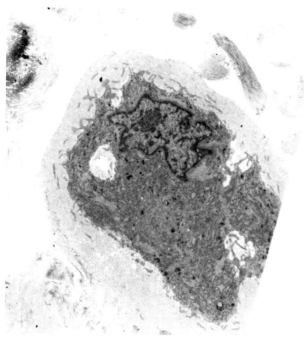

Figure 19–3. The ultrastructure of a chondrocyte surrounded by pericellular matrix shows a nucleus with an indented margin and the cytoplasm containing a fairly extensive rough endoplasmic reticulum and vacuoles. (Uranyl acetate and lead citrate, × 6500.)

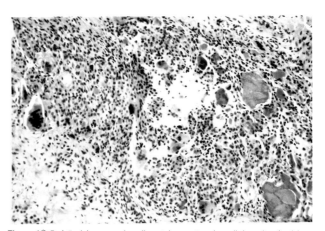

Figure 19–5. A "calcium granuloma" contains scattered small deposits of calcium, macrophages, and multinucleated giant cells. (Hematoxylin and eosin, × 100.)

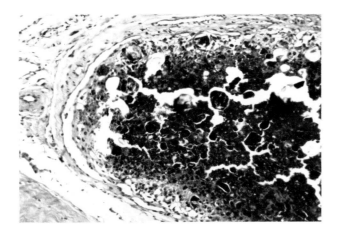

Figure 19–6. Capillary channels surround a calcific deposit. (Toluidine blue, × 100.)

leukocytes including polymorphonuclear cells and fibroblasts. Phagocytosed substance within macrophages or multinucleated giant cells can be easily discerned (Fig. 19–7). The ultrastructure of these cells shows electron-dense crystalline particles in cytoplasmic vacuoles (Fig. 19–8), but the crystals are somewhat different in appearance from those in the extracellular deposits.

Small areas representing the process of repair can be found in the general vicinity of calcification, showing considerable variation in appearances. Granulation tissue with young fibroblasts and newly formed capillaries (Fig. 19–9) contrasts with well-formed scars with vascular channels and maturing fibroblasts that are in the process of alignment along the long axis of the tendon fibers (Fig. 19–10).

Calcific deposits in the subacromial bursa also tend to be multifocal (Fig. 19–11). Cellular reaction is seldom seen around the bursal deposits.

Pathogenesis

Codman[20] proposed that degeneration of the tendon fibers precedes calcification. The fibers become necrotic, and dystrophic calcification follows. Degeneration of fibers of the rotator cuff tendons because of

"wear-and-tear" effect and aging has been postulated or demonstrated by many investigators. Obviously, these two causes are interrelated. It is reasonable to assume that the rotator cuff tendons suffer a "wear-and-tear" effect because the glenohumeral joint is not only a universal but probably the most used joint of the body. Studies performed in Sweden seem to indicate that stress and strain induced by work involving the arm can lead to supraspinatus tendinitis.[40] However, there are no indications that even a worker engaged in heavy manual labor would develop calcifying tendinitis in time, and Olsson[67] has shown that the cuff tendons from the dominant arm show no more evidence of degeneration than those from the contralateral arm.

Aging is considered to be the foremost cause of degeneration in cuff tendons. Brewer[14] believes that with aging there is a general diminution in the vascularity of the supraspinatus tendon along with fiber changes. The well-delineated bundles of collagen or the fascicles that constitute the distinctive architecture of the tendon show the most conspicuous age-related changes that begin at the end of the fourth or the fifth decade.[67] The majority of the fascicles undergo thinning and fibrillation which is defined as a degenerative process characterized by splitting and fraying of the fibers. The thinned fascicles show irregular cellular arrangement, and the fragmented fibers are often hy-

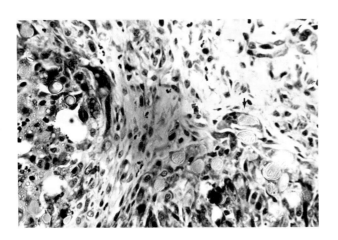

Figure 19–7. Macrophages and multinucleated giant cells contain phagocytosed substance *(arrow)*. (Toluidine blue, × 250.)

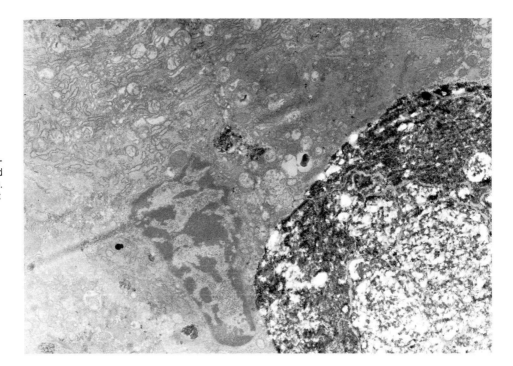

Figure 19–8. The ultrastructure of a macrophage shows apparently phagocytosed electron-dense material in the cytoplasm. (Uranyl acetate and lead citrate, × 11,500.)

pocellular. The intervening connective tissue that carries the blood vessels between the fascicles may appear increased when contrasted with the volume of the fascicles. In our experience, it is difficult to ascertain the numerical decrease in vessels, but more vessels with thicker walls are consistently found in the cuff tendons of aged individuals.

Since calcifying tendinitis seldom affects persons before the fourth decade, it can be argued that a primary degeneration of tendon fibers is responsible for the subsequent deposition of calcium. Following Codman's[20] suggestion of the degenerative nature of calcifying tendinitis, subsequent investigators have found ample histological evidence for the sequence of degeneration, necrosis, and calcification. According to McLaughlin,[54] the earliest lesion is focal hyalinization of fibers that eventually become fibrillated and get

detached from the surrounding normal tendon. Continued motion of the tendon grinds the detached, curled-up fibers into "wen-like substance," consisting of necrotic debris on which calcification occurs. This sequence of events was demonstrated experimentally by MacNab[51] in the course of investigations on the effects of interruption of vascular supply to the tendo Achillis of rabbits.

AUTHORS' OPINION

In our opinion, however, the self-healing nature of calcifying tendinitis and the various aspects of its pathology are not characteristic of a degenerative disease. We believe that the process of calcification is actively mediated by cells in a viable environment,[84, 95, 98] and

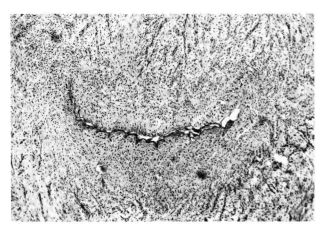

Figure 19–9. Granulation tissue is almost completely replacing the area previously occupied by calcific deposits. A speck of calcium is still visible *(arrow)*. The central portion shows amorphous precipitate. (Hematoxylin and eosin, × 40.)

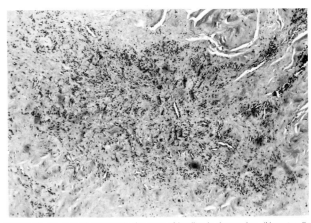

Figure 19–10. A scar represents the area of healing in the tendon. (Hematoxylin and eosin, × 40.)

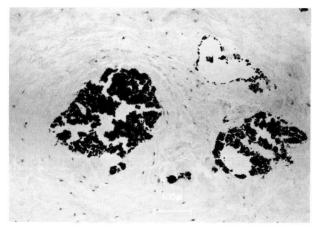

Figure 19–11. Multiple foci of calcific deposits in the subacromial bursa do not show any cellular reactions. (Hematoxylin and eosin.)

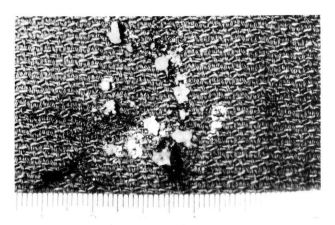

Figure 19–13. The calcium removed from a patient during the formative phase has a granular aspect.

Resorptive Phase

Following a variable period of inactivity of the disease process ("resting period" in the schema), the spontaneous resorption of calcium is heralded by the appearance of thin-walled vascular channels at the periphery of the deposit. Soon after, the deposit is surrounded by macrophages and multinucleated giant cells that phagocytose and remove the calcium. This is the last step in the calcific stage, which we have termed the "resorptive phase." If an operation is performed at this stage, the calcific deposit is a thick, white, cream-like or toothpaste-like material (Fig. 19–14). Simultaneously with the resorption of calcium, granulation tissue containing young fibroblasts and new vascular channels begin to remodel the space occupied by calcium. As the scar matures, fibroblasts and collagen eventually align along the longitudinal axis of the tendon. We have termed this stage "postcalcific." Figure 19–15 outlines the correlation between pathogenesis, morphologic findings, and symptoms during the various stages of calcifying tendinitis.

Although the pathogenesis of the calcifying process can be reasonably constructed from morphological studies, it is difficult to resolve what triggers the fibrocartilaginous transformation in the first place.

we propose the following concept for the evolution of the disease, which can be divided into three distinct stages: (1) precalcific, (2) calcific, and (3) postcalcific (Fig. 19–12).

Formative Phase

In the precalcific stage, the site of predilection for calcification undergoes fibrocartilaginous transformation. In the ensuing calcific stage, calcium crystals are deposited primarily in matrix vesicles which coalesce to form large areas of deposits.[84] For the convenience of description, we have used the term "formative phase" to denote this initial period of the calcific stage.[98] If the patient undergoes surgery at this stage, the deposit appears chalk-like (Fig. 19–13) and has to be scooped out for removal. At this time, the area of fibrocartilage with the foci of calcification is generally devoid of vascular channels. The fibrocartilage is gradually eroded by the enlarging deposit.

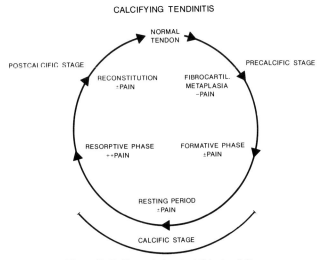

Figure 19–12. The evolution of calcifying tendinitis.

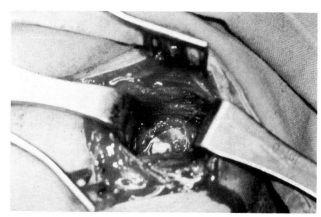

Figure 19–14. After opening of the deposit, which was in the resorptive phase, a cream-like fluid emerged under pressure; it can be seen in the wound margins.

THE PATHOPHYSIOLOGY, MORPHOLOGICAL ALTERATIONS AND SYMPTOMS
DURING VARIOUS PHASES

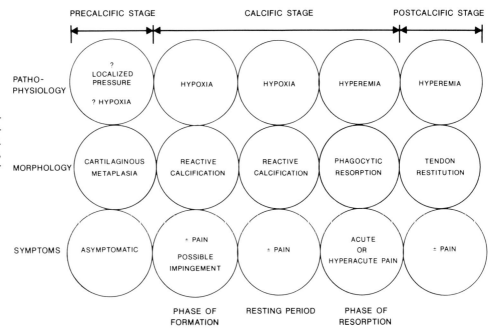

Figure 19–15. The pathophysiology, morphological alterations, and symptoms during various stages of calcifying tendinitis. In the course of evolution of the disease, the stages are likely to overlap one another.

Codman[20] suggested tissue hypoxia as the primary etiological factor. This still remains an attractive hypothesis because of the peculiarity of the tendon vasculature and shoulder mechanics. We have recently found that there is an increased frequency of HLA-Al in patients with calcifying tendinitis, indicating that these individuals may be genetically susceptible to the condition.[90]

Clinical Presentation

We would like to emphasize strongly that an understanding of the pathogenetic mechanism of calcifying tendinitis is essential for the clinical evaluation and management of this disease entity. There is a tendency to assume that the disease begins with acute symptoms and progresses to a chronic state. Our understanding of the disease is entirely to the contrary. We believe that the initial stage of formation of the deposit which lacks vascular and cellular reaction is likely to cause few symptoms or nondebilitating discomfort because the intratendinous tissue tension is hardly raised by the deposit. Thus, the disease generally begins with chronic symptoms, if any at all. Larger deposits can lead to impingement against the coracoacromial ligament, a fact already observed by Baer[5] in 1907 during surgery. During the later phase of calcium resorption, on the other hand, exudation of cells along with vascular proliferation must enlarge the tissue space considerably and thus produces a raised intratendinous pressure causing pain. The pain is probably further exacerbated as the increased volume of the tendon impinges upon

the unyielding structures that limit the subacromial compartment.

In fact, the subclinical nature of the formative phase of calcification has been recognized by many authors. Codman[20] stated that "the usual history is not acute pain at the beginning." Wilson[105] noted that many patients might know about a calcium deposit in one or both shoulders for months or years prior to an acute attack. Pinals and Short[75] wrote: " . . . calcium deposition precedes rather than follows the development of an acute attack of calcific periarthritis and the attack is accompanied by disintegration and gradual disappearance of the deposit." Similarly, Gschwend and associates[36] felt that the calcification is often symptomless at the beginning, whereas its disappearance is associated with pain.

It is therefore evident that we are not dealing with two unrelated disease processes, an acute and a chronic calcific tendinitis, but a disease cycle. Lippmann[48] described a phase of increment followed by a short, self-limited phase of disruption. Each phase has its characteristics. During the phase of increment, the symptoms were described as being mild, the consistency of the deposit was said to be hard and chalky, and no inflammation was noted. During the phase of disruption, the pain was severe, the consistency allowed tapping, and radiographs showed a fluffy deposit. Lippmann concluded that failure to identify the phase of the cycle resulted in crediting "useless therapeutic measures with magical healing power and, on the other hand, led to the performance of needless surgical procedures."

The clinical presentation depends on the acuteness of symptoms. Simon[91] is of the opinion that a definite relationship exists between the intensity of symptoms and their duration. They can last up to two weeks when they are acute, three to eight weeks when they are subacute, and three months or more when they are chronic. Pendergrass and Hodes[73] observed that the acute symptoms subside in one to two weeks, even in the absence of treatment. It is also known that symptoms may change rapidly.

During the subacute and chronic phases, patients complain of pain or tenderness. They are usually able to localize the point of maximum tenderness. Irradiation of pain is the rule, the insertion of the deltoid being the most frequent site of pain referral. Referred pain was seen in 42.5 per cent of the patients of De Sèze and Welfling.[24] The radiation of pain occurred more often into the arm than toward the neck. Wrede[107] and many authors after him found that clinical symptoms are often absent. Usually the range of motion is decreased by pain, the patients cannot sleep on the affected shoulder, and often they complain of an increase in pain during the night. A painful arc of motion between 70 and 110 degrees has been described by Kessel and Watson,[44] but they were unable to classify these patients into any of their three types of the painful arc syndrome (posterior, anterior, and superior). In 97 patients with this syndrome, they found 12 instances of calcification. Patients often have the sensation of catching when going through the arc of motion. This is most probably due to a localized impingement. This, in turn, leads to a loss of the scapulohumeral rhythm. Impingement between calcium deposit and coracoacromial ligament during abduction has already been noted by Baer[5] and by Wrede.[107] A further sign of long-standing symptoms of calcifying tendinitis is the atrophy of both spinati muscles. Although some authors reported the presence of swelling and redness on clinical examination, we were never able to find these signs.

During the acute phase, the pain is so intense and excruciating that patients refuse to move their shoulders. De Sèze and Welfling[24] feel that this severe pain leads to a locking. Any attempt at mobilization of the glenohumeral joint will be resisted by the patient. Patients hold their arms close to their bodies in internal rotation.

Although we have described the involvement of the bursa in painful shoulder syndromes,[84] its involvement in various phases of calcifying tendinitis has not been documented in detail.

During the chronic phase, the subacromial bursa is not the site of a widespread reaction. Only in the presence of impingement is a zone of hyperemia noted around the calcium deposit (Fig. 19–16). Carnett[16] noted that bursitis forms a minor and infrequent feature.

During the acute phase bursitis is said to be a source of pain. Yet during surgery the bursal reaction is minimal and often limited to a localized hyperemia (Fig. 19–17). This reaction is usually not severe enough to cause a bursal thickening. In fact the calcific deposit

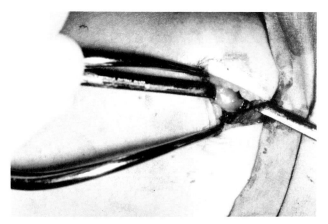

Figure 19–16. Intraoperative photograph after opening of the bursal cavity. The whitish area of a deposit during the formation phase is surrounded by slight bursal hyperemia.

often shines through the deep or visceral layer of the bursa. Litchman and colleagues[49] also noted the absence of bursal inflammation. Many authors state that rupture of the deposit into the bursa causes a crystalline type of bursitis and consequently pain. De Sèze and Welfling[24] followed 12 patients with ruptures of the deposit into the bursa. Only eight showed symptoms. In our histological specimens we could observe synovial cells resorbing calcium. No inflammatory reaction, in particular no leukocytes or lymphocytes, accompanied this resorptive process. It seems therefore probable that the edema and the proliferation of cells and vessels causes an increased intratendinous pressure which is the cause of pain rather than a bursitis. This impression seems to be confirmed by intraoperative observations during the acute phase. Upon incision of the deposit, the content spurts out under pressure.

In 41 operated patients we have correlated the symptoms with radiological findings and consistency of the deposit. Of 31 patients with chronic symptoms, 24 had radiographic signs compatible with formation, and 29 had chalk-like granular calcium deposits. Of 10 patients with acute symptoms, 8 had radiographic signs

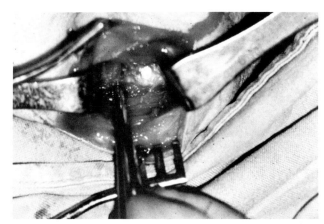

Figure 19–17. Intraoperative photograph of a patient during the resorptive phase. The whitish deposit shines through the bursal wall, which is locally hyperemic.

typical of resorption, and 9 exhibited a toothpaste-like consistency of their deposit.

Should calcifying tendinitis be considered a systemic disease as Pinals and Short[75] have speculated? There is no good evidence despite the high incidence of calcifications occurring at other sites. With the exception of an increased incidence of HLA Al in patients with calcifying tendinitis, all other laboratory tests are normal.[90] An associated illness was never reported,[49] and Gschwend and associates[36] were unable to prove an association with diabetes or gout, although this had been repeatedly suspected by various authors but never documented. A relationship to occupation must be suspected, given the high incidence of clerical workers observed by us and other investigators. Litchman and colleagues,[49] on the other hand, stated that no relationship to occupation could be found.

The incidence of frozen shoulder or contracture following calcifying tendinitis is not entirely clear. We could only observe a single instance of this syndrome. Lundberg[50] reported seeing 24 patients with calcification among 232 patients with frozen shoulders. This does not point toward a strong correlation between calcifying tendinitis and frozen shoulder.

Radiology

Calcium deposits in calcifying tendinitis are localized inside a tendon. They are usually not in continuity with or extending into the bone. They must be clearly distinguished from stippled calcifications seen at the tendon insertion in cases of arthropathies.

In all cases of suspected calcification of tendons, a

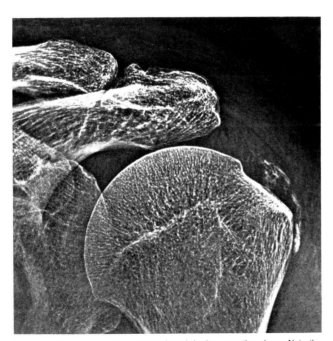

Figure 19–18. Xerogram of a calcium deposit in the resorptive phase. Note the presence of calcific material in the bursa.

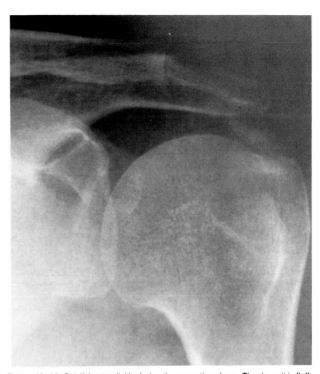

Figure 19–19. Calcifying tendinitis during the resorptive phase. The deposit is fluffy and ill defined.

radiograph must be taken. The radiological assessment is also important during follow-up examinations. It permits assessment of changes in density and in extent.

Initial radiographs should include an anteroposterior film in neutral rotation and in internal and external rotation. Deposits in the supraspinatus are readily visible on films in neutral rotation, whereas deposits in the infraspinatus and teres minor are best seen in internal rotation. Calcifications in the subscapularis occur only in rare instances, and a radiograph in external rotation will show them well. Axillary views are rarely indicated. Scapular views, however, will help to determine whether a calcification causes an impingement. Ruptures into the bursa will show as a crescent-like shadow overlying the actual calcification and extending over the greater tuberosity, outlining well the extent of the bursa (Fig. 19–18). Despite an extensive literature search, we were unable to find reports on the use of and possible indications for computed tomography (CT) and magnetic resonance imaging (MRI).

Calcium deposits in the acute or resorptive phase are often barely visible on radiographs (Fig. 19–19). In these cases a xerogram is helpful (see Fig. 19–18). We suspect that computerized radiography may give similar results.

Bursograms have not been shown to be of great value in our hands.[96] Arthrograms have been performed and usually show a distinct delineation between deposit and joint cavity. We believe that they are indicated only in exceptional instances, especially when a tear is suspected.

Radiographs not only allow confirmation of the absence or presence of calcium deposits, they also permit proper localization. Besides, the extent, delineation, and density can be well appreciated.[101]

DePalma and Kruper[22] described two radiological types. Type I has a fluffy, fleecy appearance, and its periphery is poorly defined. It is usually encountered in acute cases. An overlying crescent-like streak indicates rupture into the bursa which occurs only in this type. Type II is more or less discrete and homogeneous. Its density is uniform and the periphery well defined. This type is seen in subacute and chronic cases. Moreover, DePalma and Kruper[22] reported that in 52 per cent of their patients the calcification was seen as a single lesion.

De Sèze and Welfling[24] observed that in the presence of acute pain the deposit was less dense and the margins not well defined. In chronic cases, on the other hand, the margins were well defined, and the calcification was dense. They described the following radiological sequence in acute cases. First, a fluffy, ill-defined intratendinous deposit is followed by calcific material in the bursa only, and finally, no calcific material can be seen at all. We feel, however, that calcific material can often be seen in both bursa and tendon, that the calcific material disappears rather rapidly from the bursa, and that often a faintly visible shadow remains in the tendon for some time.

Our observations confirm those of DePalma and Kruper[22] and of de Sèze and Welfling.[24] During the formative or chronic phase, the deposit is dense and well defined and of homogeneous density (Fig. 19–20). During the resorptive or acute phase, the deposit is fluffy, cloud-like, and ill defined, and its density is irregular (see Fig. 19–17). Perforations into the bursa have been observed only during the latter phase.

Most authors agree that radiological evidence of degenerative joint disease is usually lacking. This, of course, holds true mostly for patients in the fourth and fifth decades of life. In three of our patients in the sixth decade, we observed acromioclavicular osteophytes.

Bony changes at the insertion of the supraspinatus into the greater tuberosity can sometimes be seen after resorption of the deposit. Whether this occurs more often after intraosseous extension of the calcium deposit into bone, as has been suggested, is difficult to confirm.

Calcifications seen in arthropathies have a quite different appearance. They are stippled and overlie the bony insertion. They are always accompanied by degenerative bony or articular changes. Moreover, the acromiohumeral compartment or interval is always narrowed. These calcium deposits constitute dystrophic calcifications; they must be clearly separated from the reactive intratendinous calcifications.

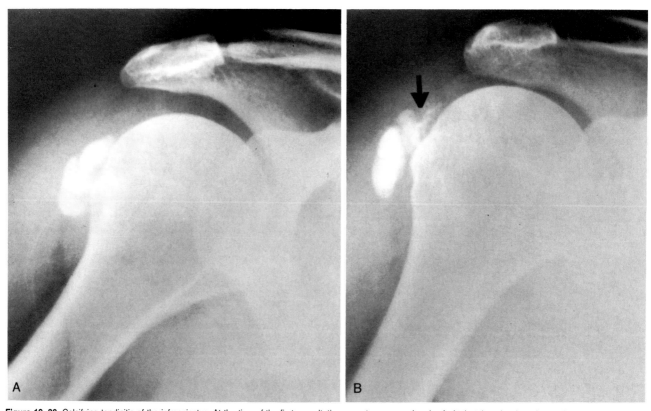

Figure 19–20. Calcifying tendinitis of the infraspinatus. At the time of the first consultation, symptoms were chronic. *A,* At that time the deposit was dense, homogeneous, and well defined. *B,* Four months later the patient reported acute pain of spontaneous onset. Note the beginning of resorption. The arrow points to an area of decreased density with irregular margins.

The use of ultrasonography in cases of calcifying tendinitis is limited since in the presence of significant calcifications, ultrasonography cannot show a small tear.[21] After rupture of the deposit into the bursa, Crass was able to demonstrate a crater-like defect in the supraspinatus.[21]

Laboratory Investigations

There are no abnormalities of calcium and phosphorus metabolism. Therefore, serum values are within normal limits. Also, the alkaline phosphatase is normal. There is no increase in the number of white blood cells, and the erythrocyte sedimentation rate is normal.

In our attempts to distinguish further between degenerative and reactive tendinopathies, we proceeded with tissue typing in 50 patients with calcifying tendinitis and compared the results with those of 36 patients with a tear of the rotator cuff and with 982 controls.[90] HLA-Al was present in 50 per cent of patients with calcifications, in 27.8 per cent of patients with tears, and in 26.7 per cent of controls. There is statistically significant difference between patients suffering from calcifying tendinitis and those having a tear, the p value being .0025.

During screening of patients with calcifications, the serum glucose values and the level of uric acid and iron should be determined.

Complications

Although the calcification starts inside the tendon it may extend into the muscle or bone. DePalma and Kruper[22] noted that in cases of osseous penetration, the point of entry was to be found at the sulcus, the interval between articular surface and tendon insertion. They observed that intraosseous deposits were always in continuity with intratendinous calcifications. In their experience, a bony involvement led to protracted symptoms; deposits in these patients were resistant to conservative measures, and he advocated surgical removal.

Bicipital tendinitis may complicate calcifying tendinitis. It occurred in 16 out of 136 patients reported by DePalma and Kruper.[22]

As stated before, frozen shoulder may occur in association with calcification. It was seen by DePalma and Kruper[22] in 7 out of 94 patients. They felt that frozen shoulder was due to an inflammatory process whereby adhesions occur between cuff and humeral head.

Rupture of the deposit into the bursa cannot be regarded as a complication. Complete tears, however, must be included, and to our knowledge, they have been reported only by Patte and Goutallier,[70] who observed a rupture of the deposit into the glenohumeral joint, seen only in the type they call diffuse calcification.

Complications from surgery must be of little importance, for they have not been reported. Careful attention must be paid to spare the axillary nerve during the splitting of the deltoid. Postoperative wound infection has not been seen by us, and all wounds healed without undue delay.

Recurrence of calcification after surgical removal has been observed by us in one out of 127 operated patients. In other patients where the deposit was not removed in its entirety, the spontaneous disappearance of the deposit was rather slow.

Differential Diagnosis

Here again we wish to insist on a proper distinction between reactive and dystrophic calcifications. In calcifying tendinitis, the major part of the deposit is situated inside the tendon without being either in continuity or in contact with bone. Dystrophic calcifications, on the other hand, are part of a degenerative process with concomitant radiological evidence of osteoarthritis and a rotator cuff tear, leading to a narrowing of the interval between humeral head and acromion. These calcifications are small and stippled and sit just over the greater tuberosity.

Treatment

Treatment varies according to the training and expertise of the treating physician. In general, rheumatologists seem to favor a conservative approach more often than surgeons. It also depends on the acuteness of symptoms and on the patience of doctor and patient. Some of the impatience is understandable since no one knows how long the disease in its chronic phase will last or when the calcification will spontaneously disappear.

NONOPERATIVE

Gschwend and co-workers[36] estimate that at least 90 per cent of patients are treated conservatively. In a series of 100 patients reported by Litchman and colleagues,[49] only one underwent surgery.

All authors agree to the need for adequate physiotherapy. Range of motion and pendulum exercises and, later on, muscle strengthening exercises are recommended. In acute cases, gentle attempts at mobilization are preceded by the local application of ice, whereas local heat is recommended in chronic cases. Infrared treatments should be understood as a local application of heat. Ultrasonography is said to be able to mobilize the calcium crystals, but no randomized study proving its value could be found by Griffin and Karselis.[34] Griffin and Karselis[34] observed pain relief, thought to result from a physiological rise in tissue temperature. The main aim of physiotherapy is the decrease of muscle spasm and the prevention of stiffness. Relief of pain can sometimes be obtained by placing the arm on a pillow in abduction.[16] The treatment regimen outlined is indicated mostly in chronic cases.

In acute cases, easing pain becomes a priority. Patterson and Darrach[71] and later Lapidus[47] recommended needling and injection of local anesthetics. Repeated perforations seem to decrease the intratendinous pressure. An added lavage may also help to remove part of the deposit, but it is effective only in the presence of radiological evidence of resorption. The site of needle insertion is based on the site of maximum tenderness and radiographic localization. Although these injections had to be repeated in some patients two or three times, Harmon[49] reported that they led to excellent results in 78.9 per cent of more than 400 patients. DePalma and Kruper's[22] results were less good; they obtained 61 per cent good, 22 per cent fair, and 17 per cent poor results.

Some authors suggest adding a corticosteroid preparation to local treatment. Gschwend and colleagues[36] note that its action is short, and its effect exclusively symptomatic. Dhuly and associates[25] showed that corticosteroids inhibit vascular proliferation, local hyperemia, and macrophage activity. Lippmann[48] warns that corticosteroids abort the activity that produces disruption and that they return the deposit to a static phase. Harmon[39] felt that the addition of corticosteroids did not accelerate the process of resorption but did reduce the muscle spasm. Murnaghan and McIntosh[63] treated 27 patients with xylocaine injections alone and 24 with hydrocortisone and could not find a difference in results. During the acute phase, analgesics are absolutely necessary to calm the often excruciating pain. Nonsteroidal anti-inflammatory drugs are recommended by many authors. No randomized study, however, could be found documenting its salutary effect on the process of resorption.

RADIATION

Radiotherapy has enjoyed an important place in the treatment of calcifying tendinitis. Milone and Copeland[57] treated 136 patients with radiotherapy. They concluded that "patients with the acute syndrome experience the most favorable response." Out of 54 patients, 49 had excellent and good results, whereas only 15 out of 24 patients with chronic pain obtained the same degree of relief. Results in patients with chronic symptoms fell to 33 per cent in Young's[108] and Chapman's[17] series. Out of 609 patients reported by Harmon,[39] 79 received radiotherapy. Of these, 28 needed surgical excision at a later date. Plenk[76] concluded that radiotherapy was ineffective. In a series of 38 patients, he radiated 21 and interposed a shield between the source of radiation and the shoulder in 17. The calcium deposit disappeared in 67 per cent of the shielded and in 44 per cent of radiated patients. He gained the impression that in acute cases radiation delayed resorption in five out of nine patients, whereas in shielded patients the deposit persisted in only one out of eight patients. In this context, Gschwend and colleagues'[36] sarcastic remark that in acute cases any form of treatment is successful is noteworthy. "Therapy cannot hinder the success," they conclude.

SURGERY

Bosworth[11, 12] expressed the opinion of many surgeons when he wrote that the quickest and most dependable way of ridding patients of large and troublesome deposits is by open surgery. Vebostad[102] obtained excellent and good results with surgery in 34 out of 43 patients. Litchman and colleagues[49] feel that prolonged waiting in the chronic group leads to adhesive capsulitis and frozen shoulder. This view is not commonly shared. Gschwend and associates[36] formulated the following operative indications:

1. Progression of symptoms.
2. Constant pain interfering with activities of daily living.
3. Absence of improvement of symptoms after conservative therapy.

They reported excellent and good results in 25 out of 28 subjects. Moseley[60] restricts the indication in recommending surgery for large deposits in the mechanical phase. He, like most other authors, is in favor of conservative treatment for acute cases. DePalma and Kruper[22] reported 96 per cent good and only 4 per cent fair results after surgery. The time of recovery following surgery is surprisingly long. In DePalma and Kruper's[22] series, 53 per cent recovered in 2 to 6 weeks, and in an additional 30 per cent, it took 5 to 10 weeks. We reported similar results.[53]

Surgical Techniques

Discussing the surgical technique, Gschwend and colleagues[35, 36] recommend a muscle-splitting approach but warn against a deltoid detachment. They are in favor of a resection of the coracoacromial ligament. Vebostad[102] could not find an improvement in results when he performed a partial resection of the acromion which, according to his description, seems to have consisted of an anterior acromioplasty. Occasionally, serial vertical tendon incisions become necessary when the deposit is not readily identifiable.

Another surgical approach has been shown by Ellman.[28] He performed bursoscopy and emptied the calcific deposit. It seemed that the consistency of the calcified mass was cream- or toothpaste-like.

Following surgery, early mobilization is recommended. If a sling is worn, it must be removed at regular intervals for exercises.

Authors' Preferred Method of Treatment

Our therapeutic approach is based mainly on the severity of symptoms. Of course, the radiological aspect of the deposit will also be taken into consideration (Fig. 19–21).

Since it is our firm belief that symptoms during the formative phase are chronic or even absent and that the acute symptoms accompany the process of resorption, we will first state our management during the formative phase. Patients with subacute symptoms are classified as belonging to the formative phase unless the radiographs show evident signs of resorption.

During the formative phase we favor a conservative approach. Surgical removal is the exception and done only when an adequate conservative approach has failed and when the symptoms interfere with either work or the activity of daily living.

CONSERVATIVE MEASURES

The patient is instructed to do a daily program of exercises to maintain the full mobility of the glenohumeral joint. We also instruct the patient to position his arm in abduction as often as possible. This can be achieved by placing the arm on the backrest of a chair or on a seat beside him or her. While lying down, a pillow should be placed in the axilla. Application of moist heat is also suggested if the symptoms are subacute. Diathermy may be included. Although ultrasound is used occasionally in our physiotherapy department and some patients have commented on its beneficial effect, we have seen no evidence that this treatment modality accelerates the disappearance of calcium deposits.

Local intrabursal corticosteroid injections are never done in the presence of chronic symptoms. Only in the presence of impingement causing subacute symptoms do we give one intrabursal corticosteroid injection mixed with xylocaine. Needling of dense, homogeneous deposits has never been attempted. Attempts at lavage have not been successful in our hands. This is not surprising, given the chalk-like consistency of the deposit.

Nonsteroidal anti-inflammatory drugs are not prescribed when the symptoms are chronic but are given for 1 week to 10 days when subacute symptoms are present. Analgesics are rarely indicated.

Patients are assessed clinically and radiologically every four weeks. In cases where the outcome of conservative treatment is not satisfactory and the patient meets our criteria for surgical intervention, the indication is discussed with the patient. Should the patient consent, the operation is done on a short-stay basis in the hospital. History and physical as well as all laboratory tests and radiographs (chest and affected shoulder) are done one week prior to surgery. On the day of surgery, the patient is admitted to our short-stay unit and discharged the same day following surgery. Before discharge, the patient will be seen by the physiotherapist to assure that a proper postoperative exercise program is followed.

SURGICAL TECHNIQUE

Removal of calcium deposits is done under general anesthesia. The patient is in a supine position, and a sandbag is placed under the affected shoulder. We make sure that the side of the patient to be operated on is as close to the edge of the table as possible. The arm is free-draped to assure full mobilization of the arm during surgery. We use the skin incision recommended by Neer,[64] going from the acromion to the coracoid process. The deltoid fibers are bluntly separated. A stitch to protect the axillary nerve in the distal part near the deltoid splitting has not been found necessary. The deltoid muscle is not detached from the acromion. The bursa is then opened and the edges retracted with army-navy retractors. The bursal wall is inspected. The coracoacromial ligament is then identified and cleaned of all overlying soft tissues. Care is taken to visualize the posterior edge of the ligament. The state of the ligament is recorded. Although described by Watson,[103] we have never observed a thickening. The narrowness of the interval between rotator cuff and ligament is then tested, usually using the little finger. Introduction of this finger is made easier through longitudinal traction of the arm. While the finger is in place, the arm is rotated and lifted in position between flexion and abduction. The undersurface of the acromion is also palpated. If the space between ligament and rotator cuff is "tight," it is usually necessary to proceed with only a partial resection of the ligament; an anterior acromioplasty is definitely the exception. Before proceeding with the partial resection, a curved hemostat is introduced into the bursa under the ligament; it exits exactly at the posterior border of the ligament. The use of the hemostat prevents a lesion of the artery, which is just behind the ligament. We warn against a blind division of the ligament. Following partial resection of the

SYMPTOM	THERAPY	EFFECTS
CHRONIC PAIN	CONSERVATIVE	MAINTENANCE OF ROM AND OF STRENGTH
	AVOID CORTISONE SURGERY, IF UNSUCCESSFUL AND IF INTERFERENCE WITH WORK AND ADL	
ACUTE PAIN	NEEDLING AND LAVAGE	DECOMPRESSION
	SINGLE CORTISONE INJECTION	HYPEREMIA ↓ PHAGOCYTOSIS ↓
	PENDULUM AND ROM EXERCISES	AVOIDANCE OF FROZEN SHOULDER
SUBSIDING PAIN	REST IN ABDUCTION	RELIEVE STRETCH PRESSURE ↓ BLOOD FLOW ↑
	ROM AND STRENGTHENING EXERCISES	AVOIDANCE OF FROZEN SHOULDER AND OF MUSCLE WEAKNESS
	AVOID CORTISONE	

Figure 19–21. Outline of our treatment approach. (ROM = range of motion.)

ligament, the inspection of the rotator cuff and its covering bursal wall is easy. External and internal rotation of the arm will permit inspection of the entire rotator cuff. If a bursal reaction is present, its localization and extent are recorded. It is usually limited to a hyperemic reaction around the calcific deposit, which shines through the bursal wall. The tendon is then incised in the direction of its fibers, and the calcific mass is curetted. We usually proceed then with a limited resection of the frayed tendon edges, which are usually sites of calcium incrustation. Sometimes more than one deposit is present, necessitating separate tendon incisions. A proper preoperative radiograph is of great importance for the determination not only of location but also of the number of deposits. If no calcium can be seen during inspection, small incisions are made at the site of suspected calcifications as determined by radiography.

After removal of the deposit, a copious lavage is done. The shoulder is moved through its full range of motion, the tendon edges are approximated, and the wound is closed in layers. A sling is applied after surgery. We hasten again to add that this sling must be removed at least four times a day for pendulum and range-of-motion exercises. The sling is completely removed after three days. We encourage patients to keep the arm in abduction as often as possible. If the postoperative pain is severe, local ice packs should be applied. We have never resorted to postoperative corticosteroid injections.

INJECTION TECHNIQUE

During the phase of resorption when the symptoms are acute or in the presence of subacute symptoms when radiographs indicate ongoing resorption, we attempt a lavage of the deposit with two 18-gauge needles. A local anesthetic (xylocaine 2 per cent without epinephrine) is used to freeze the sites of needle placement, and 5 ml are injected into the bursa. The site of lavage is based on the site of tenderness and on radiographic localization. If the lavage is not successful, the needling usually helps to decrease the intratendinous pressure. At the end of lavage or needling, we always proceed with an intrabursal corticosteroid injection when the pain is excruciating. This injection will not be repeated.

The patient is instructed to apply ice and to do pendulum exercises. Analgesics are prescribed. Although we always instruct the patient to take nonsteroidal anti-inflammatory drugs for one week, we have no absolute proof of their beneficial effect. After the first treatment, the patient will be asked to report back three or four days later. As soon as the symptoms decrease, usually after one week, the patient is referred to physiotherapy for range-of-motion and strengthening exercises. Radiographs are taken four weeks after the first visit. They nearly always show a considerable decrease in, if not disappearance of, the deposit.

Ultrasound has not been used by us during the resorptive phase.

We have not observed a single case of frozen shoulder or adhesive capsulitis in patients treated in this fashion. One case with this syndrome, however, was seen in consultation. This patient had been treated with systemic corticosteroid medication and a sling for six weeks.

Although at the beginning of our intensive involvement with calcifying tendinitis we have operated during the acute phase, we feel now that surgery is not indicated at a time when nature attempts, and usually succeeds with, removal of the calcific deposit.

Concluding Remarks

The success of management of patients with calcifying tendinitis depends on a thorough understanding of the disease process. Obviously, formation of the deposit must precede its resorption. Moreover, clinical observations leave no doubt that spontaneous resorption always takes place, the moment of resorption being the only question.

Factors responsible for the fibrocartilaginous metaplasia and ensuing calcification, as well as those triggering the resorptive process, are far from being known. Their elucidation should be the goal of future research.

Experimental reproduction of localized tendon calcification has not been too successful. Attempts were made at the level of the rotator cuff, using a plastic mold under the supraspinatus. This foreign body as well as the surgical trauma never led to changes compatible with calcifying tendinitis. Selye[89] published results obtained with his calciphylaxis model which led to tendon calcification in only one strain of mice. Besides, there is no question that calciphylaxis constitutes a systemic metabolic disease and not a localized disease process. We have recently obtained specimens of tendon and ligament calcification of inbred tiptoe-walking Yoshimura (TWY) mice from the Japanese Research Council. The sections show cartilaginous metaplasia in ligaments and tendons followed by calcification around chondrocytes.

References

1. Ali SY: Crystal induced arthropathy. *In* Verbruggen G and Veys EM (eds): Degenerative Joints, Vol 2. New York: Elsevier, 1985.
2. Anderson HC: Electron microscopic studies of induced cartilage development and calcification. J Cell Biol *35*:81–101, 1967.
3. Anderson HC: Vesicle associated with calcification in the matrix of epiphyseal cartilage. J Cell Biol *41*:59–72, 1969.
4. Anderson HC: Calcific diseases. Arch Pathol Lab Med *107*:341–348, 1983.
5. Baer WS: The operative treatment of subdeltoid bursitis. Johns Hopkins Hosp Bull *18*:282–284, 1907.
6. Baird LW: Roentgen irradiation of calcareous deposits about the shoulder. Radiology *37*:316–324, 1941.

7. Bateman JE: The Shoulder and Neck. Philadelphia: WB Saunders Company, 1978.

8. Bergemann D, and Stieda A: Uber die mit Kalkablagerungen einhergehende Entzündung der Schulterschleimbeutel. Münch Med Wschr 52:2699–2702, 1908.

9. Bonucci E: Fine structure and histochemistry of "calcifying globules" in epiphyseal cartilage. Z Zellforsch 103:192–217, 1970.

10. Booth RE, Jr, and Marvel JP, Jr: Differential diagnosis of shoulder pain. Orthop Clin North Am 6:353–379, 1975.

11. Bosworth BM: Calcium deposits in the shoulder and subacromial bursitis: a survey of 12,122 shoulders. JAMA 116:2477–2482, 1941.

12. Bosworth BM: Examination of the shoulder for calcium deposits. J Bone Joint Surg 23:567–577, 1941.

13. Brenckmann E, and Nadaud P: Le traitement des calcifications périarticulaires de l'épaule par radio thérapie. Arch d'Electric Med 40:27–29, 1932.

14. Brewer BJ: Aging of the rotator cuff. Am J Sports Med 7:102–110, 1979.

15. Brickner WM: Shoulder disability: stiff and painful shoulder. Am J Surg 26:196–204, 1912.

16. Carnett JB: The calcareous deposits of so-called calcifying subacromial bursitis. Surg Gynecol Obstet 41:404–421, 1925.

17. Chapman JF: Subacromial bursitis and supraspinatus tendinitis; its roentgen treatment. Calif Med 56:248–251, 1942.

18. Codman EA: On stiff and painful shoulders. Boston Med Surg J 154:613–620, 1906.

19. Codman EA: Bursitis subacromialis, or periarthritis of the shoulder joint. Publications of the Mass Gen Hospital Boston 2:521–591, 1909.

20. Codman EA: The Shoulder. Boston: Thomas Todd, 1934.

21. Crass JR: Current concepts in the radiographic evaluation of the rotator cuff. CRC Crit Rev Diagn Imaging 28:23–73, 1988.

22. DePalma AF, and Kruper JS: Long term study of shoulder joints afflicted with and treated for calcific tendinitis. Clin Orthop 20:61–72, 1961.

23. DePalma A: Surgery of the Shoulder, 2nd ed. Philadelphia: JB Lippincott, 1973.

24. De Sèze S, and Welfling J: Tendinites calcifiantes. Rhumatologie 22:5–14, 1970.

25. Dhuly RG, Lauler DP, and Thorn GW: Pharmacology and chemistry of adrenal glucocorticosteroids. Med Clin North Am 57:1155–1165, 1973.

26. Dieppe P: Crystal deposition disease and the soft tissues. Clin Rheum Dis 5:807–822, 1979.

27. Duplay S: De la périarthrite scapulohumerale et des raideurs de l'épaule qui en sont la consequence. Arch Gen Med 513:542, 1872.

28. Ellman H: The controversy of arthroscopic vs. open approaches to shoulder instability and rotator cuff disease. Fourth open meeting of the American Society of Shoulder and Elbow Surgeons. American Academy of Orthopedic Surgeons, Atlanta, Georgia, 1988 Symposium.

29. Faure G, and Daculsi G: Calcified tendinitis: a review. Ann Rheum Dis 42[Suppl]49–53, 1983.

30. Faure G, Netter P, Malaman B, et al.: Scanning electronmicroscopic study of microcrystals implicated in human rheumatic diseases. Scanning Microsc (3):163–176, 1980.

31. Friedman MS: Calcified tendinitis of the shoulder. Am J Surg 94:56–61, 1957.

32. Ghormley JW: Calcareous tendinitis. Surg Clin North Am 4:1721–1728, 1961.

33. Glatthaar E: Zur Pathologie der Periarthritis humeroscapularis. Dtsch Z Chir 251:414–434, 1938.

34. Griffin EJ, and Karselis TC: Physical agents for physical therapists. In Ultrasonic Energy, 2nd ed. Springfield, IL: Charles C Thomas, 1982.

35. Gschwend N, Patte D, and Zippel J: Die Therapie der Tendinitis calcarea des Schultergelenkes. Arch Orthop Unfallchir 73:120–135, 1972.

36. Gschwend N, Scherer M, and Lohr J: Die Tendinitis calcarea des Schultergelenks. Orthopade 10:196–205, 1981.

37. Halverson PB, McCarty DJ, Cheung HS, and Ryan LM: Milwaukee shoulder syndrome. Ann Rheum Dis 43:734–741, 1984.

38. Harbin M: Deposition of calcium salts in tendon of supraspinatus muscle. Arch Surg 18:1491–1512, 1929.

39. Harmon HP: Methods and results in the treatment of 2580 painful shoulders. With special reference to calcific tendinitis and the frozen shoulder. Am J Surg 95:527–544, 1958.

40. Herberts P, Kadefors R, Hogfors C, and Sigholm G: Shoulder pain and heavy manual labor. Clin Orthop 191:166–178, 1984.

41. Howorth MB: Calcification of the tendon cuff of the shoulder. Surg Gynecol Obstet 80:337–345, 1945.

42. Jones GB: Calcification of the supraspinatus tendon. J Bone Joint Surg 31B:433–435, 1949.

43. Jozsa L, Baliut BJ, and Reffy A: Calcifying tendinopathy. Arch Orthop Traumat 97:305–307, 1980.

44. Kessel L, and Watson M: The painful arc syndrome. J Bone Joint Surg 59B:166–172, 1977.

45. Key LA: Calcium deposits in the vicinity of the shoulder and other joints. Ann Surg 129:737–753, 1949.

46. Kozin F: Painful shoulder and the reflex sympathetic dystrophy syndrome. In McCarty DJ (ed): Arthritis and Allied Conditions, 10th ed. Philadelphia: Lea & Febiger, 1985.

47. Lapidus PW: Infiltration therapy of acute tendinitis with calcification. Surg Gynecol Obstet 76:715–725, 1943.

48. Lippmann RK: Observations concerning the calcific cuff deposits. Clin Orthop 20:49–60, 1961.

49. Litchman HM, Silver CM, Simon SD, and Eshragi A: The surgical management of calcific tendinitis of the shoulder. Int Surg 50:474–482, 1968.

50. Lundberg J: The frozen shoulder. Acta Orthop Scand [Suppl]119:1–59, 1969.

51. Macnab I: Rotator cuff tendinitis. Ann Royal Coll Surg 53:271–287, 1973.

52. McCarty DJ, Halverson PB, Carrera GF, et al: "Milwaukee Shoulder": Association of microspheroids containing hydroxyapatite crystals, active collagenase, and neutral proteas with rotator cuff defects. I. Clinical aspects. Arthritis Rheum 24:464–473, 1981.

53. McKendry RJR, Uhthoff HK, Sarkar K, and St George-Hyslop P: Calcifying tendinitis of the shoulder: prognostic value of clinical, histologic and radiologic features in 57 surgically treated cases. Rheumatology 9:75–80, 1982.

54. McLaughlin HL: Lesions of the musculotendinous cuff of the shoulder. III. Observations on the pathology, course and treatment of calcific deposits. Ann Surg 124:354–362, 1946.

55. McLaughlin HL: Selection of calcium deposits for operation—the technique and results of operation. Surg Clin North Am 43:1501–1504, 1963.

56. Meyer AW: Chronic functional lesions of the shoulder. Arch Surg 35:646–674, 1937.

57. Milone FP, and Copeland MM: Calcific tendinitis of the shoulder joint. AJR 85:901–913, 1961.

58. Moschkowitz E: Histopathology of calcification of the spinatus tendons associated with subacromial bursitis. Am J Med Sci 149:351–361, 1915.

59. Moseley HF: Shoulder Lesions, 3rd ed. Edinburgh: Churchill Livingstone, 1960.

60. Moseley HF: The natural history and clinical syndromes produced by calcified deposits in the rotator cuff. Surg Clin North Am 43:1489–1494, 1963.

61. Moseley HF: The results of nonoperative and operative treatment of calcified deposits. Surg Clin North Am 43:1505–1506, 1963.

62. Moseley HF, and Goldie I: The arterial pattern of the rotator cuff of the shoulder. J Bone Joint Surg 45B:780–789, 1963.

63. Murnaghan GF, and McIntosh D: Hydrocortisone in painful shoulder. Controlled trial. Lancet 21:798–800, 1955.

64. Neer CS II: Impingement lesions. Clin Orthop 173:70–77, 1983.

65. Neer CS II, Craig EV, and Fukuda H: Cuff-tear arthropathy. J Bone Joint Surg 65A:1232–1244, 1983.

66. Nutton RW, and Stothard J: Acute calcific supraspinatus tendinitis in a three year old child. J Bone Joint Surg 69B:148, 1987.

67. Olsson O: Degenerative changes of the shoulder and their

connection with shoulder pain. Acta Chir Scand [Suppl] *181*:1–110, 1953.

68. Ozaki J, Fuijimoto S, Nakagawa Y, et al.: Tears of the rotator cuff of the shoulder associated with pathological changes in the acromion. J Bone Joint Surg *70A*:1224–1230, 1988.

69. Painter CF: Subdeltoid bursitis. Boston Med Surg J *156*:345–349, 1907.

70. Patte D, and Goutallier D: Calcifications. Rev Chir Orthop *74*:277–278, 1988.

71. Patterson RL, and Darrach W: Treatment of acute bursitis by needle irrigation. J Bone Joint Surg *19*:993–1002, 1937.

72. Pedersen HE, and Key JA: Pathology of calcareous tendinitis and subdeltoid bursitis. Arch Surg *62*:50–63, 1951.

73. Pendergrass EP, and Hodes PJ: Roentgen irradiation in treatment of inflammations. AJR *45*:74–106, 1941.

74. Perugia L, and Postacchini F: The pathology of the rotator cuff of the shoulder. Ital J Orthop Haematol *11*:93–105, 1985.

75. Pinals RS, and Short CL: Calcific periarthritis involving multiple sites. Arthritis Rheum *9*:566–574, 1966.

76. Plenk HP: Calcifying tendinitis of the shoulder. Radiology *59*:384–389, 1952.

77. Rathbun JB, and Macnab J: The microvascular pattern of the rotator cuff. J Bone Joint Surg *52B*:540–553, 1970.

78. Remberger K, Faust H, and Keyl W: Tendinitis calcarea. Klinik, Morphologie, Pathogenese und Differentialdiagnose. Pathologe *6*:196–203, 1985.

79. Rothman RH, Marvel JP, Jr, and Heppenstall RB: Anatomic considerations in the glenohumeral joint. Orthop Clin North Am *6*:341–352, 1975.

80. Rothman RH, and Parke WW: The vascular anatomy of the rotator cuff. Clin Orthop *41*:176–186, 1965.

81. Ruttimann G: Über die Häufigkeit röntgenologischer Veränderungen bei Patienten mit typischer Periarthritis humeroscapularis und Schultergesunden. Inaugural dissertation, Zurich 1959.

82. Sandstrom C: Peritendinitis calcarea: common disease of middle life: its diagnosis, pathology and treatment. AJR *40*:1–21, 1938.

83. Sandstrom C, and Wahlgren F: Beitrag zur Kenntnis der "Peritendinitis calcarea" (sog. "Bursitis calculosa") speziell vom pathologisch-histologischen Gesichtspunkt. Acta Radiol [Stockh] *18*:263–296, 1937.

84. Sarkar K, and Uhthoff HK: Ultrastructural localization of calcium in calcifying tendinitis. Arch Pathol Lab Med *102*:266–269, 1978.

85. Sarkar K, and Uhthoff HK: Ultrastructure of the subacromial bursa in painful shoulder syndromes. Virchows Archiv *400*:107–117, 1983.

86. Schaer H: Die Duplay'sche Krankheit. Med Klin *35*:413–415, 1939.

87. Schaer H: Die Periarthritis humeroscapularis. Ergebn Chir Orthop *29*:211–309, 1936.

88. Seifert G: Morphologic and biochemical aspects of experimental extraosseous tissue calcification. Clin Orthop *69*:146, 1970.

89. Selye H: The experimental production of calcific deposits in the rotator cuff. Surg Clin North Am *43*:1483–1488, 1963.

90. Sengar DPS, McKendry RJ, and Uhthoff HK: Increased frequency of HLA-A1 in calcifying tendinitis. Tissue Antigens *29*:173–174, 1987.

91. Simon WH: Soft tissue disorders of the shoulder. Frozen shoulder, calcific tendinitis, and bicipital tendinitis. Orthop Clin North Am *6*:521–539, 1975.

92. Steinbrocker O: The painful shoulder. *In* Hollander JE (ed): Arthritis and Allied Conditions, 8th ed. Philadelphia: Lea & Febiger, 1972.

93. Stieda A: Zur Pathologie der Schultergelenkschleimbeutel. Arch Klin Chir *85*:910–924, 1908.

94. Thornhill TS: The painful shoulder. *In* Kelley WN, Harris ED, Shaun R, and Sledge CB (eds): Textbook of Rheumatology, 2nd ed. Philadelphia: WB Saunders, 1985.

95. Uhthoff HK: Calcifying tendinitis, an active cell-mediated calcification. Virchows Arch Path Anat *366*:51–58, 1975.

96. Uhthoff HK, Hammond DI, Sarkar K, et al.: The role of the coracoacromial ligament in the impingement syndrome: a clinical, radiological and histological study. Int Orthop *12*:97–104, 1988.

97. Uhthoff HK, Loehr J, and Sarkar K: The pathogenesis of rotator cuff tears. *In* Takagishi N (ed): The Shoulder. Tokyo: Professional Postgraduate Services, 1986, pp 211–212.

98. Uhthoff HK, Sarkar K, and Maynard JA: Calcifying tendinitis. Clin Orthop *118*:164–168, 1976.

99. Uhthoff HK, Lohr J, Hammond I, and Sarkar K: Aetiologie und Pathogenese von Rupturen der Rotatorenmanschette. *In* Helbig B, and Blauth W (eds): Schulterschmerzen und Rupturen der Rotatorenmanschette. Berlin: Springer-Verlag, 1986, pp 3–9.

100. Uhthoff HK, and Sarkar K: Tendopathia Calcificans. Beitr Orthop Traumat *28*:269–277, 1981.

101. Uhthoff HK, Sarkar K, and Hammond I: Die Bedeutung der Dichte und der Schärfe der Abgrenzung des Kalkschattens bei der Tendinopathia calcificans. Radiologe *22*:170–174, 1982.

102. Vebostad A: Calcific tendinitis in the shoulder region. A review of 43 operated shoulders. Acta Orthop Scand *46*:205–210, 1975.

103. Watson M: The impingement syndrome in sportsmen. *In* Bateman JE, and Welsh RP (eds): Surgery of the Shoulder. Philadelphia: BC Decker, 1984, pp 140–142.

104. Welfling J, Kahn MF, Desroy M, et al.: Les calcifications de l'épaule. II. La maladie des calcifications tendineuses multiples. Rev Rheum *32*:325–334, 1965.

105. Wilson CL: Lesions of the supraspinatus tendon. Degeneration, rupture and calcification. Arch Surg *46*:307–325, 1943.

106. Wolfgang GL: Surgical repairs of the rotator cuff of the shoulder. J Bone Joint Surg *56A*:14–26, 1974.

107. Wrede L: Uber Kalkablagerungen in der Umgebung des Schultergelenkes und ihre Beziehungen zur Periarthritis humeroscapularis. Langenbecks Arch Klin Chir *99*:259–272, 1912.

108. Young BR: Roentgen treatment for bursitis of shoulder. AJR *56*:626–630, 1946.

The Biceps Tendon

Wayne Z. Burkhead, Jr., M.D.

The tendon of the long head of the biceps brachii is the proverbial stepchild of the shoulder. It has been blamed for numerous painful conditions of the shoulder from arthritis to adhesive capsulitis. Kessell[114] described the tendon as "somewhat of a maverick, easy to inculpate but difficult to condemn." Its function has been often misunderstood. It has been tenodesed, translocated, pulled through drill holes in the humeral head, and debrided with an arthroscope, oftentimes with marginal results. Lippmann[125] likened the long head of the biceps to the appendix: "An unimportant vestigial structure unless something goes wrong with it."

Charles S. Neer II and Charles A. Rockwood, Jr. have stressed the fact that 95 to 98 per cent of patients with a diagnosis of biceps tendinitis have, in reality, a primary diagnosis of impingement syndrome with *secondary* involvement of the biceps tendon. They have condemned routine biceps tenodesis.

This chapter will present a historical perspective, review the pertinent anatomy, attempt to explain the function of the long head of the biceps, and present a review of current concepts on the etiology, diagnosis, and management of lesions of the biceps tendon.

Historical Review

Hippocrates[96] was the first to call attention to the possibility of pathological displacement of muscle and tendons in dislocations. Accurate depictions of the anatomy of the biceps region and intertubercular groove appeared in the 1400s (Fig. 20–1A). Traumatic injuries to the bicipital region are depicted in a German wound manikin in the 1500s (Fig. 20–1B). The first reported case of dislocation of the tendon of the long head of the biceps brachii muscle was in 1694 by William Cowper in a book entitled *Myotoma Reformata*.[48] In his case, a woman who was wringing clothes felt something displace in her shoulder. Three days after the injury he examined her and noticed a depres-

sion of the external part of the deltoid, accompanied by rigidity in the lower biceps and an inability to extend the forearm. He reduced it by manipulation, and the patient at once recovered the use of the arm. This miraculous recovery is seldom seen in my practice in patients with painful and stiff shoulders; although the recognition of this injury was accepted by Boerhaave and Bromfield,[29] Cowper's observation became subject to suspicion, because of his plagiarism of the Dutch anatomist Godfried Bidloo.[24] Before Cowper's description, most reported cases of biceps injury were undoubtedly a result of direct trauma, most likely as depicted in Figure 20–1B. In 1803, Monteggia[161] reported a second case resembling that of Cowper, except that the dislocation was habitual. From that time until 1910, numerous additional clinical reports appeared.[85, 87, 186, 197, 198] It was not until 1841 that Soden[212] reported a case that was clinically proven at necropsy. Hueter[102] described clearly the signs and symptoms of lesions of this tendon.

However, there was controversy. Jarjavey,[107] discussing cases in 1867, felt that most of the symptoms were related to subacromial bursitis and that simple luxation did not exist. Some authors[13, 29] believed that the lesion was secondary to arthritis or concomitant problems. Callender[31] mentioned one case of recurring dislocation in which the tendon could not be retained in the groove because of fibrous tissue. Duplay[58–60] described "periarthrite scapulo-humerale." It is evident from his work that this included tendinitis of the biceps. McClellan[139] discussed the function of the biceps tendon:

Furthermore, the long tendon of the biceps muscle which is lodged below the tuberosities pierces the capsular ligament and passes over the head of the humerus to the top of the glenoid cavity, strengthens the upper anterior part of the joint and prevents the head of the humerus from being brought against the acromion, processing the normal upward movements of the arm. In fact it is mainly by the normal position of this tendon, assisted somewhat by atmospheric pressure, that the head of the humerus is retained in its natural position.

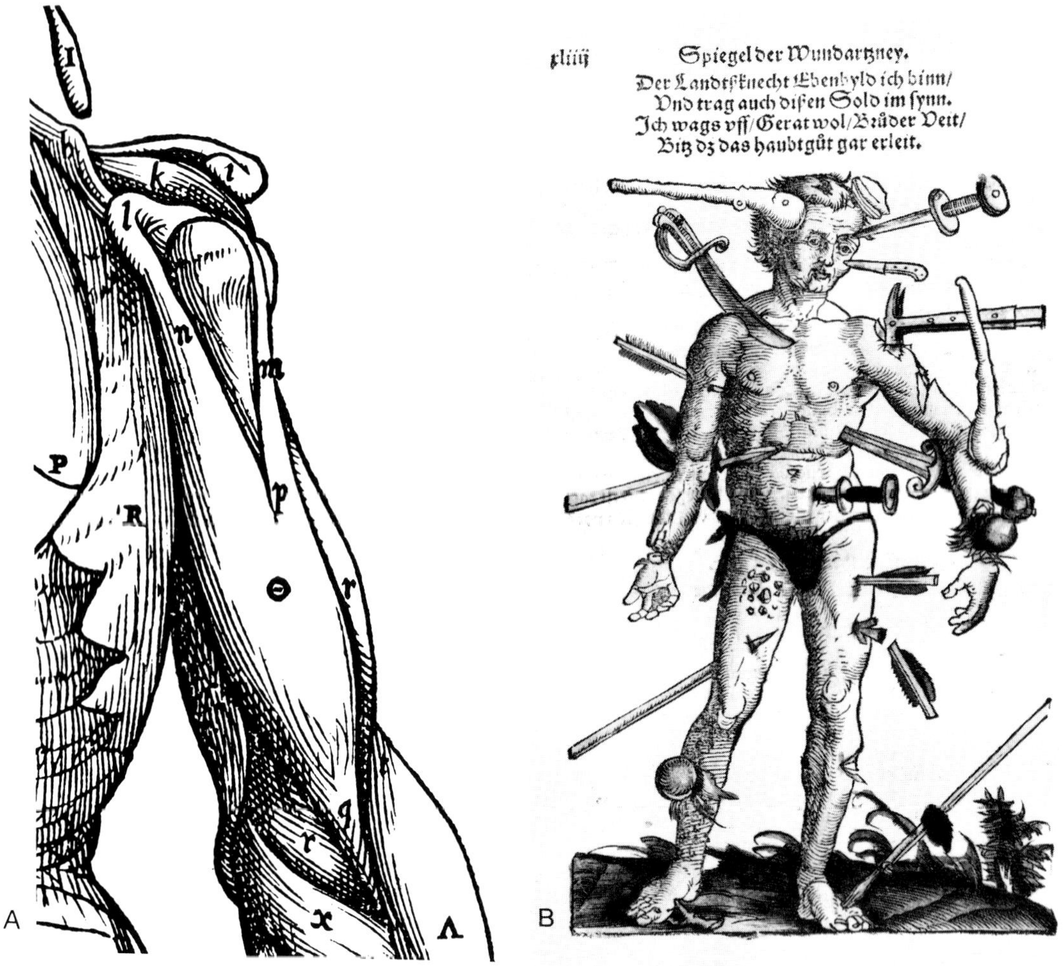

Figure 20–1. A, Close-up of the three tendons of the biceps brachii: short head (N), long head (M), distal tendon (Q). (From the Sixth Plate of Muscles. Possibly by Jan Stevenz van Calcar [Flemish ca. 1499–1550]. From Andreas Vesalius, DeHumani Corporis Fabrica. Basel: Johames Oporinus, 1543). B, Probable mechanism of injury to the biceps prior to Cowper's description. Notice the saber-type incision in the opposite shoulder. (Anonymous wound manikin, 1517. From von Gersdorff H: Feldthbuch der Wundartzney. Strasbourg: Hans Schotten, 1540.) (Reprinted with permission from Karp D: ARS Medica: Art, Medicine, and the Human Condition. Philadelphia, Copyright © 1985, the University of Pennsylvania Press.)

Bera[23] in 1910 felt that osteitis reduced the height of the lesser tuberosity and led to instability. In the 1920s, valuable contributions were made by Meyer.[145–152] He discussed his observations based on a total of 59 incidences of spontaneous dislocation of the long head of the tendon and on 20 examples of complete rupture. He was the first to describe the supratubercular ridge (Fig. 20–2); he also described degenerative changes on the undersurface of the acromion, in the acromioclavicular joint, and in the coracoacromial ligament. Meyer concluded that attrition, particularly following the use of the extremity in abduction and external rotation, led to a gradual destruction of the capsule proximal to and in the region of the lesser tuberosity. As a consequence of the weakness of the capsule, dislocation ensued.

According to Schrager,[205] F. Pasteur,[187] then medical colonel of the military hospital at Val de Gras, recognized the condition of bicipital tendinitis in all its aspects, described it fully, and raised it to the status of a distinct clinical entity. In 1934, the specificity of the diagnosis of biceps tendinitis was questioned by Codman,[43] who wrote, "Personally, I believe that the sheath of the biceps is less apt to be involved than are other structures. I have never proved its involvement in a single case. I think that the substance of the tendon of the supraspinatus is most often involved." In the 1940s, Lippmann,[124, 125] Tarsy,[218] and Hitchcock and Bechtol[97] believed that bicipital tendinitis was an important cause of shoulder pain, and all described operations for the relief of symptoms. In 1950, DePalma[51] described degenerative changes in the tendon that occurred with aging and reported on both operative and conservative management. Although he was grateful that more surgeons were recognizing the disorder (bicipital tendinitis), he felt that many were still reluctant to give this disorder the importance it deserved. Based on gross and microscopic examination in 78 cases, he concluded that bicipital groove tenosynovitis is the most common cause of the painful and

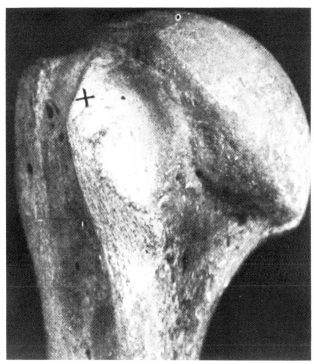

Figure 20–2. Original photograph of the supratubercular ridge taken by Meyer. (Reproduced with permission from Gilcreest EL: Dislocation and elongation of the long head of the biceps brachii. Analysis of six cases. Ann Surg *104*:118–138, 1936.)

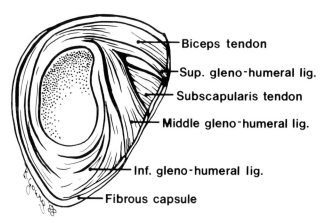

Figure 20–3. The biceps tendon is seen inserting on the superiormost portion of the glenoid labrum. Its origin may be simple, bifurcated, or trifurcated.

stiff shoulder. In 1972, Neer[166] described the anterior impingement syndrome, pointing to anterior acromial spurring with thickening and fibrosis of the coracoacromial ligament, causing impingement wear on the rotator cuff and biceps tendon. He pointed out a close association between ruptures of the biceps tendon and rotator cuff tears.

Although the pendulum, over the past 14 years, has swung away from primary bicipital tendinitis and isolated biceps tendon instability, O'Donohue[178] reported on surgical techniques for treating the subluxating biceps tendon in the athlete. Neviaser[177] recommended tenodesis of the biceps at the time of acromioplasty and excision of the distal clavicle as part of the four-in-one arthroplasty, and in 1987, Post[194] presented a series of patients with primary bicipital tenosynovitis.

It has been almost 300 years since Cowper[48] described his first case, and controversy over the importance of this lesion still exists.

Anatomy

The long head of the biceps brachii originates at the supraglenoid tubercle and glenoid labrum in the superiormost portion of the glenoid (Fig. 20–3). It is a long tendon (9 cm) that can be bifurcated or trifurcated at its origin. In a study by Habermeyer,[86] the biceps was found to originate off the supraglenoid tubercle in 20 per cent and off the superior posterior labrum in 48

per cent and 28 per cent had origins from both of these structures. The cross-sectional characteristics of the long head of the biceps change during its course, 8.5 × 7.8 mm at its origin, 4.7 × 2.6 mm in the area of strongest demand (the entrance to the sulcus), and 4.5 × 2.8 mm at the musculotendinous junction. It courses obliquely across the top of the humeral head into the intertubercular groove or sulcus. The tendon continues down the ventral portion of the humerus, becoming musculotendinous near the insertion of the deltoid. The angle formed by a line from the bottom of the groove to a central point on the humeral head is constant and corresponds precisely to the retrotorsion angle measured from the epicondyles[86] (Fig. 20–4).

The biceps tendon is intra-articular but extrasynovial. The proximal layer of synovial sheath reflects back on itself to form a visceral sheath (Fig. 20–5). The sheath, which communicates directly with the glenohumeral joint, ends in a blind pouch at the end of the bicipital groove. Many authors and texts have stated that there is an intra-articular and groove portion to the biceps tendon and that it becomes extra-articular

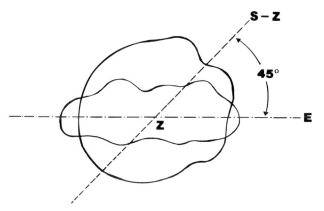

Figure 20–4. A line (S–Z) drawn through the center of the bottom of the bicipital groove, intersecting with a line drawn across the humeral condyles (E), accurately depicts the retroversion of the humeral head. (Redrawn from Habermeyer P, Kaiser E, Knappe M, et al: Functional anatomy and biomechanics of the long biceps tendon. Unfallchirurg *90*(7):319–329, 1987.)

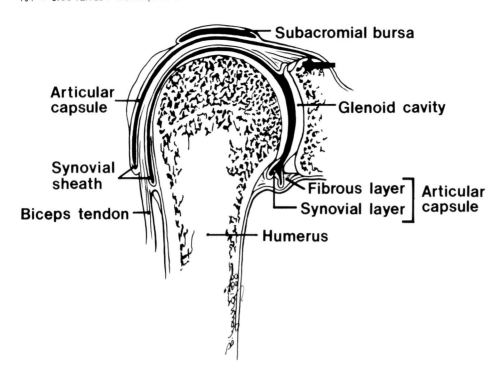

Figure 20–5. This figure illustrates both the insertion of the biceps onto the superior glenoid labrum as well as the supraglenoid tubercle *(black arrow)*, and the reflection of the synovial sheath, which maintains the tendon as an extracapsular structure while it is on its intra-articular course.

at the insertion of the capsule. In reality, as is discussed later under functional anatomy, the humeral head glides up and down on the biceps tendon so that at some point (i.e., the extremes of abduction), there is only a very small portion of tendon that is intra-articular, while at others (i.e., adduction and extension), the intra-articular portion is longer. The extra-articular component of the biceps begins distal to the synovial sheath. The muscle along with the short head of the biceps forms a common distal tendon (Fig. 20–6) that inserts in the bicipital tuberosity of the radius. Occasionally, a third muscle belly is present. The blood supply to the muscle of the long head of the biceps is via the brachial artery. The anterior circumflex artery in particular supplies the biceps tendon in the groove.[86] The nerve supply to the biceps is via the musculocutaneous nerve stemming from C5 to C7.

Mercer[144] and Gilcreest[73] measured the tensile strength of the biceps tendon as from 150 to 200 pounds.

SOFT TISSUE RESTRAINT

The tendon of the long head of the biceps is restrained at several levels along its course in the arm. In its anatomical position, the intra-articular portion of the biceps tendon runs underneath the coracohumeral ligament that lies between and strengthens the interval between the subscapularis and supraspinatus, the so-called rotator interval. It is an integral part of the cuff and capsule and can be distinguished only by sharp dissection.[180] The most important feature in retention of the biceps tendon in this area is that portion of the capsule of the shoulder joint thickened by the coracohumeral ligament and edges of subscapularis and supraspinatus tendons that bridge the tuberosities in the uppermost portion of the sulcus (Figs. 20–7 and 20–8). *This portion of the capsule is the first and chief obstacle to a medial dislocation of the tendon, and Meyer*[145, 150] *found that in all of his cases of dislocation it had been torn or stretched.* Codman,[43] in commenting on Meyer's work, stated that in his opinion, "displacement of the tendon is a result of rupture at that portion of the musculotendinous cuff, which is inserted into the inner edge of the intratubercular notch."

Paavolainen and colleagues,[180] in a study on soft tissue restraint to dislocation of the biceps, were unable to dislocate the tendon medially over the lesser tuberosity in the intact specimen. Transection of the intertubercular transverse ligament allowed for no appreciable lateral or medial movement of the tendon. However, when the portion of the rotator cuff above the lesser tuberosity was additionally transected, the tendon could be easily displaced medially, over and beyond the lesser tuberosity, taking a new course across the tendon of the subscapularis muscle. Further dissection down the groove showed that the restraint to dislocation of the tendon in the groove was the medial portion of the coracohumeral ligament close to its insertion on the lesser tuberosity. Traditional teaching was that the biceps tendon is held in place within the sulcus by means of the transverse humeral ligament (Fig. 20–9). Meyer[145] disputed this, finding that this structure was either too weak or entirely absent. The chief structure containing the tendon within the groove below the top of the tuberosity is the tendinous expansion from the insertion of the sternocostal portion of the pectoralis major, the falsiform ligament[1] (see Fig.

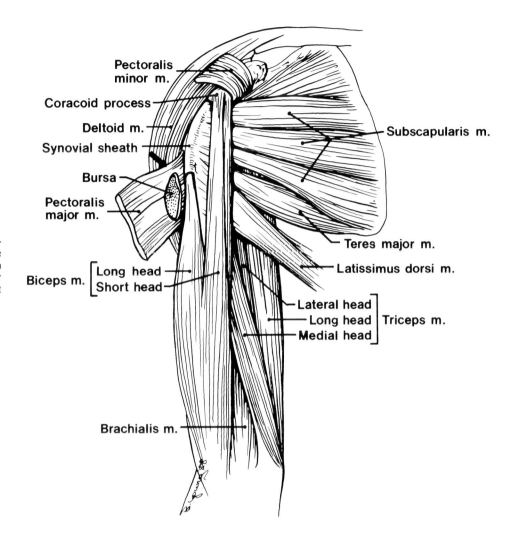

Figure 20–6. General anatomic relationships of the long head of the biceps. Note how the pectoralis major and falsiform ligament *(large black arrow)* cross over the tendon and help to stabilize it after it exits the groove.

Pectoralis minor m.
Coracoid process
Deltoid m.
Synovial sheath
Bursa
Pectoralis major m.
Biceps m. { Long head / Short head }
Subscapularis m.
Teres major m.
Latissimus dorsi m.
Lateral head / Long head / Medial head } Triceps m.
Brachialis m.

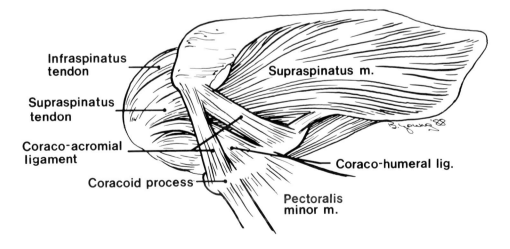

Infraspinatus tendon
Supraspinatus tendon
Coraco-acromial ligament
Coracoid process
Supraspinatus m.
Coraco-humeral lig.
Pectoralis minor m.

Figure 20–7. The coracohumeral ligament serves to reinforce the capsule in the rotator interval. The capsule, along with the edges of the supraspinatus and subscapularis, stabilize the tendon as it leaves the sulcus.

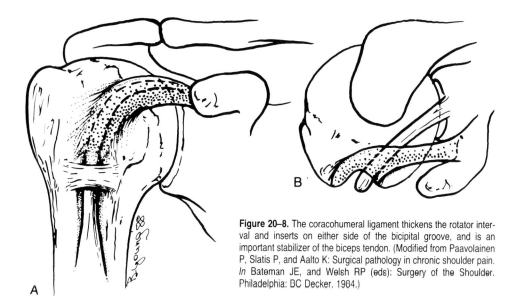

Figure 20–8. The coracohumeral ligament thickens the rotator interval and inserts on either side of the bicipital groove, and is an important stabilizer of the biceps tendon. (Modified from Paavolainen P, Slatis P, and Aalto K: Surgical pathology in chronic shoulder pain. *In* Bateman JE, and Welsh RP (eds): Surgery of the Shoulder. Philadelphia: BC Decker, 1984.)

20–6). It forms a margin with the deep aspect of the main tendon and is attached to both lips of the groove, blending above with the capsule at the shoulder joint.

OSSEOUS ANATOMY

The bicipital groove (Fig. 20–10) is formed between the lesser and greater tuberosities. The medial wall is made up of the lesser tuberosity, while the lateral wall is the edge of the greater tuberosity. A cadaver and radiographic study of the bicipital groove has been done by Cone and colleagues.[15] They measured the medial wall angle, width, and depth of the intertubercular groove (Fig. 20–11). The mean value for the medial wall angle was 56 degrees (range 40 to 70 degrees). The width of the intertubercular sulcus was measured in two locations on the bicipital groove view. The top width was determined as the distance between the medial and lateral lips of the intertubercular sulcus. The middle width was measured between the walls of the intertubercular sulcus, a point equal to half of the depth of the sulcus. There were wide differences in width measurements in this study, but the ratio of the width was constant at 1.6 from the top to the middle distance. They found the average depth of the groove

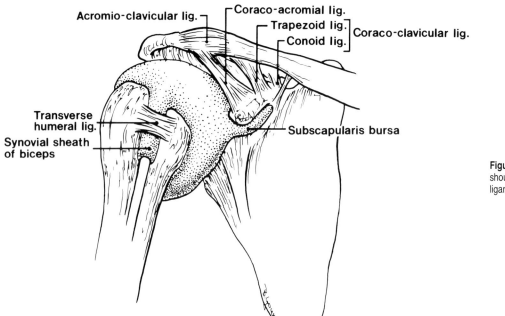

Figure 20–9. The ligaments around the shoulder. Meyer[145] found the transverse ligament to be too weak or entirely absent.

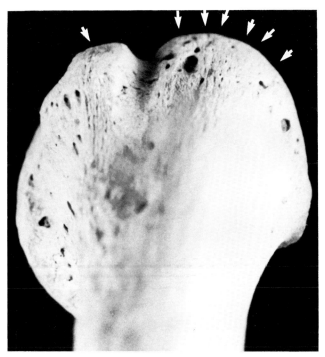

Figure 20–10. The bicipital groove is made up of the walls of the lesser tuberosity *(small arrow)* and greater tuberosity *(multiple arrows)*. (Reproduced with permission from Cone RO, Danzig L, Resnick D, and Goldman AB: The bicipital groove: radiographic, anatomic, and pathologic study. Am J Roentgenol *41*:781–788, 1983. Copyright © Am Roentgen Ray Soc 1983.)

to be 4.3 mm, range 4 to 6 mm. Variability of the medial wall angle confirms previous studies by Hitchcock and Bechtol[97] and Habermeyer and associates.[86] Hitchcock and Bechtol[97] found that the medial wall angle was 90 degrees in 10 per cent, 75 degrees in 35 per cent, 60 degrees in 34 per cent, 45 degrees in 13 per cent, 30 degrees in 6 per cent, and 15 degrees in 2 per cent (Fig. 20–12). They also noted a strong correlation between lower medial wall angles and subluxation and dislocation of the biceps tendon. Haber-

meyer[86] agrees that the angle also correlated with the probability of subluxation of the long head of the biceps tendon. Cone and colleagues,[45] however, found no correlation between the incidence of subluxation and low medial wall angles.

COMPARATIVE ANATOMY

Hitchcock and Bechtol,[97] using specimens from the Museum of Natural History in Chicago, have outlined the changes in relationship of the scapula and bicipital groove from the quadruped to the erect biped (Fig. 20–13). There has been a progressive anteroposterior flattening of the thorax. This results in an increased angle that the scapula forms with the thorax and a relative lateral displacement of the scapula. Humans have a relatively short forearm, which, along with the scapular position, necessitates greater medial rotation of the humerus in order for the hand to reach the midline. The anteroposterior flattening of the thorax and the short forearm were compensated for, but only incompletely, by torsion of the humerus. In the quadruped opossum, the biceps tendon takes a straight course through the bicipital groove and is an effective abductor of the arm in the forward plane. However, in humans, the tendon is lodged against the lesser tuberosity where a supratubercular ridge or shallow groove can traumatize the tendon. Humans are unique among the primates in presenting marked variations (see Fig. 20–12B) in the configuration of the bicipital groove.

The human arm was derived from the foreleg of the quadruped, the latter devised to bear weight and to be swung in a pendulum fashion. With the development of upright posture by man, the upper limb had to be moved away from the body, not only against its own weight but also against the weight of other objects. This short power arm has to act against a long lever arm, producing unfavorable mechanical conditions leading to tendinitis of the rotator cuff and biceps.

Figure 20–11. Measurements taken by Cone and associates, including the medial wall angle as well as the width and depth of the bicipital groove. MW = medial wall angle; Le = lesser tuberosity; Gr = greater tuberosity; D = depth of groove; W = width of groove. (Reproduced with permission from Cone RO, Danzig L, Resnick D, and Goldman AB: The bicipital groove: radiographic, anatomic, and pathologic study. Am J Roentgenol *41*:781–788, 1983. Copyright © Am Roentgen Ray Soc 1983.)

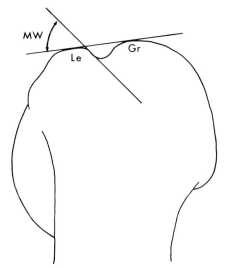

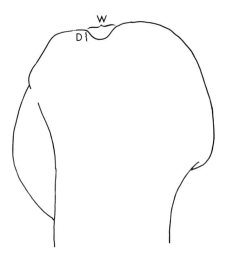

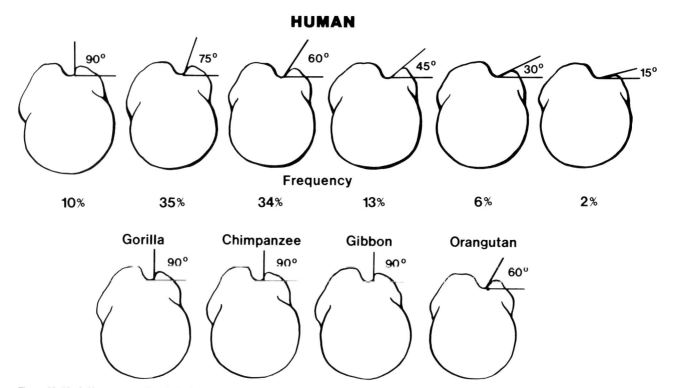

Figure 20–12. *A*, Humans are unique in having variations in the bicipital groove. *B*, The groove of the biceps in primates is constant within the species. (Modified and redrawn from Hitchcock HH, and Bechtol CO: Painful shoulder. Observations on the role of the tendon of the long head of the biceps brachii in its causation. J Bone Joint Surg *30A*:263–273, 1948.)

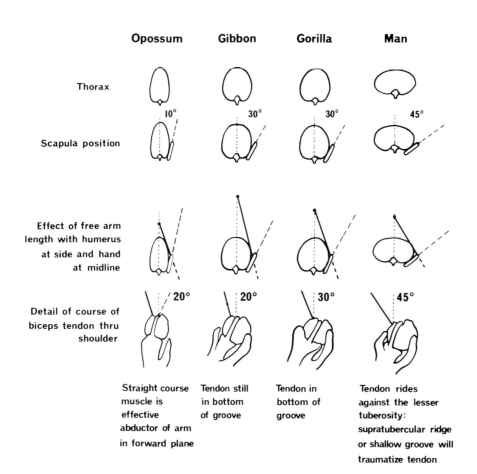

Figure 20–13. Progressive changes in anteroposterior flattening of the thorax, scapular position, and migration of the biceps tendon from the quadruped to the biped. (Modified from Hitchcock HH, and Bechtol CO: Painful shoulder. Observations on the role of the tendon of the long head of the biceps brachii in its causation. J Bone Joint Surg *30A*:263–273, 1948.)

DEVELOPMENTAL ANATOMY

During the ninth week of gestation, the limbs undergo rotation. The upper limb rotates dorsally at the elbow. This rotation is reflected in the shoulder as humeral retroversion, which averages 35 degrees. This rotation, in essence, leaves the biceps tendon behind on the anterior aspect of the shoulder in the groove and requires that the biceps cross the joint obliquely at a 30- to 45-degree angle, rather than proceeding in a straight line laterally as in the quadrupeds.

The development of the glenohumeral joint is similar to that of other synovial joints in the human body. According to Gardner,[70] it involves two basic processes. Initially, there is a formation of an inner zone between the two developing bones of the joint, followed by the creation of cavities by enzymatic action. The inner zones often comprise three layers, a chondrogenic layer on either side of a looser layer of cells. The joint capsule and many of the intra-articular structures, such as the synovial membrane, the ligaments, the labrum, and the biceps tendon, form from this inner zone of tissue. Giuliani and associates[78] confirmed that the tendon of the long head of the biceps brachii arises in continuity with the anlage of the glenoid labrum. At approximately seven weeks of gestation, the joint is well formed, the humeral head is spherical, and the tendons of the infraspinatus, subscapularis, and biceps as well as the glenoid labrum can be seen (Fig. 20–14).

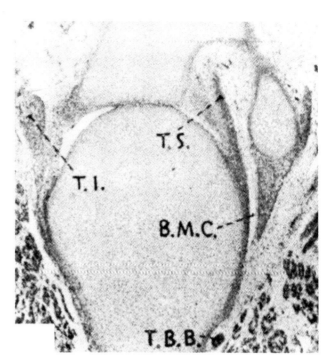

Figure 20–14. At approximately seven weeks' gestation, the joint is well formed and the humeral head is spherical. The biceps tendon (TBB) is clearly seen in the groove. This picture is taken before rotation occurs; the biceps tendon will eventually assume a position less lateral than shown here. The other structures in this picture are the tendon of the infraspinatus (TI), the subscapularis (TS), and the bursa of the coracobrachialis (BMC). (Reproduced with permission from Gardner E, and Gray DJ: Prenatal development of the human shoulder and acromioclavicular joint. Am J Anat 92:219, 1953.)

PATHOLOGICAL ANATOMY

Many authors[51–55] believe that tenosynovitis is the chief cause of pain with bicipital tendinitis and leads to an altered tendon sheath gliding mechanism. They describe gradual pathological changes in the area of the biceps tendon, including, initially, capillary dilatation and edema of the tendon with progressive cellular infiltration of the sheath and synovium and the development of filmy adhesions between the tendon and the tendon sheath. In the chronic stage, there is fraying and narrowing of the biceps tendon with minimal to moderate synovial proliferation and fibrosis and, ultimately, replacement of the tendon fibers by fibrous tissue and organization of dense fibrous adhesions between the tendon, passing through the bicipital groove and across the joint. The biceps tendon passes directly under the critical zone of the supraspinatus tendon. Claessens and Snoek[40] have also described microscopic changes that can be found in the tendon, including atrophic irregular collagen fiber, fissurization and shreading of tendon fibers, fibrinoid necrosis, and a productive inflammatory reaction with an increase in fibrocytes (Fig. 20–15). Macroscopic changes in cadaver studies by DePalma[51–55] and Claessens[39, 40] revealed tendinitis with shreading of the tendon fibers by osteophytes, adhesions between the synovial sheaths and between the tendon and its osteofibrous compartment, subluxation or dislocation of the tendon, and rupture of the tendon with retraction of the distal portion or adhesion of the distal portion to the sulcus. Although it was common belief that the tendon, when it dislocates, always displaced medially to the lesser tuberosity riding *over* the subscapularis tendon (Fig. 20–16B), Petersson[189] in his study found only one case such as this. In the majority of cases in his series, internal degeneration of the subscapularis in the region of the lesser tuberosity had occurred, allowing the tendon to dislocate medially under the subscapularis (Fig. 20–16C). Similar pathological findings were described by DePalma (Fig. 20–17).

The biceps tendon and its enveloping synovial sheath are bound to be affected by inflammatory or infectious processes of the glenohumeral joint owing to their anatomical location and course. Therefore, tenosynovitis of the biceps accompanies septic arthritis of the shoulder as well as rheumatic inflammation, osteoarthritis, and crystalline arthritis. The clinical syndrome in these cases is dominated by the articular pathology. In the past, biceps rupture has been reported to occur in conjunction with tuberculous and luetic infection.

Osseous Pathoanatomy

The shape of the groove has been implicated frequently in the pathogenesis of biceps tendon rup-

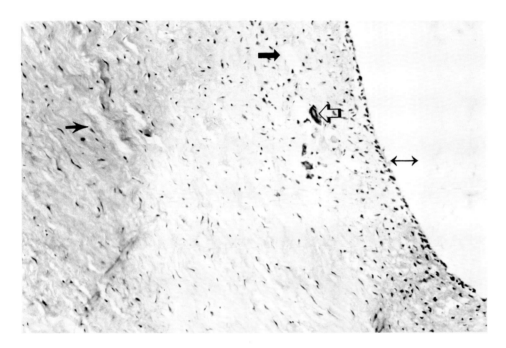

Figure 20–15. Pathology in a degenerative biceps tendon. The *double arrow* indicates the synovial membrane; the *open arrow* points to dystrophic calcification; the *closed arrow* marks total loss of fibers; the *arrowhead* indicates fissuring in the collagen with a disorderly collagen pattern. A productive inflammatory reaction with an increase in fibrocytes is seen in the lower right corner.

Figure 20–16. *A,* The normal relationship of the biceps tendon in the groove covered by the transverse ligament. *B,* Rupture of the transverse ligament and subluxation of the biceps tendon out of the groove, with the tendon lying anterior to the subscapularis muscle. *C,* Intratendinous disruption of the subscapularis found in the majority of cases by Petersson, in which the subscapularis insertion degenerates and the tendon subluxates beneath the muscle tendon belly. The subscapularis tendon may have attachment to the greater tuberosity through the coracohumeral and transverse ligaments. (Modified from Petersson CJ: Degeneration of the gleno-humeral joint: an anatomical study. Acta Orthop Scand *54:*277–283, 1983.)

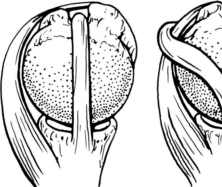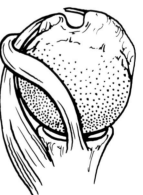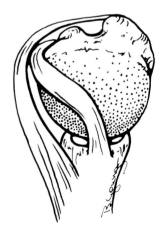

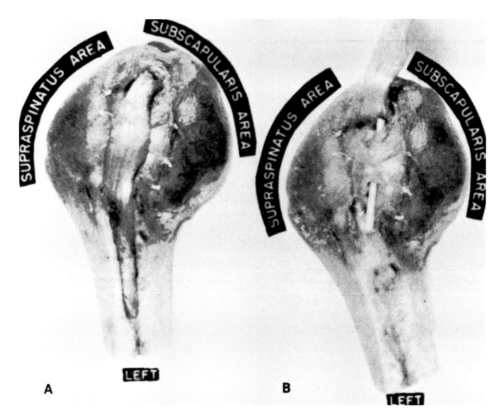

Figure 20–17. Obliteration of the bicipital groove by inflammation, with subluxation of the tendon lying in a fascial sling made by the insertion of the subscapularis. (Reproduced with permission from DePalma A: Surgery of the Shoulder, 2nd ed. Philadelphia: JB Lippincott, 1983.)

A   B

tures.[51–54, 86, 97] A shallow flattened groove (Fig. 20–18) is commonly associated with subluxation or dislocation of the biceps tendon, and a narrow groove with a sharp medial wall and an osteophyte at the aperture is associated with bicipital tendinitis and rupture (Fig. 20–19). Spurs on the floor of the groove may erode the tendon (Fig. 20–20). Although these groove abnormalities may contribute to bicipital tendon problems, it is more likely that some are changes in response to pathology of the soft tissues around the shoulder. In all of the degenerative conditions around the shoulder, soft tissue changes precede bony changes, i.e., in the impingement syndrome, fibrosis, bursitis, and tendinitis precede the formation of spurring in the anterior acromion. Synovitis and cartilage degeneration precede the spurs in the acromioclavicular joint. It seems logical that changes in the bicipital groove and its opening follow changes in the tendon, capsule, ligaments, and synovium around it.

BONY ANOMALIES

Bony anomalies and variations have been proposed as a cause of subluxation and tendinitis of the biceps tendon. The supratubercular ridge has been described by Meyer[145] as a ridge that extends forward and downward from the region of the articular cartilage to the upper and dorsal portions of the lesser tuberosity (Fig. 20–21). Its incidence, according to Cilley,[33] is 17.5 per cent out of 200 humeri. The ridge, when present,

decreases the depth of the sulcus and diminishes the effectiveness of the tuberosity as a trochlea. Meyer believed that the ridge pushed the biceps tendon against the transverse ligament, favoring dislocation.

In Hitchcock and Bechtol's[97] series, the supratubercular ridge was found to be markedly developed in 8 per cent and moderately developed in 59 per cent. Hitchcock and Bechtol[97] found a direct correlation with the supratubercular ridge and spurs on the lesser tuberosity (medial wall spurs). In their series, medial wall spurs were found in approximately 45 per cent of patients with a supratubercular ridge. When there was no supratubercular ridge, only 3 per cent of the humeri showed spurs on the lesser tuberosity (Fig. 20–21C). They concluded that the spurs on the lesser tuberosity were spurs reactive to pressure from the biceps tendon being pressed up against the tuberosity by the supratubercular ridge.

A supratubercular ridge was found in approximately 50 per cent of patients by Cone and colleagues[45] but did not correlate very well with the presence of bicipital groove spurs. They thought that the medial wall spur was related more to a traction enostosis, i.e., reactive bone formation at the site of a tendon or ligament insertion of the transverse humeral ligament. In one specimen, the transverse humeral ligament was completely ossified, converting the bicipital groove into a bony tunnel. They agree with DePalma that the presence of bony spurs on the *floor* of the bicipital groove is related to chronic bicipital tenosynovitis (Fig. 20–22).

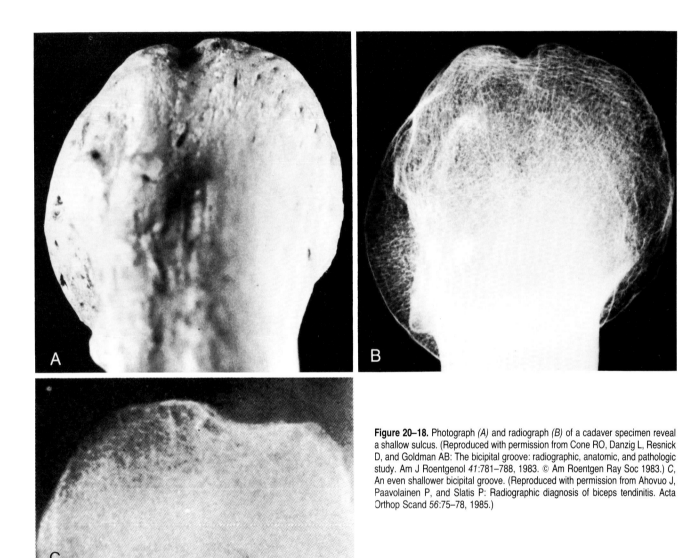

Figure 20–18. Photograph *(A)* and radiograph *(B)* of a cadaver specimen reveal a shallow sulcus. (Reproduced with permission from Cone RO, Danzig L, Resnick D, and Goldman AB: The bicipital groove: radiographic, anatomic, and pathologic study. Am J Roentgenol *41*:781–788, 1983. © Am Roentgen Ray Soc 1983.) *C,* An even shallower bicipital groove. (Reproduced with permission from Ahovuo J, Paavolainen P, and Slatis P: Radiographic diagnosis of biceps tendinitis. Acta Orthop Scand *56*:75–78, 1985.)

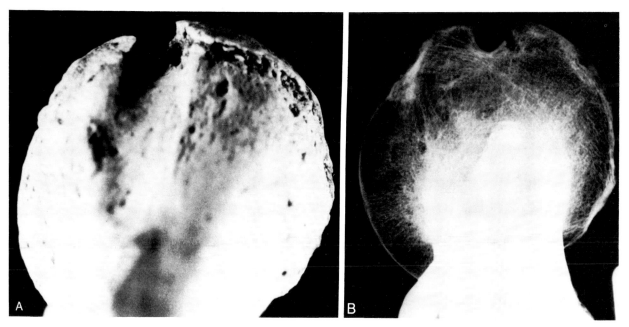

Figure 20–19. Pathological specimen *(A)* and groove radiograph *(B)* of the bicipital groove with a 90-degree medial wall angle and medial osteophyte at the aperture, seen commonly with bicipital tendinitis and rupture. (Reproduced with permission from Cone RO, Danzig L, Resnick D, and Goldman AB: The bicipital groove: radiographic, anatomic, and pathologic study. Am J Roentgenol *41*:781–788, 1983. © Am Roentgen Ray Soc 1983.)

Figure 20–20. *A*, A large bony spur is seen in the floor of the groove. A corresponding defect is present in the biceps tendon. *B*, The tendon has been replaced in the groove. (Reproduced with permission from DePalma A: Surgery of the Shoulder, 2nd ed. Philadelphia: JB Lippincott, 1983.)

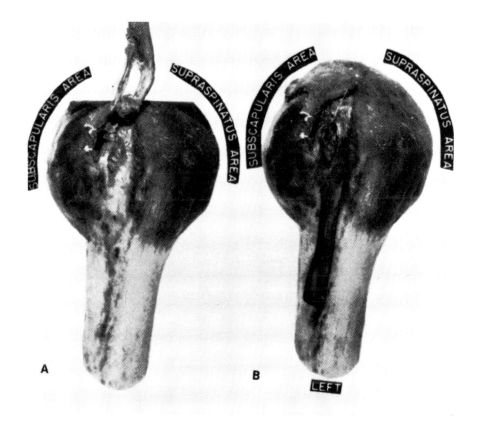

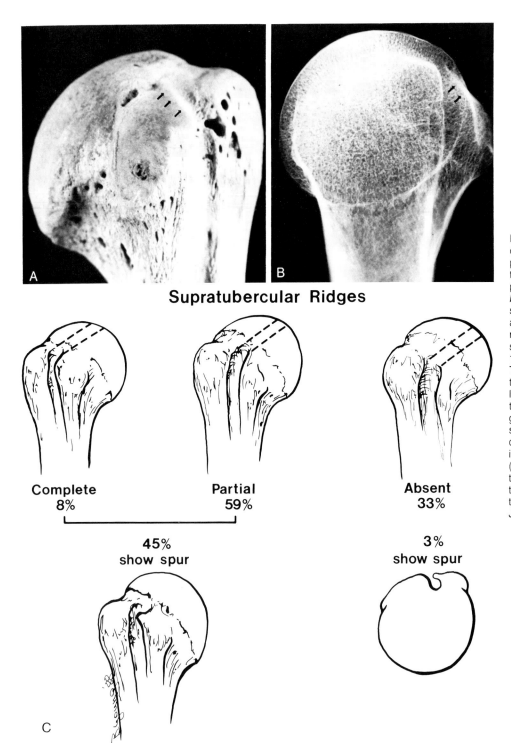

Figure 20–21. *A,* Externally rotated view of a cadaveric specimen showing the supratubercular ridge *(black arrows). B,* Internally rotated radiograph showing a prominent supratubercular ridge *(small black arrows).* (Reproduced with permission from Cone RO, Danzig L, Resnick D, and Goldman AB: The bicipital groove: radiographic, anatomic, and pathologic study. Am J Roentgenol *41*:781–788, 1983. © Am Roentgen Ray Soc 1983.) *C,* This illustrates the presence of the supratubercular ridge (seen extending from the lesser tuberosity, altering the angle of the biceps tendon) and narrowing of the groove, both partial and complete in the specimens of Hitchcock and Bechtol. Medial wall spurs are much more common in specimens with supratubercular ridges. (Redrawn from Hitchcock HH, and Bechtol CO: Painful shoulder. Observations on the role of the tendon of the long head of the biceps brachii in its causation. J Bone Joint Surg *30A*:263–273, 1948.)

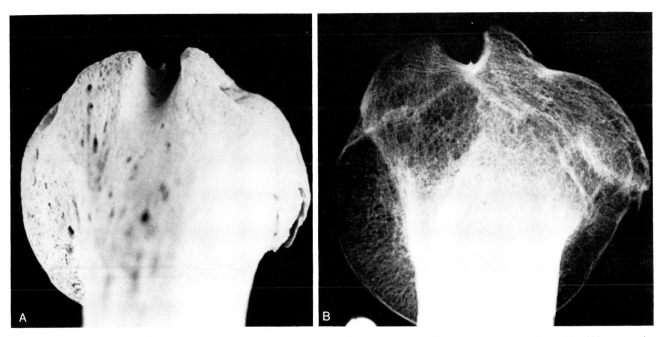

Figure 20–22. *A,* A bicipital groove floor spur thought by Cone and colleagues to be significant in biceps tendinitis as opposed to the medial wall spur, which was seen in a number of normal specimens. *B,* Groove radiograph of the same structure. (Reproduced with permission from Cone RO, Danzig L, Resnick D, and Goldman AB: The bicipital groove: radiographic, anatomic, and pathologic study. Am J Roentgenol *41:*781–788, 1983. © Am Roentgen Ray Soc 1983.)

Function of the Biceps Tendon

FUNCTIONAL ANATOMY

Lippmann[124, 125] and Hitchcock and Bechtol,[97] making observations while operating under local anesthetic, observed that it is not the tendon that slides in the groove, but the humerus that moves on the fixed tendon during motions of the shoulder. From adduction to complete elevation of the arm, a given point in the groove moves along the tendon for a distance of as much as 1½ inches. In order to facilitate this motion, the synovial pouch (see Fig. 20–2 and 20–5) extends from the shoulder joint to line the intertubercular groove for the greater part of its extent. Below this bursa, the tendon glides through its peritendineum. Motion of the humerus on the tendon occurs in all movements of elevation, whether it be forward flexion or abduction. If the arm is internally rotated at the shoulder, the tendon works against the medial wall of the groove, and the lesser tuberosity acts as a pulley. When the arm is in full external rotation, the tendon occupies the floor of the groove, and its more proximal portion exercises pressure on the head of the humerus. Therefore, it was originally believed that only in external rotation did the long head act directly on the shoulder as a head depressor and enhance somewhat the power of abduction of this joint. A vector diagram has been used by Lucas[129] to establish the resultant force of the biceps as that of depressing the head (Fig. 20–23). Figure 20–24 illustrates how the biceps acts as a static head depressor, preventing migration of the

humeral head into the acromion by the pull of the deltoid.

The function of the biceps at the elbow has been well worked out, and there is general agreement that the biceps brachii is a strong supinator of the forearm and a weak flexor at the elbow. Debate continues, however, on the exact function of the biceps at the shoulder level. Most anatomy texts regard the biceps as a weak flexor of the shoulder.[98] Studies on function of the biceps tendon can be divided into two broad categories: direct observation and electromyographic (EMG) studies.

Direct Observation

Lippmann,[124, 125] in studying cadaver and operating room material, noted that motion of the long biceps tendon with reference to the humerus was passive and occurs only when the shoulder joint is moved. He observed that motion of the biceps tendon in the bicipital groove could not be produced by contraction or relaxation of the biceps muscle when the shoulder is held immobile in any position. Any motion of the shoulder joint, however, entails motion of the biceps tendon in the groove. Elevation of the arm in internal rotation causes minimal excursion of the tendon, while in external rotation, maximum excursion occurs. With the arm in the position of full abduction, 1.3 cm of tendon remained in the shoulder joint. Five cm of tendon is in the shoulder joint when the arm is depressed and externally rotated. This yields an overall excursion of 3.7 cm. Therefore, Lippmann believed that the tendon should not be considered as two-part,

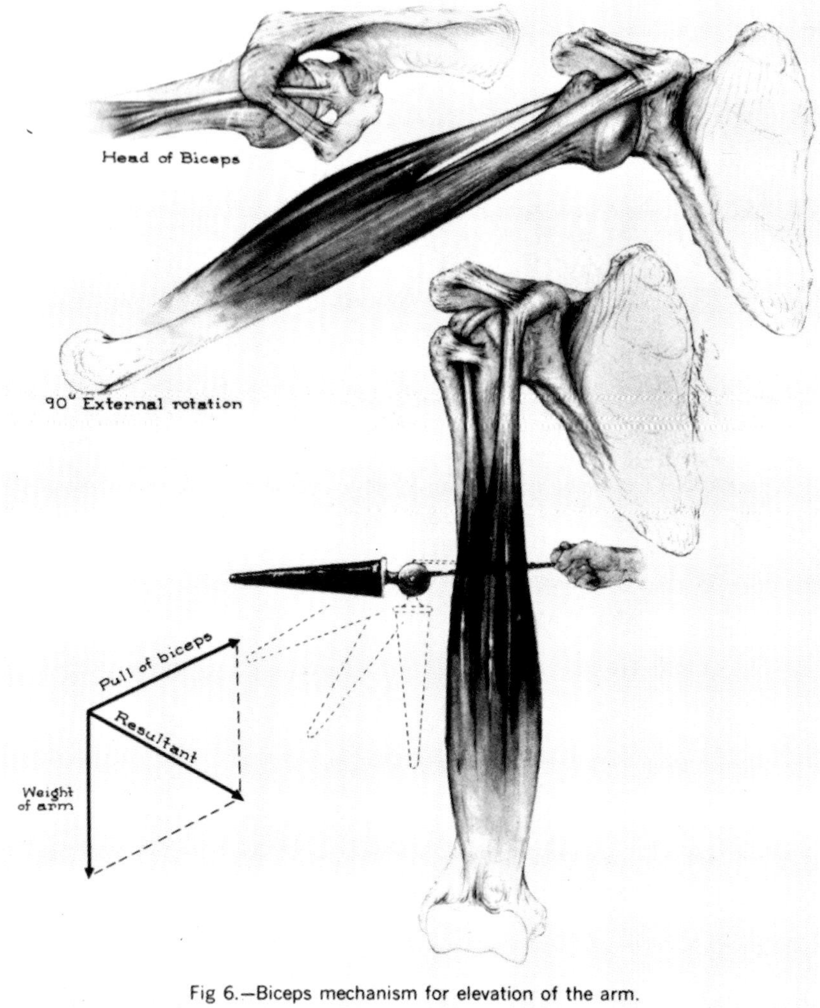

Head of Biceps

90° External rotation

Pull of biceps

Resultant

Weight of arm

Fig 6.—Biceps mechanism for elevation of the arm.

Figure 20–23. Artist conception and vector diagram of the resultant force of the biceps tendon. (Reproduced with permission from Lucas DB: Biomechanics of the shoulder joint. Arch Surg *107*:425–432, 1973. Copyright 1973, American Medical Association.)

Figure 20–24. From this illustration it is evident that the biceps tendon is at least a static head depressor. Given the line of pull and the resultant vector, it is an active head depressor, though undoubtedly a weak one as is shown by the percentage of recruitment on EMG analysis. (Redrawn from Habermeyer P, Kaiser E, Knappe M, et al: Functional anatomy and biomechanics of the long biceps tendon. Unfallchirurg *90*(7):319–329, 1987.)

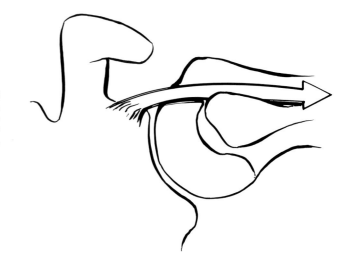

i.e., an intracapsular and a groove portion, because of this movement of the humeral head along the tendon (Fig. 20–25).

Meyer[151] observed that the humeral head during the beginning of abduction slides up on the tendon for a distance of half an inch and then slides back down during progressive abduction. Again, this observation was made while operating on patients under local anesthetic. Hitchcock and Bechtol[97] confirmed the earlier findings of Meyer[151] and Lippmann[125] that the humerus moved on the tendon rather than the tendon moving through the groove.

Rowe[204] states that in chronic rupture of the rotator cuff, the head depressor responsibility of the biceps tendon increases, and the tendon is often found to be hypertrophied. Bush[30] noted an increased depressor effect of the tendon when it was transplanted laterally for repairing cuff defects.

Andrews and colleagues[9] observed the biceps tendon and superior glenoid labrum complex arthroscopically during electrical stimulation of the biceps. They noted definite superior lifting of the labrum and compression of the glenohumeral joint. They observed that the biceps is in this respect a "shunt muscle of the shoulder" and does help stabilize the glenohumeral joint during throwing. Its primary role during throwing, they agree, is still the deceleration of the elbow, and it is this sudden deceleration that leads to the tearing of the superior glenoid labral complex by the biceps tendon.

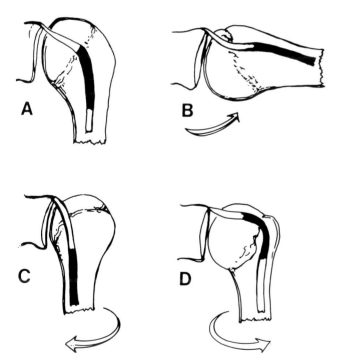

Figure 20–25. Lippmann found by direct observation under a local anesthetic that the biceps tendon slid freely in its sheath upon motion of the shoulder. Motion of the tendon in its groove appears only with motion of the shoulder joint. At any given position, a different amount of the biceps tendon can be found within the joint. (Modified from Lippmann RK: Bicipital tenosynovitis. NY State J Med 90:2235–2241, 1944. Copyright by the Medical Society of the State of New York.)

I have observed that during the treatment of four-part fractures, if a portion of the groove is maintained and the biceps returned to its groove, there is an increase in anteroposterior and inferosuperior stability. The replaced humeral head also seems to track more normally in the glenoid.

Electromyographic Evaluation

Basmajian[14] was a pioneer in evaluating the musculoskeletal system, including the shoulder, with integrated function and dynamic spectrum EMG analysis. He reported both heads of the biceps to be active during shoulder flexion, with the long head being most active.[16] Habermeyer and associates[86] have performed EMG analysis, while Cybex testing was performed on normal individuals. Clear EMG activity was seen in the biceps during abduction, its peak being found at 132 degrees of abduction. Interestingly, they found the muscle to be active even with the arm in neutral rotation, i.e., the biceps is active in abduction even when the arm is not externally rotated. In flexion, they found the main activity recorded during the first 90 degrees. The biceps was active in external but not internal rotation. The effectiveness of the long head of the biceps is greater in external rotation when tension on it is maximal. In arm adduction and internal rotation, the long head was always inactive, while the short head was active in half of the cases of adduction and only seldom active in internal rotation. The biceps was totally inactive in extension.

Laumann[120–122] has divided by percentage the contribution of various muscles around the shoulder to shoulder flexion. Based on his work, he estimated that the biceps contributes approximately 7 per cent of the power of flexion.

Furlani and colleagues,[68] in studying electromyographic participation of the biceps in movements of the glenohumeral joint, found that in flexion with an extended elbow, performed with and without resistance, both the long and short heads of the biceps brachii were active in the majority of cases. In abduction without resistance, the biceps was inactive, while the addition of resistance increased the activity to 10 per cent.

Ting and coworkers[219] have performed EMG analysis on the long head of the biceps on patients with rotator cuff tears. In all of their patients, an EMG record was expressed as percentage of the activity recorded during maximal effort. They correlated their data with operative findings as well. They found that during both shoulder abduction and flexion, four out of the five subjects tested demonstrated a significantly greater degree of EMG activity in the biceps tendon in the extremity with a torn cuff compared with that in the contralateral uninjured shoulder. In addition, all shoulders with compromised rotator cuffs proved to have a significantly larger tendon than those of controls, confirming the observations of Rowe.[204] Ting and colleagues[219] suggested that the lateral head of the biceps may be a greater contributor to abduction and flexion in the compromised shoulder than in the normal shoulder and that concomitant enlargement of the tendon may indicate a use-induced hypertrophy. They therefore recommended not sacrificing the intracapsular portion of the tendon for graft material or tenodesing the tendon indiscriminantly in the groove as a routine part of rotator cuff repair and acromioplasty.

Recently, the biceps' contribution to the shoulder during throwing has been evaluated by Jobe and associates[108] and Perry.[188] In these studies, biceps function correlated with motion occurring at the elbow and not in the shoulder. A relatively stable elbow position during acceleration was accompanied by marked reduction in the muscle's intensity. During follow-through, the need for deceleration of the rapidly extending elbow and pronating forearm was accompanied by peak biceps action. They showed no activity in the biceps muscle during the act of throwing, except when the elbow was active. Peak activity was only 36 per cent of its maximum capacity. With a 9-cm^2 cross section and only half of the muscle related to the long head, the humeral force is small. In Perry's words: "It seems doubtful that the long head (biceps tendon) is a significant stabilizing force at the glenohumeral joint." Glousman and associates,[79] on the other hand, have reported increased activity in the biceps during the throwing act in patients with unstable shoulders. Therefore, it seems that the biceps takes on more importance if the primary stabilizers are injured.

SUMMARY

It appears from a review of the literature that, based on the finding of consistent EMG activity with shoulder flexion and abduction independent of elbow flexion and given the resultant force of the biceps muscle, the biceps tendon does have a weak active head depressor effect. Based on its anatomical position, it serves as a superior checkrein to humeral head excursion and therefore at the very least acts as a static head depressor. As long as the tendon is located in its groove, the humeral head will slide up and down on the tendon and on the glenoid face in the normal fashion. With tears of the rotator cuff and medial subluxation of the biceps tendon, this checkrein effect is lost.

The tendon's activity seems to increase in pathological states of the shoulder such as rotator cuff tears and shoulder instability, as evidenced by increased EMG activity as well as observation of hypertrophy. Based on these findings, I cannot recommend that it be routinely tenodesed at the time of acromioplasty or used as a free graft for performing rotator cuff repairs.

Classification of Bicipital Lesions

Classification of biceps lesions has been historically divided into biceps tendinitis and biceps instability. By far, the most common of these is secondary bicipital tendinitis, i.e., bicipital tendinitis secondary to an intra-articular problem such as rheumatoid or osteoarthritis or, more commonly, biceps tendinitis secondary to the impingement syndrome with concomitant irritation or tears of the rotator cuff.

The pathological entity of primary biceps tendinitis has been likened to de Quervain's tenosynovitis by Lapidus,[118] with thickening and stenosis of the transverse ligament and sheath and narrowing of the tendon underneath the sheath. DePalma[51–55] has shown that the severity of the process is governed by duration of the condition and the age of the patient. Post[193] has found consistent inflammation within the intertubercular portion of the tendon with proliferative tenosynovitis, characterized by inflammation and irregularity of the walls of the groove. The intra-articular portion of the biceps is always normal. Codman[43] stated that biceps tendinitis was a rare entity, while DePalma[51–55] related that it was the most common cause of stiff and painful shoulder. Even so, 39 per cent of DePalma's operative cases had associated disorders. Crenshaw and Kilgore[49] were also proponents of the concept of primary biceps tendinitis, although in their series 40 per cent of the patients had associated lesions in the cuff or glenohumeral joint. They go on to state that whether or not the biceps tendon and its sheath become involved primarily or secondarily is not important, but that the tenosynovitis was the chief cause of pain and limitation of motion in pericapsulitis.

Many authors[53, 54, 166–169, 193, 194] believe that the pathology seen in the biceps is directly related to its intimate relationship with the rotator cuff. As they pass under the coracoacromial arch, both are involved in the impingement syndrome.

Although the diagnosis of primary bicipital tendinitis, i.e., biceps tendinitis in the absence of impingement, was more common in the 1940s, 50s, and 60s, it is made less frequently by shoulder surgeons today. Because the changes described are a common occurrence in other tendons that have to pass through a fibro-osseous tunnel, such as the tendons in the first dorsal compartment of the wrist or the flexor tendons of the hand, and because this entity has been described in pathological specimens by well-respected orthopedic surgeons in the past and present, I am sure that it exists, but I do not think it is very common. It should be regarded as a diagnosis of exclusion. The clinical entities that must be excluded before the diagnosis is made are discussed later in the section on differential diagnosis.

Slatis and Aalto[211] have offered what appears to be a useful clinical classification of biceps lesions. It is based on the pathoanatomy and appears to have some prognosticating significance based on their review. It is as follows:

TYPE A: IMPINGEMENT TENDINITIS

This is the most common cause of bicipital tendinitis (Fig. 20–26). It is encountered in conjunction with the

TYPE A: IMPINGEMENT TENDINITIS

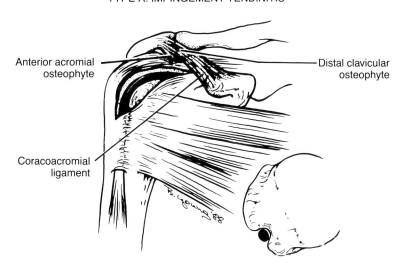

Anterior acromial osteophyte

Distal clavicular osteophyte

Coracoacromial ligament

Figure 20–26. Type A impingement tendinitis. Rupture of the rotator cuff exposes the tendon to compression between the acromion above and the humeral head below. The tendon lies normally in its groove. (Modified from Paavolainen P, Slatis P, and Aalto K: Surgical pathology in chronic shoulder pain. *In* Bateman JE, and Welsh RP (eds): Surgery of the Shoulder. Philadelphia: BC Decker, 1984.)

impingement syndrome and tears of the rotator cuff, especially those located in the anterior part of the cuff. With elevation and rotation of the arm, the now exposed biceps tendon is impinged between the head of the humerus, the acromion, and the coracoacromial ligament (Fig. 20–27). The synovium is not usually inflamed. Fraying of the tendon is seldom seen and is mostly confined to the intertubercular groove.

TYPE B: SUBLUXATION OF THE BICEPS TENDON

Normally the tendon of the long head of the biceps lies in the intertubercular groove, surrounded by the synovial pouch (Fig. 20–28). On elevation of the arm, the intra-articular portion of the tendon is only a few centimeters long, but on extension, this length increases to about 4 cm. Since the tendon is fixed at the superior glenoid rim, the head of the humerus must move against the tendon on elevation and extension. Paavolainen and associates[180] feel strongly that the gliding mechanism of the tendon is guided by the coracohumeral ligament. A lesion at the medial portion of the ligament disturbs the normal gliding mechanisms, and the tendon can gradually displace medially. The lesion may be isolated but is usually concomitant with moderate or massive tears extending into the anterior part of the cuff. A fully displaced bicipital tendon lies in the sling of the ruptured cuff and may in the early phases slip in and out of the groove, but as the sulcus gradually fills with scar tissue, the groove becomes shallower and finally the tendon remains in a medially dislocated position.

Impingement area

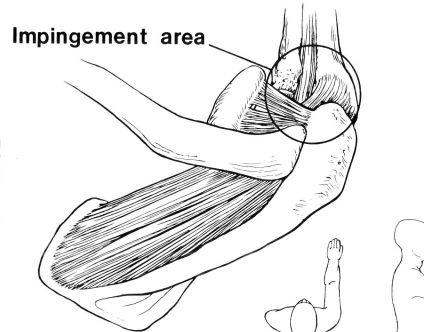

Figure 20–27. When the arm is forward flexed, the impingement area, i.e., the groove, biceps tendon, and anterior cuff, comes in contact with the coracoacromial arch. The longer the acromial process, the more likely the biceps will be involved. (Courtesy of Charles A. Rockwood, Jr., M.D.)

TYPE B: SUBLUXATION

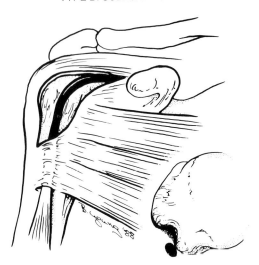

Figure 20–28. Type B subluxation of the biceps. A tear in the medial portion of the coracohumeral ligament causes subluxation and medial displacement of the tendon from the bicipital groove. Note filling of the groove with fibrous tissue. (Modified from Paavolainen P, Slatis P, and Aalto K: Surgical pathology in chronic shoulder pain. *In* Bateman JE, and Welsh RP (eds): Surgery of the Shoulder. Philadelphia: BC Decker, 1984.)

TYPE C: ATTRITION TENDINITIS

Attrition tendinitis corresponds most closely to the entity previously described as primary bicipital tendinitis (Fig. 20–29). In these cases, the synovial reaction is impressive and includes edema, swelling, and intense erythema. The intertubercular area of the tendon was frequently frayed and thin, whereas the intra-articular portion, as a rule, was unaffected by the nearby reaction. According to Paavolainen and Slatis,[181] this type of bicipital tendinitis seems to be the most painful and is apparently the most common cause of complete rupture of the tendon.

In the attrition type of tendinitis, local new bone reaction and adhesion formation causes stenosis of the bicipital groove, leading to attrition of the tendon of the long head of the biceps. In attrition tendinitis a spur frequently is visible on the groove view of the humerus.

Incidence

In 1934, DePalma[51–55] stated that tenosynovitis of the long head of the biceps brachii muscle is the most common antecedent of painful and stiff shoulders. He believed that this was true of both younger and older age periods of life. In the series by DePalma[52] in 1954, the lesion was encountered in 77 men and 98 women, ranging in age from 16 to 69 years, the highest incidence being between 45 and 55 years. Bilateral involvement was observed in 8 per cent of the cases. The more severe lesions were found in the older decades

of life, where more severe degenerative changes prevail. In 61.2 per cent of the cases, bicipital tenosynovitis was a localized pathological process without involvement of the surrounding tissue. In 38.8 per cent of the cases, the inflammatory process noted in the biceps tendon and sheath was part of a generalized chronic inflammatory process. In DePalma's[51–55] series, he felt that bicipital tenosynovitis was the initiating agent in 80 per cent of the cases of frozen shoulder and, regardless of the cause, bicipital tenosynovitis was always a concomitant of the frozen shoulder.

According to McCue[140] and O'Donohue,[178] biceps tendinitis and subluxation are common causes of anterior shoulder pain in throwing athletes. It is more common in football quarterbacks because of the weight of the ball and the need for additional pushing action and in softball pitchers because of forceful supinator strain with arm and forearm flexion. Lapidus[118] identified 89 patients with tendinitis of the long head of the biceps in a total of 493 patients treated for shoulder pain, an incidence of 18 per cent. Paavolainen and Slatis[181] reported on patients who had failed to respond to conservative care and were referred to a shoulder center. A preoperative diagnosis of bicipital tendinitis was made prior to arthrotomy in 38 of 126, or 30 per cent. Postoperatively with a direct inspection of the biceps tendon, the incidence was much higher, rising to 54 per cent of the operative specimens showing some evidence for biceps tendinitis. In patients with cuff ruptures, the incidence was 31 of 51, or 60 per cent. If the rotator cuff was intact (no full-thickness tear), the incidence was approximately 50 per cent. Although the cuff was "intact" at surgery, most of these cuffs did show some evidence of degeneration, edema, and signs of Stage I and II impingement.

TYPE C: ATTRITION TENDINITIS

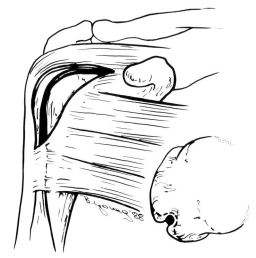

Figure 20–29. The cuff is exposed to show the pathology of constriction of the biceps tendon within the groove. Local formation of new bone and connective tissue causes stenosis of the bicipital groove, leading to attrition of the tendon of the long head of the biceps.

Medial dislocation of the biceps tendon occurred in 12 of 51 cases with the cuff ruptured and 9 of 75 cases when the cuff was intact, yielding an overall incidence of dislocation of 17 per cent. Frank ruptures of the biceps tendon were seen in 8 of the 126 patients, or 5 per cent.

As bicipital tenosynovitis oftentimes occurs with a concomitant impingement syndrome, it remains a very common cause of anterior shoulder pain. However, as an isolated entity, i.e., primary bicipital tenosynovitis, it is much less common.

Etiology

Although the majority of biceps tendon dislocations occur secondarily, as the result of chronic impingement with attrition wear by the anterior acromion on the anterior cuff and coracohumeral ligament,[73–77, 145–152, 166–169] acute traumatic dislocation of the tendon of the biceps has been described. Abbott and Saunders[1] in 1939 presented six cases with operative findings. Four occurred from falls with direct blows to the shoulder or from indirect force from falls on the outstretched hands. Two occurred during heavy lifting. All but one of these patients had a concomitant injury to the rotator cuff as well.

DePalma[51–54] and later Michele[153] divided the etiology by the age group of the patient. In the younger age group, anomalies of the bicipital groove together with a repeated trauma are the major factors in initiating the syndrome. In the older age group, degenerative changes in the tendon are the predominant etiological factor.

Like most other musculoskeletal problems, the etiology is most likely multifactoral. Chief among the causes is the anatomical location of the tendon, juxtaposed as it is to the rotator cuff and coracoacromial arch, leading to impingement wear and tendinitis. The blood supply of the tendon has been studied by Rathbun and Macnab[200] and shown to be diminished, with a critical zone similar to that seen in the supraspinatus (Fig. 20–30). In abduction, there is a zone of avascularity in the intracapsular portion of the tendon felt to be caused by pressure from the head of the humerus, the so called "wringing out" phenomenon. Occupational causes also exist since patients who do repetitive overhead lifting and throwing are more prone to ruptures, elongations, and dislocations of their biceps. Meyer[145–152] reasoned that capsular defects leading to problems with the biceps resulted from repeated and continual use of the arm in a position of marked abduction and external rotation. Borchers[26] and later DePalma[51–55] explained spontaneous ruptures within the groove on the basis of osteophytic excrescences there, which eventually wear away the tendon. Etiological factors based on the variations in the groove have been previously discussed.

Prevention

Prevention of biceps injuries in workers and athletes entails the same type of preventive rehabilitation that is used in athletes for their rotator cuff, i.e., warm-up passive stretching, strengthening, and avoidance of painful activities during the time of symptoms. Strengthening should include all the muscles of the

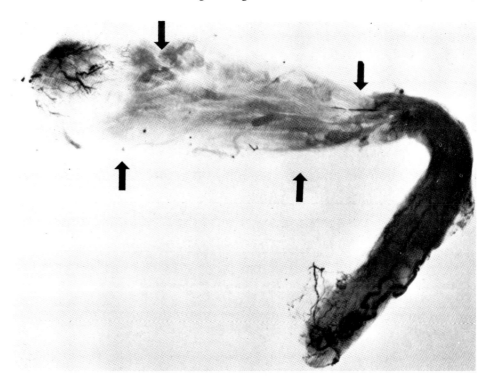

Figure 20–30. Zone of relative avascularity seen in the biceps. (Reproduced with permission from Rathbun JB and Macnab I: The microvascular pattern of the rotator cuff. J Bone Joint Surg 52B:540–553, 1970.)

rotator cuff to improve the force couple and decrease impingement. The parascapular muscles should also be rehabilitated. The better balanced shoulder musculature will prevent or at least decrease the vicious circle of impingement tendinitis, irritation, and muscle weakness, which is followed by altered biomechanics, subluxation, and further impingement. Persons who do manual labor with heavy lifting or repetitive overhead work, such as carpenters, should probably spend as much time stretching before undertaking their jobs as a football and baseball player spend before undertaking theirs. Stretching of the biceps tendon is maximal when the shoulder is fully extended and externally rotated and the elbow is fully extended as well.

Careful pre-employment screening and testing, including muscular strength, could be used, and any deficits noted could be corrected with exercise before beginning a job that requires heavy lifting or overhead use of the arm. The scapular lateral outlet view and the 30-degree caudal tilt x-ray view could possibly be used to prevent people at risk for impingement from taking jobs that would put their shoulders at risk for injury.

Clinical Presentation of Bicipital Lesions

There is no substitute in any medical condition for an accurate history and physical examination. This is especially true of subtle lesions of the shoulder such as biceps tendinitis, instability, and impingement syndrome. In this section, the historical and specific clinical features of bicipital tendinitis and instability are presented; in the section on differential diagnosis, a more thorough history and physical examination of the shoulder is reviewed.

Patients with bicipital tendinitis usually present with chronic pain in the proximal anterior area of the shoulder. The pain sometimes extends down the arm into the region of the biceps muscle belly. It can, like pain from impingement syndrome, radiate to the deltoid insertion as well. There is no radiation into the neck or distally beyond the biceps. In most cases, there is no history of major trauma, although, as has been stated previously, acute trauma can predispose to bicipital tendinitis rupture or dislocation. Typically, the patient is young or middle aged with a history of use of the arm in repetitive actions, particularly overhead. The pain is less intense at rest and worse with use. Neviaser[170] states that there is no significant night pain, while Simon[210] believes that nocturnal exacerbation is common. In my experience all painful conditions of the shoulder are worse at night because of compression loading and because the supine position places the shoulder at or below the level of the heart. Rolling over on the involved shoulder further increases the problem by decreasing the venous return from the upper extremity. The pain from calcific tendinitis of the biceps is of such great intensity that the patient often walks the floor. Bicipital tendinitis is frequently seen in patients who participate in the following sports: swimming, tennis, and golf, and sports that involve throwing. In each of these activities, the rotation of the humerus at or above the level of the horizontal brings the tuberosities, the intervening groove, biceps tendon, and rotator cuff in direct contact with the anterior acromion and coracoacromial ligament.

Biceps instability is suggested by a pain pattern similar to the above. It is seen most commonly in throwing athletes. Motion is often accompanied by a palpable snap or pop at a certain position in the arc of rotation. The patient indicates pain in the front of the shoulder, usually reproduced by raising the arm to 90 degrees. Biceps rupture appears frequently with acute pain and sometimes an audible pop in the shoulder. Over the next several days, the patient will notice a change in contour of the arm and ecchymoses.

PHYSICAL EXAMINATION

Physical examination reveals point tenderness in the biceps groove, which is best localized with the arm in about 10 degrees of internal rotation.[138] With the arm in this position, the biceps tendon should be facing directly anteriorly and located three inches below the acromion[138] (Fig. 20–31). The point tenderness in this area, i.e., 3 inches below the anterior acromion, should move with rotation of the arm. It often disappears as the lesser tuberosity and groove rotate internally under the short head of the biceps and coracoid. The tender-

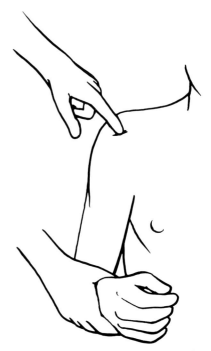

Figure 20–31. Metsen[138] has found that the biceps tendon can be palpated directly anteriorly with the arm in 10 degrees of internal rotation. This is the same position utilized before performing deAnquin's and Lippmann's tests (described in the text).

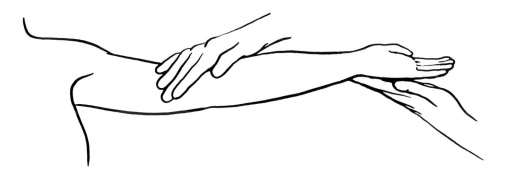

Figure 20–32. Speed's test. The biceps resistance test is performed with the patient flexing the shoulder against resistance, with the elbow extended and the forearm supinated. Pain referred to the biceps tendon area constitutes a positive test.

ness of subdeltoid bursitis is generally more diffuse and should not move with arm rotation. The tenderness seen with impingement is often diffuse and accompanied by tenderness in the arm, acromion, coracoacromial ligament, and coracoid process. However, it should not move with rotation. This "tenderness in motion" sign is, in my opinion, the most specific for bicipital lesions. It does not, however, differentiate biceps instability from tendinitis. Many authors have stated that the biceps can be felt subluxating out of the groove. It is difficult to discern whether what one is feeling is actually a subluxating tendon or the muscle bundles of the deltoid rolling up underneath one's finger as it is pressed against the humerus. Anyone who has looked at the biceps surgically should have trouble thinking that he or she is actually palpating the tendon, especially in a well-muscled individual. There may be slight restriction of abduction and internal rotation. This loss of motion is usually due to pain and not to capsular constricture and should improve with local anesthetic injection. There is pain with abduction and internal rotation, abduction and external rotation, and resisted forward flexion of the shoulder. Several tests have been reported to aid in the diagnosis. There are, however, no data as to the sensitivity or specificity of any of these tests in patients with shoulder pain. The most important question when performing provocative tests on any part of the musculoskeletal system is "Does this maneuver specifically reproduce the patient's pain?" Selective injection with obliteration of pain is an extremely important part of clinical evaluation of the shoulder. There is no substitute for clinical experience, repeated examination, selective injection, and a cautious approach to anterior shoulder pain. Many poor results from surgery in this region come from a surgical procedure's being performed too early, directed only at the biceps lesion. Repeated examination may show evolution of an impingement syndrome, adhesive capsulitis, or evidence of glenohumeral instability. The following tests have been described by authors in the past in isolating lesions in the biceps tendon:

1. Speed's test[77] (Fig. 20–32). The patient flexes the shoulder against resistance while the elbow is extended and the forearm supinated. The pain is localized in the bicipital groove.

2. Yergason's sign[235] (Fig. 20–33). This test is per-

formed with the patient's elbow flexed. The patient is asked to forcibly supinate against resistance. Pain referred to the front and inner aspect of the shoulder in the bicipital groove constitutes a positive sign. Post[194] found an incidence of 50 per cent positivity with this sign in patients with primary bicipital tendinitis.

3. Biceps instability test[1] (Fig. 20–34). Dislocation of the tendon, complete or incomplete, may be differentiated from peritendinitis by the test of Abbott and Saunders.[1] After full abduction of the shoulder, the arm, which is held in complete external rotation, is slowly brought down to the side in the plane of the scapula. A palpable and even audible and sometimes

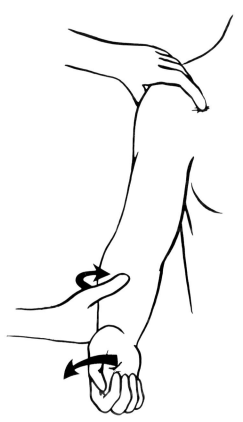

Figure 20–33. Yergason's sign. With the arm flexed, the patient is asked to forcefully supinate against resistance from the examiner's hand. Pain referred to the anterior aspect of the shoulder in the region of the bicipital groove constitutes a positive test.

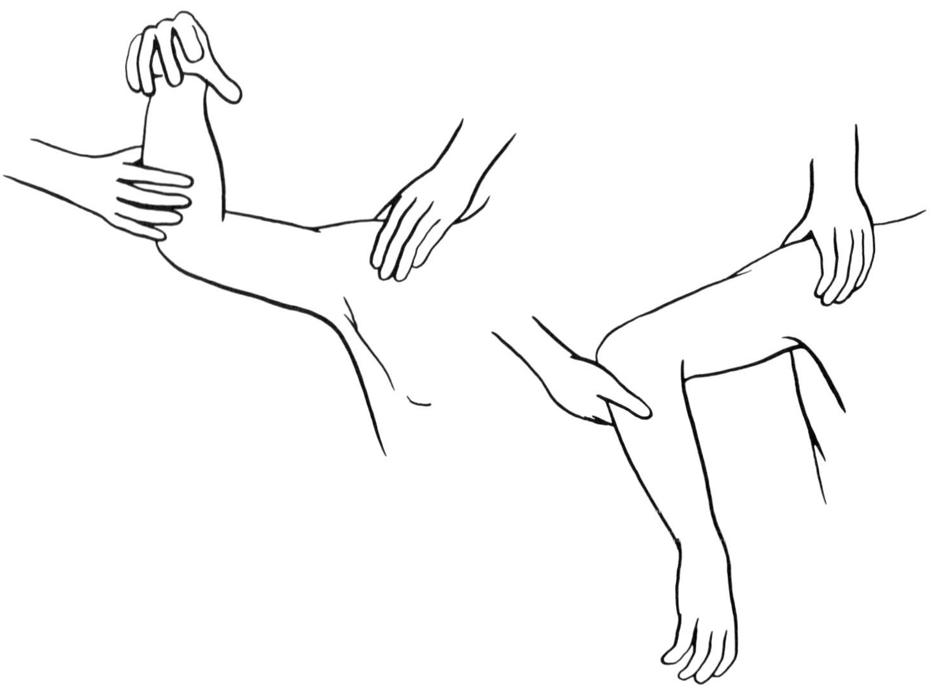

Figure 20–34. Biceps instability test (described by Abbott and Saunders'). During palpation of the biceps in the groove while taking the arm from an abducted externally rotated position to a position of internal rotation, a palpable or audible painful click is noted as the biceps tendon is forced against or over the lesser tuberosity.

painful click is noted as the biceps tendon, now forced against the lesser tuberosity, becomes subluxated or dislocated from the groove.

4. Ludington's test[131] (Fig. 20–35). In Ludington's test the patient is asked to put his or her hands behind the head. In this position of abduction and external rotation, the patient is asked to flex his biceps isometrically, and the pain is that of the bicipital groove in tendinitis. If the examiner's finger is in the groove at the time of the contraction, subluxation can sometimes be felt. Subtle differences in the contour of the biceps in cases of elongation are best noted in this fashion.

5. deAnquin's test[216] (Fig. 20–36). The arm is rotated with the examiner's finger on the most tender spot. There is immediate pain as the tendon glides beneath the finger.

6. Lippmann's test[124] (see Fig. 20–31). Lippmann's test produces pain, and the tendon is displaced from one side to the other by the probing finger and released. This is done about three inches from the shoulder joint, with the elbow flexed at a right angle. I think we are more often rolling up the deltoid muscle with this test and the biceps is not palpated.

7. Hueter's sign.[102] Hueter's sign is positive when flexion of the supinated forearm (primarily a biceps function) is less forceful than flexion of the pronated forearm.

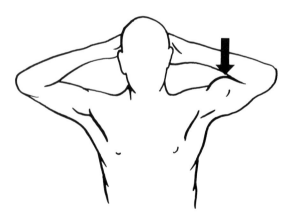

Figure 20–35. Ludington's test. The patient is asked to put his or her hands behind the head and flex the biceps. The examiner's finger can be in the bicipital groove at the time of the test. Subtle differences in the contour of the biceps are best noted with this maneuver. In this illustration the patient has a ruptured biceps at the left shoulder.

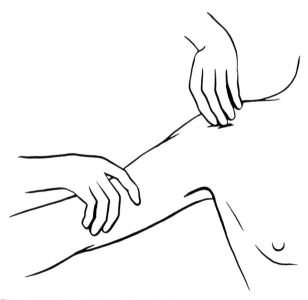

Figure 20–36. DeAnquin's test. The patient's arm is rotated while the examiner has his or her finger in the most tender spot in the bicipital groove. A positive test occurs in biceps tendinitis when the patient feels pain as the tendon glides beneath the finger.

Physical examination in patients with complete biceps rupture is much less subtle (Fig. 20–37) because of the obvious deformity that develops. There is a hollowness in the anterior portion of the shoulder accompanied by balling up of the biceps below the midbrachium. In these patients it is important to look specifically for cuff atrophy because tears in the biceps in the older population are frequently associated with attrition-type tears in the rotator cuff preceding the biceps rupture. These may or may not have been symptomatic prior to the bicipital rupture, but it is not uncommon for the patient to have a history of being treated in the remote past for "bursitis."

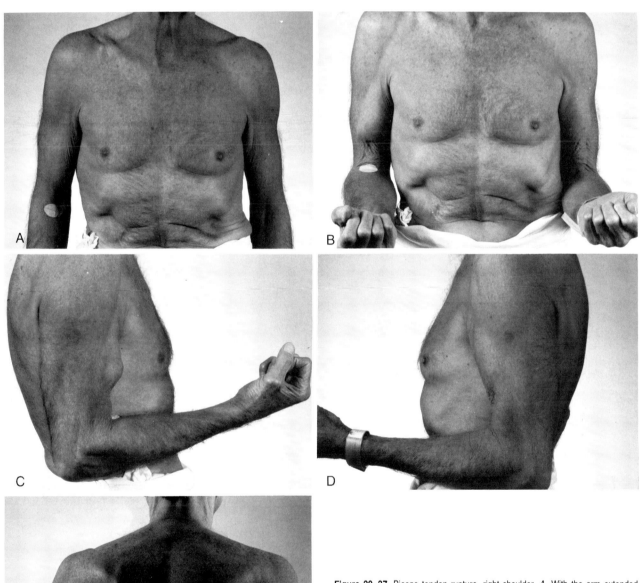

Figure 20–37. Biceps tendon rupture, right shoulder. A, With the arm extended, one notices only a hollowness about the anterior aspect of the shoulder. B, With flexion, rupture of the long head of the biceps tendon becomes obvious. C, Lateral view of biceps tendon rupture, right shoulder. D, Same patient, normal side for comparison. E, Note the marked wasting from associated chronic rotator cuff disease in this patient with clinical biceps rupture.

Associated Conditions

The following are associated conditions and are discussed under differential diagnosis:

1. Impingement syndrome.
2. Adhesive capsulitis.
3. Rheumatoid and osteoarthritis.
4. Glenohumeral instability.
5. Coracoid impingement syndrome.
6. Thoracic outlet/brachial plexopathy/plexitis.
7. Peripheral nerve entrapment, cervical radiculopathy.

CONCOMITANT INJURIES

One should remain alert for a wide range of lesions in a biceps rupture. These include extensive damage to the rotator cuff and variable degrees of brachial plexus stretch, which are occasionally seen in association with biceps rupture and almost invariably occur as the result of a fall on the posteriorly outstretched arm in an elderly patient. There is the occasional associated anterior dislocation of the shoulder. Humeral fractures and fracture dislocations can occur. The biceps can become interposed and block reduction of both fractures and dislocations.[101, 106, 141] An extensive area of ecchymoses of the chest associated with the injury should tip one off that the biceps tendon rupture is not an isolated injury. In isolated biceps ruptures, the swelling and ecchymoses should be limited to the brachium.

Diagnostic Tests

PLAIN FILM RADIOLOGY

Frequently, routine plain films of the shoulder are normal in biceps tendinitis. This has led to the development of special views for the biceps groove and the use of other imaging techniques to evaluate the biceps tendon.

Fisk Method

The Fisk method[65] (Fig. 20–38A) has the patient hold the cassette and lean over the table. The biceps groove is marked, and the central beam is perpendicular to the groove.

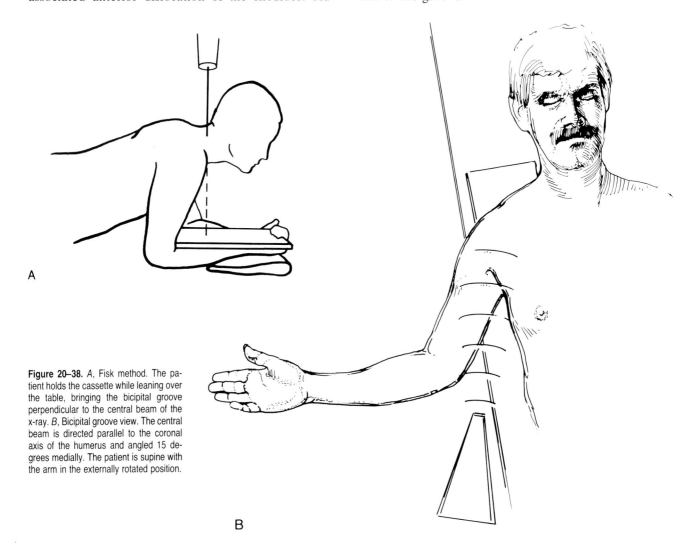

Figure 20–38. A, Fisk method. The patient holds the cassette while leaning over the table, bringing the bicipital groove perpendicular to the central beam of the x-ray. B, Bicipital groove view. The central beam is directed parallel to the coronal axis of the humerus and angled 15 degrees medially. The patient is supine with the arm in the externally rotated position.

A

B

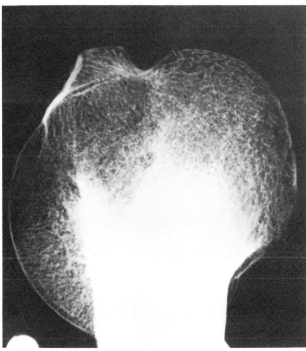

Figure 20–39. Normal bicipital groove projection. (Reproduced with permission from Cone RO, Danzig L, Resnick D, and Goldman AB: The bicipital groove: radiographic, anatomic, and pathologic study. Am J Roentgenol *41*:781–788, 1983. © Am Roentgen Ray Soc 1983.)

Bicipital Groove View

In the bicipital groove view described by Cone and colleagues[45] (Fig. 20–38*B*), the patient is supine, with the arm in external rotation. The central beam is directed parallel to the coronal axis of the humerus and angled 15 degrees medially. The film cassette is held perpendicular to the superior aspect of the shoulder. Using the radiographs, the medial wall angle, the width, presence or absence of bicipital groove spurs, coexisting degenerative changes in the greater or lesser tuberosity, and the presence or absence of a supratubercular ridge can be determined (Fig. 20–39). In a study by Ahovuo[4] in which radiographic findings were correlated with the surgical findings, half of the patients with surgically proven bicipital tendinitis had degenerative changes in the walls of the groove. In patients with attrition tendinitis, the groove had a depth of 4.8 mm or more or an inclination of 58 degrees or more. A shallow groove was seen more frequently with bicipital dislocation.

Two additional views that are helpful in differential diagnosis of biceps tendinitis are the caudal tilt view[707] radiograph and the outlet view of Neer and Poppen.[169] The caudal tilt radiograph is a standing anteroposterior view of the shoulder with a 30-degree caudal tilt to the x-ray beam (Fig. 20—40*A*). With this technique, the degree of anterior acromial prominence or spurring can be appreciated. The outlet view is a trans-scapular radiograph done with a 10-degree caudal tilt. The easiest way to take this radiograph is with the patient standing with the spine of the scapula perpendicular to the cassette. The x-ray beam should be parallel to the spine but with a 10-degree caudal tilt (Fig. 20–40*B*). These views should be done routinely to avoid the most common problem seen with biceps lesions today—a failure to relieve the underlying cause of the bicipital lesion, i.e., coracoacromial arch impingement syndrome.

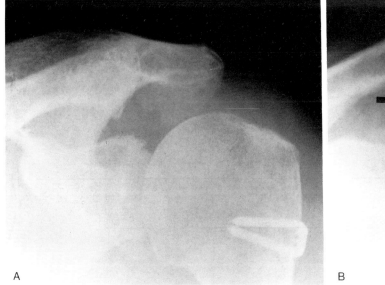

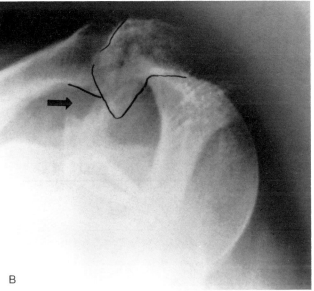

A   B

Figure 20–40. *A,* Thirty-degree caudal tilt radiograph reveals anterior acromial spurring with the "shark's tooth" appearance. The patient had undergone a biceps tenodesis but continued to have pain following the surgery. His pain was completely relieved and function was greatly improved by acromioplasty and rotator cuff repair. *B,* An outlet view of the same patient demonstrating a Type III acromion with marked inferior spurring and narrowing in the supraspinatus outlet. (The film is somewhat underexposed; the lines were added to aid in reproduction.)

ARTHROGRAPHY

Shoulder arthrography can provide information on the state of the biceps tendon. Many shallow grooves contain a normal tendon.[4] Whether or not a shallow groove on plain films is associated with a dislocation of the biceps can be determined by an arthrogram. Sometimes the dislocation is obvious in the anteroposterior view (Fig. 20–41). In other patients a groove view must be performed with the contrast instilled to make the diagnosis.[90, 92, 93] Second, in biceps tendinitis, there may be loss of sharp delineation of the tendon.[90] In rheumatoid arthritis, irregularities in the sheath of the biceps tendon may be caused by synovitis. However, in the study by Ahovuo,[4] the arthrogram showed no difference in the filling of the tendon sheath between patients with surgically verified biceps tendinitis and those with a normal tendon. Arthrography in patients with biceps tendinitis shows that the cuff is intact but the bicep is poorly outlined, has a thickened sheath, or is elevated at its origin.[172, 174] When adhesive capsulitis exists, the biceps sheath, like the subscapularis recess and dependent axillary fold, contracts (Fig. 20–42). The tendon and bicipital groove can also be assessed with computed tomographic (CT) arthrography (Fig. 20–43).

ULTRASONOGRAPHY

The use of ultrasonography to evaluate the long head of the biceps has recently become popular.[4, 154]

When comparing arthrography with sonography of the biceps, Middleton and colleagues[154] found that while sonography and arthrography were equally successful in facilitating the evaluation of the bony anatomy of the bicipital groove, sonography gave a *superior* image of the biceps tendon within the groove (Fig. 20–44A). Not only can the tendon be visualized in the groove but also the intra-articular portion and that portion just distal to the groove can be visualized (Fig. 20–44B,C). In Middleton's study, 16 patients were found to have biceps tendon sheath effusions or swelling detected by sonography (Fig. 20–44D); 15 of these patients had associated pathological conditions elsewhere in the joint. The majority of these were rotator cuff tears.

It has been previously documented that the biceps tendon sheath often does not fill when a rotator cuff tear is present.[170–177] This occurs either from an associated tendinitis or contracture of the capsule or from the fact that the dye leaks out of the joint through the tear in the supraspinatus before enough pressure is generated to force the dye into the bicipital groove. Since arthrograms often do not disclose a biceps tendon or sheath abnormality in many of the patients in which ultrasound was positive, Middleton[154] concluded that sonography is the imaging method of choice in patients with suspected biceps tendon lesions.

Author's Comment: The sonogram is an excellent noninvasive test for biceps and cuff lesions. It is, however, very examiner dependent, and if equivocal, arthrography should be performed. A positive sonogram like the clinical entity of biceps rupture itself should also make one suspicious that rotator cuff pathology coexists.

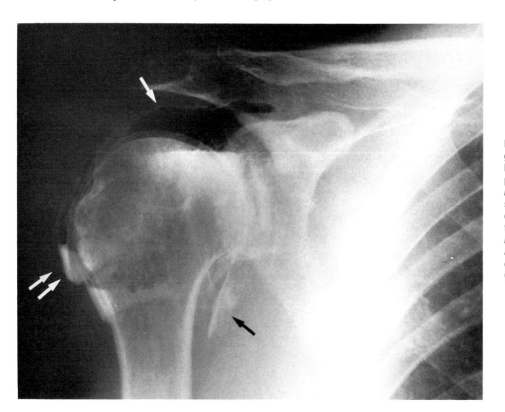

Figure 20–41. Anteroposterior arthrogram revealing medial dislocation of the biceps tendon, as indicated by the medial position of the biceps sheath *(black arrow)*. This patient also sustained a massive rupture of the rotator cuff at the time of the injury. Note the presence of air in the subacromial bursa *(single white arrow)* and contrast medium *(double white arrow)* in the subdeltoid bursa. (Courtesy of Guerdon Greenway, M.D. and Robert Chapman, M.D.)

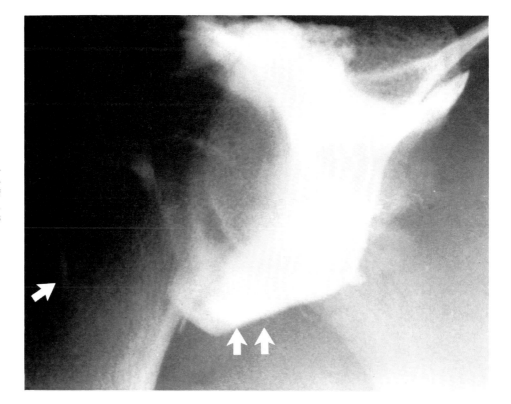

Figure 20–42. The arthrogram in adhesive capsulitis frequently will show nonfilling of the bicipital groove because of constriction in the bicipital sheath *(arrow)*. This is similar to the restriction that occurs in the axillary recess *(double arrows)*.

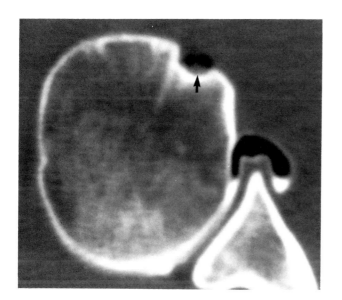

Figure 20–43. The bicipital tendon is seen *(black arrow)* seated in the groove on a CT arthrogram.

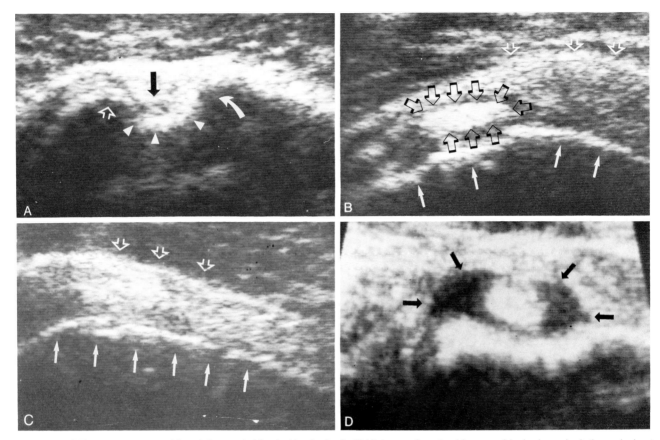

Figure 20–44. *A,* Transverse sonogram of the anterior aspect of the shoulder showing the bicipital groove *(arrowheads)* as a semicircular depression in the proximal part of the humerus formed by the lesser tuberosity medially *(open arrow)* and the greater tuberosity laterally *(curved arrow).* The biceps tendon is seen as an echogenic ellipse within the groove *(black arrow). B,* Sonogram perpendicular to the long axis of the intra-articular portion of the biceps tendon *(open black arrowheads),* seen between the subscapularis anteriorly and the supraspinatus posteriorly. The deep surface of the deltoid muscle is shown by *open white arrowheads* and the humeral head by *solid white arrowheads. C,* On longitudinal scans, the biceps tendon appears as an echogenic band sandwiched between the upper portion of the humeral head *(solid arrows)* and the lower portion of the deltoid *(open white arrows). D,* Transverse sonogram of the distal part of the biceps tendon showing biceps sheath effusion *(arrows)* surrounding the biceps tendon. (Reproduced with permission from Middleton WD, Reinus WR, Tetty WG, et al: Ultrasonographic evaluation of the rotator cuff and biceps tendon. J Bone Joint Surg *68*(3):440–450, 1986.)

MAGNETIC RESONANCE IMAGING (MRI) SCAN

The MRI scan can visualize the normal biceps tendon both intra-articularly and in the groove and can accurately predict the presence of rotator cuff tears and impingement tendinitis in the supraspinatus.[113, 150] Unfortunately, it is expensive and, as a screening test for bicipital lesions, not cost effective. As the technology advances, surface coils improve, and as the cost comes down, it may be the test of choice in the future to help the clinician manage shoulder problems.

ARTHROSCOPY

Arthroscopy can be useful in evaluating chronic shoulder pain, especially anterior shoulder pain which has escaped diagnosis after a careful history, physical, and diagnostic examination.[8, 9, 179, 231] Lesions of the biceps and the superior labral complex have been well described by Andrews[9] and others and may mimic bicipital tendinitis. Numerous conditions cause anterior shoulder pain. Chief among them are anterior instability, impingement syndrome, labral tears without instability, and bicipital tendinitis. Using the arthroscope, the subtle anterior and posterior glenoid labral tears and cartilaginous humeral head defects can be visualized; these are not always seen on CT scan. Lesions of the intra-articular portion of the biceps can also be appreciated.

Complications

The most common complication of biceps tendon rupture or dislocation is, as has been emphasized previously, the failure to recognize a disruption of the rotator cuff. The majority of rotator cuff tears are secondary to chronic impingement wear and tendinitis. Some patients will sustain an acute massive cuff avulsion as the result of trauma. Although the results of cuff debridement and decompression are impressive in terms of pain relief and range of motion, if the patient is young (less than 60 years of age) and wants to maintain a strong shoulder for use above the horizontal, an early diagnostic work-up and aggressive surgical approach is preferred.

Adhesive capsulitis can follow a number of painful conditions about the shoulder. Since biceps tendinitis has been previously associated with adhesive capsulitis, early recognition of this condition and treatment with anti-inflammatory agents, moist heat, and early, gentle patient-directed range-of-motion exercises may aid in preventing or shortening this often painful, long process.

Nontreatment of biceps ruptures especially in the elderly, is accepted by many patients and physicians. Very few of these individuals note any dysfunction related to the biceps rupture itself. Predictably, patients with bicipital rupture who have an intact brachialis muscle will have no decrease in flexion strength at the elbow. Loss of supination strength has been estimated by Warren and associates to be between 10 and 20 per cent with Cybex testing.[227, 228]

Differential Diagnosis

As in any other clinical entity, differential diagnosis in bicipital tendinitis or subluxation should begin with an accurate history and physical. Because tendinitis of the long head of the biceps usually occurs secondary to another condition and primary bicipital tendinitis is a diagnosis of exclusion, the other clinical entities which can mimic or be associated with this entity must be remembered. They are impingement syndrome, adhesive capsulitis, rheumatoid and osteoarthritis, glenohumeral instability, coracoid impingement syndrome, thoracic outlet syndrome or brachial plexopathy/plexitis, peripheral nerve entrapment, and cervical radiculopathy.

One pertinent historical feature is the mechanism of injury. This should include the amount and direction of force applied, whether it was direct or indirect, and in what position the arm was at the time of application of the force. Was the onset insidious? Has there been a gradual loss of motion over several months? Had the patient engaged in any unusual overhead activity before the onset of symptoms? Has the patient had an injury to the shoulder before or been treated for "bursitis"? Has the patient engaged in activities that required overhead use of the arm such as swimming, throwing, or tennis? What makes the pain better; what makes the pain worse? Where does the patient feel the pain most in his shoulder? Does activity improve or exacerbate the painful phenomenon? Inspection for atrophy of the deltoid, infraspinatus, suprasinatus, and trapezius, swelling, and obvious biceps ruptures should be performed. The patient should be examined from the front, the side, and the back and comparison with the other side made. Physical examination should include cervical spine range of motion and detailed neurovascular examination including deep tendon reflexes, sensation, strength testing, and specific physical tests for thoracic outlet syndrome. Range of motion of the shoulder should be examined. Both the active and passive range of forward flexion, abduction, external rotation, internal rotation, and extension should be noted. The relative contribution of glenohumeral and scapulothoracic joint motion should be assessed. Anterior apprehension testing as well as anterior, posterior, and inferior drawer test should be performed. The examiner should look for the impingement sign[166] and the impingement reinforcement sign of Hawkins.[93] The acromioclavicular joint is palpated, and a compression test or hug test, specific for acromioclavicular joint arthritis, is performed. Specific areas of point tenderness over the anterior acromion, coracoacromial ligament, and coracoid are noted. The biceps tendon is palpated in the groove, anteriorly at a position of approximately 10 degrees of internal rotation, 4 to 6 cm distal to the acromion (see Fig. 20–31). A helpful point in determining whether this is the tendon and groove area is to see if the point of tenderness moves with rotation of the humerus. A diffuse bursitis will not move, while an inflamed biceps will. The point of tenderness of bicipital tendinitis may completely disappear underneath the coracoid upon marked internal rotation. The diagnosis of primary bicipital tendinitis must be arrived at by exclusion of the other, more common, causes of anterior shoulder pain.

BICEPS TENDINITIS VERSUS IMPINGEMENT SYNDROME

Biceps tendinitis usually occurs secondary to the impingement syndrome and only rarely exists as an isolated entity. To differentiate primary bicipital tendinitis from impingement tendinitis, selective injection with a local anesthetic is helpful. In patients with impingement syndrome without bicipital involvement, the pain is located more proximally, with tenderness primarily on the anterior acromion, coracoacromial ligament, and supraspinatus tendon insertion. The impingement sign and impingement reinforcement signs are positive. In patients with an impingement syndrome, the injection of lidocaine (Xylocaine) into the subacromial space usually relieves all of the patient's pain. In patients who have an associated bicipital tendinitis, there is pain distally in the groove, the subacromial injection does not relieve all of their pain, and they continue to have pain over the bicipital groove. Further injection of Xylocaine into the sheath with obliteration of pain confirms the associated bicipital tendinitis. It is important to remember that the subdeltoid bursa, which covers the groove, is continuous with the subacromial bursa, and inadvertent injection into this area will anesthetize the subacromial bursa. Therefore, I always inject the subacromial bursa first, doing it from the lateral or posterolateral corner of the acromion to avoid inadvertent injection of

Xylocaine into the groove. Only if subacromial injection has absolutely no effect on the patient's pain while isolated biceps injection relieves all pain and restores 100 per cent of their motion, will I make a clinical diagnosis of primary bicipital tendinitis.

The technique of injection is described by Kerlin[113] in which the patient is placed supine with the arm over the table. The elbow is bent and the shoulder extended with the arm in external rotation, decreasing the distance from the groove to the surface. The biceps tendon is located anteriorly, and a mark is made on the skin. The area is prepared in a sterile fashion and injected. It is extremely important, especially if corticosteroids are used, that the injection be into the sheath and not into the tendon proper. Direction of the needle superiorly tangential to the tendon should hopefully eliminate this complication. There must be an easy flow of fluid; if any resistance is felt, the needle should be repositioned. Because of the anatomy of the sheath and its communication with the joint, I use a very low volume of local anesthetic, only 2 to 3 ml of 1 per cent Xylocaine during the biceps ablation test.

Claessens and Snoek[40] thought that intra-articular injection of an anesthetic is important in differentiating rotator cuff tendinitis from bicipital tendinitis. Although this is true of bursal side lesions, undersurface tears of the rotator cuff will be anesthetized with this technique as well. Radiographs, sonography, and arthrography should be used to confirm one's clinical impression.

ANTERIOR SHOULDER INSTABILITY

The pain associated with anterior subluxation of the glenohumeral joint will be noted in the anterior portion of the shoulder. At the same time, patients may often have pain posteriorly from capsular stretching. The pain is episodic in nature and associated with a palpable and audible clunk, such as has been described previously from medial dislocation in the biceps. The pain generally lasts for several days after a major subluxation episode. If the brachial plexus is inflamed and stretched, pain and paresthesias can be experienced transiently or in varying degrees for several weeks or months. The mechanism of injury described for both of these conditions is very similar in that they most commonly occur with forced abduction and external rotation. The differential diagnosis can be even more confusing if anterior shoulder instability and impingement syndrome coexist, which is not uncommon. A derangement in the glenohumeral joint leading to weakness in the short rotators and secondary impingement is seen frequently in patients with recurrent subluxation.

Historically, patients with pure instability have pain for only a few days after a subluxation episode unless impingement syndrome or brachial neuritis coexists. Therefore, it is relatively easy to differentiate this problem from pure bicipital tendinitis. When differ-

entiating this problem from subluxation of the biceps tendon, provocative tests are helpful. In anterior shoulder instability, the maximum point of apprehension and clicking should be in 90 degrees of abduction and maximum external rotation, i.e., a positive apprehension sign. Pain in the anterior part of the shoulder occurs as the humeral head translates across the torn glenoid labrum. Pain can also be felt posteriorly at this time, secondary to cuff stretching. In the patient with a subluxating biceps tendon, the pain is not maximal until the arm is brought down from the position of maximum abduction and external rotation and the click occurs as the examiner begins to internally rotate the arm, i.e., biceps instability test. Yergason's and Speed's signs should be negative in patients with anterior shoulder instability but positive if the biceps is inflamed. Special roentgenographic views for shoulder instability should be employed (see Chapter 5 on radiology of the shoulder). The CT arthrogram can be extremely helpful in demonstrating lesions of the anterior cartilaginous labrum in patients with instability. The biceps tendon can be visualized within its groove on CT arthrography.

If, after the above studies, the diagnosis remains unclear, arthroscopy can be performed. Glenohumeral arthroscopy allows one to visualize directly the anterior labrum as well as the intra-articular portion of the biceps tendon, the aperture of the sulcus, and the surrounding cuff tissue.

GLENOID LABRUM TEARS WITHOUT INSTABILITY

Glenoid labrum tears without instability, such as those that occur in the superior one-third of the labrum in close proximity to the biceps, can demonstrate symptoms similar to those of subluxation of the biceps tendon. These superior labrum tears can occur in baseball players and other throwing athletes and frequently show symptoms very similar to those of a subluxating bicipital tendon or a rotator cuff tear (see Chapter 26 on shoulder injuries in athletes). An audible or palpable clunk occurs as the tear flips in and out of the joint impinging on the humeral head during rotation above the horizontal. A high index of suspicion for this lesion should be present if one is dealing with a throwing athlete with shoulder pain. These patients sometimes have more pain with release because of the deceleration effect of the biceps pulling on the torn labrum. CT arthrography will occasionally miss this lesion, and the best way to differentiate this problem from subluxating biceps tendon is by glenohumeral arthroscopy.

ADHESIVE CAPSULITIS

Patients with adhesive capsulitis frequently have tenderness in the anterior aspect of the shoulder in the region of the bicipital groove and anterior portion of the subdeltoid bursa.

In evaluating patients with painful and stiff shoulders who have direct areas of point tenderness over the bicipital groove, I will inject this with Xylocaine, initially without cortisone, to see what effect this has on motion and how much of a fixed capsular contracture is present. If one injects and infiltrates the tendon sheath with 2 to 3 ml of Xylocaine and the patient's pain is obliterated but there is no appreciable change in motion, one can be sure one is dealing with an adhesive capsulitis or frozen shoulder and not just a painful stiff shoulder from biceps tendinitis. If injection into the biceps region eliminates pain and motion returns in full, a bicipital tendinitis exists. Whether it is part of the impingement syndrome can be determined by clinical examination and subacromial injection.

GLENOHUMERAL ARTHRITIS

Early arthritis of the glenohumeral joint frequently presents as anterior shoulder pain with limited range of motion. Since the biceps tendon is an intra-articular structure, it will be involved with any process within the joint. Inflammatory changes occur in the visceral layer of the synovium of the biceps recess as they do in the subscapular and axillary recess. Plain radiography may show spurs off the proximal humerus with a ring osteophyte and flattening of the glenoid. Prior to the development of obvious osseous spur formation, double contrast arthrography can reveal thinning of the articular cartilage.

CORACOID IMPINGEMENT SYNDROME

Warren[227, 228] and Gerber[71] have described the role of the coracoid process in the chronic impingement syndrome and have noted similarity in symptoms to biceps tendinitis and instability. Based on CT scan data, Gerber[71] has calculated the normal coracoid-to-humeral distance (8.6 mm) and noted that it is decreased in patients (average 6.7 mm) with coracoid impingement syndrome. The syndrome has been described in patients with an excessively long or laterally placed coracoid process and in those who have had bone block and osteotomy procedures for instability. Symptoms of coracoid impingement are dull pain in the front of the shoulder with referral to the front and upper arm, occasionally extending into the forearm. The pain is consistently brought about by forward flexion and internal rotation or abduction or internal rotation. In contrast to the more common type of impingement, forward flexion was most often painful between 120 and 130 degrees, rather than full forward flexion. The diagnosis is established clinically by obliteration of the patient's pain by subcoracoid injection.

The importance of consideration of this entity before performing surgery on the biceps tendon is pointed out by Dines and associates;[57] they report a series in which one-third of their failures from biceps tenodesis were related to undiagnosed coracoid impingement syndrome.

THORACIC OUTLET SYNDROME

Thoracic outlet syndrome frequently presents with some anterior shoulder pain. It is generally associated with paresthesias into the distribution of the lower trunk of the plexus, i.e., the ulnar two fingers. Neck pain, parascapular pain, and radiation into the pectorals are not uncommon. The body habitus may be asthenic with a long neck and round back or endomorphic with pendulous breasts. The shoulders slope forward and downward owing to rhomboid, levator, and trapezius weakness. Provocative tests for thoracic outlet syndrome, such as Wright's maneuver, Adson's test, or Roo's overhead grip test, will be positive when Yergason's, Speed's, and the impingement tests are all negative or equivocal. Subacromial and bicipital injections should not alleviate pain completely. Cervical spine series looking specifically for cervical ribs as well as Doppler examination and EMGs are useful adjuncts to clinical testing. However, the diagnosis remains a clinical one.

BRACHIAL NEURITIS

Viral brachial plexitis (syndrome of Parsonage and Turner) is an extremely painful condition that frequently presents with anterior shoulder pain. Early in the course of this condition, which usually follows a viral illness, pain exceeds neurological findings, and one may be fooled into thinking that one is dealing with an acute calcific tendinitis. Later, numbness and weakness with obvious atrophy become prominent. The course is variable.

PERIPHERAL NERVE ENTRAPMENT/CERVICAL RADICULOPATHY

The common syndromes of peripheral nerve entrapment, i.e., carpal tunnel, ulnar neuritis, and posterior interosseous nerve entrapment, may all present with anterior shoulder pain that is referred and can potentially be confused with bicipital tendinitis. Cervical radiculopathy, especially C5–C6, can also mimic primary shoulder lesions. Careful and repeated neurological examination followed by EMG and nerve conduction velocity tests can help distinguish among these entities. In patients with persistent anterior shoulder pain, especially if it is typical of neurogenic pain, in whom the work-up for primary shoulder pathology is negative and neurological examination is unrevealing, one must consider the possibility that one is dealing with a tumor in the apex, the mediastinum, or diaphragm region.

Treatment of Bicipital Lesions: Review of Conservative Treatment

Bromfield[29] in 1773 discussed the technical aspects of reducing biceps tendon dislocation. Tendinitis treatment was initially discussed by Schrager[205] in the 1920s. Recommendations during the 1920s and 1930s included morphine, sudden traction, diathermy, massage, faradization, and light and x-ray treatment. Milgram[156-159] and later Lapidus[118] were proponents of procaine hydrochloride (Novocain) infiltration and aspiration of the calcific deposits in cases of acute calcific tendinitis.

DePalma[53] initially treated bicipital tenosynovitis conservatively with hydrocortisone injection directly into the tendon, under the transverse ligament, and noted improvement in 10 of 18 cases. He recommended, as a rule, three or four 1-ml injections into the tendon under the transverse ligament at weekly intervals. It is apparent now from data by Kennedy[112] that this interval is too frequent, the injection should be only into the tendon sheath, and the tendon itself should not be directly injected. In conservatively treated patients he noted excellent results in 29 per cent, good in 45 per cent, fair in 9 per cent, and poor in 16 per cent.

Results of Nonoperative Treatment of Biceps Rupture

There is slight functional deficit after disruption of the long head of the biceps tendon. After a period of conservative care, including range of motion exercise, moist heat, and strengthening, most patients have relatively normal strength and flexion and only minimal loss of supination power.[100-105] Carroll and Hamilton[32] studied 100 patients who had a rupture of the biceps brachii as a result of forced extension. Follow-up function was ascertained by the patient's ability to lift weights. They believed that a patient could return to work earlier and suffered no residual disability from conservative treatment. Treated conservatively, the patients in their series returned to work on an average of four weeks. It was thought that a conservative approach should be adopted in treating this type of injury. Warren,[227] using Cybex testing in 10 patients with chronic biceps rupture, failed to reveal any statistically significant loss of elbow flexion and only 10 per cent loss of elbow supination.

Review of Operative Treatment

Surgical treatment of the biceps tendon received little attention prior to Gilcreest[74] in 1926. He was the first to suggest suturing the stump of the tendon to the coracoid process and described intracapsular, intertubercular, and labral junction ruptures of the tendon. In 1939 Abbott and Saunders[1] reviewed six cases of surgical treatment of biceps dislocations. Their procedure involved stabilizing the biceps tendon, with half of the tendon drilled through drill holes, leaving the intracapsular portion intact. In their review, four of the six patients required reoperation for pain, and all patients had some pain, weakness, and limited range of motion, even after a second operation. Poor results from their procedure stemmed from two problem areas: (1) the procedure as described prevents the normal upward and downward motion of the humerus on the bicipital tendon; (2) more attention was paid to the biceps lesion, with not enough attention to the cuff rupture and impingement area. The one patient in their series who did have a good result had the biceps replaced into the groove and the fibrous roof reconstructed.

Lippmann[124, 125] recommended tenodesis of the long head of the biceps to the lesser tuberosity (Fig. 20–45) to shorten the course of frozen shoulder. He strongly believed, based on 12 operated cases, that periarthritis, or frozen shoulder, was caused by tenosynovitis of the long head of the biceps.

Hitchcock and Bechtol[97] in 1948 described tenodesis of the biceps tendon within the groove with an osteal

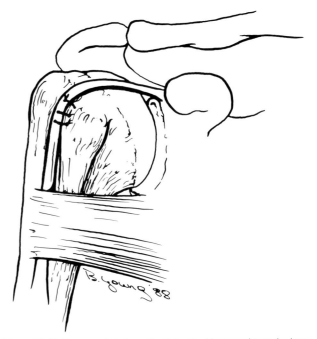

Figure 20–45. Lippmann technique of suturing the biceps tendon to the lesser tuberosity for adhesive capsulitis.

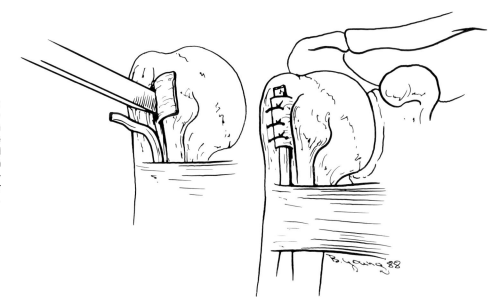

Figure 20–46. Hitchcock procedure. With an osteotome, a bed is made in the intertubercular groove by elevating a portion of the floor from the outside inward. The tendon is roughened and then sutured beneath this osteal periosteal flap with heavy nonabsorbable sutures. The transverse humeral ligament is laid down over the tendon and the osteal periosteal flap.

periosteal flap (Fig. 20–46), and Hitchcock's name has become synonymous with tenodesis in the groove. According to the authors, extensive fixation of the long head of the biceps tendon to the floor of the intratubercular groove in the manner they described greatly expedites convalescence, promotes loss of pain, and promotes rapid functional recovery. However, they supplied no objective data to support this statement, describing primarily case results and stating that, in 26 such cases, the results have been most satisfactory. The authors recognized the association of other lesions, such as ruptures of the rotator cuff. Their main concern was that peritendinitis of the biceps tendon not be overlooked and not the converse, i.e., overlooking rotator cuff pathology when biceps symptoms predominate.

In 1954, DePalma and Callery[52] reported on 86 cases of bicipital tenosynovitis treated operatively, the bulk of which were treated with suture into the coracoid process (Fig. 20–47). Shortly before publication several patients had tenodesis of the tendon in the groove, with a staple for fixation. The rationale cited for changing was that the three-prong staple provided firm fixation of the tendon and that tenodesis in the groove eliminated much of the dissection on the anterior aspect of the shoulder joint, necessary to expose the coracoid process. Of the 86 cases, only 59 were available for follow-up, with an average of 27 months. Twenty-three were complicated by frozen shoulder. Excellent results were achieved in 64 per cent, good results in 16 per cent, fair results in 8 per cent, and poor results in 10 per cent, i.e., 80 per cent of the patients achieved an excellent or good result. Analysis of the poor results revealed errors in diagnosis, technique, and reflex sympathetic dystrophy.

Michele[153] in 1960 described the keystone tenodesis. In this technique, a rectangular block of bone, including the bicipital groove, is removed. The bone is decorticated. The bony trough is prepared for insertion

and exit of the tendon by placement of two semilunar holes at the central poles at the sites of the remaining portions of the intertubercular sulcus. The tendon and sheath of the biceps are replaced into the defect created and then the bone block replaced. The periosteum is sutured back to secure the bony block in place. Michele

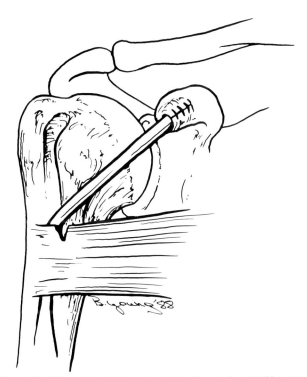

Figure 20–47. Tenodesis of the long head of the biceps to the coracoid process. This procedure was initially described by Gilcreest and popularized by DePalma. It involves medial dissection and potential denervation of the deltoid if done through a deltoid-splitting approach. It also theoretically changes the long head from a static head depressor to an active head elevator. (Modified from Crenshaw AH, and Kilgore WE: Surgical treatment of bicipital tenosynovitis. J Bone Joint Surg 45:1496–1502, 1966.)

reported on 16 cases in which roentgenograms demonstrated persistence of the entrance and exit holes and "smooth gliding of the biceps through the holes." Maneuverability was complete in all directions and asymptomatic. There was no recurrence of symptoms.

In 1966 Crenshaw and Kilgore[49] reported on the surgical treatment of bicipital tendinitis. They used the Hitchcock procedure in most of their cases, performing a total of 65 Hitchcock, 5 DePalma, and 3 Lippmann procedures. Relief of moderate to severe pain was good in 90 per cent of patients, while 2 per cent of the patients continued to complain of "mild, nagging pain." Restoration of motion in their series was often disappointing, with only 85 per cent of normal at follow-up. Interestingly, half of the patients who had good motion before surgery actually lost motion after the Hitchcock procedure. One has to wonder what the addition of an acromioplasty would have done to these results.

Keyhole tenodesis (Fig. 20–48) of the biceps origin was described by Froimson and Oh[67] for the treatment of rupture, instability, and tendinitis of the biceps in 1974. They reported on 12 shoulders in 11 patients, with an average follow-up of 24 months. They report satisfactory results in all of their patients but state that the patients with tenosynovitis enjoyed less than excellent results because of associated pericapsulitis. The advantages cited by the authors include: (1) the procedure avoids hardware and undue medial dissection; (2) the procedure removes the remnant of the biceps tendon, allowing motion of the humeral head and avoiding intra-articular derangement; and (3) the inherent stability of their method gives one confidence to begin early, gentle range of motion of both the shoulder and elbow.

Dines, Warren, and Inglis[57] commented on surgical treatment of lesions of the long head of the biceps in 1980. Seventeen patients had tenodesis of the long head of the biceps into the humeral head via the keyhole technique and three had transfixion of the tendon into the coracoid. In addition, excision of the coracoacromial ligament was performed in 14 of 20 of their patients. They had 6 failures out of the 20 patients (33 per cent). Revision surgery was required for four of six patients. In four failures in the tendinitis group, three were found to have an impingement syndrome. One had a typical anterior impingement, and two patients had coracoid impingement. The other patient was later noted to have glenohumeral instability. The patients who did well in their series were older patients, averaging 41 years of age. In those patients, excision of the coracoacromial ligament was part of the operation. However, it is their recommendation now that an acromioplasty as well as a coracoacromial ligament release be performed. In patients who were found to have coracoid impingement, coracoid osteotomy later relieved their pain. The most salient recommendation and lesson from this review is that at the time of surgical exposure, if biceps tenodesis is planned, the subacromial space and the inter-relation of the cora-

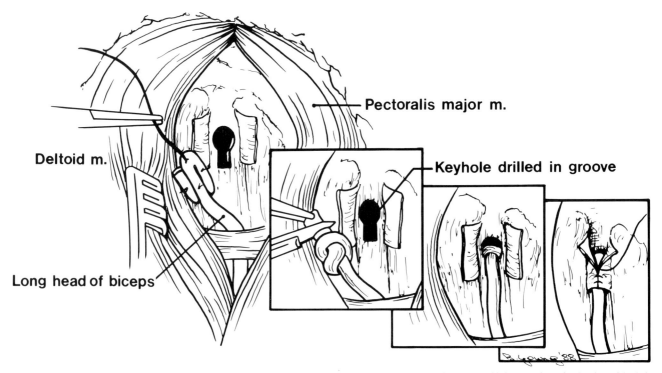

Figure 20–48. Keyhole tenodesis as described by Froimson. The biceps tendon is rolled into a thick ball in the proximal stump; this is sutured together in a knot. A keyhole is made in the groove using a dental bur. The tendon is then inserted into the keyhole and the transverse ligament repaired over the tendon with nonabsorbable suture. Post has recommended marking the groove and the tendon with methylene blue prior to incision of the tendon in order to determine the normal tension of the tendon postoperatively. (Modified from Froimson AI, and Oh I: Keyhole tenodesis of biceps origin at the shoulder. Clin Orthop 112:245–249, 1974.)

coacromial arch to the tendon must be observed. Careful preoperative evaluation as well as examination under anesthesia will reveal concomitant anterior instability. It was their impression that isolated inflammation of the long head of the biceps is an infrequent finding unless injury to the biceps tendon in the groove has occurred and that the entity of the subluxating biceps tendon is still questionable. They state, "The role of the biceps tendon in the production of shoulder pain is difficult to assess and easily overestimated. Biceps tendon inflammation may be a secondary manifestation of an impingement syndrome. Unless treated, the impingement syndrome surgery will not be successful."

O'Donohue[178] presented a series of 56 cases of biceps instability treated with the Hitchcock procedure, 71 per cent reporting excellent progress, 77 per cent said they could throw satisfactorily, and 77 per cent resuming their sport. It was believed in the young, motivated athlete for whom throwing was important that this was a very worthwhile operation.

Neviaser[177] reported on the four-in-one arthroplasty for relief of chronic subacromial impingement. In his procedure all elements of the coracoacromial arch are addressed. The four-in-one arthroplasty includes anterior acromioplasty, excision of the coracoacromial ligament, excision of the distal clavicle, and biceps tenodesis. Eighty-six per cent of their 89 patients had no pain whatsoever, while 13 per cent had pain only with excessive exercise. Motion was improved in 81 per cent. Most of the early studies showing good results of biceps tenodesis had very scant and short follow-up.

Cofield[44] reviewed the long-term results of 51 patients in whom there were 54 shoulders with isolated biceps tenodesis. At six months 94 per cent felt they had benefited from the procedure; however, satisfactory results fell to 52 per cent at an average of seven years. Fifteen per cent underwent subsequent surgery, primarily cuff repairs and acromioplasty, and 33 per cent continued to have moderate to severe pain. Their impression was that isolated biceps tenodesis was not particularly efficacious in the long term.

Ogilvie-Harris[179] reported on arthroscopic findings in biceps tendon lesions. The usual lesion consisted of fraying of the tendon, with loose fronds hanging down into the joint. The fraying appeared to be greatest at the point where the biceps tendon entered the bicipital groove. The arthroscopic procedure consisted of debridement of the tendon by removing all the loose fronds, and in some cases, attempts at dilatation of the orifice through which the biceps tendon passed were made. There were 46 patients with lesions of the biceps tendon in his series. Some of them had had previous rotator cuff repairs, and the biceps tendon appeared to be adherent to the undersurface of the rotator cuff. These adhesions were freed arthroscopically, using small scissors. Of patients with isolated lesions at the biceps tendon, according to Ogilvie-Harris, "Three fourths of them did well with simple debridement."

However, he admits that the follow-up was short, being only 24 months. Four of nine patients who had the biceps tendon stuck to the undersurface of the rotator cuff after repair had "relief of symptoms" following lysis of adhesions.

In 1987, Post[194] presented 21 patients in whom the diagnosis of primary tendinitis of the long head of the biceps was made. In his cases, he excluded any with associated impingement syndrome, rotator cuff pathology, recurrent anterior shoulder instability, and repeated biceps tendon subluxation. All patients in his series had marked tenderness over the long head of the biceps, a negative impingement sign, and little or no relief of pain with subacromial injection. Fifty per cent of the cases had a positive Yergason's sign. Seventeen patients in his series underwent biceps tenodesis via the keyhole technique; four patients had a transfer to the coracoid process. In the transfer group there were two excellent and two good results. One patient required a manipulation under anesthesia. Of 17 patients who had tenodesis, there were 13 excellent results, 2 good results, and 1 failure. Two patients did require manipulation. The 1 patient who was considered a failure in this group developed symptoms and findings of an impingement syndrome postoperatively and eventually required a partial anterior acromioplasty. In the tenodesis group, there were 88.3 per cent good and excellent results. On the basis of his experience, it is Post's conviction that primary biceps tendinitis does occur as an isolated entity. Also, when it does occur, it is observed in the intertubercular groove alone.

Author's Preferred Methods of Treatment

The treatment of lesions of the biceps tendon, with the exception of acute traumatic rupture of the tendon in the young patient or in association with a massive cuff tear in an active patient, should be viewed as a continuum with prolonged (several months) conservative care and repeated evaluation. As long as the patient is making slow, gradual improvement, surgical intervention is not recommended. Surgical treatment is only indicated after a minimum of six months of conservative care. I have divided the treatment of chronic lesions using the classification of Paavolainen and associates.[180]

IMPINGEMENT TENDINITIS

Treatment of bicipital tendinitis when associated with coracoacromial arch impingement closely follows the treatment outlined by Neer in his original and follow-up articles. The stages and treatment of this clinical entity are well described in Chapter 15.

In Stage II, if symptoms remain the same after six months of active conservative treatment, I will sometimes employ glenohumeral arthroscopy to visualize the intra-articular portion of the biceps and glenoid labrum. The biceps tendon can be pulled into the joint with a probe and synovitis demonstrated if present. This obviates the need for opening the rotator interval, which prolongs recovery. Although good results from arthroscopic decompression have been reported in Stage II impingement,[61] when biceps symptoms predominate, patients often have a long acromion, and I prefer an open approach as performed by Rockwood (Fig. 20–49). It involves a removal of all of the acromion that extends anterior to the anterior border of the clavicle, i.e., an anterior acromionectomy with a straight osteotome, which is then followed by an inferior acromioplasty with a curved osteotome. The advantages of this double-cut approach are (1) it ensures adequate removal of anterior bone, (2) it allows the surgeon to better appreciate the thickness of the acromion, and (3) it avoids leaving residual anteromedial and anterolateral acromion that can still impinge (Fig. 20–50).

Biceps tenodesis is performed in Stage II only if the tendon is extremely frayed. It is important to remember that the offending structure is not the tendon itself but the overlying coracoacromial arch. When biceps tenodesis is required, which is extremely rare, the keyhole tenodesis[67] is used.

Post[193] has offered a solution to one problem I have had previously when doing a biceps tenodesis, and that is, "Under what type of tension should the biceps be tenodesed?" Should this be done in elbow flexion, extension, etc.? He recommends marking the biceps tendon and intertubercular groove with methylene blue after the bicipital groove is opened but before the intertubercular portion is cut so that after the tendon is cut, these adjacent areas can be matched again at the time of tenodesis.

In Stage III impingement, by definition, a full-thickness tear exists in the rotator cuff. These patients generally also have severe spurring of the anterior acromion and distal clavicle. Frequently, if the anterior cuff is involved, subluxation, hypertrophy, degenerative changes, or frank rupture of the biceps tendon may be present. In these patients, a formal open

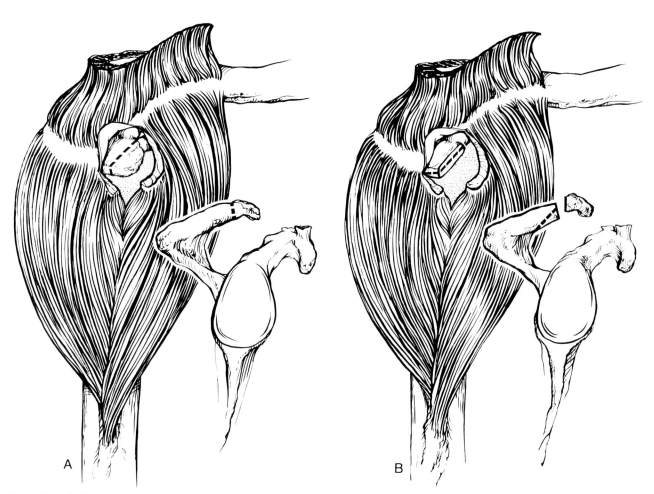

Figure 20–49. *A,* The anterior acromionectomy is shown by the dotted line. This is accomplished with a vertical cut with an osteotome. The amount of acromion removed is all bone that is anterior to the anterior border of the clavicle. *B,* The dotted line indicates the anteroinferior acromioplasty. (Courtesy of Charles A. Rockwood, Jr., M.D.)

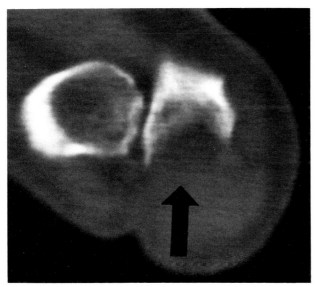

Figure 20–50. An anterior acromioplasty has been performed using a curved osteotome in a single oblique acromioplasty. This unfortunately left residual anterior acromion with residual coracoacromial ligament attached to the medial aspect *(arrow)*, as seen on this CT scan. For this reason I recommend initially an anterior acromionectomy done with a straight osteotome (as taught by Rockwood).

anterior acromioplasty and cuff repair is performed with reconstruction of the rotator cuff. If the biceps is dislocated, it is replaced in the groove, and after suturing the supraspinatus either tendon to tendon or tendon to bone, the rotator interval is closed and the edges of the subscapularis and coracohumeral ligament complex are sutured to the repaired supraspinatus,

recreating the stabilizing effect at the aperture of the tuberosities (Fig. 20–51). The biceps tendon is not tenodesed unless severe attrition wear and eminent rupture is found. No attempt is made to repair chronic ruptures (greater than six weeks) of the tendon. The patient is informed preoperatively that he or she will continue to have a bulge in the lower portion of the brachium. The intra-articular portion is removed.

TREATMENT OF BICEPS INSTABILITY

In my experience, surgically proven biceps instability is always related to a degenerative process in the cuff, restraining capsule, and coracohumeral ligament in the proximal portion of the groove. It is doubtful, I think, that the clunk felt by patients with this entity is related to actual subluxation of the biceps tendon. More commonly, the roughened edges of the cuff catch against the anterior edge of the acromion and the coracoacromial ligament, and the intervening thickened bursa causes the palpable crepitus in this region. As with impingement tendinitis, primary attention should be placed on repair of the rotator cuff as well as performing a thorough decompression of the coracoacromial arch. It has been well established that the main stabilizer of the biceps tendon is the musculotendinous cuff and the coracohumeral ligament. These structures can be injured acutely or by the mechanisms previously described, and a fixed or recurrent subluxation of the biceps tendon can occur. If the history of injury is acute and the patient is under 65, early

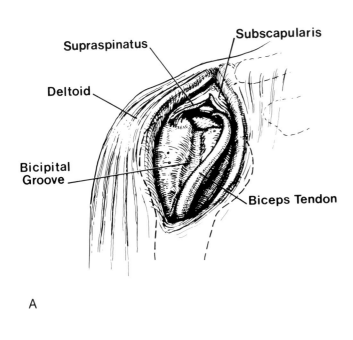

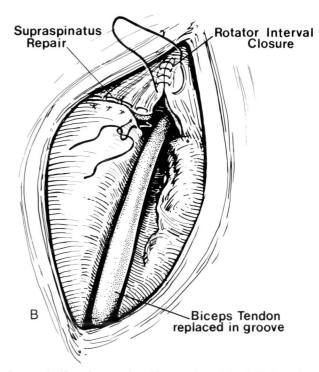

Figure 20–51. *A,* Rotator cuff tear and dislocated biceps tendon. *B,* The rotator cuff has been repaired into a bony trough and the rotator interval closed with the tendon replaced in the groove.

sonography is recommended to diagnose this condition and to evaluate the status of the rotator cuff. If the biceps is dislocated, I recommend early open reduction of the tendon with reconstruction of the fibrous roof, combined with an acromioplasty procedure (see Fig. 20–51). It is important to remember that once one has made the diagnosis of a dislocated biceps tendon, one has also made a diagnosis of rupture of a portion of the rotator cuff. Whereas in the older (over 65) age group, this can be accepted and treated conservatively, younger (less than 50) patients will fare better if the tendon is replaced and the fibrous roof reconstructed. Again, unless there is severe pre-existing attrition wear in the biceps tendon and rupture appears imminent, I do not recommend tenodesis for fixed subluxation or dislocation of the biceps unless it is impossible to reconstruct the fibrous roof.

TREATMENT OF ATTRITION TENDINITIS

These are patients in whom subacromial injection offers absolutely no improvement in the pain, but pain and motion consistently respond to local anesthetic injections into the bicipital groove region. These patients generally respond to the judicious use of rest, aspirin or nonsteroidal anti-inflammatory agents, moist heat, and gentle patient-directed exercises. The judicious use of corticosteroids by injection can also be helpful. Because the injection of steroids into the tendon can produce disruption of collagen, I do not recommend steroid injection into the tendon. The injection should be into the bicipital sheath and should require only minimal pressure on the syringe and a low volume of fluid, i.e., 2 to 3 ml of Xylocaine and 1 ml of water-soluble steroid should be used. The technique of injection has been described previously under differential diagnosis. The point of maximal tenderness is determined, and I try to inject with a cephalic tilt on the needle to try to get the needle into the sheath, skiving tangentially to avoid direct injection into the tendon. There have been numerous case reports of tendon ruptures temporally and causally related to corticosteroid injections. These include the patellar and Achilles' tendons and tendons of the flexors and extensors of the hand as well as the long head of the biceps. Although some tendons, especially those in the older patient with systemic disease or attrition tendinitis, may rupture as a result of the disease process, there is a strong suggestion that the use of injection into the tendon contributes to tendon degradation. Kennedy and Willis[112] have shown collagen necrosis as well as disorganization and loss of normal parallel collagen arrangement in Achilles' tendons injected with corticosteroids. This is accompanied by a 35 per cent loss of failure strength at approximately 48 hours postinjection. The failure strength at the tendon returns at approximately two weeks; however, ultrastructural changes in the tendon itself do not completely revert for six weeks. Because of this, the patients are asked to avoid any strenuous activity for three weeks. In my own experience, I have injected patients with steroids at the very most only every six weeks and have limited myself to a total of three injections. Injections have been shown to be more efficacious than a placebo or naproxen (Naprosyn) in the treatment of chronic shoulder pain and are equivalent to the use of indomethacin (Indocin).[221, 222] Unfortunately, some patients with this problem cannot tolerate nonsteroidal anti-inflammatory agents in the doses required. An injection will frequently make him or her more comfortable and shorten the course of the illness.

If the patient fails to respond to conservative care over a 6- to 12-month period, surgery is recommended. Since the results of isolated biceps tenodesis have not been spectacular in the long term and impingement syndrome has developed after biceps tenodesis, I routinely perform an anterior acromioplasty and coracoacromial ligament excision at the same time.

TREATMENT OF ISOLATED BICEPS RUPTURE IN PATIENTS UNDER THE AGE OF 50

In younger, active patients, particularly those involved in overhead sports or weight-lifting, a sudden overload can result in an isolated biceps rupture. This may be within the muscle tendon junction, rather than the long head tendon. Physical examination and ultrasonography of the biceps should be able to isolate the point of rupture. Sonography of the rotator cuff should be employed to determine the status of the rotator cuff. If physical examination is consistent with an acute rupture and the sonogram is equivocal or negative, an arthrogram can be used. In these patients with high functional expectations an early repair is the best alternative. If the rupture is musculotendinous or at the transverse ligament and sonography is negative for a cuff tear, I recommend early repair using a Bunnell-type weave suture through a deltopectoral incision. This is the only group of patients in whom I would use the deltopectoral approach rather than the superior acromioplasty approach. The other group of patients who I feel are candidates for tenodesis or repair are those whose work requirements involve repetitive forceful supination.

TREATMENT OF ACUTE BICIPITAL RUPTURE IN PATIENTS OVER THE AGE OF 50

If the patient is inactive physically, I prefer a wait-and-see attitude. I recommend rest, anti-inflammatory medications, and moist heat for 2 to 3 weeks. During this time, the patient is instructed in keeping the shoulder motion free and easy by passive motions. If the patient is physically active, an early aggressive diagnostic work-up should be performed. I generally start with sonography. If this is equivocal, an arthrogram should be performed. One will generally find an "acute" cuff tear as well as the biceps tendon rupture. Many of these patients will have had symptoms of "bursitis" in the past, and some have had corticosteroid injections. Others in this group of patients have had no shoulder pain, but clearly at the time of surgery, degenerative changes are present in the biceps tendon and in the adjacent rotator cuff. I prefer a two-incision approach in all these cases (Fig. 20–52A). If a tear is present in the rotator cuff, an anterior acromioplasty with cuff repair and bicipital tenodesis is performed. The biceps tendon is exposed through a separate incision over the sulcus (Fig. 20–52B). The subcutaneous tissue is incised, and frequently upon entering the fascia, edema and old hemorrhage will be evacu-

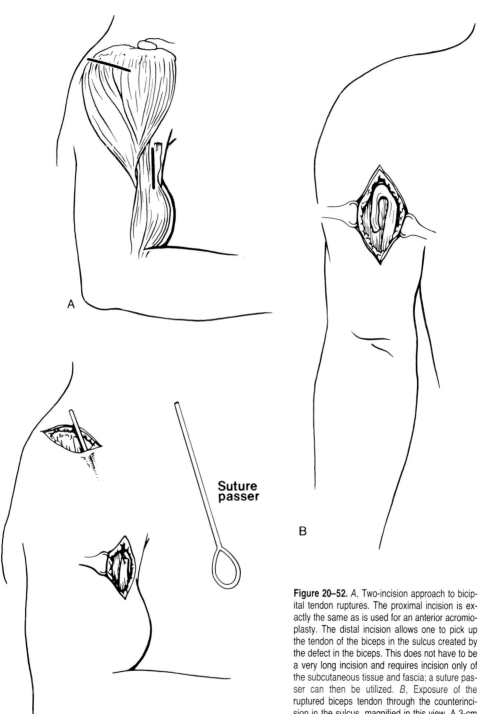

Figure 20–52. *A*, Two-incision approach to bicipital tendon ruptures. The proximal incision is exactly the same as is used for an anterior acromioplasty. The distal incision allows one to pick up the tendon of the biceps in the sulcus created by the defect in the biceps. This does not have to be a very long incision and requires incision only of the subcutaneous tissue and fascia; a suture passer can then be utilized. *B*, Exposure of the ruptured biceps tendon through the counterincision in the sulcus, magnified in this view. A 3-cm incision is all that is required to pick up the end of the tendon in this region. *C*, A suture passer is utilized to bring the tendon into the proximal wound for tenodesis or repair.

Suture passer

ated. The tendon is found curled up in this area. Using a suture-passer, passed down from above through the bicipital groove and into the lower wound, the tendon is advanced into the superior wound (Fig. 20–52C). A biceps tenodesis into the groove is then performed. After suturing the tendon in the groove, I make sure that I can extend the elbow fully without significant tension being generated on the repair so that early elbow extension can be performed.

POSTOPERATIVE CARE

Unless there is some tension on the cuff repair with the arm at the side, I will use a Velcro elastic immobilizer postoperatively for three weeks. The patient is encouraged to take the elbow out and gently flex and extend it passively with the opposite hand the night of the surgery. Gentle pendulum exercises are initiated on the first postoperative day. Passive flexion performed by the patient (with his other arm), nurse, or therapist is begun on the second postoperative day. Because holding on to a pulley handle requires some active contraction of the biceps, I generally instruct a family member in gentle, passive forward flexion and external rotation. At one month, the pulley can safely be used and gentle, active elbow flexion begun. Strengthening of the repaired cuff, deltoid, and biceps generally begins at two months and becomes more vigorous at three months. Patients usually can return to work at jobs that require some lifting at approximately six months.

Summary

Because of its unique anatomical position, variations in local anatomy, and, most important, its relationship to the coracoacromial arch, the biceps tendon is secondarily involved in painful conditions about the shoulder.

The biceps tendon appears to function both as a dynamic and static head depressor. Although the former is weak, both depressor effects of the biceps tendon appear to increase in pathological conditions about the shoulder. Because of this, routine tenodesis of the biceps at the time of uncomplicated acromioplasty or the incorporation of the biceps tendon as a free graft into a rotator cuff repair is not recommended by the author.

Although the bicipital sheath is involved with the same inflammatory process as the rest of the synovium in adhesive capsulitis, biceps tendinitis is not the initiating factor in most cases of adhesive capsulitis. The loss of the gliding mechanism of the biceps is not the primary cause of loss of motion in this entity.

The major retaining factor for the biceps tendon in the groove is the coracohumeral ligament and the rotator cuff, proximal to the groove. Therefore, because of this and its intimate relationship to the coracoacromial arch, whenever one considers the diagnosis of biceps pathology, one should also consider the diagnosis of impingement of the rotator cuff. Whenever possible, subluxation of the biceps should be treated with replacement of the tendon into the groove and reconstruction of the rotator cuff combined with subacromial decompression.

Isolated biceps tenodesis is not recommended. The addition of an anterior acromioplasty with excision of the coracoacromial ligament adds little morbidity to surgery on the biceps tendon and improves the results. Recognition that the diagnosis of isolated biceps tendon pathology is a diagnosis of exclusion, coupled with long-term conservative care for painful conditions about the shoulder, can often obviate the need for surgery and improve the results if surgical procedures are required.

References

1. Abbott LC, and Saunders LB de CM: Acute traumatic dislocation of the tendon of the long head of biceps brachii; report of 6 cases with operative findings. Surgery 6:817–840, 1939.
2. Abbott LC, and Lucas DB: The function of the clavicle: its surgical significance. Ann Surg 140:583–597, 1954.
3. Adams R: Abnormal Conditions of the Shoulder-Joint, Cyclopaedia of Anatomy and Physiology, Vol. 4. London: Longman, 1847–1849, p 595.
4. Ahovuo J: The radiographic anatomy of the intratubercular groove of the humerus. Eur J Radiol 2:83, 1985.
5. Ahovuo J, Paavolainen P, and Slatis P: Radiographic diagnosis of biceps tendinitis. Acta Orthop Scand 56:75–78, 1985.
6. Ahovuo J, Paavolainen P, and Slatis P: Diagnostic value of sonography in lesions of the biceps tendon. Clin Orthop 202:184–188, 1986.
7. Anciaux-Ruyssen A, and Claessens H: L'arthrographic de l'epaule. J Belge Radiol 39:837, 1956.
8. Andrews J, and Carson W: Shoulder joint arthroscopy. Orthopedics 6:1157–62, 1983.
9. Andrews J, Carson W, and McLeod W: Glenoid labrum tears related to the long head of the biceps. Am J Sports Med 13:337–341, 1985.
10. Anglesio B: Osteotomia per omero varo. Arch Orthop 46:417–428, 1930.
11. Ashurst J: The Principles and Practice of Surgery. Philadelphia: H. C. Lea, 1871, p 287.
12. Baker BE, and Bierwagen D: Rupture of the distal tendon of the biceps brachii. J Bone Joint Surg 67(3):414–417, 1985.
13. Baer WS: Operative treatment of subdeltoid bursitis. Bull Johns Hopkins Hosp 18:282–284, 1907.
14. Basmajian JV, Latif MA: Integrated actions and function of the chief flexors of the elbow. J Bone Joint Surg 39A:1106–1118, 1957.
15. Basmajian JV: Muscles Alive, 4th ed. Baltimore: Williams & Wilkins, 1978.
16. Basmajian JV: Muscles Alive, 5th ed. Baltimore: Williams & Wilkins, 1985.
17. Bateman JE: The Shoulder and Environs. St. Louis: CV Mosby, 1944.
18. Bateman JE: The Shoulder and Neck. Toronto: WB Saunders, 1978.

Acknowledgments ■ The author would like to thank Karen Lozano very much for her valuable help and tremendous patience in preparing this manuscript.

19. Bateman JE: The Shoulder and Neck, 2nd ed. Philadelphia: WB Saunders Company, 1978.
20. Becker DA, and Cofield RH: Biceps brachii tenodesis for chronic tendinitis. Long term followup. Orthop Trans 210:447, 1986.
21. Bedi SS and Ellis W: Spontaneous rupture of the calcaneal tendon in rheumatoid arthritis after local steroid injection. Ann Rheum Dis 29(5):494–495, 1970.
22. Bennett GE: Shoulder and elbow lesions of professional baseball pitcher. JAMA 117:510–514, 1941.
23. Bera A: Syndrome commun, rupture, elongation, luxation du tendon du long biceps. Paris: These, 1910–1911.
24. Bidloo G: Anatomia Humani Corporis. Amstelodami, 1685.
25. Booth RE, and Marvel JP: Differential diagnosis of shoulder pain. Orthop Clin North Am 6:353–379, 1975.
26. Borchers E: Die ruptur der sehne des langen biceps kopfes. Beitr Klin Chir 90:635–648, 1914.
27. Bossuet: Two Cas de Luxation du Tendon de la Longue Portion du Biceps Brachii. Bull Soc Anat Phys 28:154, 1907.
28. Brickner WM: JAMA 69:1237–1243, 1918.
29. Bromfield W: Chirgical Observations and Cases. London: 1773, p 76.
30. Bush LF: The torn shoulder capsule. J Bone Joint Surg 57A:256, 1975.
31. Callender GW: Dislocation of muscles and their treatment. Br Med J July 13, 1878.
32. Carroll RE, and Hamilton LR: Rupture of biceps brachii—a conservative method of treatment. J Bone Joint Surg 49A:1016, 1967.
33. Cilley: Quoted by Meyer AW. Arch Surg 17:493–506, 1928.
34. Clark DD, Ricker JH, and MacCollum MS: The efficacy of local steroid injection in the treatment of stenosing tenovaginitis. Plast Reconstr Surg 51(2):179–180, 1973.
35. Clark KC: Positioning in Radiography, Vol. 1, 9th ed. London: William Heinemann Medical Books Ltd., 1973.
36. Claessens H: De pijnlijke schouder. Belg T Geneesk 1050, 1956.
37. Claessens H, and Anciauz-Ruyssen A: L'arthrographie de l'epaule. Acta Orthop Belg 3–4:289, 1956.
38. Claessens H, and Brosgol M: Rapport: Les lesions traumatiques des parties molles de l'epaule. Acta Orthop Belg 2:97, 1957.
39. Claessens H, and Biltris R: Diagnostic differentiel entre les lesions de la coiffe musculotendineuse et celles de la longue portion du biceps. J Belge Rheumatol Med Phys 20:53, 1965.
40. Claessens H, and Snoek H: Tendinitis of the long head of the biceps brachii. Acta Orthop Belg 38:1, 1972.
41. Claessens H, and Veys E: Les arthrites et l'arthrose de l'articulation scapulohumerale. J Belge Rheumatol Med Phys 72:73, 1965.
42. Codman EA: The supraspinatus syndrome. Boston Med Surg J 150:371–374, 1904.
43. Codman EA: The Shoulder. Boston: Thomas Todd, 1934.
44. Cofield RH, and Becker D: Surgical tenodesis of the long head of the biceps brachii for chronic tendinitis. Presented at the 53rd Annual Meeting of the American Academy of Orthopaedic Surgeons, New Orleans, Louisiana, February 21, 1986.
45. Cone RO, Danzig L, Resnick D, and Goldman AB: The bicipital groove: radiographic, anatomic, and pathologic study. AJR 41:781–788, 1983.
46. Conti V: Arthroscopy in rehabilitation. Orthop Clin North Am 10(3):709–711, 1979.
47. Cooper A: A Treatise on Dislocations and Fractures of the Joints. Boston: Lilly, Wait, Carter & Hendee, 1832, p 407.
48. Cowper W: Myotomia Reformata. London: 1694, p 75.
49. Crenshaw AH, and Kilgore WE: Surgical treatment of bicipital tenosynovitis. J Bone Joint Surg 48A:1496–1502, 1966.
50. Day BH, Govindasamy N, and Patnaik R: Corticosteroid injections in the treatment of tennis elbow. Practitioner 220(1317):459–462, 1978.
51. DePalma AF: Surgery of the Shoulder. Philadelphia: JB Lippincott, 1950.
52. DePalma AF, and Callery GE: Bicipital tenosynovitis. Clin Orthop 3:69–85, 1954.
53. DePalma AF: The painful shoulder. Postgrad Med 21:368–376, 1957.
54. DePalma AF: Surgical anatomy of the rotator cuff and the natural history of degenerative periarthritis. Surg Clin North Am 43:1507–1520, 1963.
55. DePalma AF: Surgery of the Shoulder, 2nd ed. Philadelphia: JB Lippincott, 1983.
56. Despates H: Gaz Hebd 15:374–378, 1878.
57. Dines D, Warren RF, and Inglis AE: Surgical treatment of lesions of the long head of the biceps. Clin Orthop 164:165–171, 1982.
58. Duplay S: Arch Gen Med 2:513–542, 1872.
59. Duplay S, and Reclus P: Traite de Chirurgie, Vol. 1. Paris: G. Masson, 1880–1882, p 825.
60. Duplay S: On scapulo-humeral periarthritis. (Paris Clinical Lectures.) Med Presse, 69:571–573, 1900.
61. Ellman H: Arthroscopic subacromial decompression. Society of American Shoulder and Elbow Surgeons, New Orleans, 1986.
62. Ennevaara K: Painful shoulder joint in rheumatoid arthritis: clinical and radiologic study of 200 cases with special reference to arthrography of the glenohumeral joint. Acta Rheumatol Scand [Suppl] 2:11–116, 1967.
63. Ewald: Traumatic ruptures usually due to arthritis deformans or other diseases of shoulder. Munch Med Wchnschr 74:2214–2215, 1927.
64. Fenlin JM Jr, and McShane RB: Conservative open anterior acromioplasty. Orthop Trans, J Bone Joint Surg 11(2):229–230, 1987.
65. Fisk C: Adaptation of the technique for radiography of the bicipital groove. Radiol Technol 37:47–50, 1965.
66. Freeland AE, and Higgins RW: Anterior shoulder dislocation with posterior displacement of the long head of the biceps tendon. Arthrographic findings. A case report. Orthopedics 8(4):468–469, 1985.
67. Froimson AI, and Oh I: Keyhole tenodesis of biceps origin at the shoulder. Clin Orthop 112:245–249, 1974.
68. Furlani J: Electromyographic study of the m. biceps brachii in movements at the glenohumeral joint. Acta Anat (Basel) 96(2):270–284, 1976.
69. Gainer BJ, Piotrowski G, Truhl J, et al.: The throw: biomechanics and acute injury. Am Sports Med 8:114–118, 1980.
70. Gardner E, and Gray DJ: Prenatal development of the human shoulder and acromioclavicular joint. Am J Anat 92:219–276, 1953.
71. Gerber C, Terrier F, and Ganz R: The role of the coracoid process in the chronic impingement syndrome. J Bone Joint Surg 67B:703–708, 1985.
72. Gerster AG: Subcutaneous injuries of the biceps brachii, with two new cases and some historical notes. NY Med J 27:487–502, 1878.
73. Gilcreest EL: Rupture of muscles and tendons, particularly subcutaneous rupture of the biceps flexor cubiti. JAMA 84:1819–1822, 1925.
74. Gilcreest EL: Two cases of spontaneous rupture of the long head of the biceps flexor cubiti. Surg Clin North Am 6:539–554, 1926.
75. Gilcreest EL: The common syndrome of rupture, dislocation and elongation of the long head of the biceps brachii. An analysis of one hundred cases. Surg Gynecol Obstet 58:322–339, 1934.
76. Gilcreest EL: Dislocation and elongation of the long head of the biceps brachii. Analysis of six cases. Ann Surg 104:118–138, 1936.
77. Gilcreest EL, and Albi P: Unusual lesions of muscles and tendons of the shoulder girdle and upper arm. Surg Gynecol Obstet 68:903–917, 1939.
78. Giuliani P, Scarpa G, Marchini M, and Nicoletti P: Development of scapulohumeral articulation in man, with special reference to its relation to the tendon of the long head of the biceps muscle of the arm. Arch Ital Anat Embriol 82(1):85–98, 1977.
79. Glousman R, Jobe FW, Tibone JP, et al: Dynamic EMG analysis of the throwing shoulder with glenohumeral instability.

80. Godsil RD, Jr, and Linschied RL: Intratendinous defects of the rotator cuff. Clin Orthop 69:181–188, 1970.
81. Goldman AB: Shoulder Arthrography. Boston: Little, Brown, 1981, pp 239–257.
82. Goldman AB, and Ghelman B: The double contrast shoulder arthrogram. A review of 158 studies. Radiology 127:658–663, 1978.
83. Goldthwait JE: An anatomic and mechanical study of the shoulder joint, explaining many of the cases of painful shoulder, many of the recurrent dislocations and many of the cases of brachial neuralgias or neuritis. Am J Orthop Surg 6(4):579–606, 1909.
84. Green JS: Dislocation of the long head of the biceps flexor cubiti muscle. Virginia Med Monthly 4:106, 1877–1878.
85. Guermonprez, and Michel A: Posterior luxation of shoulder. Rupture of lesser tuberosity, rupture and luxation of tendon of long head of biceps. Recovery. Bull Soc Anat Paris 4:1890.
86. Habermeyer P, Kaiser E, Knappe M, et al.: Functional anatomy and biomechanics of the long biceps tendon. Unfallchirurg 90(7):319–329, 1987.
87. Haenisch GF: Fortsch Rontgenstrahl 15:293–300, 1910.
88. Ha'eri GB, and Maitland A: Arthroscopic findings in the frozen shoulder. J Rheumatol 8:149–152, 1981.
89. Ha'eri GB, and Wiley AM: Advancement of the supraspinatus muscle in the repair of ruptures of the rotator cuff. J Bone Joint Surg 63A:232–238, 1981.
90. Haggart GE, and Allen HA: Painful shoulder: Diagnosis and treatment with particular reference to subacromial bursitis. Surg Clin North Am 15:1537–1560, 1935.
91. Hall-Craggs EC: Anatomy as a Basis for Clinical Medicine. Baltimore: Urban & Schwartzberg, 1985, p 111.
92. Hammond G, Torgerson W, Dotter W, and Leach R: The painful shoulder. Am Acad Orthop Surg Instructional Course Lectures. St. Louis: CV Mosby, 1971, pp 83–90.
93. Hawkins RJ, and Kennedy JC: Impingement syndrome in athletes. Am J Sports Med 8:151–158, 1980.
94. Heikel HVA: Rupture of the rotator cuff of the shoulder. Acta Orthop Scand 39:477–492, 1968.
95. Herberts P, Kadefors R, Andersson G, and Petersen I: Shoulder pain in industry: an epidemiological study on welders. Acta Orthop Scand 52:299–306, 1981.
96. Hippocrates: Quoted by Duplay, Reclus and Garrison.
97. Hitchcock HH, and Bechtol CO: Painful shoulder. Observations on the role of the tendon of the long head of the biceps brachii in its causation. J Bone Joint Surg 30A:263–273, 1948.
98. Hollinshead WH: Anatomy For Surgeons, Vol. 3. New York: Harper & Row, 1969, p 325.
99. Hollinsworth GR, Ellis RM, and Hattersley TS: Comparison of injection techniques for shoulder pain: results of a double blind, randomized study. Br Med J 287(6402):1339–1341, 1983.
100. Horowitz MT: Lesions of the supraspinatus tendon and associated structures. Investigation of comparable lesions in the hip joint. Arch Surg 38:990–1003, 1939.
101. Howard HJ, and Eloesser L: Treatment of fractures of the upper end of the humerus: an experimental and clinical study. J Bone Joint Surg 16:1–29, 1934.
102. Hueter C: Zur Diagnose der Verletzungen des M. Biceps Brachii. Arch Klin Chir 5:321–323, 1864; and also Grundriss der Chirurgie, vol. 2, p 735.
103. Ingelbrecht: Arch Franco-Belges Chir 29:922–923, 1926.
104. Inman VT, and Saunders JB de CM: Observations on the function of the clavicle. Calif Med 65:158–166, 1946.
105. Inman VT, Saunders JB de CM, and Abbott LC: Observations on the function of the shoulder joint. J Bone Joint Surg 26:1–30, 1944.
106. Janecki CJ, and Barnett DC: Fracture dislocation of the shoulder with biceps interposition. J Bone Joint Surg 61A:1–143, 1979.
107. Jarjavey JF: Luxation du tendon du biceps humeral et des tendons des peroniers lateraux. Gaz Hebd. Med (Paris) 4:325–327, 357–359, 387–391, 1867.
108. Jobe FW, Tibone JE, Perry J, et al.: An EMG analysis of the shoulder in throwing and pitching. A preliminary report. Am J Sports Med 11:3–5, 1983.
109. Jobe FW, and Jobe CM: Painful athletic injuries of the shoulder. Clin Orthop 173:117–124, 1983.
110. Jobe FW, Moines DR, Tibone JE, et al.: An EMG analysis of the shoulder in pitching. A second report. Am J Sports Med 12:218–220, 1984.
111. Jungmichel D, Winzer J, and Lippoldt G: Tendon rupture of the biceps muscle of the arm and its treatment with special reference to the key hole operation. Beitr Orthop Traumatol 33(5):226–232, 1986.
112. Kennedy JC, and Willis RB: The effects of local steroid injections on tendons: a biomechanical and microscopic correlative study. Am J Sports Med 4(1):11–21, 1976.
113. Kerlin RK: Throwing injuries to the shoulder. In Zarins B, Andrews JR, and Carson WG (eds): Injuries to the Throwing Arm. Philadelphia: WB Saunders, 1985, p 114.
114. Kessel L, and Watson M: The painful arch syndrome. Clinical classification as a guide to management. J Bone Joint Surg 59B:166–172, 1977.
115. Kieft GJ, Bloem JL, Rozing PM, and Obermann WR: Rotator cuff impingement syndrome. MR imaging. Radiology 166:211–214, 1988.
116. Killoran PJ, Marcove RL, and Freiberger RH: Shoulder arthography. AJR 103:658–668, 1968.
117. Kneeland JB et al.: MR imaging of the shoulder: diagnosis of rotator cuff tears. AJR 149:333–337, 1987.
118. Lapidus PW, and Guidotti FP: Local injection of hydrocortisone in 495 orthopedic patients. Ind Med Surg 26(5):234–244, 1957.
119. Lapidus PW: Infiltration therapy of acute tendinitis with calcification. Surg Gynecol Obstet 76:715–725, 1943.
120. Laumann U: Decompression of the subacromial space: an anatomical study. In Bayley I, and Kellel L (eds): Shoulder Surgery. Berlin: Springer-Verlag, 1982, pp 14–21.
121. Laumann U: Kinesiology of the shoulder joint. In Kolbel R, Bodo H, and Blauth W (eds): Shoulder Replacement. New York: Springer-Verlag, 1987.
122. Laumann U: Decompression of the subacromial space: an anatomical study. In Bayley I, and Kessel L (eds): Shoulder Surgery. Berlin: Springer-Verlag, 1982, pp 14–21.
123. Levitskii FA, and Nochevkin VA: Plastic repair of the tendon of the long head of the biceps muscle. Vestn Khir 130(3):92–94, 1983.
124. Lippmann RK: Frozen shoulder, periarthritis, bicipital tenosynovitis. Arch Surg 47:283–296, 1943.
125. Lippmann RK: Bicipital tenosynovitis. NY State J Med 44:2235–2240, 1944.
126. Lloyd-Roberts GC: Humerus varus. Report of a case treated by excision of the acromion. J Bone Joint Surg 35B:268–269, 1953.
127. Logal R: Rupture of the long tendon of the biceps brachii muscle. Clin Orthop 2:217–221, 1976.
128. Loyd JA, and Loyd HA: Adhesive capsulitis of the shoulder: arthrographic diagnosis and treatment. South Med J 76:879–883, 1983.
129. Lucas DB: Biomechanics of the shoulder joint. Arch Surg 107:425–432, 1973.
130. Lucas LS, and Gill JH: Humerus varus following birth injury to the proximal humeral epiphysis. J Bone Joint Surg 29:367–369, 1947.
131. Ludington NA: Am J Surg 77:358, 1923.
132. Lundberg BJ: The frozen shoulder. Acta Orthop Scand 119:1–59, 1969.
133. Lundberg BJ: Glycosaminoglycans of the normal and frozen shoulder joint capsule. Clin Orthop 69:279–284, 1970.
134. Lundberg BJ: The frozen shoulder: clinical and radiographical observations, the effect of manipulation under general anesthesia, structure and glycosaminoglycans content of the joint capsule. Local bone metabolism. Acta Orthop Scand 119:1–49, 1969.
135. Lundberg BJ, and Nilsson BE: Osteopenia in the frozen shoulder. Clin Orthop 60:187–191, 1968.

136. Macnab I: Rotator cuff tendinitis. Ann Roy Coll Surg Engl 53:271–287, 1973.
137. Makin M: Translocation of the biceps humeri for flail shoulder. J Bone Joint Surg 59(4):490–491, 1977.
138. Matsen F, and Kirby R: Office evaluation and management of shoulder pain. Orthop Clin North Am 13(3):45, 1982.
139. McClellan: Textbook of Surgery, 1892.
140. McCue FC III, Zarins B, Andrews JR, and Carson WG: Throwing injuries to the shoulder. In Zarins B, Andrews JR, and Carson WG (eds): Injuries to the Throwing Arm. Philadelphia: WB Saunders, 1985, p 98.
141. McLaughlin HL: Lesions of musculotendinous cuff of shoulder; observations on pathology, course and treatment of calcific deposits. Ann Surg 124:354, 1946.
142. McLaughlin HL: Dislocation of the shoulder with tuberosity fracture. Surg Clin North Am 43:1615–1620, 1963.
143. Meagher DM, Pool R, and Brown M: Bilateral ossification of the tendon of the biceps brachii muscle in the horse. JAVMA, 174(3):283–285, 1979.
144. Mercer A: Partial dislocations: consecutive and muscular affections of the shoulder joint. Buffalo Med Surg J 4:645–652, 1859.
145. Meyer AW: Spolia anatomica. Absence of the tendon of the long head of the biceps. J Anat 48:133–135, 1913–1914.
146. Meyer AW: Anatomical specimens of the unusual clinical interest. II. The effect of arthritis deformans on the tendon of the long head of the biceps brachii. Am J Orthop Surg 13:86–95, 1915.
147. Meyer AW: Unrecognized occupation destruction of the tendon of the long head of the biceps brachii. Arch Surg 2:130–144, 1921.
148. Meyer AW: Further observations upon use destruction in joints. J Bone Joint Surg 4:491–511, 1922.
149. Meyer AW: Further evidences of attrition in the human body. Am J Anat 34:241–267, 1924.
150. Meyer AW: Spontaneous dislocation of the tendon of the long head of the biceps brachii. Arch Surg 13:109–119, 1926.
151. Meyer AW: Spontaneous dislocation and destruction of the tendon of the long head of the biceps brachii. Arch Surg 17:493–506, 1928.
152. Meyer AW: Chronic functional lesions of the shoulder. Arch Surg 35:646–674, 1937.
153. Michele AA: Bicipital tenosynovitis. Clin Orthop 18:261, 1960.
154. Middleton WD, Remus WR, Totty WG, et al: Ultrasonographic evaluation of the rotator cuff and biceps tendon. J Bone Joint Surg 68(3):440–450, 1986.
155. Middleton WD et al.: High resolution MR imaging of the normal rotator cuff. AJR 148:559–564, 1987.
156. Milgram JE: Pathology and treatment of calcific tendinitis and bursitis of the shoulder. Scientific exhibit, American Academy of Orthp Surg, 1939 meeting.
157. Milgram JE: Bursitis—pathology and treatment of calcific tendinitis and bursitis by aspiration and vascularization. Med Rev Mex 125:283–305, 1945.
158. Milgram JE: Shoulder anatomy. Instructional Courses Volume. American Academy of Orthopedic Surgeons, pp 55–68, Chicago, January 1946.
159. Milgram JE: Aspiration of bursal deposits (quoted by Crowe, Harold). Bull Am Acad Orthop Surg p 11, April 1963.
160. Minami M, Ishii S, Usui M, and Ogino T: A case of idiopathic humerus varus. J Orthop Trauma Surg 20:175–178, 1975.
161. Monteggia GB: Instituzioni Chirurgiche. Milan: G. Truffi, T.V., 1829–1830, p 179; also Part II, 1803, p 334.
162. Moseley HF: Rupture of supraspinatus tendon. Can Med Assoc J 41:280–282, 1939.
163. Moseley HF: Shoulder Lesions. Springfield, IL: Charles C Thomas, 1945, pp 58–65.
164. Moseley HF, and Goldie I: The arterial pattern of the rotator cuff of the shoulder. J Bone Joint Surg 45B:780–789, 1963.
165. Moseley HF, and Overgaard B: The anterior capsular mechanism in recurrent anterior dislocation of the shoulder: morphological and clinical studies with special reference to the glenoid labrum and the glenohumeral ligaments. J Bone Joint Surg 44B:913–927, 1962.
166. Neer CS II: Anterior acromioplasty for the chronic impingement syndrome in the shoulder. J Bone Joint Surg 54A:41–50, 1972.
167. Neer CS, and Marberry TA: On the disadvantages of radical acromionectomy. J Bone Joint Surg 63A:416–419, 1981.
168. Neer CS II: Impingement lesions. Clin Orthop 173:70–77, 1983.
169. Neer CS II, and Poppen NK: Supraspinatus outlet. Orthop Trans J Bone Joint Surg 11(2):234, 1987.
170. Neviaser JS: Adhesive capsulitis of the shoulder. A study of the pathological findings in periarthritis of the shoulder. J Bone Joint Surg 27:211–222, 1945.
171. Neviaser JS: Surgical approaches to the shoulder. Clin Orthop 91:34, 1973.
172. Neviaser JS: Arthrography of the Shoulder. Springfield, IL: Charles C Thomas, 1975.
173. Neviaser JS, Neviaser RJ, and Neviaser TJ: The repair of chronic massive ruptures of the rotator cuff of the shoulder by use of a freeze-dried rotator cuff. J Bone Joint Surg 60A:681, 1978.
174. Neviaser RJ: Lesions of the biceps and tendinitis of the shoulder. Orthop Clin North Am 11:343–348, 1980.
175. Neviaser RJ, and Neviaser TJ: Lesions of the musculotendinous cuff of the shoulder: diagnosis and management. In A.A.O.S. Instructional Course Lectures. St. Louis: CV Mosby, 1981, pp 239–257.
176. Neviaser TJ, and Neviaser RJ: Lesions of the long head of the biceps tendon. Instr Course Lect 30:250–257, 1981.
177. Neviaser TJ, Neviaser RJ, and Neviaser JS: The four in one arthroplasty for the painful arc syndrome. Clin Orthop 163:107, 1982.
178. O'Donohue D: Subluxating biceps tendon in the athlete. Clin Orthop 164:26, 1982.
179. Ogilvie-Harris DJ, and Wiley AM: Arthroscopic surgery of the shoulder: a general appraisal. J Bone Joint Surg 68B:201–207, 1986.
180. Paavolainen P, Bjorkenheim JM, Slatis P, and Paukku P: Operative treatment of severe proximal humeral fractures. Acta Orthop Scand 54:374–379, 1983.
181. Paavolainen P, Slatis P, and Aalto K: Surgical pathology in chronic shoulder pain. In Bateman JE, and Welsh RP (eds): Surgery of the Shoulder. Philadelphia: BC Decker, 1984.
182. Packer NP, Calvert PT, Bayley JIL, and Kessel L: Operative treatment of chronic ruptures of the rotator cuff of the shoulder. J Bone Joint Surg 65B:171–175, 1983.
183. Painter CF: Subdeltoid bursitis. Boston Med Surg J 156:345–349, 1907.
184. Pappas AM, Goss TP, and Kleinman PK: Symptomatic shoulder instability due to lesions of the glenoid labrum. Am J Sports Med 11:279–288, 1983.
185. Parkhill CS: Dislocation of the long head of the biceps. Internat J Surg 10:132, 1897.
186. Partridge R: The case of Mr. John Soden. Communication to the Royal and Chirurgical Society of London, July 6, 1841.
187. Pasteur F: Les algies de L'epaule et la physiotherapie. La tenobursite bicipitale. J Radiol Electrol 16:419–429, 1932.
188. Perry J: Muscle control of the shoulder. In Rowe C (ed): The Shoulder. New York: Churchill Livingstone, 1988, p 26.
189. Petersson CJ: Degeneration of the gleno-humeral joint: an anatomical study. Acta Orthop Scand 54:277–283, 1983.
190. Petersson CJ: Spontaneous medial dislocation of the tendon of the long biceps brachii. Clin Orthop 211:224–227, 1986.
191. Petri M, Dobrow R, Neiman R, et al: Randomized, double-blind, placebo-controlled study of the treatment of the painful shoulder. Arthritis Rheum 30(9):1040–1045, 1987.
192. Pinzur M, and Hopkins G: Biceps tenodesis for painful inferior subluxation of the shoulder in adult acquired hemiplegia. Clin Orthop 206:100–103, 1986.
193. Post M, Silver R, and Singh M: Rotator cuff tear. Diagnosis and treatment. Clin Orthop 173:78–91, 1983.
194. Post M: Primary tendinitis of the long head of the biceps. Paper presented at the Closed Meeting of the Society of American Shoulder and Elbow Surgeons, Orlando, Florida, 1987.
195. Postacchini F: Rupture of the rotator cuff of the shoulder

associated with rupture of the tendon of the long head of the biceps. Ital J Orthop Traumatol 12(2):137–149, 1986.

196. Postacchini F, and Ricciardi-Pollini T: Rupture of the short head tendon of the biceps brachii. Clin Orthop 124:229–232, 1977.

197. Postgate J: Displacement of long tendon of biceps. Med Times, n.s. III, p 615, London, 1851.

198. Pouteau C: Melanges de Chirurgie. Lyons: G. Regnault, 1760, p 433.

199. Quinn CE: Humeral scapular periarthritis. Observations on the effects of x-ray therapy and ultrasound therapy in cases of "frozen shoulder." Ann Phys Med 10:64–69, 1967.

200. Rathbun JB, and Macnab I: The microvascular pattern of the rotator cuff. J Bone Joint Surg 52B:540–553, 1970.

201. Resnick D: Shoulder arthrography. Radiol Clin North Am 19:243–253, 1981.

202. Rockwood C, Burkhead W, and Brna J: Anterior acromial morphology in relation to the caudal tilt radiograph (unpublished).

203. Rothman RH, and Parke WW: The vascular anatomy of the rotator cuff. Clin Orthop 41:176–182, 1965.

204. Rowe CR (ed): The Shoulder. New York. Churchill Livingstone, 1988, p 145.

205. Schrager VL: Tenosynovitis of the long head of the biceps humeri. Surg Gynecol Obstet 66:785–790, 1938.

206. Schutte JP, and Hawkins RJ: Advances in Shoulder Surgery. Orthopedics 10:1725–1728, 1987.

207. Seeger LL, Ruszkowski JT, and Bassett LW, et al: MR imaging of the normal shoulder: anatomic correlation. AJR 148:83–91, 1987.

208. Sheldon PJH: A retrospective survey of 102 cases of shoulder pain. Rheum Phys Med 11:422–427, 1972.

209. Simmonds FA: Shoulder pain: with particular reference to the "frozen" shoulder. J Bone Joint Surg 31B:426–432, 1949.

210. Simon WH: Soft tissue disorders of the shoulder. Frozen shoulder, calcific tendinitis, and bicipital tendinitis. Orthop Clin North Am 6:521–538, 1975.

211. Slatis P, and Aalto K: Medical dislocation of the tendon of the long head of the biceps brachii. Acta Orthop Scand 50:73–77, 1979.

212. Soden J: Two cases of dislocation of the tendon of the long head of the biceps. Med Chir 24:212, 1841.

213. Soto-Hall R, and Haldeman KO: Muscles and tendon injuries in the shoulder region. Calif Western Med 41(5):318–321, 1934.

214. Stanley E: Observations relative to the rupture of the tendon of the biceps at its attachment to the edge of the glenoid cavity. Med Gaz 3:12–14, 1828–1829.

215. Stanley E: Rupture of the tendon of the biceps at its attachment to the edge of the glenoid cavity. Med Gaz 3:12, 1829.

216. Steindler A: Interpretation of pain in the shoulder. AAOS Instructional Course Lecture. Ann Arbor: J. W. Edwards, 1958, p 159.

217. Stevens HH: The action of short rotators on normal abduction of arm, with a consideration of their action on some cases of subacromial bursitis and allied conditions. Am J Med 138:870, 1909.

218. Tarsy JM: Bicipital syndromes and their treatment. NY State J Med 46:996–1001, 1946.

219. Ting A, Jobe FW, Barto P, et al: An EMG analysis of the lateral biceps in shoulders with rotator cuff tears. Third Open Meeting of the Society of American Shoulder and Elbow Surgeons, California, 1987.

220. Treves F: Surgical Applied Anatomy. Philadelphia: H. C. Lea's Son & Co., 1883.

221. Valtonen EJ: Subacromial triamcinolone, mexacetonide and methylprednisolone injections in treatment of supra spinatus tendinitis. A comparative trial. Scand J Rheumatol (Suppl) 16:1–13, 1976.

222. Valtonen EJ: Double acting betamethasone (celestone chronodose) in the treatment of supraspinatus tendinitis: a comparison of subacromial and gluteal single injections with placebo. J Intern Med Res 6(6):463–467, 1978.

223. Veisman IA: Radiodiagnosis of subcutaneous ruptures of the biceps tendons. Ortop Traumatol Protez 31(7):25–29, 1970.

224. Verbrugge J, Claessens H, and Maex L: L'arthrographie de l'epaule. Acta Orthop Belg 3–4:289, 1956.

225. Vigerio GD, and Keats TE: Localization of calcific deposits in the shoulder. AJR 108:806–811, 1970.

226. Volkmann R: Luxationen der Muskeln und Sehnen. Billroth Pitha's Handb Allgemeinen Speciellen Chir 2:873, 1882.

227. Warren RF: Lesions of the long head of the biceps tendon. AAOS Instr Course Lect 34:204–209, 1985.

228. Warren RF, Dines DM, Inglis AE, and Pavlos H: The coracoid impingement syndrome. Read at Second Meeting of the Society of American Shoulder and Elbow Surgeons, American Academy of Orthopaedic Surgery, New Orleans, February 19–20, 1986.

229. White JW: A case of supposed dislocation of the tendon of the long head of the biceps muscle. Am J Med Soc 87:17–57, 1884.

230. White RH, Paull DM, and Fleming KW: Rotator Cuff tendinitis: comparison of subacromial injection of a long acting corticosteroid versus oral indomethacin therapy. J Rheumatol 13(3):608–613, 1986.

231. Wiley AM, and Older MW: Shoulder arthroscopy: investigations with a fiberoptic instrument. Am J Sports Med 8:31–38, 1980.

232. Winterstein O: On the periarthritis humero-scapularis and on the rupture of the long biceps tendon. Arch Orthop Unfallchir 63(1):19–22, 1968.

233. Withrington RH, Girgis FL, and Seifert MH: A placebo-controlled trial of steroid injections in the treatment of supraspinatus tendinitis. Scand J Rheumatol 14(1):76–78, 1985.

234. Wolfgang GL: Surgical repair of tears of the rotator cuff of the shoulder. J Bone Joint Surg 56A:14–26, 1974.

235. Yergason RM: Rupture of biceps. J Bone Joint Surg 13:160, 1931.

CHAPTER

21

Frozen Shoulder

J. Patrick Murnaghan, M.D.

In this chapter, *frozen shoulder* is a descriptive term used to indicate a clinical syndrome wherein the patient has a restricted range of active and passive glenohumeral motion for which no other cause can be identified.

One of the major stumbling blocks for most physicians in coming to grips with frozen shoulder syndrome is the confusing terminology. Initially, periarthritis of the shoulder was used as an all-encompassing term to describe painful shoulders for which the symptoms could not be explained on the basis of arthritis of the glenohumeral joint.[32] With an improved understanding of the different pathological processes occurring about the shoulder, the broad term of periarthritis has been further resolved into its component parts. In the early literature, calcifying tendinitis, adhesive subacromial bursitis, biceps tendinitis, supraspinatus tendinitis, and partial tears of the rotator cuff were all included under the broad heading of periarthritis of the shoulder. Such a grouping together of heterogenous clinical disorders makes the interpretation of published clinical findings and the results of treatment very difficult.

The terms adhesive capsulitis, capsulitis, and periarthritis of the shoulder are used at times with a meaning synonymous with frozen shoulder. In this chapter, the term frozen shoulder will indicate the clinical syndrome defined above and such terms as adhesive capsulitis and irritative capsulitis will be used to describe subsets of patients as defined in the text.

Exclusion criteria for frozen shoulder in its most pure form include patients with shoulder arthritis, fractures, dislocations, cervical spondylosis, neuromuscular disease, and referred pain.[14] Specific exclusions also take into account other intrinsic shoulder pathology, such as subacromial impingement, supraspinatus tendinitis, calcifying tendinitis, and tendinitis of the long head of the biceps. These latter conditions can usually be excluded based on history and clinical examination.[25]

Unfortunately there is often an overlap of symptom complexes. Frozen shoulder syndrome may coexist with other types of shoulder pathology, making the exact diagnosis more difficult to identify. Binder and associates found that 40 per cent of their patients with frozen shoulder had pain on resisted active shoulder movements, suggesting that these patients had an element of tendinitis as well.[7]

Historical Review

The painful stiff shoulder has been the subject of many investigations over the years as authors have tried to elucidate a cause for this disabling condition.

Duplay was one of the first to theorize that the pathology in these shoulders was in the periarticular tissues, rather than a type of arthritis of the glenohumeral joint. He coined the term "periarthrite scapulo humerale."[32] The primary pathology was thought to be in the subacromial bursa. The recommended treatment was manipulation under anesthesia to overcome the joint stiffness.

Dickson and Crosby associated the clinical syndrome of periarthritis of the shoulder with a remote focus of infection or glandular dysfunction. They observed that the prognosis was the same in calcifying or noncalcifying tendinitis, which were both considered under the broad heading of periarthritis of the shoulder.[31]

Codman initially attributed the pathology of these painful, stiff shoulders to adhesions in the subacromial bursa. He later changed his opinion and used the term "uncalcified tendinitis" to describe the pathology. Codman expressed some frustration with this disorder when he described these patients as a class of cases which he found "difficult to define, difficult to treat and difficult to explain . . . from the point of view of pathology."[19]

Lippman theorized that tenosynovitis of the long head of the biceps was the basic pathological condition in the frozen shoulder syndrome in agreement with Pasteur.[95] He attributed the eventual clinical improvement to scarring around the biceps tendon sheath with progressive tethering of the biceps tendon in the bicipital groove.[66]

Neviaser concluded that the essential pathology in frozen shoulder was a thickening and contraction of the shoulder joint capsule. The capsule later became adherent to the humeral head but could be readily separated from the cartilage using a suitable elevator and with minimal bleeding. He described microscopic evidence of reparative inflammatory changes in the capsule. He felt the term "adhesive capsulitis" better described the pathology of the frozen shoulder.[82]

Moseley emphasized the variety of causes of frozen shoulder. He believed that with time the term "periarthritis" would eventually be resolved into its component parts, allowing for more specific treatment plans.[79]

Withers made a clinical distinction between "irritative capsulitis" and the more restricted stage of "adhesive capsulitis," based on an examination under anesthesia. He likened the role of the subacromial bursa to that of the peritoneum. He commented that peritoneum-like tissues are rarely the site of primary pathology but reflect changes in adjacent tissues.[133]

Steinbroker described shoulder hand syndrome as an idiopathic association of pain and swelling of the hand with an ipsilateral painful stiff shoulder. With time, the shoulder stiffness would resolve, but there would be ongoing stiffness, flexion deformities, and trophic changes in the hand and fingers.[119]

Simmonds reported on the tight inelastic tissues around the shoulder joint. He believed that the pathological changes in frozen shoulder were due to degeneration and focal necrosis of the supraspinatus tendon. With revascularization, the tendon pathology could resolve. With an inadequate vascular response, the tendon would continue to degenerate, developing tears of varying size, or a secondary biceps tendinitis could develop.[116]

McLaughlin emphasized the many different causes of frozen shoulder and stressed the need to treat the primary cause. He cautioned against closed manipulation of the shoulder, based on his experience with manipulation following surgical exposure. He observed that the subscapularis tendon and the anterior joint capsule tore routinely during forced manipulation.[75]

DePalma proposed that muscular inactivity was a major etiological factor in frozen shoulders. He also implicated bicipital tendinitis as a predisposing factor. The restrictions to joint motion were attributed to intra- and extracapsular adhesions. For patients who failed to respond to the usual treatment protocols, he recommended detaching the intrascapular long head of biceps and moving it to the coracoid.[28]

Meulengracht and Schwartz found an association between frozen shoulder and Dupuytren's contracture in 18 per cent of their 78 patients. They also noted an association with thyroid disorders in 27 per cent of their 78 patients.[77]

Coventry defined periarthritis of the shoulder as pain and stiffness in the shoulder. He recognized three distinct forms of periarthritis: (1) pain with minimal stiffness, (2) pain with marked stiffness (frozen shoulder), and (3) shoulder-hand syndrome. Coventry theorized that there had to be a combination of three factors for the clinical syndrome to manifest itself: (1) pain in the shoulder, (2) a period of disuse, and (3) a peculiar constitutional and emotional state that he labeled periarthritic personality.[22]

Quigley stated whimsically that the observed personality changes in frozen shoulder patients could be "as often the result of the painful shoulder as they were the cause." Based on his experience he coined the term "checkrein shoulder" to describe a subgroup of patients in whom he noted a good prognosis. On examination, this subgroup of patients had a sharp and definite block to passive glenohumeral abduction at about 45 degrees and only about 50 per cent of normal humeral rotation. The distinguishing feature that these patients had in common was that during manipulation under anesthesia, a definite audible and palpable release was noted, followed by a free range of motion. Patients with these characteristic findings had a shorter history of disease and less subsequent pain and stiffness.[98]

Harmon in a study of patients with frozen shoulder concluded that the common denominator in recovery was "motivation and physical capability to stretch, actively exercise and withstand a certain amount of physical discomfort." He believed that functional use of the arm was the only known method to restore the inelastic joint capsule to a more resilient state.[46]

Kopell and Thompson theorized that entrapment of the suprascapular nerve could give a deep discomfort in the shoulder with clinical dysfunction similar to frozen shoulder. They recommended surgical release of the suprascapular nerve as it passes underneath the superior transverse scapular ligament.[59]

Johnson reported on the increased incidence of frozen shoulders in patients receiving treatment for tuberculosis in sanitoria. He associated the increased incidence of frozen shoulder in this patient group with the prolonged bedrest used in the treatment of these debilitated patients. He recommended regular arm exercises as a preventive measure.[52]

Neviaser described the typical arthrographic findings of frozen shoulder patients. He observed a marked decrease in joint volume, with an obliteration of the axillary fold and subscapular bursa. The biceps tendon sheath was visualized in all but 18 per cent of cases with adhesive capsulitis. Neviaser recommended arthrography as the most important diagnostic test to separate true adhesive capsulitis (frozen shoulder) from other causes of painful stiff shoulders.[83]

Andren and Lundberg described favorable results using a joint distention technique to relieve shoulder pain in patients with mild to moderately stiff and painful shoulders. They used sequential distention of the joint, using increasing volumes of fluid until rupture of the capsule occurred. Return of motion often lagged behind the pain relief. The joint distentions were well tolerated, and thus, repeat injections could be done where needed.[2]

Lundberg, in a major study of frozen shoulder, observed that "there is no condition which quite resembles frozen shoulder." He was unable to identify any causative constitutional factor. He observed that a specific age group was predisposed to develop frozen shoulder. A period of inactivity also seemed to be a significant contributing factor. At operation, he reaffirmed the microscopic findings of fibrosis and fibroplasia of the joint capsule but found no significant changes in the synovial lining.[69]

Macnab suggested an autoimmune mechanism for the diffuse capsulitis seen in frozen shoulder. He postulated a response to degenerative changes in the rotator cuff tendons and recommended a trial of short-term systemic steroids before considering manipulation.[71]

Hazleman, reviewing retrospectively the outcome of several forms of treatment of frozen shoulder, found no difference in clinical results between treatment with physiotherapy, manipulation under anesthesia, or hydrocortisone injections.[47]

Bridgman identified an increased incidence of frozen shoulder in patients with diabetes mellitus. Those patients who were insulin dependent were particularly predisposed. He also commented on the higher incidence of bilateral shoulder involvement in diabetics.[11]

Lee and colleagues were some of the first to use a controlled clinical trial to assess treatment outcomes. In their patient groupings, exercises had a beneficial effect on the outcome.[62]

Lee and colleagues used multivariate analysis to assess four different treatment protocols. Three of the four patient groups that received exercises as one component of their treatment had similar outcomes. The one group that had received analgesics alone had an inferior outcome over the six-week duration of the follow-up.[63]

De Seze noted that frozen shoulder (capsulite retractile) was often associated with other shoulder disorders: tendinitis, impingement, and calcifying tendinitis. He emphasized the need for a careful evaluation of the patient to come to an accurate diagnosis. Treatment of the underlying disorder was needed as well as addressing the restricted passive range of shoulder motion.[29]

Reeves, in a follow-up study of patients with idiopathic frozen shoulder syndrome, noted that the duration of the recovery phase had a direct relationship to the duration of the stiffness phase. He also questioned the classical teaching as to the duration of symptoms. In his series, patients' symptoms did not resolve on average until 2.5 years.[103]

Bruckner and Nye reported on a prospective study of patients who developed frozen shoulder in a neurosurgical unit. The combination of shoulder immobilization, a specific age group, and an associated depressive personality were identified as significant risk factors.[12]

Binder, Bulgen, Hazleman, and colleagues reported extensively on their experience in a series of controlled prospective clinical studies of patients with frozen shoulders. Their patients were carefully selected and thoroughly investigated. Treatment protocols were compared with those of a control group. Their investigations questioned the use of many previously accepted treatment protocols which did not offer a predictably better outcome than the patients' doing their own pendulum exercises on a regular basis several times each day. These investigators have further emphasized the need for well-designed, controlled prospective studies to test the efficacy of commonly used treatment protocols.[7–9, 14]

R. J. and T. J. Neviaser reported an arthroscopic documentation of the changes in adhesive capsulitis previously diagnosed by arthrography. Four stages of arthroscopic findings were described. These authors stressed the importance of an individualized treatment plan matched to the patient's clinical staging in the overall course of frozen shoulder.[86–88]

At present, we seem to know more about what frozen shoulder is not than what it is. Frozen shoulder is a clinical grouping of symptoms and signs which are readily recognized. However, when specifics as to motion, pathology, and recovery are sought, there seems to be few answers on review of the literature.

Anatomy

It is important when considering frozen shoulder to include the overall shoulder girdle complex and not concentrate solely on the glenohumeral joint. The scapula articulates indirectly with the trunk, linked through the clavicle and its associated articulations at the acromioclavicular and sternoclavicular joints. The scapula is both moved and stabilized on the chest wall by its muscle attachments to the trunk and adjacent thoracic wall. Scapulothoracic and glenohumeral movements occur simultaneously as the arm is used away from the side.[51] With normal subjects in abduction, about two-thirds of the elevation of the arm is attributed to the glenohumeral joint, the remainder occurring at the scapulothoracic space.[39] There is considerable individual variation. The scapulothoracic and glenohumeral contributions to combined elevation are also related to the load carried by the arm.[96]

The glenohumeral joint is enclosed by the joint capsule. The capsule of the shoulder joint is normally a loose structure whose surface area is almost twice that of the humeral head.[57] The capsule attaches around the perimeter of the glenoid and spans across to attach to the anatomical neck of the humerus, except inferiorly where the attachment is about 1 cm distal to the articular margin. At the upper end of the bicipital groove, the capsule bridges the gap between the greater and lesser tuberosities as the transverse humeral ligament.[61] The tendons of the rotator cuff adjacent to the joint capsule thicken the capsule anteriorly, superiorly, and posteriorly. The glenohumeral ligaments are further areas of thickening of the joint capsule, best seen when the joint capsule is viewed from inside the joint. The inferior capsule, however, is not supported by adjacent muscles and tendons, leaving a lax double fold of capsule which forms the inferior recess (Fig. 21–1). This inferior redundant fold of capsule is normally present while the arm is at the side but disappears as the arm is taken up into forward elevation or abduction owing to stretching of the inferior capsule (Fig. 21–2).

In the normal shoulder there may be two or three joint recesses that can be seen at arthrography or arthroscopy. Anteriorly, a synovial recess is usually present between the superior and middle glenohumeral ligaments and is called the subscapular bursa. The inferior recess is the area of redundant inferior capsule that forms a lax, pouch-like fold when the arm is at the side. Posteriorly, an out-pouching deep to the infraspinatus muscle may occur, known as the infraspinatus bursa.

The synovial membrane lines the capsule and is in continuity with the subscapularis bursa anteriorly and the inferior recess inferiorly. It may also communicate with the infraspinatus bursa.[61] The synovium also invests the long head of the biceps and is reflected around the biceps tendon as it passes deep to the transverse humeral ligament into the bicipital groove. The biceps tendon sheath may extend for a distance of 5 cm beyond the transverse ligament, down the bicipital groove, especially when the arm is in abduction, the arm position where the least amount of biceps tendon is within the joint[79] (see Fig. 21–2).

Histologically, the capsule consists of bundles of

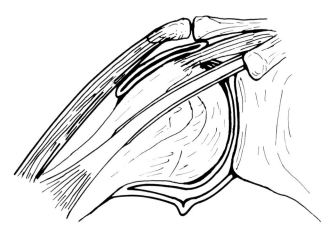

Figure 21–2. The redundant inferior recess is placed under tension as the arm is taken into abduction or forward elevation.

Type 1 collagen aligned with the axis of tensile strength of the capsule. There are comparatively few fibrocytes.[53, 69] Synovial cells are loosely attached to the inner surface of the capsule. The fibrous capsule is moderately strong when tested under tension load. The electron microscopic examination does not show any structural differences between the shoulder capsule and other joint capsules.[53]

Pathology

Nicholson noted in patients with frozen shoulder that, during active elevation, the scapula usually moved excessively in upward rotation to compensate for the loss of glenohumeral motion. On clinical examination, he consistently found the inferior glide of the humerus to be the most restricted of the accessory movements of the shoulder.[89]

Much of our current understanding of the pathology of frozen shoulder is due to the work of J. S. Neviaser, who coined the term *adhesive capsulitis* to describe a contracted, thickened joint capsule that seemed to be drawn tightly around the humeral head with a relative absence of synovial fluid. He also noted cellular changes of chronic inflammation with fibrosis and perivascular infiltration in the subsynovial layer of the capsule consistent with a reparative inflammatory process. The synovial layer itself did not show any specific abnormality.[82]

McLaughlin, at the time of operative release of frozen shoulders, found in 10 per cent of his cases a nonspecific proliferative synovitis. He observed that the capsular folds and pouches were obliterated by adhesions of the adjacent synovial surfaces (Fig. 21–3). The rotator cuff muscle bellies were contracted, fixed, and inelastic. McLaughlin noted that the biceps tendon sheath was frequently involved. Few adhesions were identified in the subacromial bursa.[75]

Simmonds described a local increase in vascularity in the joint capsule. He thought that the tight, inelastic

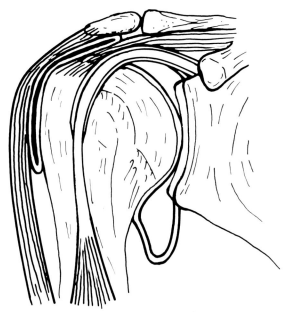

Figure 21–1. Schematic cross-section of the glenohumeral joint showing the unsupported inferior capsule, which makes a redundant fold (inferior recess) with the arm at the side.

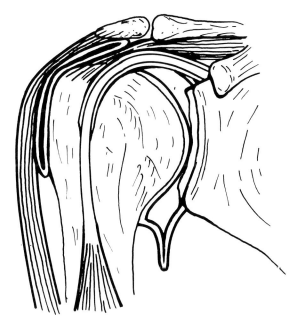

Figure 21–3. A schematic cross-section of the shoulder showing adhesions of adjacent surfaces of the inferior recess as one possible explanation for the restricted range of motion in frozen shoulder.

characteristics of the capsular tissue extended out into the soft tissues around the shoulder. He postulated that a chronic inflammatory reaction in the supraspinatus tendon was the underlying cause.[116]

Macnab later postulated that a partial loss of blood supply in the area of insertion of the supraspinatus tendon could initiate degeneration of the collagen in the tendon. The localized degeneration of the collagen was then theorized to induce an autoimmune response. Macnab felt that the round cell infiltrate and pyroninophilic lymphoid cells found in the capsule at open surgical release of the shoulder could be interpreted as being an autoimmune response.[71, 72] Other authors have found conflicting results in their efforts to identify an immunological disorder.[13, 15] Recent reports have failed to identify any statistically significant clinical or laboratory evidence for an immunological basis for this condition.[57, 140]

Reeves commented that no acute inflammatory changes were seen in the synovium when shoulders were exposed at open manipulation. He also observed little bleeding during open manipulation, even when the capsule was torn by the manipulation.[102]

Lundberg confirmed the absence of intra-articular adhesions in his operative observations and at cinearthrography.[69, 70] On histological examination he found the synovial cells largely unchanged. Lundberg reported seeing a more compact, dense collagen layer in the shoulder capsule. These findings were confirmed at electron microscopic examination showing a more compact arrangement of collagen fibers but no differences in structure or periodicity of the fibers. The glycosaminoglycans' distribution in the shoulder capsule had the characteristics of a repair reaction.[69]

The reported pathological findings are generally non-specific and have failed to indicate a cause for the macroscopic capsular changes.

Diagnostic Criteria

There is little consensus on the specifics of which restrictions of shoulder motion are needed to qualify as frozen shoulder syndrome. How much loss of motion is required? In which planes of motion are the restrictions most important? What is the functional significance of these measured losses of shoulder mobility? These questions remain unanswered. The normally mobile shoulder is crucial to the function of the upper extremity, allowing the arm to be positioned widely in space away from the body.

Shoulder motion is a three-dimensional activity. Describing a single plane or multiple individual planes of motion makes it difficult to convey to the reader the restrictions experienced by each individual patient. Several authors have tried to develop mathematically based composite scores to combine multiple planes of motion into a value that will allow meaningful inter-patient comparisons.[14, 63]

There is a wide variation in the degree of restriction of shoulder motion used by different authors to make the diagnosis of frozen shoulder. Table 21–1 summarizes the published criteria for the diagnosis of frozen shoulder.

Lundberg included patients with painful, stiff shoulders who on physical examination had a loss of shoulder motion localized to the glenohumeral joint and whose total elevation was 135 degrees or less.[69] The clinical criteria used by Rizk and associates are very specific. These authors restricted the diagnosis of frozen shoulder to patients who met the following criteria: (1) a passive combined abduction of less than 100 degrees (60 per cent of normal), (2) less than 50 degrees of external rotation (55 per cent of normal), (3) less than 70 degrees of internal rotation (75 per cent of normal), and (4) less than 140 degrees of forward elevation (80 per cent of normal).[107] Neviaser and Kay both believed that patients should have shoulder abduction restricted to less than 90 degrees to fit the criteria for diagnosis.[55, 84, 85] Quigley insisted that patients have less than 45 degrees (40 per cent) of glenohumeral abduction and less than 50 per cent of normal rotation with the arm at the side.[98, 99] Bruckner and Nye believed that a loss of 20 per cent of glenohumeral abduction and a loss of 40 degrees of external rotation in patients who had night pain were sufficient criteria for the diagnosis of frozen shoulder.[12] Binder and associates included only those patients with a restriction of all active and passive shoulder movements who had a reduction of external rotation of at least 50 per cent. They also required that the patient have shoulder pain for at least one month and that there be an associated sleep disturbance secondary to night pain.[7] The criteria used by Lloyd-Roberts and col-

Table 21–1. CRITERIA FOR DIAGNOSIS OF FROZEN SHOULDER SYNDROME

Author(s)	Specified Shoulder Ranges of Motion				Elevation	Other Criteria
	Abduction	Rotation				
		External	Internal	Total		
Lundberg[69]	<135° combined				<135° combined	Pain, loss of motion localized to glenohumeral joint
Rizk et al[106]	<100° combined	<50%	<70%		<140° combined	
Neviaser[84, 85]	<90° combined					Very restricted capsular volume on arthrogram
Kay[55]	<90° combined			+/−		Painful stiff shoulder
Quigley[98, 99]	<45° glenohumeral			<50%		
Bruckner and Nye[12]	<70° glenohumeral	<60%				
Binder et al[9]		<50%				Some restriction of all shoulder movements, pain longer than 1 month, night pain
Lloyd-Roberts et al[67]		<50%				Pain for 3 months, cannot lie on the affected side
Kessel et al[57]						Spontaneous onset, progressive loss of glenohumeral motion, no identifiable systemic illness, normal radiographs

leagues for inclusion were patients with shoulder pain for at least three months who were unable to lie on the affected shoulder. They insisted that each patient should have lost at least 50 per cent of normal external rotation measured with the arm at the side.[67] Kessel and colleagues reserved the diagnosis of frozen shoulder for those patients who experienced spontaneous onset of shoulder pain accompanied by increasingly severe limitations of glenohumeral movements. These patients could not have any identifiable general illness, and the radiographs had to be entirely normal.[58]

In my practice, I include those patients with a typical history of progressive shoulder pain and stiffness for whom no other cause of the symptoms can be found. I pay particular attention to restricted external rotation and forward elevation. The measured range of motion will depend on the stage of disease at which the patient is assessed. In patients with a typical history, I include patients with less than 30 degrees of external rotation, forward elevation less than 130 degrees, and combined abduction less than 120 degrees. The limitation of internal rotation is quite variable.

Classification

Within the overall group of patients with a diagnosis of frozen shoulder, several authors have attempted to define subgroups by classifying their patients using criteria that they judged to be relevant. If successful, such a classification could identify more homogenous sets of patients, thus simplifying treatment choices and making outcomes more predictable. The criteria and subgroups are summarized in Table 21–2.

Lundberg separated patients who met the motion and pain requirements into two groups, which he labelled *primary frozen shoulder* and *secondary frozen shoulder*. Patients who had no findings in the history,

on clinical examination, or on review of x-rays that could explain the decrease in shoulder motion were classified as having a *primary frozen shoulder*. Patients who developed restricted shoulder motion after a traumatic injury were classified as having a *secondary frozen shoulder*.[69]

Kay used a clinical classification based on the degree of restriction of shoulder motion. He chose the term *early capsulitis* to describe those patients who had restricted shoulder motion but whose combined shoulder abduction was still greater than 90 degrees. He reserved the term *frozen shoulder* for patients with less than 90 degrees of combined shoulder abduction.[55]

Withers classified his patients based on findings on examination under anesthesia. *Irritative capsulitis* was the term used for patients who had the characteristic shoulder pain and stiffness but who were found at examination under anesthesia to have a full range of shoulder motion. He restricted the term *adhesive capsulitis* to patients who had clinical findings similar to those of the above group; however, their range of motion when examined under anesthesia was as restricted as while awake. Withers found this distinction useful from a treatment decision standpoint.[133]

Reeves used arthrographic criteria to classify his patients. The *post-traumatic stiff shoulder* group at arthrography had a decreased joint volume and abnormal filling of the subscapularis bursa. In this group, the arthrographic findings in the area of the biceps tendon sheath were usually normal. The second group of patients designated as having *frozen shoulder* had a more restricted arthrogram showing a markedly decreased joint volume. In this group there was no filling at arthrography of the subscapularis bursa, the biceps tendon sheath, or the inferior recess. Reeves felt that the lesser restricted patients had a better response to treatment.[102]

Helbig and colleagues, who also used arthrographic criteria, separated their patients into three radiological

Table 21–2. CLASSIFICATIONS OF FROZEN SHOULDER

Basis for Classification	Subgroups			Author(s)
Degree of restriction of range of motion	*Early Capsulitis* Combined shoulder abduction over 90 degrees	*Frozen Shoulder* Less than 90 degrees of combined shoulder abduction		Kay[55]
Findings at examination under anesthesia	*Irritative Capsulitis* Characteristic pain and stiffness, but under anesthesia full range of motion	*Adhesive Capsulitis* Some pain and stiffness but ROM just as restricted under anesthesia as while awake		Withers[133]
History of associated events or illnesses	*Primary Frozen Shoulder* No other explanation	*Secondary Frozen Shoulder* Post-traumatic		Lundberg[69]
Arthrographic findings	*Post-Traumatic Stiff Shoulder* Decreased joint volume, abnormal filling of subscapularis bursa, normal biceps tendon sheath	*Frozen Shoulder* Marked decrease in joint volume, no filling of subscapularis bursa, axillary recess, or biceps tendon sheath		Reeves[102]
Arthrographic findings and clinical criteria	*Group 1* Moderate stiffness, slightly defective filling of axillary recess, pear-like restriction of capsule	*Group 2* Further loss of motion, axillary recess almost obliterated, restricted suscapularis bursa, lateral adhesion of capsule	*Group 3* Complete loss of subscapularis bursa	Helbig et al[48]
Arthrographic findings and clinical criteria	*Painful Stiff Shoulders* Moderately restricted joint volume, combined shoulder abduction greater than 90 degrees	*Adhesive Capsulitis* Similar pain but combined shoulder abduction less than 90 degrees, markedly restricted joint volume		Neviaser[84, 85]

groups based on a qualitative assessment of the degree of capsular restriction. They concluded that the level of disability before manipulation had little or no effect on the final outcome.[48]

J. S. Neviaser used a combination of arthrographic and clinical criteria to better classify patients with frozen shoulders. Those presenting with a combined shoulder abduction greater than 90 degrees and a moderately restricted joint volume at arthrography (10 to 12 ml) were designated as having *painful stiff shoulders*. Patients with similar pain but whose combined shoulder abduction was less than 90 degrees and whose arthrograms demonstrated a markedly restricted joint volume (5 to 10 ml) were classified under the heading of *adhesive capsulitis*. Neviaser observed that the less involved shoulders responded well to physiotherapy, whereas the *adhesive capsulitis* group often required manipulation.[84, 85]

AUTHOR'S COMMENTS

I find the use of the primary and secondary classification of Lundberg to be useful in planning treatment, but one must realize that this classification is not necessarily useful in predicting outcome. The primary and secondary terminology allows the identification of more homogenous patient groups, thus permitting more meaningful analyses.

There appears to be value in making a distinction between those patients with mild involvement and those more severely restricted if meaningful conclusions are to be obtained from further studies. The variable restriction of shoulder motion on presentation in patients with a typical history makes a definition of

specific motion criteria for the diagnosis of frozen shoulder elusive at this time. An agreement to use a standard examination technique measuring the same planes of motion in future investigations is the only way that the question of whether or not specific motion criteria exist will be answered. The measurement techniques described by Clarke and associates using a modified hydrogoniometer allow reproducible measurements with good interexaminer correlation.[18] Devices to measure three-dimensional shoulder motion would be a further refinement, but such technology is not yet available.

The use of arthrography as the basis for establishing a definitive diagnosis would appear justified in the context of doing clinical research, but arthrography is not necessarily justified as part of a routine investigation in clinical practice.[74]

Some standardization of inclusion criteria would be most helpful when trying to make comparisons between different investigators. In recent articles, there is a consensus that patients with arthritis, hemiplegia, or other significant musculoskeletal disorders should not be classified with frozen shoulder as their primary diagnosis.

Incidence

The lack of universally accepted criteria for frozen shoulder creates problems in identifying the incidence. Another relative problem is the changing normal range of shoulder motion with age and sex. In general, males have less motion than females, with discrepancies between investigators as to which specific movements are most affected. There is also a tendency to lose motion with advancing years, thus the need for age-matched controls.[1, 14, 18] Murray and colleagues, however, found similar ranges of motion amongst men and women of two age groups.[81] Which arm is dominant does not appear to be a factor.[14, 18]

Having clearly defined the diagnostic criteria for primary frozen shoulder (see Classification), Lundberg estimated the incidence of this condition to be at least 2 per cent in the general population.[69] Bridgman reviewed outpatients attending medical clinics (n = 600) and specifically excluded diabetics, who made up the comparison group (n = 800). To diagnose frozen shoulder, he insisted that the patients have shoulder pain of at least three months' duration and sufficient pain to awaken the patient at night. All patients had to have a limitation of shoulder motion and specifically a loss of at least 50 per cent of external rotation. When these criteria were met, he reported the incidence of frozen shoulder symptoms as 2.3 per cent among nondiabetics, compared with 10.8 per cent in the diabetics.[11] Pal and colleagues examined nondiabetic hospital staff and persons accompanying patients to clinics in search of signs and symptoms of frozen shoulder (n = 75). They identified the incidence of frozen shoulder to be 5 per cent in nondiabetics, compared with an incidence of 19 per cent in their diabetic clinic population (n = 109).[94] Sattar identified a 3 per cent incidence of frozen shoulder in controls (n = 100), compared with a 19 per cent incidence in diabetics (n = 100).[113]

Mechanism of Injury

The pathomechanics of frozen shoulder are poorly understood. The autoimmune theory has been proposed, but conclusive evidence has not been found as yet.[15, 57, 59, 140]

A relationship to myofascial pain syndrome has been proposed. A syndrome of active trigger points about the shoulder, specifically within the subscapularis muscle, has been suggested as a possible cause of the frozen shoulder syndrome.[124] Trigger points are defined as locally tender, self-sustaining, hyperirritable foci located in skeletal muscle or its associated fascia. The trigger points are also characteristically related to a zone of referred pain when the trigger point is stimulated. The trigger points may be activated by a sudden overload of muscle or by chronic repetitive strains. Once activated, perpetuating factors may be responsible for the chronicity of the pain. Another characteristic of the myofascial pain syndrome is palpable bands of muscle fibers that undergo a local twitch response when the trigger point is stimulated with a snapping palpation.[60, 118, 136]

Travell and others theorize that the subscapularis trigger points exert an influence on the sympathetic vasomotor activity, leading to hypoxia of the periartic-ular tissues. It is further theorized that the hypoxia leads to local proliferation of fibrous tissue about the shoulder capsule, resulting in the clinical picture of frozen shoulder syndrome.[124]

Predisposing Factors

PERIOD OF IMMOBILITY

Common to most patients presenting with frozen shoulder is a period during which the shoulder has been relatively immobile.[28, 44, 52, 85, 117] The reasons for the period of immobility are diverse: pain after overuse, a flare-up of cervical spondylosis, minor shoulder trauma, etc. In a prospective study on a neurosurgical unit, Bruckner and Nye noted a 25 per cent incidence of frozen shoulder, five to nine times the incidence in the general population. In their patient group, the positive risk factors could all be associated with a period during which normal shoulder mobility was prevented for a variety of reasons.[12]

Binder and colleagues found that 50 per cent of patients received no advice about the care of their painful shoulder from the primary care physician on initial assessment. Of those receiving some advice, 75 per cent were told to rest the shoulder, and only 25 per cent were told to exercise the shoulder gently.[9]

The period of immobility seems to be an important factor in the development of frozen shoulder. This information needs to be more widely disseminated. Appropriate education of primary care physicians should be helpful, with the aim of minimizing the incidence of this disabling condition.

SPECIFIC AGE GROUP

Frozen shoulder occurs during a specific age range. Except in diabetic patients, frozen shoulder is uncommon below the age of 40 years or over the age of 70 years.[12, 46, 69, 77, 80, 103] Patients are usually middle-aged, with the mean age for males being slightly greater than that of females (55 years versus 52 years).[69]

DIABETES MELLITUS

There is a higher than normal association between frozen shoulder and diabetes mellitus.* The incidence of frozen shoulder in the general population is 2 to 5 per cent, while among diabetics it is 10 to 20 per cent.[11, 65, 94, 113] Diabetic patients who are insulin dependent have a higher incidence of frozen shoulder (36 per cent), with a markedly increased frequency of bilateral shoulder involvement (up to 42 per

*See references 11, 37, 65, 69, 78, 94, 113, 134, 139.

cent).[11, 37, 78] When a new patient presents with bilateral frozen shoulders, investigations to exclude diabetes mellitus should be undertaken. Diabetics who have cheiroarthropathy (waxy thickening and induration of the skin and connective tissues associated with flexion contractures of the fingers) and frozen shoulder may have an even higher incidence of bilateral shoulder involvement (77 per cent).[37] Patients with frozen shoulder and diabetes mellitus are more likely to have long-standing diabetes and advanced diabetic retinopathy.[78, 94] Diabetic patients who have been insulin dependent for more than 10 years have a more serious risk of developing shoulder symptoms persisting for more than two years.[78] There is a significant incidence of ongoing disability in these patients despite treatment.[37, 113]

TRAUMA

The association of frozen shoulder with major trauma to the shoulder or other parts of the upper extremity is recognized. The association with minor trauma which may be forgotten is difficult to document and may be overlooked.[19, 31, 75] Frozen shoulder is best prevented in cases of axillary node dissection, as in other surgery around the shoulder, by careful attention to postoperative exercises by the surgeon, nurses, and physiotherapists.[75]

CERVICAL DISC DISEASE

Lundberg and others report an increased incidence of frozen shoulder in patients with degeneration of the intervertebral discs of the cervical spine.[69, 76, 138] The peak incidence of cervical disc degeneration coincides with the peak incidence of frozen shoulder.[54]

THYROID DISORDERS

An association of frozen shoulder with hyperthyroidism has been reported.[31, 77, 135, 139] The shoulder disorder frequently resolves when the hyperthyroidism is corrected.[93]

INTRATHORACIC DISORDERS

Johnston reported an increased incidence of frozen shoulder in patients treated in sanitoria for tuberculosis. The clinical course of frozen shoulder in tuberculosis patients was noted to be generally mild.[52] An association between frozen shoulder and emphysema and chronic bronchitis was reported by Saha.[111] Bronchogenic carcinoma in the upper lobe of the lung may be associated with a frozen shoulder syndrome.[33, 75, 83] Ischemic heart disease has a long-standing association with frozen shoulder.[4, 34, 75, 139] Changes in the philosophy of management of cardiac patients toward more ambulatory care have greatly diminished the incidence of frozen shoulder in these patients in recent years.

INTRACRANIAL PATHOLOGY

Patients with hemiplegia, cerebral hemorrhage, and cerebral tumors have been shown to be at increased risk of developing frozen shoulder.[10, 12, 139] Bruckner and Nye questioned whether these predisposing neurological conditions all had in common a period during which normal spontaneous shoulder motion was prevented.[12]

PERSONALITY DISORDER

Coventry chose the term *periarthritic personality* to describe one component of a three-part theory on the pathogenesis of frozen shoulder in a group of patients with painful, stiff shoulders. He observed that most patients had "a peculiar emotional constitution in which they were unable to tolerate pain, expected others to get them well and refused to take any personal initiative in their recovery."[22] Quigley believed that the abnormal emotional state might be secondary to the shoulder condition, rather than the cause.[98] Others have observed that psychological factors and the inability to adapt predispose to the development of a frozen shoulder syndrome.[90]

Tyber, a psychiatrist, reported on 55 patients with painful shoulder syndromes whom he treated with lithium and amitriptyline; he observed good results.[125] From an orthopedic perspective, however, he was treating a mix of shoulder problems, making the clinical relevance of the results more difficult to interpret.

Wright and Haq found no evidence of a characteristic personality disorder using the Maudsley Personality Inventory when 148 patients with symptoms consistent with frozen shoulder were compared with controls.[139] Fleming and colleagues examined the personality profiles of 56 patients, using the Middlesex Hospital Questionnaire. They found that females had significantly increased somatic anxiety levels compared with controls.[38] Bruckner and Nye, in their analysis of 20 patients with frozen shoulder on a neurosurgical unit, using the same Middlesex Hospital Questionnaire, found a significant increase in depression indices when compared with controls.[12]

It would appear from the above that when subjected to scrutiny, a specific periarthritic personality type is difficult to identify. The role of psychological factors should be considered, at best, a secondary factor in the management of these patients.

Clinical Examination

Frozen shoulder is a symptom complex associated with a measurable restriction of passive motion of the shoulder. A complete physical examination of the upper extremities, spine, and trunk is necessary to rule out other intrinsic and extrinsic causes of shoulder disability. A careful assessment of the cervical spine is needed to rule out local pathology in the neck as a possible source of shoulder pain. An examination of the sternoclavicular and acromioclavicular joints is necessary to identify other possible local causes of shoulder discomfort and explain the reluctance on the part of the patient to move the shoulder.

The minimum examination of shoulder range of motion as recommended by the Society of American Shoulder and Elbow Surgeons must include:

1. Measurement of passive forward elevation, with the patient supine, measured as the angle between the arm and the thorax.

2. Passive external rotation with the arm at the side measured as the angle between the forearm and the sagittal plane with the elbow flexed to 90 degrees.

3. Active forward elevation, standing or sitting, measured as the angle between the arm and the trunk in the sagittal plane.

4. Active internal rotation measured as the level of spinous process that the patient can reach behind the back with the tip of the thumb of the affected arm.

5. Active abduction in the plane of the scapula measured as the angle between the arm and the trunk.

Further information can be obtained by assessing glenohumeral movement independent of scapulothoracic motion. To measure glenohumeral motion in forward elevation and abduction, the scapula should be stabilized against the chest wall by using direct pressure on the axillary border of the scapula. While assessing glenohumeral rotation in internal and external rotation, one hand can be used to stabilize the scapula and clavicle, thus eliminating most movement at the scapulothoracic space.

An examination of muscle strength in the different planes of shoulder motion is helpful. Resisting specific muscle actions may uncover a tendinitis component to the shoulder symptoms.[25]

Such an examination, performed routinely at each visit, allows documentation of the initial restrictions and any progress or lack thereof during follow-up.

Clinical Presentation

Because frozen shoulder is a symptom complex rather than a specific diagnostic entity, a high index of suspicion is needed on hearing the clinical presentation to make the appropriate diagnosis. Not all patients are typical, but an awareness of the typical clinical course of idiopathic or primary frozen shoulder and secondary frozen shoulder is desirable.

PRIMARY FROZEN SHOULDER

This is a unique condition that rarely recurs in the same shoulder.[31, 44, 69, 77] In most patients only one shoulder is affected. Subsequent involvement of the other shoulder may occur in up to 20 per cent of patients.[69, 106, 112]

There are classically three stages to the clinical course of primary, or idiopathic, frozen shoulder.

Painful Phase

A good clinical history is fundamental to making the diagnosis of frozen shoulder. There is often a gradual onset of diffuse shoulder pain, which the patient has difficulty localizing anatomically or temporally. Patients will frequently describe a progressive onset of shoulder pain lasting for a period of weeks to months prior to seeking orthopedic consultation. The pain is usually worse at night, exacerbated by lying on the affected side. It may be the first episode of shoulder pain, or the patient may have recognized a similar condition in the opposite shoulder.

It is during this painful phase that patients are most anxious. The duration of the painful phase is variable, lasting from two to nine months.[103] As the patient uses the arm less and less, there is usually less discomfort, with the patient taking some satisfaction in the false belief that he or she is doing the best thing for the shoulder. It is often difficult to obtain a history of a precipitating event.

Stiffening Phase

The painful phase of frozen shoulder is usually followed by a slowly progressive loss of shoulder movement. This phase may last 4 to 12 months.[103] The restrictions to shoulder movement are noted by the patient as an inability to use the arm away from the side in activities of daily living such as dressing, washing hair, or personal hygiene. The functional restrictions do not consistently coincide with the objectively measured shoulder motion. Patients may complain of an inability to use the arm in activities such as swinging a racquet or golf club, reaching out for a telephone, removing a wallet from a back pocket, or reaching for an object in the back seat of the car. The inability to reach to the back of the head or to the interscapular area of the back is more frequently expressed by female patients.

Shoulder movement is often restricted in a characteristic pattern with loss of external rotation, internal rotation, and abduction[25] (Fig. 21–4). Most patients will have a moderate restriction of external rotation with the arm at the side, i.e., less than 30 degrees. Internal rotation is often limited to the point that the patient is unable to raise the tip of the thumb up the back past the spinous process of L2. The arm may be quite restricted in abduction, allowing less than 110 degrees of combined shoulder abduction.

Approximately 10 per cent of patients will present with negligible glenohumeral movement. There are atypical patterns of loss of motion, such as a predominant loss of internal rotation, which add to the mystery of these frozen shoulder patients.

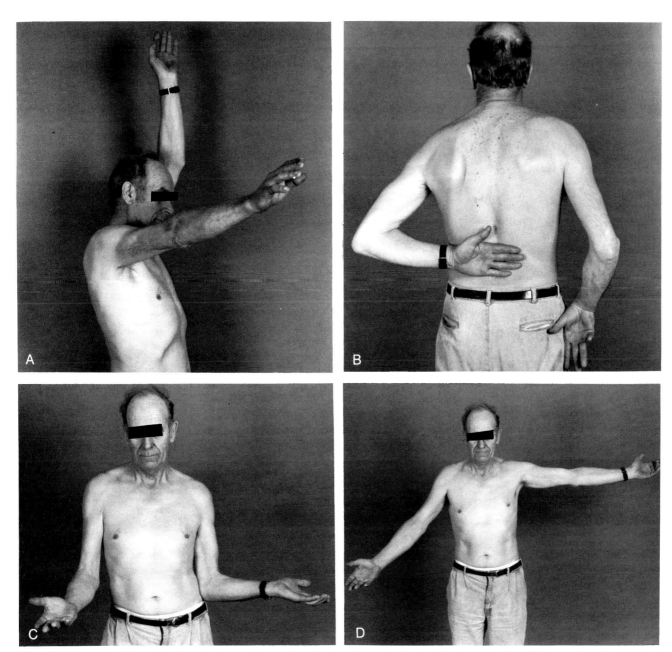

Figure 21-4. A typical restriction of shoulder motion in a patient presenting with primary frozen shoulder. *A*, Active forward elevation of 75 degrees. Note the extension of the trunk, which must be accounted for in recording measurements. *B*, Active internal rotation with the tip of the thumb shown at approximately the T12 spinous process. *C*, Active external rotation, the same as passive external rotation, measured here as 10 degrees. *D*, Active abduction, seen here as 35 degrees with no lateral shifting of the trunk.

Patients often experience a dull aching shoulder and periscapular pain punctuated by sharp pains which occur when the arm comes to the end of its free range of motion. During the period of moderate restriction of shoulder motion, reaching suddenly to grab a swinging door or to catch a falling object is an episode vividly described by the patient as being particularly painful. The pain subsides in most cases as the motion is gradually regained. The pain threshold is variable among patients and does not correlate with a fixed percentage of overall shoulder motion. As a stretching program begins, the pain in most cases gradually subsides to a more tolerable level. It may take weeks or months for all discomfort to resolve.

Thawing Phase

The final phase described as thawing, or the gradual regaining of shoulder motion, is very variable. The time course of this phase is measured in weeks or months rather than days. As motion slowly increases, there is a progressive lessening of the discomfort, which comes as a great relief. The time course of return of shoulder motion is quite unpredictable. It will often take six to nine months for patients to regain a good functional range of motion and to be free of aching discomfort. For others, symptoms may unexplicably resolve over a period of four to six weeks.

Without specific treatment, shoulder motion is regained as a gradual process, with patients reporting progress as they achieve functional milestones such as being able to tuck in a shirt or blouse behind their back, wash their hair, or achieve a more natural golf swing. Some patients continue to have quite a restricted range of shoulder motion when measured objectively, but when asked, they themselves feel that they are back at a full functional level.[7]

SECONDARY FROZEN SHOULDER

In these patients a precipitating event can be identified. There may have been a recent or remote episode of shoulder pain possibly related to overuse. A localized shoulder pain suggesting subacromial bursitis or tendinitis may have occurred at the outset and the initial pain resolved or continued as a lingering, aching discomfort. Frozen shoulder may develop after soft tissue trauma or a fracture. Such injuries may be anatomically at the shoulder or remote from it. A history of an upper extremity fracture followed by a full-blown clinical frozen shoulder is fortunately seen less frequently now because of an increasing emphasis by physicians on early shoulder movement after injuries to the upper extremity.

A painful shoulder condition such as a partial-thickness tear of the rotator cuff may be the precipitating event. A nonspecific brachialgia that in retrospect was of cervical spine origin may be misinterpreted by the patient as intrinsic shoulder pain and be mistreated by a period of self-imposed shoulder immobilization. A painful inflammatory condition of the shoulder joint or adjacent soft tissues, whatever the cause, may be the triggering incident.

In patients with a secondary frozen shoulder, the previously described three phases of frozen shoulder may not always be recognizable.

DURATION OF SYMPTOMS

The classical teaching has been that the clinical syndrome of frozen shoulder is a self-limiting disorder lasting 12 to 18 months.[42, 44, 69, 126, 133] More recent results cast doubt on the accuracy of earlier predictions of a transient problem with few, if any, long-term consequences (Fig. 21–5).

An optimistic outlook was presented by Withers, who advised an initial period of rest followed by an exercise program and reported achieving a normal, painless range of motion by 14 weeks in most patients (n = 20).[133] In a follow-up of 226 patients, Watson Jones observed that only 5 per cent failed to regain 150 degrees of abduction within six months by doing a three-minute exercise routine each hour.[126]

Lloyd-Roberts and associates reported less favorable

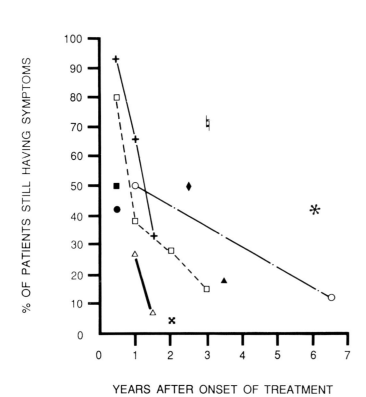

- ▲ BINDER ET AL. (7)
- ● BULGEN ET AL. (14)
- ✱ CLARKE ET AL. (18)
- ✕ GREY (42)
- ■ HARMON (46)
- + LLOYD ROBERTS ET AL. (67)
- □ MEULENGRACHT ET AL. (77)
- △ QUIN (101)
- ◆ REEVES (103)
- ○ SANY ET AL. (112)
- ♮ SIMMONDS (116)

YEARS AFTER ONSET OF TREATMENT

Figure 21–5. Distribution of patients with persisting symptoms after initial assessment. The classical view that frozen shoulder is a self-limiting disorder that runs its course in 12 to 18 months is brought into question by longer, more critical follow-up studies.

results with a group of 27 patients who received non-specific treatments, of whom only 44 per cent were better at one year and 33 per cent had not recovered by 18 months.[67] A longer duration of symptoms has been reported by Meuelengracht and colleagues who, at an average of three years follow-up, found 23 per cent of their patients (n = 65) had persisting pain and an ongoing limitation of shoulder movements.[77] Reeves reported on 41 patients who were followed for 5 years; of these, 61 per cent failed to achieve a return of shoulder range of motion equal to the opposite side. Of the restricted group, 12 per cent had a severe restriction and 88 per cent continued with a mild persistent disability. The mean duration of symptoms was 30 months with a range of 12 to 42 months.[103] Several studies have reported ongoing shoulder disability up to 10 years after the onset of frozen shoulder.[7, 18, 103, 112, 116]

Patients in general are poor judges of their own shoulder motion, often underestimating their restrictions and overestimating their recovery.[7, 18, 112] At follow-up, shoulder motion is often less than that of the normal contralateral shoulder or less than that of age- and sex-matched controls.[7, 9, 14, 18] Seven to 42 per cent of patients continue to have moderate restriction in shoulder motion up to 5 years following the onset of shoulder pain.[7, 18, 103] A measurable restriction in the range of motion at follow-up was present in 39 to 76 per cent of patients.[7, 112, 116]

The effect of duration of symptoms before treatment on the final clinical outcome remains controversial. Early presentation by the patient for medical treatment has been reported as being associated with a shorter disease course.[47, 103] Binder and associates noted a more rapid rate of recovery in patients who presented early.[7] Helbig and associates observed that the degree of disability before treatment had no influence on final outcome.[48] Dominant arm involvement has been reported as a good prognostic indicator, while other factors, such as patient occupation and the treatment program used, did not achieve statistical significance when analyzed as to their effect on outcome.[7, 18]

Investigations

HEMATOLOGICAL AND BIOCHEMICAL INVESTIGATIONS

The routine blood work, including hemoglobin, white cell count, smear, and differential, in patients presenting with a classic picture of frozen shoulder is usually normal.[106] Routine serum biochemistry is also within normal limits unless there is some other underlying disorder. When the history and physical examination are consistent with frozen shoulder and both the shoulder radiographs and the routine blood work are normal, no further investigations are usually required.

The erythrocyte sedimentation rate (ESR) may be normal; it has been reported elevated in up to 20 per cent of cases.[7, 77, 101, 109] More recent series, however, report no significant increase in the ESR in patients with frozen shoulder.[57, 140] Fearnley and colleagues suggested that patients with a raised ESR responded better to corticosteroids, but this has not been reported by others.[36]

An association between HLA-B27 histocompatibility antigen and patients having frozen shoulder has been reported. However, when more patients were analyzed, no increased incidence of HLA-B27 in patients with frozen shoulder could be confirmed.[13, 16] Other authors have reported that the incidence of HLA-B27 is not increased in the frozen shoulder population.[108, 115, 117, 140]

Bulgen and associates reported on an investigation of 40 patients with clinical signs of frozen shoulder who had shown an increase in immune complex levels, including C-reactive protein and impaired cell-mediated immunity. Tests to measure these values eight months following the onset of the shoulder disorder showed a tendency for the values to return to normal levels.[15]

The autoimmune hypothesis of Macnab is appealing, but there is no conclusive evidence to support the presence of an immune deficiency state nor an autoimmune process at this time.[139]

RADIOLOGY

It is important to obtain a complete series of shoulder x-rays to rule out other abnormalities about the shoulder which may mimic frozen shoulder. A minimum examination consists of a set of orthogonal views of the shoulder. An anteroposterior projection, taken at right angles to the plane of the scapula, can be used to obtain two views of the proximal humerus, one with the humerus in internal rotation and the other in external rotation. These views give a good visualization of the proximal humerus and surrounding soft tissues. An axillary view will help exclude dislocation, fracture, and locking osteophytes. Special attention should be paid to reviewing the films to seek other possible causes for the shoulder pain and limitation of motion.

Shoulder radiographs are usually normal in patients with frozen shoulder.[8] A mild to moderate osteopenia may be seen in those patients who have had a prolonged period of restricted range of motion.[104] Minor degenerative changes of the humeral head in the area of the greater tuberosity (19 per cent) or a narrowing of the subacromial space (12 per cent) have been reported.[8]

RADIONUCLIDE SCANNING

Bone scans with technetium-99m pertechnetate often show an increased uptake in patients with frozen shoulder. Wright and colleagues noted a favorable association between an increased pertechnetate uptake about the shoulder and a rapid response to corticosteroid injections.[137] Stodell and associates reported an association between an increased technetium-99m pertechnetate uptake and subjective pain levels, but they could not make a similar association when technetium-99m methylene diphosphonate scans were used.[122] Binder and associates observed that over 90 per cent of their patients had an increased uptake on the diphosphonate scans, with 29 per cent having more than a 50 per cent increase in uptake compared with the opposite shoulder. Binder and associates, however, could not find any association between the bone scan findings and the duration of symptoms, the initial severity of disease, the arthrographic findings, or the eventual recovery.[8]

ARTHROGRAPHY

Kernwien and colleagues observed a restricted joint volume at arthrography in patients with frozen shoulder.[56] The early descriptions of the characteristic shoulder arthrography findings in frozen shoulder by J. S. Neviaser have allowed a better understanding of the underlying shoulder joint pathology without having to resort to surgical exposure. He described as typical the combination of a decreased joint volume, an irregular joint outline, and variable filling of the bicipital tendon sheath[83] (Fig. 21–6). The reduction in the shoulder joint capsule capacity to less than 10 to 12 ml and the variable lack of filling of the axillary fold and subscapular bursa are the currently accepted characteristic findings.* A good correlation has been reported between the clinical range of shoulder motion and the

severity of capsular retraction at arthrography.[48, 69, 84, 88, 102] In an effort to quantitate the capsular contraction, authors have recorded the volume of fluid that can be injected at the time of arthrography. The volumes have been correlated to the restriction of range of shoulder motion.[69, 84, 102]

The biceps tendon sheath is outlined arthrographically in the majority of cases of adhesive capsulitis, but the extent of filling is variable.[68, 83] Reeves observed that there was no filling of the biceps tendon sheath in those patients with a moderate reduction in joint volume.[102]

Arthrography has also been used to document tearing of the joint capsule during manipulation under anesthesia.[2, 69, 102] The tears of the capsule allow dye to escape into the extracapsular space, but no tears of the rotator cuff tendons themselves following manipulation under anesthesia were noted in an extensive study by Lundberg.[69]

In the clinical research setting, selecting patients by the characteristic findings at arthrography is one factor in attempting to objectively standardize the patient groups.[68, 76, 88] Arthrography is an invasive investigation, and its routine use in the investigation of patients presenting with the typical history and clinical findings of frozen shoulder needs further assessment.[74] In two series, no correlation between the arthrographic findings and treatment outcome could be found.[8, 68] When clinical findings are well documented, there remains a puzzling group of patients (6 to 20 per cent) who have a normal arthrogram.[13, 69, 83]

The author's indications for shoulder arthrography in the management of frozen shoulder are limited. The

---

*See references 2, 48, 68, 69, 83–85, 102, 128.

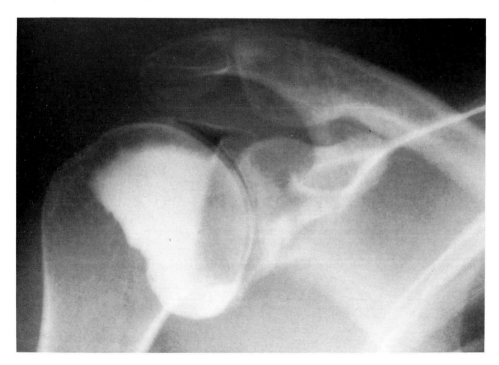

Figure 21–6. Arthrogram showing a restricted joint volume with an irregular margin. No filling of the bicipital tendon sheath can be seen on this projection.

shoulder arthrogram is a source of additional information in situations where there is a failure of improvement of the patient's condition following a specified treatment program or when some question exists as to the exact shoulder pathology.

ARTHROSCOPY

With experience gained from arthroscopic examination of the knee, shoulder arthroscopy saw its initial development in the late 1970s and early 1980s.[30, 43, 130]

The use of the arthroscope to examine patients with painful, stiff shoulders is technically demanding.[87, 88, 131] The early investigators reported seeing a contracted anterior joint capsule, but no intra-articular adhesions were visualized.[30, 43] A mild to moderate synovitis with areas of increased vascularity and obliteration of the subscapularis bursa was also described.[30, 43, 131] Visualization of the inferior capsular recess may be difficult owing to the limited external rotation found in these patients. There remains a controversy of interpretation as to what is happening in the inferior recesses of the shoulder capsule. Some believe that the axillary pouch may be deformed but deny seeing obliteration of the recess.[30, 43, 130] Neviaser reports seeing adhesions in the dependent folds of the capsule whenever there is a significant restriction of motion of the shoulder.[87]

In an investigational study, Neviaser defined four stages of arthroscopic changes in adhesive capsulitis: Stage 1, a mild reddened synovitis; Stage 2, acute synovitis with adhesions of the dependent folds of the synovial lining; Stage 3, maturation of adhesions; and Stage 4, chronic adhesions. The staging was used as a guide to treatment planning.[87]

When patients underwent arthroscopy after manipulation of the shoulder under anesthesia, a consistent tear of the inferior capsule was visualized.[87, 91]

The role of shoulder arthroscopy in the diagnosis and treatment of frozen shoulder is not yet established.[86]

Complications

In the majority of cases, frozen shoulder syndrome is a self-limiting disorder that resolves with time. There may be a residual loss of objectively measured shoulder motion. Some loss of shoulder motion occurs in up to 70 per cent of patients, but represents only a functional problem in 10 to 15 per cent of patients. A few patients continue to have a stiff, painful shoulder.[7, 18, 103, 112, 116] Some patients continue to have persistent pain for which other modalities of pain management have to be explored.

The complications of greatest concern are those of over treatment. The potential complications of manipulation, including dislocation and fracture, must be weighed against the possible benefits. There is also a risk of stretching the brachial plexus and other peripheral nerves when the arm is manipulated into abduction.

There is a small risk of infection with intra-articular injections. The use of both nonsteroidal anti-inflammatory drugs and systemic steroids has inherent risks of potential systemic complications.[23]

Differential Diagnosis

Frozen shoulder needs to be distinguished from other causes of painful, stiff shoulders[24, 35] (Table 21–3). A good clinical history and a careful physical examination can rule out many of the alternative diagnoses. The soft tissue examination techniques of Cryiax, based

Table 21–3. DIFFERENTIAL DIAGNOSIS OF FROZEN SHOULDER

Trauma
  Fractures of shoulder region
  Other fractures anywhere in upper extremity
  Shoulder dislocation, especially a missed posterior dislocation
  Hemarthrosis of shoulder secondary to contusion
Other Soft Tissue Disorders about the Shoulder
  Tendinitis of rotator cuff
  Tendinitis of long head of biceps
  Subacromial bursitis
  Impingement
  Shoulder-hand syndrome
  Fibrositis
  Soft tissue neoplasm
  Suprascapular nerve entrapment
  Thoracic outlet syndrome
  Neuralgic amyotrophy—Parsonage-Turner syndrome
  Polymyalgia rheumatica
Joint Disorders
  Degenerative arthritis of acromioclavicular joint
  Degenerative arthritis of glenohumeral joint
  Inflammatory arthritis—Monarticular/polyarticular
  Septic arthritis
  Neuropathic arthritis, e.g., syringomyelia, diabetes
  Crystalline arthritis—gout, pseudogout
  Hemophilic arthritis
  Osteochondromatosis
Bone Disorders
  Avascular necrosis—osteonecrosis
  Metastatic tumor
  Primary bone tumor, including multiple myeloma
  Paget's disease
  Osteomalacia
  Hyperparathyroidism
Cervical Spine Disorders
  Cervical spondylosis
  Cervical disc herniation
  Neoplasm
  Infection
Intrathoracic Disorders
  Diaphragmatic irritation
  Pancoast tumor
  Myocardial infarction
  Esophagitis
Abdominal Disorders
  Gastric ulcer
  Cholecystitis or cholelithiasis
  Subphrenic abscess
Psychogenic

on the effects on symptoms of tension in the soft tissues, are often useful in clarifying the diagnosis.[25, 26] Radiological and laboratory tests are helpful to further exclude other conditions.

With the clinical presentation of shoulder pain, a blockage to external rotation and an overall limitation of shoulder motion can superficially be likened to a frozen shoulder; however, one must rule out the possibility of a missed dislocation of the shoulder, especially a posterior dislocation. Appropriate radiographs, specifically an axillary view, should conclusively determine whether the humeral head is articulating with the glenoid.

Patients with acute tendinitis or bursal inflammation may have restrictions of both active and passive range of motion of their shoulder. The history of onset should raise suspicions as to the correct diagnosis. Injection of the subacromial bursa with a local anesthetic will usually greatly improve the passive range of motion in the tendinitis-bursitis group while having little or no effect on the range of motion of the frozen shoulder patients.

A large calcific deposit may on occasion cause both an active and a passive block to shoulder motion. Shoulder radiographs taken to display the subacromial space with the humerus in internal and external rotation should detect such a calcification. It is important to note that calcifying tendinitis occurs with equal frequency in patients with or without frozen shoulder.[69, 129, 137]

Abnormal scapulothoracic mobility may be seen in a few clinical situations which could be mistaken for frozen shoulder. Multiple rib fractures adjacent to the scapulothoracic space may be associated with restricted excursion of the scapula. Prolonged post-traumatic shoulder immobilization may also be a factor in restricting scapulothoracic motion. Chest wall deformities, including those related to scoliosis, may restrict scapulothoracic motion. Congenital abnormalities, such as Klippel-Feil and Sprengel deformities, are potential causes of restricted scapulothoracic motion. Poor posture over a prolonged period may in turn restrict scapular motion.[110] These abnormalities should be identified by a thorough history and physical examination. Radiographs will document the obvious deformities if present.

Osteochondromatosis or other causes of intra-articular loose bodies may present as a painful, stiff shoulder. The typical catching or locking episodes may allow these patients to be identified. A careful review of radiographs, looking for loose bodies, may be helpful. Other investigations, including arthrography or arthroscopy, may be indicated where the diagnosis is unclear.

A painful acromioclavicular joint may also mimic a frozen shoulder and should be suspected when the clinical findings reveal a localized tenderness over the acromioclavicular joint. The question of whether the acromioclavicular pathology is primary or secondary needs to be addressed. A restricted range of motion of the glenohumeral joint may be accompanied by increased movement at the scapulothoracic interspace as the patient tries to move the arm.[89] These added stresses on the acromioclavicular joint are a potential source of inflammation and pain.[46, 75, 138] A 1-ml injection of 1 per cent lidocaine into the acromioclavicular joint should relieve all the symptoms in a primary acromioclavicular disorder. Where there is partial relief of pain but no improvement in range of motion, one should look beyond the acromioclavicular joint for the cause of symptoms.

Inflammatory arthritis associated with rheumatoid or rheumatoid-like arthritis, ankylosing spondylitis, or psoriatic arthritis should be considered when assessing painful, stiff shoulders. The possibility of septic arthritis should also be considered. A search for other clinical signs and a careful choice of laboratory investigations will usually corroborate the diagnosis of a systemic inflammatory condition.

Primary glenohumeral degenerative arthritis, post-traumatic arthritis, or neuropathic arthropathy (as seen with syringomyelia) may all have clinical symptoms similar to those of frozen shoulder. In the early stages of arthritis, the restricted range of motion and the dull, poorly localized pain are quite similar to the symptoms found in patients with frozen shoulder syndrome. However, with a careful history, physical examination, and radiographic evaluation, these patients should be easily differentiated from patients with frozen shoulder.

Avascular necrosis or osteonecrosis, whatever the cause, may present with symptoms of pain and restricted range of motion that may mimic frozen shoulder.[23] The history and characteristic radiological findings of avascular necrosis of the humeral head should allow the clinician to distinguish between these two diagnoses.

As in most patients in the sixth decade or older who present with a localized skeletal pain, a primary or secondary malignancy must be ruled out. Radiographic imaging and a bone scan are helpful in evaluating this possibility. Screening blood work and a clinical search for a primary source is appropriate. A biopsy is often the best source of diagnostic information if a specific lesion is identified in the shoulder region.

Referred pain should also be considered in the differential diagnosis. Pain from the cervical spine radiating to the shoulder and upper arm may be the event that precedes the onset of shoulder pain and stiffness. Identifying the neck as a source is important in planning treatment so as to avoid further exacerbations of the cervical spondylosis. Pain referred from a bronchogenic tumor of the apex of the lung is another possible cause of shoulder pain and subsequent restriction of shoulder movement.[33, 75, 83] Pain referred to the shoulder may originate from intrathoracic and intra-abdominal disorders, which need to be ruled out in the history and physical examination. Further investigations may be dictated by information gathered in the initial and subsequent patient interviews and examinations.

Reflex sympathetic dystrophy and frozen shoulder have many common features. Shoulder hand syndrome is a type of reflex sympathetic dystrophy involving the upper extremity and is characterized by a painful disability of the shoulder associated with diffuse swelling, exquisite tenderness, and vasomotor changes in the hands and digits of the same extremity.[114, 119, 120] Spotty demineralization of the bones may occur. Later, trophic changes of the skin may become more noticeable. In general, the treatment of shoulder hand syndrome is initially an exercise program, and if unsuccessful, a series of sympathetic nerve blocks should be administered. Sympathetic nerve blocks may have to be repeated on several occasions to obtain lasting relief.[120]

The clinical condition known as fibrositis has been redefined considerably in the last 20 years. The term fibrositis is now restricted to a specific condition characterized by widespread soft tissue pain and aching, without apparent cause, associated with multiple areas of local tenderness. The diagnostic criteria require that at least 7 of 14 identified potential tender points be sensitive to palpation. The pain of fibrositis tends to be chronic and may be associated with morning fatigue and stiffness. Poor sleep is often an associated symptom. Cold, weather change, and emotional stress all have an exacerbating effect, whereas increased physical activity seems to have a beneficial effect. The treatment is a long-term undertaking. Education of the patient as to the diagnosis and its long-term management is most important. Low-dose amitriptyline is effective in reducing pain, fatigue, and tender point sensitivity. A recreational aerobic exercise program also tends to be beneficial.[136]

Hysteria and malingering should be included here for completeness in a differential diagnosis of frozen shoulder, but such diagnoses can only be made very hesitantly in this group of patients. The lack of a specific history or unique clinical findings in frozen shoulder means that the diagnosis should be continuously questioned, and the examiner should look for other potentially more serious causes of the shoulder symptoms.

Treatment

The objectives of treatment in frozen shoulder are to relieve discomfort and restore motion and thereby restore function. As in other medical conditions where the pathophysiology is poorly understood, many different forms of treatment are used empirically in the management of frozen shoulder syndrome (Table 21–4). The choice of treatment is based on the clinical findings and the stage at which the patient seeks treatment. Treatment is continuously modified, depending on the individual's response to a particular treatment modality.

Table 21–4. TREATMENT ALTERNATIVES FOR FROZEN SHOULDER

Prevention
General Measures
  Pain control: analgesia, NSAIDs, heat, ice, TENS
  Exercises
    Instruction and encouragement
    Warm-up exercises:
      pendulum
      pulley
    Passive stretching:
      Auto-assisted
      Physiotherapist directed
      Ultrasound
    Strengthening within available range
    Encourage functional use within range
Mobilization Techniques
  Accessory movements
Local Injection
  Paired steroid injections: joint and bursa
  Intra-articular steroid injection
  Other injection techniques
Myofascial Approach to Treatment
  Spray and stretch
  Trigger point injections
Distention Brisement
  Distention arthrography
Manipulation
  Manipulation under anesthesia
  Manipulation and steroid injection
  Manipulation and oral steroids
  Manipulation under local anesthesia
Other Treatments
  Oral corticosteroids
  Prolonged traction
  Stellate ganglion block
  Radiotherapy
Surgical Treatment
  Arthroscopic freeing up of adhesions
  Open surgical release

PREVENTION

The primary consideration in treatment should be prevention. The incidence of frozen shoulder related to trauma in the upper extremity is much less frequent now than it was previously. The current insistence that patients move their arms, including the elbow and shoulder, early after any injury to the upper extremity is felt to be a major factor in avoiding the frozen shoulder syndrome. Education of primary caregivers would be helpful so that patients might be advised on first contact with a physician to avoid prolonged immobilization of their shoulders, even though there may be persisting discomfort. Binder and associates on questioning their patients found that 50 per cent received no advice from the primary care physician on the need for early motion. Of those getting advice, 75 per cent were told to rest the shoulder, whereas only 25 per cent were told to exercise the shoulder gently.[9]

GENERAL MEASURES

Efforts to obtain pain relief by rest, analgesia, or transcutaneous electrical nerve stimulation (TENS) are useful in the early stages of frozen shoulder.[9, 106] Salicylate and nonsalicylate analgesics are effective. It may be necessary to use preparations containing codeine during acute flare-ups. Nonsteroidal anti-inflammatory drugs are often used empirically, but when questioned, patients found the nonsteroidal agents less helpful than nonsalicylate analgesics.[9] Starting pendulum exercise movements as soon as possible is advised. Patients doing regular exercises did consistently better than patient groups receiving analgesics only.[63] Short periods of exercise, i.e., two or three minutes every one to two hours, are recommended.[9, 126] It must be stressed to the patient by all persons participating in a patient's care that the patient's participation in the exercise program is crucial to its success.[64]

PHYSIOTHERAPY

Physiotherapy modalities, such as the application of heat or ice, short-wave diathermy, and infrared or ultrasound, have not been shown to have benefit on their own.[14] Each of these modalities can help in pain control and muscle relaxation. Physiotherapists perform a major role as teachers, instructing patients about the natural history of their condition as well as outlining suitable exercises. Ongoing encouragement of the patient by the therapist is invaluable in difficult cases. The exercises are modified in keeping with ongoing feedback from the physiotherapist.

Hazleman reported on a group of patients treated with physiotherapy who had pain relief equivalent to those treated with injections or manipulation. In the physiotherapy group, 54 per cent were cured or improved; however, 28 per cent experienced an exacerbation of their pain with physiotherapy.[47] Rizk and associates reported on a patient group receiving a combination of physiotherapy treatment modalities of whom only 60 per cent achieved pain-free sleep by four to five months.[106]

Ultrasound in dosages of 0.5 to 2 watts per square centimeter has been used for its thermal effect and to increase tissue extensibility. Ultrasound treatments have not been found to offer any advantage over heat and exercises when outcome was assessed by pain scores at two and three months follow-up and the time required for full recovery.[101]

STRETCHING EXERCISES

As pain is brought under control, a stretching program is initiated in forward elevation, external rotation, and internal rotation. Patients have to be motivated to participate in such an exercise program. All patients have to be able to withstand some physical discomfort, which is part of any stretching exercise program.[20] I prefer to avoid stretching into abduction initially since many patients will develop impingement-like symptoms until the joint becomes supple enough

to allow the humeral head to slide under the coracoacromial arch.

STRENGTHENING EXERCISES

As the range of glenohumeral motion returns, a strengthening program within the available range of motion is initiated. Active assisted exercises can be followed by antigravity eccentric strengthening in forward elevation. Pulleys are a useful mechanical assist here. I prefer to start the antigravity exercises with the patient supine, loading the shoulder eccentrically and progressing later to lifting the arm from the side as a concentric strengthening exercise.[50] The patient can then advance to a light-resistance strengthening program, progressing as tolerated over time to a more intensive strengthening program. The aim of the strengthening program is to restore equal function to both upper extremities.[46]

MOBILIZATION TECHNIQUES

Mobilization of the glenohumeral joint by performing passive oscillatory movements of the joint surfaces has been recommended as another treatment modality in frozen shoulder syndrome.[73] The techniques used depend on the patient's presentation and whether the treatment is for pain control, stiffness, or both. The accessory glenohumeral movements of gliding, rolling, and distraction are performed in the pain-free part of the joint range of motion. The same accessory movements are done at the end of the physiological range as a stretching exercise to overcome stiffness.[73] The force, direction, and amplitude of the therapeutic movements are continually modified, based on the subjective and objective response of the patient.[89] Nicholson, in a controlled study, compared patients doing mobilizations and active exercises with patients doing only active exercises. Of all motions tested, passive abduction was the only motion that was significantly better in the mobilization group. There was no significant difference in pain scores between the two patient groups up to four weeks after starting treatment.[89]

INJECTION

In attempting a more direct therapeutic approach to the local pathology in frozen shoulder, several injection protocols have been used. The rationale for this treatment is based on observations that steroid injections have a strong local anti-inflammatory effect.[27] The common injection protocols will be reviewed.

Paired Injections

Richardson reported the results of a blind, controlled, multicenter study of 37 patients with frozen shoulder who received two injections of 25 mg of prednisolone acetate, one into the bursa and the other into the glenohumeral joint, on the initial visit and again at two weeks. These patients were compared with controls receiving injections of normal saline. No difference in outcome was noted when the treatment groups were assessed as to pain and movement at the two- and six-week follow-up examinations. When Richardson monitored attempted intra-articular injections by arthrography, he noted the inability of most physicians to successfully inject into the markedly retracted shoulder joint.[105] His findings are consistent with those of Weiss and colleagues who described the use of an arthrogram to better determine the anatomical landmarks to be used for subsequent intra-articular injections. A technically satisfactory arthrogram could not be achieved in 12 per cent of their patients.[128]

Roy and associates reported on 55 patients with 60 painful, stiff shoulders who were treated with paired injections of 20 mg of methyl prednisolone acetate injected both into the glenohumeral joint and the subacromial bursa weekly to a maximum of three paired injections. In this group, 80 per cent of patients had their pain abolished by two weeks, and 95 per cent were pain free at four weeks. By eight weeks, 73 per cent achieved 150 degrees of abduction, and 53 per cent achieved 45 degrees of external rotation. Eight per cent of the patients were considered to be treatment failures because they continued to have a limited range of motion and aching discomfort.[109]

Less impressive results were reported by Bulgen and colleagues who studied 11 patients receiving paired injections of 20 mg of methyl prednisolone acetate into the glenohumeral joint and the subacromial bursa for three weekly injections. The control group consisted of eight patients who were taught only pendulum exercises and given nonsalicylate analgesics and mild sedation. At the six-month follow-up, when pain and range of motion were assessed, no difference was noted between the two patient groups. Of the injection group, only 36 per cent were pain free at 8 weeks, and only 18 per cent achieved 150 degrees of shoulder abduction by 10 weeks.[14]

Intra-articular Injections

In a study of 80 patients divided into 4 groups, Lee and associates observed that among the intra-articular injection group there was no significant difference in the final range of motion when compared with the patients who did exercises only.[62]

Lee and associates reported on 15 patients receiving the combined treatment of an intra-articular injection of hydrocortisone and exercises who were compared with three other groups. There was no demonstrable advantage to the injection and exercises patients when compared with those receiving heat and exercises. The intra-articular hydrocortisone and exercise group fared better than the analgesic group (controls), but there was no significant difference in outcome up to six

weeks from the time of injection among the three treatment groups.[63]

Williams and associates followed a group of patients who were given three weekly intra-articular injections of 50 mg of hydrocortisone acetate and compared them with a group of patients receiving stellate ganglion blocks. All patients were shown an exercise program and were allowed to use nonsteroidal anti-inflammatory medications. At the 12-week follow-up, using a subjective assessment, half of the patients felt they were improved by 75 per cent, one-quarter improved by 25 per cent, and one-quarter were unchanged. The observed changes in range of motion paralleled the patients' own assessment. At the four-week and three-month follow-up, there was no significant difference between the treatment groups.[132]

Hollingsworth and associates reported on 43 patients with the clinical findings of frozen shoulder syndrome who were divided between two treatment arms. One group (n = 23) received intra-articular injections, and the other group (n = 20) had injections of tender points about the shoulder. The injections consisted of 40 mg methyl prednisolone acetate and 1 per cent lidocaine. These patients were assessed at one week; if no relief was obtained, the alternative (cross-over) injection was given. Overall, 26 per cent of the frozen shoulder group were considered to have benefited from an intra-articular injection, while none of the tender point injections were beneficial in patients with frozen shoulder.[49]

Thomas and colleagues, using an intra-articular injection of 50 mg of hydrocortisone acetate, reported at three-month follow-up a good improvement in the range of motion in only 13 per cent of patients and a substantial improvement in day pain scores in 47 per cent.[123]

The use of intra-articular injections have theoretical merits, but the evidence is equivocal. In patients with moderately stiff shoulders for whom the pain is a major impediment to exercise, an intra-articular injection repeated on one or two occasions, if needed, seems justified. The steroid injections have not been shown to improve the rate of return of shoulder motion.[68, 100]

Other Injection Techniques

Murnaghan and colleagues compared regional infiltration of the shoulder joint capsule with 25 mg of hydrocortisone acetate with injections of 2 per cent lidocaine in the absence of a control group. Both treatments were felt to be beneficial, but the hydrocortisone did not seem to offer any real advantage.[80]

Injection of 40 mg of methylprednisolone into the area of maximum tenderness was not successful in relieving pain and clinical signs in 20 patients with frozen shoulder.[49] Multiple injections with a variety of steroid preparations injected into combinations of the subacromial bursa, the posterior pericapsular structures, and the long head of the biceps were reviewed by Steinbrocker. He reported that 66 per cent of his patients had pain relief after one or two visits and 66 per cent went on to achieve 85 per cent or better of normal function within six weeks.[121]

MYOFASCIAL APPROACH TO TREATMENT

Trigger points in the subscapularis muscle have been theorized to be a source of shoulder pain and restricted range of motion. These patients with restricted elevation, external rotation, and abduction have been found to have trigger points within the muscle belly of the subscapularis muscle accessible to palpation only when the scapula is abducted.[124]

In the context of the myofascial trigger point approach to musculoskeletal disorders, the subscapularis trigger points cause associated trigger points to develop in the other shoulder muscles, especially the pectoralis major and minor, the latissimus dorsi, and the triceps.[124] Kraft noted that the peak age for frozen shoulder syndrome is the same as that of myofascial pain syndrome.[60] A careful examination is required to identify the muscular origin as the cause of the restricted range of motion of the shoulder. Trigger points are identified by palpation of the anterior aspect of the abducted scapula. Light to moderate pressure on specific firm bands of muscle fibers reproduces the patient's pain over the posterior shoulder, occasionally radiating distally as far as the wrist.[124]

The recommended treatment is to use a local vapocoolant spray, swept upward over the area of the axilla including the veterbral and dorsal surfaces of the scapula, in association with stretching of the glenohumeral joint into abduction and external rotation. Travell cautions that these stretching procedures may precipitate trigger points in the antagonist muscles. The spray and stretch is followed immediately by a local application of heat and active range of motion exercises.[124]

The injection of trigger points with procaine is the procedure recommended if the spray and stretch techniques fail. Travell and colleagues recommend using a No. 22 spinal needle for injecting the trigger points. The injection site is identified by the onset of the typical referred pain or a local twitch response in the subscapularis muscle as the needle first enters the active trigger point. The injection is then followed by a spray and stretch program, followed by hot packs to the anterior aspect of the shoulder.[124]

I am not aware of any controlled studies comparing these techniques with nontreatment or with more conventional treatment modalities.

DISTENTION ARTHROGRAPHY OR BRISEMENT

Distention of the shoulder joint at the time of arthrography by progressive injections of fluid may have a beneficial effect.[2, 21, 92, 102] During distention arthrography, using serial injections, progressively more fluid is injected, generating intra-articular pressures of 1000 to 1500 mm Hg.[102] In patients with frozen shoulder and a very restricted joint volume, the capsule often ruptures at these pressures in the area of the subscapularis bursa or the biceps tendon sheath.[2, 102]

In shoulders in which there is still a demonstrable subscapularis bursa at arthrography, the joint volume can usually be distended by serial injections, with pressures in the range of 1200 to 1800 mm Hg. However, there is only a small margin of safety between joint distention and biceps tendon sheath rupture. Arden and colleagues observed that it is necessary to achieve moderate joint distention for a more favorable outcome.[2]

Distention arthrography is reported to be most useful in patients with slight to moderately restricted shoulders.[2, 102] Pain relief may occur without significant change in the range of motion.[2] Older has observed that distention alone facilitates a patient's exercise program but, of its own, does not relieve pain or increase range of motion.[92] Distention arthrography can be repeated in an effort to get further improvement as there is little postdistention pain.[2] Reeves noted the recovery course was longer when distention arthrography was compared with manipulation.[102]

MANIPULATION

Manipulation under anesthesia as treatment for the painful, stiff shoulder has been a source of much controversy in orthopedic surgery.[28, 29, 64] The goal of treatment by manipulation of painful, stiff shoulders is to shorten the symptomatic course of the disease.[44, 46] Lundberg noted an increased rate of return of shoulder mobility after manipulation, but there was no effect on the total duration of the disease.[69]

Manipulation of the shoulder should be considered only in those patients with long-standing restricted range of motion who have failed to improve with a supervised treatment program. Such a program would include one or more of the following: analgesics, anti-inflammatory medications, exercises, steroid injections, or physiotherapy. For shoulder manipulation to be successful, the patient must be cooperative and capable of intellectually and physically carrying on with the required postmanipulation exercise program. The patient must be aware of the treatment alternatives and the risks of manipulation. The important risks include fractures about the shoulder, fractures of the shaft of the humerus, dislocation of the shoulder, postmanipulation pain, hemarthrosis, tearing of the joint capsule, tearing of the rotator cuff, and traction injury to nerves about the shoulder.

The recommended technique of shoulder manipulation for patients with frozen shoulder generally requires a general anesthetic or brachial plexus block. The aim is to manipulate the shoulder to regain glenohumeral motion, using controlled forces applied by using a short lever arm, i.e., the surgeon's manipulating hand held well above the elbow close to the shoulder joint. Helbig and associates caution against abrupt tearing of capsular structures and advise the judicious application of force, tempered by the response of the shoulder to the applied force.[48] Most authors prefer to stretch the inferior capsule first, taking care to stabilize the scapula while the arm is abducted.[45, 98] The scapula can be stabilized by the surgeon pushing it against the chest wall or by an assistant gripping the axillary border of the scapula as the arm is abducted. Downward pressure over the acromion can have the same effect. The shoulder can then be manipulated into external rotation and internal rotation in an effort to obtain the greatest range of motion to the limit of safety.[67, 98] The definite audible and palpable release of resistance that may be experienced on manipulation is thought by some to be a good prognostic sign.[46, 58, 98, 99] While under anesthesia, the motion should not be forced if the tissues seem to offer unyielding resistance.[69] A repeat manipulation, if necessary, can be done in an effort to achieve a final range of motion sequentially, in stages, without exceeding the safety limit of stretching the shoulder capsule.[44, 46, 48]

Postmanipulation care is most important. Patients may be reluctant to move their shoulders into full abduction for several days following the manipulation. Neviaser described a postmanipulation treatment plan that involved three to five days in the hospital with the arm supported at 90 degrees of abduction and encouraged early range of motion. Ongoing support of the arm in 90 degrees of abduction at night for three weeks is recommended.[87]

Contraindications to manipulation of the shoulder under anesthesia for the management of frozen shoulder include (1) frozen shoulders that result from a shoulder dislocation or fracture of the proximal humerus; (2) patients who have moderate bone atrophy on shoulder radiographs; and (3) patients who are unable to cooperate with the required postmanipulation exercise program. A relative contraindication to manipulation is patients who are in the acute and irritable phase of frozen shoulder.[67]

Reports of the results of shoulder manipulation are variable; figures show from 26 to 81 per cent of patients being significantly better at three months postmanipulation and 70 per cent improved at six months.[20, 46, 48, 67, 99, 102] No well-controlled studies were found that substantiated claims of superiority for this method of treatment. Kessel and colleagues felt that patients with symptoms lasting more than six months before treatment had a more dramatic response to manipulation than those with symptoms of less than six months.[58] The relationship of duration of symptoms to outcome is not supported in other series.[45, 48, 67]

At manipulation, the joint capsule is torn in a significant proportion of cases. DePalma and others have observed the tearing of the shoulder capsule when manipulation was carried out under direct observation.* The most frequent capsular tear follow-

ing manipulation is along the inferior capsule, but tears have also been observed to involve the intra-articular long head of the biceps and the subscapularis tendon.[28, 76, 102] Recurrent hemorrhagic effusion or hematomas may also occur.[48, 69] Other potential complications, such as a fracture of the humerus or a shoulder dislocation, have been reported infrequently.[45, 99] The potential for injury is always present, and suitable precautions must be taken.

MANIPULATION AND STEROID INJECTION

Several authors have recommended injecting the shoulder joint with a corticosteroid preparation at the time of manipulation in an effort to diminish postmanipulation pain and inflammation. These authors report improvement of their patients, with 33 to 83 per cent recovery at three months, using a wide variety in evaluation techniques.[45, 48, 55, 67, 98, 123]

MANIPULATION AND SYSTEMIC STEROIDS

Systemic steroids have been used in conjunction with manipulation. The steroids did not diminish the postmanipulation pain. Bayley believed that there was some benefit in hastening recovery of range of motion in flexion and external rotation, but no statistical significance was reported.[5] Lloyd-Roberts and colleagues observed that systemic steroids were without clear benefit.[3] If possible, one should consider an alternative treatment to avoid the risk of systemic steroids.[77]

MANIPULATION UNDER LOCAL ANESTHESIA

Manipulation of the shoulder with local anesthesia injected with or without arthrographic control has been advocated.[40, 68, 127] Pain relief was observed in 60 to 78 per cent of the patients, and a return of normal functional range of shoulder motion occurred in 61 to 70 per cent.[68, 127] Weiser's results show a strong inverse correlation between the degree of disability at onset and the outcome of this treatment method.[127]

OTHER CLOSED TREATMENT TECHNIQUES

Oral Corticosteroids

Systemic steroids have been recommended for use in frozen shoulder syndrome for their anti-inflammatory effect.[71] Binder and associates noted a more rapid initial recovery when compared with controls, but by five months follow-up, there was no distinguishable difference between the patient groups.[9] The potential side effects of this mode of treatment need to be taken into consideration in planning treatment.[23]

---

*See references 2, 6, 28, 31, 67, 76, 91, 97, 102.

Traction

Rizk and colleagues have reported on a manipulative technique using traction to bring the humerus into abduction. A transcutaneous electrical nerve stimulator (TENS) unit was used for pain control. The technique involved 15 minutes of traction in progressive abduction repeated up to 8 times on each of 28 physiotherapy visits over an 8-week period. They reported that pain relief and range of motion were improved when compared with improvement in patients receiving more conventional physiotherapy.[106]

Radiotherapy

Radiotherapy for the treatment of frozen shoulder in North America is of historical interest as it has not been conclusively shown to be of significant benefit. Its use has been discontinued because potentially less dangerous treatment modalities offer results at least as good. In one series, 200 patients were given 1200 rads over 10 weeks; when reviewed at 3 months, 70 per cent were better, and 12 were considered failures.[141] Coventry believed that radiotherapy did not have much effect on chronic forms of frozen shoulder.[22] Angiolini and colleagues used x-ray therapy for frozen shoulder in a series of 605 patients; dosages of up to 1800 rads were used. The pain resolved and function of the affected shoulder was restored in 55 per cent while 27 per cent were improved.[3] In a review of patients receiving x-ray therapy, Quin could find no advantage of radiotherapy over heat treatment and exercises, when assessed by outcome at two and three months and the time required for full recovery.[101]

Stellate Ganglion Block

Stellate ganglion blocks have been used on the premise that frozen shoulder is a type of autonomic dysfunction. When compared with other treatment modalities, a stellate ganglion block offers no advantages.[131]

SURGICAL TREATMENT

Arthroscopic Surgery

Neviaser made no attempt to treat the joint contracture arthroscopically.[86, 87] Ogilvie-Harris and colleagues have performed an arthroscopically controlled release of tight anterior capsular structures. They report favorable results in a small group of patients.[91]

Open Surgical Release

Because of the inconsistent results of closed manipulation of the shoulder and the unpredictable tearing of capsular structures at manipulation, McLaughlin advised open mobilization of the shoulder with release of the subscapularis tendon, excision of the intra-articular portion of the biceps tendon, and release of joint adhesions by blunt dissection.[76] In postfracture or postoperative stiff shoulders, it may also be necessary to free up the subdeltoid/subacromial space as well as the space between the coracoid and the subscapularis muscle. Others recommend looking at and possibly releasing the coracohumeral ligament, which, if contracted, may act as a block to external rotation.[28, 64]

In planning treatment, it is prudent to restrict the use of manipulation to those few patients who have failed to respond to other, less invasive treatment measures.[20, 31] For the patient with very little glenohumeral motion and diminished bone stock, one should consider proceeding to open surgical release of the shoulder if there is no improvement with other treatment modalities.[64, 76]

Author's Preferred Method of Treatment

At the initial assessment it is most important to obtain a complete history of the shoulder symptoms and a good functional enquiry into other medical problems that could be related, e.g., diabetes mellitus, trauma, cervical spondylosis, chest symptoms, cardiac symptoms, or systemic disorders.

I insist on recent anteroposterior and axillary radiographs of the shoulder which must be of diagnostic quality. Radiographs of the cervical spine are reviewed if indicated by the history and physical examination. An attempt is made to determine whether the presentation is that of a primary or secondary frozen shoulder. If a secondary frozen shoulder is diagnosed, concurrent treatment of the precipitating factor is also started when possible.

Where patients with pain and restricted range of motion are found early, treatment is started with salicylate analgesics, with or without codeine, and a program of pendulum exercises. The pendulum exercises are done for one to two minutes every one to two hours while the patient is awake. If the patient should awaken during the night, I suggest that pendulum exercises done for one to two minutes are often more beneficial than analgesics for the night pain.

At follow-up two or three weeks later, if pain remains a major problem, I recommend an intra-articular injection of 10 mg of triamcinolone acetonide and 1 per cent lidocaine. For this injection, I prefer a posterior approach to the glenohumeral joint using a No. 22 or No. 20 spinal needle. The humeral head guides the needle into the joint with passive external rotation. Such an injection has, in the majority of cases, given significant pain relief. If good pain relief is obtained temporarily and the pain recurs, I will repeat the injection once. Other modalities, such as TENS, spray and stretch, or trigger point injections, have been used in a few cases.

For patients who present with moderate to marked stiffness and whose pain is primarily at the end of the range of motion, I prefer to begin with a stretching program at the time of the initial visit. Patients who presented earlier with pain and whose pain has been brought under control will then follow this stretching program. All patients are instructed in pendulum exercises. Patients are encouraged to warm up before the stretching exercises by doing pendulum exercises or applying heat in the form of a hot bath, hot shower, or hot pack. The stretching exercise routine is modified from that described by Hughes and colleagues, concentrating on passive forward elevation and external rotation.[50] The forward elevation stretch is done by assisted elevation of the arm to reach up to a solid object that is just beyond reach. Patients stand on tiptoes, then lower themselves and sustain a moderate stretch adjusted to tolerance for 20 to 30 seconds. This stretching is repeated five times, and then the arm is lifted down using the opposite arm, since a free fall from the new upper limit of forward elevation can be very painful. External rotation stretch is done with the arm at the side and the elbow flexed to 90 degrees. The patient rotates the trunk with the hand fixed on the side of a door frame to stretch the anterior structures to allow further external rotation. A sustained stretch for 30 to 60 seconds is recommended. This exercise may cause elbow pain, and thus, careful instructions and monitoring are important.

Once these exercises are under way, a program of strengthening within the newly achieved range of motion is started. I recommend starting to work on forward elevation strengthening, progressing the resistance or load only when 10 repetitions are done without difficulty. Patients are asked to start strengthening in the supine position, lifting up to 3 kg. Following that, exercises can be started in a sitting position, dropping back to a load of 250 grams, before progressing as tolerated in stages up to 5 to 10 kg. External rotation strengthening is usually achieved using an elastic resistance looped around the wrists and rotating both forearms into external rotation with the arms at the side and the elbows flexed at right angles. Five repetitions holding for five seconds are done, progressing the resistance as tolerated.

At the next visit, usually two to three weeks later, the patient is again examined and the progress plotted. The exercises are reviewed and refined as needed. I then add stretching into internal rotation, initially by stretching into extension using a stick behind the back. When 15 to 20 cm of clearance is possible behind the back, the stick is discontinued, and the good arm is used to pull the hand of the affected arm up the back, progressively achieving more internal rotation. A towel in the opposite hand passed over the opposite shoulder pulling the affected hand up the back may accomplish the same effect.

Internal rotation strengthening is then started using an elastic resistance looped over a door handle. The patient rotates the arm across the opposite chest wall and holds the position for five seconds for five repetitions.

As the range of motion improves, further resistance can be added to the strengthening program in all directions. Many patients, when they achieve 150 degrees of forward elevation and 45 degrees of external rotation with internal rotation to the level of the 12th thoracic spinous process, will discontinue exercises because they feel they have achieved full function. Patients are encouraged to continue with their exercises for three to five minutes, twice daily, for another three months. When a functional range of motion is achieved, I encourage them to stretch in all directions, including abduction, to stretch wherever they feel stiff. I hold off stretching in abduction until this point because I find that many patients develop an impingement type of pain if they start stretching into abduction too early. A plausible explanation for the impingement is that the humeral head cannot glide inferiorly to clear the coracoacromial arch in the initial phases of the stretching program.

Patients who continue to have pain need to be reinterviewed and re-examined, and the physician must look for other causes of pain. If the pain is exacerbated by resisted external rotation or abduction and if the patient does not improve, I will then proceed to do an arthrogram to rule out a rotator cuff tear. Unfortunately, partial-thickness rotator cuff tears often cannot be visualized using this technique. The characteristic joint space contracture of frozen shoulder at arthrography is a reassurance that the diagnosis of frozen shoulder is correct.

Patients who fail to improve with the above program or who I judge are unable to exercise on their own are sent to a physiotherapist with a prescription for pain-relieving modalities and stretching exercises in forward elevation, external rotation, and internal rotation. Gentle stretching in other directions is often included. Ultrasound is added empirically for its thermal and possible tissue extensibility effects. Patients are reviewed after three weeks and the program is modified as needed. If the therapy is making the condition more painful for the patient, the program is modified, a new therapist is sought, or the program is discontinued on an individual basis.

Occasionally, a patient who fails to progress with a supervised stretching program is admitted to the hospital for manipulation under anesthesia. The manipulation is started in abduction, stabilizing the scapula and abducting the humerus to achieve as much motion as judged possible. The extent to which the manipulation can be pushed depends on the resistance of the tissues and the quality of the bone and soft tissues of that specific patient. Following manipulation, patients are given an intra-articular injection of 20 mg of triamcinolone acetonide. The patients start on the day of manipulation in a gentle range-of-motion program for forward elevation and external rotation, including the use of a pulley for stretching. The exercises are continued in the hospital until it is clear the patient is capable of continuing with a home exercise program. Very rarely a repeat manipulation may be undertaken when the patient rapidly loses the motion achieved at closed manipulation.

I have no personal experience with distention brisement of the shoulder capsule.

Open release of the shoulder in my hands has been restricted to post-traumatic stiff shoulders with subacromial adhesions as well as the characteristic changes in the shoulder capsule. Open release in primary frozen shoulder may be considered when there is moderate pain and persistent stiffness or when the bone quality is less than ideal, greatly increasing the risk of fracture with a closed manipulation.

It is important to keep in mind that there are no serious complications of frozen shoulder itself so that, on occasion, a judgment has to be made to accept a restricted range of motion. Many patients have functioned quite well with a moderately restricted shoulder range of motion; at times, I have chosen to accept these restrictions of range of motion rather than undertake a manipulation under anesthesia or an open surgical release in selected patients.

References

1. Allander E, Bjornsson OJ, Olafsson O, et al: Normal range of joint movements in shoulder, hip, wrist and thumb with special reference to side: a comparison between two populations. Int J Epidemiol 64:539–542, 1983.
2. Andren L, and Lundberg BJ: Treatment of rigid shoulders by joint distension during arthrography. Acta Orthop Scand 36:45–53, 1965.
3. Angiolini G, Pasquinelli V, and Putti C: La roentgenterapia nella cura della periartrite della spalla. Minerva Medica 56:504–508, 1965.
4. Askey JM: The syndrome of painful disability of the shoulder and hand complicating coronary occlusion. Am Heart J 22:1–12, 1961.
5. Bayley JIL, and Kessel L: Treatment of the frozen shoulder by manipulation: a pilot study. In Shoulder Surgery. Berlin-Heidelberg: Springer-Verlag, 1982, pp 118–123.
6. Berry H, Fernandes I, Bloom B, et al: Clinical study comparing acupuncture, physiotherapy, injection and oral anti-inflammatory therapy in shoulder-cuff lesions. Curr Med Res Opin 7:121–126, 1980.
7. Binder AI, Bulgen DY, Hazleman DL, and Roberts S: Frozen shoulder: a long term prospective study. Ann Rheum Dis 43:361–364, 1984.
8. Binder AI, Bulgen DY, Hazleman BL, et al: Frozen shoulder: an arthrographic and radionuclear scan assessment. Ann Rheum Dis 43:365–369, 1984.
9. Binder A, Hazleman BL, Parr G, and Roberts S: A controlled study of oral prednisolone in frozen shoulder. Br J Rheumatol 25:288–292, 1986.
10. Bohannon RW, Larkin PA, Smith MB, and Horton MG: Shoulder pain in hemiplegia: statistical relationship with five variables. Arch Phys Med Rehabil 67:514–516, 1986.
11. Bridgman JF: Periarthritis of the shoulder and diabetes mellitus. Ann Rheum Dis 31:69–71, 1972.
12. Bruckner FE, and Nye CJS: A prospective study of adhesive capsulitis of the shoulder in a high risk population. Q J Med 198:191–204, 1981.
13. Bulgen DY, and Hazleman BL: Letter. Lancet 2:760, 1981.
14. Bulgen DY, Binder AI, Hazleman BL, et al: Frozen shoulder: prospective clinical study with an evaluation of three treatment regimens. Ann Rheum Dis 43:353–360, 1984.
15. Bulgen DY, Binder A, Hazleman BL, and Park JP: Immunological studies in frozen shoulder. J Rheumatol 9(6):893–898, 1982.
16. Bulgen DY, Hazleman BL, and Voak D: HLA-B27 and frozen shoulder. Lancet 1:1042–1044, 1976.
17. Charnley J: Periarthritis of the shoulder. Postgrad Med J 35:384–388, 1959.
18. Clarke GR, Willis LA, Fish WW, and Nichols PJR: Preliminary studies in measuring range of motion in normal and painful stiff shoulders. Rheumatol Rehabil 14:39–46, 1975.
19. Codman EA: The Shoulder. Boston: Thomas Todd Co., 1934.
20. Connolly J, Regan E, and Evans OB: Management of the painful, stiff shoulder. Clin Orthop 84:97–103, 1972.
21. Conti V: Arthroscopy in rehabilitation. Orthop Clin North Am 10(3):709–711, 1979.
22. Coventry MB: Problem of the painful shoulder. JAMA 151:177–185, 1953.
23. Cruess RL: Corticosteroid-induced osteonecrosis of the humeral head. Orthop Clin North Am 16(4):789–796, 1985.
24. Curran JF, Ellman MH, and Brown NL: Rheumatologic aspects of painful conditions affecting the shoulder. Clin Orthop 173:27–37, 1983.
25. Cyriax J: The shoulder. Br J Hosp Med 19:185–192, 1975.
26. Cyriax J: Textbook of Orthopaedic Medicine. London: Bailliere Tindall, 1975, pp 182–184.
27. Cyriax J, and Trosier O: Hydrocortisone and soft tissue lesions. Br Med J 2:966–968, 1953.
28. De Seze S: Les epaules douloureuses et les epaules bloquees. Concours Medical 96(36):5329–5357, 1974.
29. DePalma AF: Loss of scapulohumeral motion (frozen shoulder). Ann Surg 135(2):193–204, 1952.
30. Detrisac DA, and Johnson LL: Arthroscopic shoulder anatomy. Thorofare, N.J.: Slack, Inc., 1986, pp 111–113.
31. Dickson JA, and Crosby EH: Periarthritis of the shoulder: an analysis of two hundred cases. JAMA 99:2252–2257, 1932.
32. Duplay ES: De la periarthrite scapulohumerale et des raideurs de l'epaule qui en son la consequence. Arch Gen Med 20:513–542, 1872.
33. Engleman RM: Shoulder pain as a presenting complaint in upper lobe bronchogenic carcinoma: Report of 21 cases. Conn Med 30:273–276, 1966.
34. Ernstene AC, and Kinell J: Pain in the shoulder as a sequel to myocardial infarction. Arch Intern Med 66:800–806, 1940.
35. Farbe P, Ziegler G, Perrault C, and Pallardy G: Epaules douloureuses et limitees. Concours Medical 97(10):1589–1607, 1975.
36. Fearnley ME, and Vadasz I: Factors influencing the response of lesions of the rotator cuff of the shoulder to local steroid injection. Ann Phys Med 10:53–63, 1969.
37. Fisher L, Kurtz A, and Shipley M: Association between cheiroarthropathy and frozen shoulder in patients with insulin dependent diabetes mellitus. Br J Rheumatol 25:141–146, 1986.
38. Fleming A, Dodman S, Beer TC, and Crown S: Personality in frozen shoulder. Ann Rheum Dis 35:456–457, 1976.
39. Freedman L, and Munro RR: Abduction of the arm in the scapular plane: scapular and glenohumeral movements. A roentgenographic study. J Bone Joint Surg 48:1503–1510, 1966.
40. Gilula LA, Schoenecker PL, and Murphy WA: Shoulder arthrography as a treatment modality. AJR 131:1047–1048, 1978.
41. Goldman AB, and Ghelman B: The double contrast shoulder arthrogram. A review of 158 cases. Radiology 127:655–663, 1978.
42. Grey RG: The natural history of idiopathic frozen shoulder. J Bone Joint Surg 60:564, 1978.
43. Haeri GB, and Maitland A: Arthroscopic findings in the frozen shoulder. J Rheumatol 8:149–152, 1981.
44. Haggart GE, Digman RJ, and Sullivan TS: Management of the frozen shoulder. JAMA 161:1219–1222, 1956.
45. Haines JF, and Hargadon EJ: Manipulation as the primary treatment of the frozen shoulder. J R Coll Surg Edinb. 27(5):271–275, 1982.
46. Harmon PH: Methods and results in the treatment of 2580 painful shoulders. Am J Surg 95:527–544, 1958.
47. Hazleman BL: The painful stiff shoulder. Rheumatol Rehabil 11:413–421, 1972.
48. Helbig B, Wagner P, and Dohler R: Mobilization of frozen

shoulder under general anaesthesia. Acta Orthop Belg 49:267–274, 1983.
49. Hollingworth GR: Comparison of injection techniques for shoulder pain. Br Med J [Clin Res] 287:1339–1341, 1983.
50. Hughes MA, and Neer CS: Glenohumeral joint replacement and postoperative rehabilitation. Phys Ther 55:850–858, 1975.
51. Inmann VT, Saunders JB, and Abbott LC: Observations on the shoulder joint. J Bone Joint Surg 26:1–30, 1944.
52. Johnston JTH: Frozen shoulder in patients with pulmonary tuberculosis. J Bone Joint Surg 41:877–882, 1959.
53. Kaltsas DS: Comparative study of the properties of the shoulder joint capsule with those of other joint capsules. Clin Orthop 173:20–26, 1983.
54. Kamieth H: Radiology of the cervical spine in shoulder periarthritis. Z Orthop 100:162–167, 1965.
55. Kay N: The clinical diagnosis and management of frozen shoulders. Practioner 225:164–172, 1981.
56. Kernwein GA, Roseberg B, and Sneed WA: Arthrographic studies of the shoulder. J Bone Joint Surg 39:1267–1279, 1957.
57. Kessel L: Clinical Disorders of the Shoulder. New York: Churchill Livingstone, 1982, p 82.
58. Kessel L, Bayley I, and Young A: The frozen shoulder. Br J Hosp Med 25:334–339, 1981.
59. Kopell HP, and Thompson WAL: Pain and the frozen shoulder. Surg Gynecol Obstet 109:92–96, 1959.
60. Kraft GH, Johnson EW, and Laban MM: The fibrositis syndrome. Arch Phys Med Rehabil 49:155–162, 1968.
61. Last RJ: Anatomy, Regional and Applied, 5th ed. London: Churchill Livingstone, 1972, p. 106.
62. Lee M, Haq AM, Wright V, and Longton E: Periarthritis of the shoulder: a controlled trial of physiotherapy. Physiotherapy 59:312–315, 1973.
63. Lee PN, Lee M, Haq AM, et al: Periarthritis of the shoulder: trial of treatments investigated by multivariate analysis. Ann Rheum Dis 33:116–119, 1974.
64. Leffert RD: The frozen shoulder. Instr Course Lect 34:199–203, 1985.
65. Lequesne M, Dang N, Bensasson M, and Mery C: Increased association of diabetes mellitus with capsulitis of the shoulder and shoulder-hand syndrome. Scand J Rheumatol 6:53–56, 1977.
66. Lippman RK: Frozen shoulder: bicipital tenosynovitis. Arch Surg 47:283–296, 1943.
67. Lloyd-Roberts GC, and French PR: Periarthritis of the shoulder, a study of the disease and its treatment. Br Med J 1:1569–1571, 1959.
68. Loyd JA, and Loyd HM: Adhesive capsulitis of the shoulder: arthrographic diagnosis and treatment. South Med J 76(7):879–883, 1983.
69. Lundberg BJ: The frozen shoulder. Acta Orthop Scand [Suppl] 119:1–59, 1969.
70. Lundberg BJ: Pathomechanics of the frozen shoulder and the effect of the brisement force. In Bayley J, and Kessel L (eds): Shoulder Surgery. Berlin-Heidelberg: Springer-Verlag, 1982, pp 107–110.
71. Macnab I: The painful shoulder due to rotator cuff tendinitis. RI Med J 54:367–374, 1971.
72. Macnab I: Rotator cuff tendinitis. Ann R Coll Surg Engl 53:271–287, 1973.
73. Maitland GD: Treatment of the glenohumeral joint by passive movement. Physiotherapy 69:3–7, 1983.
74. Matsen FA, and Kirby RM: Office evaluation and management of shoulder pain. Orthop Clin North Am 13(2):453–475, 1982.
75. McLaughlin HL: On the frozen shoulder. Bull Hosp Jt Dis 12:383–393, 1951.
76. McLaughlin HL: The frozen shoulder. Clin Orthop 20:126–131, 1961.
77. Meulengracht E, and Schwartz M: Course and prognosis of periarthritis humeroscapularis. Acta Med Scand 143:350–360, 1952.
78. Moren-Hybbinette I, Moritz U, and Schersten B: The clinical picture of the painful diabetic shoulder: natural history, social consequences and analysis of concomitant hand syndrome. Acta Med Scand 221:73–82, 1987.
79. Moseley HF: Shoulder Lesions. Springfield, IL: Charles C Thomas, 1945, p 66.
80. Murnaghan GF, and McIntosh D: Hydrocortisone in painful shoulder: a controlled trial. Lancet 269:798–800, 1955.
81. Murray MP, Gore DR, Gardner GM, and Mollinger LR: Shoulder motion and muscle strength of normal men and women in two age groups. Clin Orthop 192:268–273, 1985.
82. Neviaser JS: Adhesive capsulitis of the shoulder. J Bone Joint Surg 27:211–222, 1945.
83. Neviaser JS: Arthrography of the shoulder joint. J Bone Joint Surg 44:1321–1330, 1962.
84. Neviaser JS: Arthrography of the Shoulder. Springfield, IL: Charles C Thomas, 1975, pp 60–66.
85. Neviaser RJ: Painful conditions affecting the shoulder. Clin Orthop 173:63–69, 1983.
86. Neviaser RJ, and Neviaser TJ: The frozen shoulder diagnosis and management. Clin Orthop 223:59–64, 1987.
87. Neviaser TJ: Arthroscopy of the shoulder. Orthop Clin North Am 18(3):361–372, 1987.
88. Neviaser TJ: Adhesive capsulitis. Orthop Clin North Am 18(3):439–443, 1987.
89. Nicholson GG: The effects of passive joint mobilization on pain and hypomobility associated with adhesive capsulitis of the shoulder. Orthop Sports Phys Ther 6:238–246, 1985.
90. Oesterreicher W, and Van Dam G: Social psychological researches into brachialgia and periarthritis. Arthritis Rheum 6:670–683, 1964.
91. Ogilvie-Harris DJ, and Wiley AM: Arthroscopic surgery of the shoulder. J Bone Joint Surg 68:201–207, 1986.
92. Older MWJ: Distension arthrography of the shoulder joint. In Bayley J, and Kessel L (eds): Shoulder Surgery. Berlin-Heidelberg: Springer-Verlag, 1982, pp 123–127.
93. Oldham BE: Periarthritis of the shoulder associated with thyrotoxicosis. NZ Med J 29:766–770, 1959.
94. Pal B, Anderson J, Dick WC, and Griffiths ID: Limitation of joint mobility and shoulder capsulitis in insulin and non-insulin dependent diabetes mellitus. Br J Rheumatol 25:147–151, 1986.
95. Pasteur F: Les algies de l'epaule et la physiotherapie. J Radiol Electrol 16:419–426, 1932.
96. Poppen NK, and Walker PS: Forces at the glenohumeral joint in abduction. Clin Orthop 135:165–170, 1978.
97. Post M: The Shoulder. Philadelphia: Lea & Febiger, 1978, pp 281–284.
98. Quigley TB: Checkrein shoulder, a type of frozen shoulder. N Engl J Med 250:188–192, 1954.
99. Quigley TB: Indications for manipulation and corticosteroids in the treatment of stiff shoulders. Surg Clin North Am 43:1715–1720, 1969.
100. Quin EH: Frozen shoulder: evaluation of treatment with hydrocortisone injections and exercises. Ann Phys Med 8:22–25, 1965.
101. Quin EH: Humeroscapular periarthritis. Observations on the effects of x-ray therapy and ultrasonic therapy in cases of "frozen shoulder." Ann Phys Med 10:64–69, 1969.
102. Reeves B: Arthrographic changes in frozen and post traumatic stiff shoulders. Proc R Soc Med 59:827–830, 1966.
103. Reeves B: The natural history of the frozen shoulder syndrome. Scand J Rheumatol 4:193–196, 1975.
104. Resnick D: Shoulder pain. Orthop Clin North Am 14(1):81–97, 1983.
105. Richardson AT: The painful shoulder. Proc R Soc Med 68:731–736, 1975.
106. Rizk TE, Christopher RP, Pinals RS, et al: Adhesive capsulitis (frozen shoulder): a new approach to its management. Arch Phys Med Rehabil 64:29–33, 1983.
107. Rizk TE, and Pinals RS: Frozen shoulder. Sem Arthritis Rheum 11(4):440–452, 1982.
108. Rizk TE, and Pinals RS: Histocompatibility type and racial incidence in frozen shoulder. Arch Phys Med Rehabil 65:33–34, 1984.

109. Roy S, and Oldham R: Management of painful shoulder. Lancet *1*:1322–1324, 1976.
110. Russik AS: Scapulo costal syndrome. JAMA *150*:25–27, 1952.
111. Saha ND: Painful shoulder in patients with chronic bronchitis and emphysema. Am Rev Respir Dis *94*:455–456, 1966.
112. Sany J, Cillens JP, and Rousseau JR: Evolution lointaine de la retraction capsulaire de l'epaule. Revue Rhumatisme *49*(11):815–819, 1982.
113. Sattar MA, and Luqman WA: Periarthritis: another duration-related complication of diabetes mellitus. Diabetes Care 8:507–510, 1985.
114. Schwartzman RJ, and McLellan TL: Reflex sympathetic dystrophy. Arch Neurol *44*:555–561, 1987.
115. Seignalet J, Sany J, Caillens JP, and Lapinski H: Lack of association between HLA-B27 and frozen shoulder. Tissue Antigens *18*:364, 1981.
116. Simmonds FA: Shoulder pain with particular reference to the frozen shoulder. J Bone Joint Surg *31*:834–838, 1949.
117. Simon WH: Soft tissue disorders of the shoulder. Orthop Clin North Am *6*(2):521–539, 1949.
118. Simons DB: Myofascial pain syndromes: where are we? where are we going? Arch Phys Med Rehabil 69:207–212, 1988.
119. Steinbrocker O. Shoulder-hand syndrome. Am Med *3*:402–407, 1947.
120. Steinbrocker O: Frozen shoulder: present perspective. Arch Phys Med Rehabil *49*:388–395, 1968.
121. Steinbrocker O, and Argyros TG: Frozen shoulder: treatment by local injections of depot steroids. Arch Phys Med Rehabil 55:209–213, 1974.
122. Stodell MA, Nicholson R, Scot J, and Sturrock RD: Radio-isotope scanning in painful shoulder syndromes. Ann Rheum Dis *38*:496, 1979.
123. Thomas D, Williams RA, and Smith DS: The frozen shoulder: a review of manipulative treatment. Rheumatol Rehabil *19*:173–179, 1980.
124. Travell JG, and Simmons DG: Myofascial Pain and Dysfunction: Trigger Point Manual. Baltimore: Williams & Wilkins, 1983, pp 410–424.
125. Tyber MA: Treatment of the painful shoulder syndrome with amitriptyline and lithium carbonate. Can Med Assoc J *111*:137–140, 1974.
126. Watson Jones R: Simple treatment of stiff shoulders. J Bone Joint Surg *45*:207, 1963.
127. Weiser HI: Painful primary frozen shoulder mobilization under local anaesthesia. Arch Phys Med Rehabil *58*:406–408, 1977.
128. Weiss JJ, and Ting YM: Arthrography assisted intra-articular injection of steroids in treatment of adhesive capsulitis. Arch Phys Med Rehabil *59*:285–287, 1978.
129. Welfling J, Kahn MF, Desray M, et al: Les calcifications de l'epaule. Rev Rheum *32*:325–334, 1965.
130. Wiley AM, and Older MW: Shoulder arthroscopy. Am J Sports Med 8:31–38, 1980.
131. Wiley AM: Arthroscopic examination of the shoulder. *In* Bayley J, and Kessel L (eds): Shoulder Surgery. Berlin-Heidelberg: Springer-Verlag, 1982, pp 113–118.
132. Williams NE, Seifert MH, Cuddigan JHB, and Wise RA: Treatment of capsulitis of the shoulder. Rheumatol Rehabil *14*:236, 1975.
133. Withers RJW: The painful shoulder: review of one hundred personal cases with remarks on the pathology. J Bone Joint Surg *31*:414–417, 1949.
134. Withrington RH, Girgis FL, and Seeifert MH: A comparative study of the aetiological factors in shoulder pain. Br J Rheumatol *24*:24–26, 1985.
135. Wohlgethan JR: Frozen shoulder in hyperthyroidism. Arthritis Rheum *30*:936–939, 1987.
136. Wolfe F: Fibrositis, fibromyalgia, and musculoskeletal disease: the current status of the fibrositis syndrome. Arch Phys Med Rehabil 69:527–531, 1988.
137. Wright MG, Richards AJ, and Clarke MB: 99-M pertechnetate scanning in capsulitis. Lancet *2*:1265, 1975.
138. Wright V, and Haq AM: Periarthritis of the shoulder I: aetiological considerations with particular reference to personality factors. Ann Rheum Dis *35*:213–219, 1976.
139. Wright V, and Haq AM: Periarthritis of the shoulder II: radiological features. Ann Rheum Dis 35:220–226, 1976.
140. Young A: Immunological studies in the frozen shoulder. *In* Bayley J, and Kessel L (eds): Shoulder Surgery. Berlin-Heidelberg: Springer-Verlag, 1982, pp 110–113.
141. Zilberberg Ch, and Leveille-Nizerolle M: La radiographie anti-inflammatoire dans 200 cas de periarthrite scapulo-humerale. Sem Hop Paris *52*(24):909–911, 1976.

CHAPTER

22

Muscle Ruptures Affecting the Shoulder Girdle

Michael A. Caughey, M.B.
Peter Welsh, M.B.

Injury to muscle structures is exceedingly common, yet many of these injuries remain poorly described and ill defined. Most injuries are not identified as the cause of significant long-term disability unless they involve a complete disruption of the muscle or its attachments. Fortunately, this complication is much less common than when a rupture involves the tendon, for example, in rotator cuff tears. Interference with function, particularly diminution of strength, has previously been the major means of confirming muscular injury, since it is accompanied by palpable deficiency or major atrophy of the muscle substance. The exact pathological process has, however, been seldom defined because muscle strains and minor disruptions rarely require the surgical exposure that allows documentation of pathology. Recently, computed tomography (CT) and magnetic resonance imaging (MRI) have provided means not hitherto possible of visualizing muscle injuries. Whereas in the past relatively few muscle injuries in the shoulder girdle have been described, these will undoubtedly be more often recorded and more accurately described in the future.

Brickner and Milch[8] classified muscle ruptures as resulting from the following causes: (1) active contraction, (2) contraction of an antagonist, (3) increase of tearing over cohesive power, (4) asynchronic contraction, and (5) the additional muscular force of another muscle.

Basically, however, one may consider most significant muscle ruptures as occurring when an actively contracting muscle group is overloaded by the application of a resisting load or external force that exceeds tissue tolerance. When this occurs, the muscle fibers are torn and the muscle sheath is disrupted, leading to a palpable defect in the muscle. The defect can only heal by the formation of scar tissue. Effective surgical repair of muscle injury is very difficult.

General Principles of Rupture of the Musculotendinous Unit

The classic experiments of McMaster[52] demonstrated the relative strengths of a bone, muscle, tendon, bone preparation. He suspended the gastrocnemius of the amputated limb of an adult rabbit by passing a wire through the femur and attaching increasing weights to the os calcis until rupture occurred. Between 10 and 21 kg the unit ruptured. In the seven preparations successfully tested, rupture occurred at the insertion in three with associated bony avulsion, at the origin in two with bony avulsion, and once each through the muscle belly and the musculotendinous junction. McMaster could produce rupture of the tendon midsubstance only after 50 per cent of its substance had been divided. Normal tendon appears to be the strongest component of the musculotendinous unit, a finding confirmed by Cronkite.[17]

The site or rupture may be influenced by the rate of loading. Welsh and coworkers[94] in 1971, testing a tendon–bone system in the rabbit, found that lower rates of loading were associated with rupture at the tendon–bone junction, whereas at higher rates the tendon broke at the site of clamping. The strength of the tendon–bone junction was also shown to be greater with more rapid loading.

The mechanism of injury may influence the site of rupture. For example, in rupture of the pectoralis major, McEntire and associates[49] noted that direct trauma more commonly resulted in muscle belly rupture whereas indirect trauma was more likely to produce rupture distally. Similarly, whereas rupture of the long head of the biceps is common and rupture at the insertion well recognized, biceps muscle belly rupture is exceedingly rare. Yet as many as 48 complete belly ruptures were described by Heckman and Levine[34] in parachutists in whom the injury was caused by direct trauma from the static line.

The site of rupture is also influenced by anatomical factors peculiar to the shoulder. Rupture occurs most commonly in the tendons of the long head of the biceps and the rotator cuff. The intra-articular course of the former and impingement and impaired vascularity of the latter predispose them to rupture.

Ruptures of the muscles of the shoulder girdle are uncommon. The literature does not abound with reports of such involvement. This chapter presents a comprehensive overview of the subject, with an account of lesions of the pectoralis major, deltoid, triceps, biceps, serratus anterior, coracobrachialis, and subscapularis muscles.

Rupture of the Pectoralis Major

HISTORICAL REVIEW

Rupture of the pectoralis major, first described by Patissier[71] in 1822, is a relatively rare injury. A comprehensive review of the literature by McEntire and colleagues[49] in 1972 revealed only 45 cases, to which they added 11 more. However, only 22 of the 56 patients had undergone surgical exploration, and 1 was confirmed at autopsy. Thus actual confirmation of the lesion was lacking in 33 patients, and cases of congenital absence of the pectoralis major may have been represented in this group. Since that time 29 additional cases have been published in the English-language literature, of which 19 have been confirmed surgically.

ANATOMY

The pectoralis major arises in a broad sheet as two distinct heads—an upper clavicular head and a lower sternocostal head—that spread to a complex trilaminar insertion along the lateral lip of the bicipital groove. A portion of the sternocostal head spirals on itself to produce the round appearance of the anterior axillary fold, with the result that the lowermost fibers are inserted most proximally on the humerus and in a crescent into the capsule of the shoulder joint. McEntire and associates[49] attribute the infrequency of complete ruptures of the pectoralis major to the layered form of the muscle and its complex insertion.

CLASSIFICATION

Pectoralis major ruptures may be classified according to the extent and the site of rupture. Type 1 ruptures consist of a contusion or sprain; Type 2 are partial ruptures; and Type 3 are complete ruptures of the

muscle origin, muscle belly, musculotendinous junction, or tendon, or avulsion of the insertion.

The majority of cases are undoubtedly partial, but 16 of the 18 cases reported since 1972 that came to surgery were complete. In these reports the predominant lesion was an avulsion from the humerus in 9 instances; musculotendinous junction and tendinous ruptures accounted for 3 cases each; only 1 involved rupture of the muscle itself.

INCIDENCE AND MECHANISMS

Pectoralis major rupture is relatively rare, only about 85 cases having been reported in the world literature. However, McEntire and colleagues[49] were able to add 11 cases from the Salt Lake City region; they believed that the injury occurs more commonly than reports indicate. The problem has been reported exclusively in males. Although the injury has occurred in patients ranging in age from newborns to 72-year-olds, the majority occur between the ages of 20 and 40.

Pectoralis major rupture follows extreme muscle tension or direct trauma, or a combination of both. Of the 56 cases reviewed by McEntire and coworkers,[49] excessive muscle tension caused 37 injuries and direct trauma 9. A combination of the two mechanisms was the cause in 4 cases, and spontaneous rupture was reported in 3 instances. In the more recent literature, excess tension injury was the cause in 20 patients and direct injury in 2. A typical mechanism of injury is weightlifting, in particular bench presses, which accounted for 4 of the 9 cases reported by Zeman and associates.[95] An attempt to break a fall, resulting in severe force applied to a maximally contracted pectoralis major muscle, is another common mechanism of injury.

There appears also to be a correlation between the mechanism of injury and the site of rupture. Direct trauma causes tears of the muscle belly, whereas excessive tension causes avulsion of the humeral insertion or disruption at the musculotendinous junction. Wrestlers have a propensity to disrupt the muscle at its upper sternoclavicular portion.

CLINICAL PRESENTATION

In the case of an acute injury, a history of excessive muscle stress, a direct blow, or a crush injury of the shoulder region is associated with severe, sharp, and often burning pain and a tearing sensation at the site of rupture. This is a major and severe injury that is accompanied by significant swelling and ecchymosis. Immediate shoulder dysfunction is apparent.

The physical findings depend on the site of rupture. If the muscle is injured in its proximal part, the swelling and ecchymosis usually is noted on the anterior part of the chest wall on the involved side. The muscle belly retracts toward the axillary fold, causing a prominent

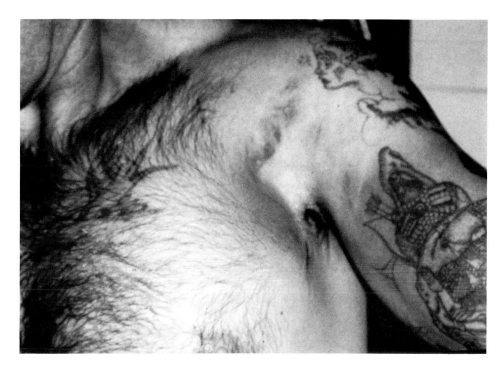

Figure 22–1. Rupture of the pectoralis major in a 30-year-old weightlifter. (Courtesy of J. J. Brownlee, M.D.)

bulge. Rupture in the distal part may cause swelling and ecchymosis in both the arm and the chest; the body of the muscle bulges on the chest, causing the axillary fold to become thin (Fig. 22–1). There is tenderness at the site of rupture, and a visible or palpable defect is usually present. Zeman and coworkers[95] described one patient in whom the tendon felt intact through to its humeral insertion. At surgery, however, a complete tear was found at the musculotendinous junction (Fig. 22–2), with an overlying fascial layer giving the impression of an intact tendon. These authors cautioned that the lack of a palpable defect in the axilla is not a reliable sign of continuity of the pectoralis major muscle. Resisted adduction and internal rotation of the arm are weak and are accom-

panied by accentuation of the defect and pain. Indeed, in cases presenting late this is the predominant sign, with the palpable defect confirmatory of the pathological process involved.

X-RAY AND LABORATORY EVALUATION

Although x-rays have generally failed to reveal any bony abnormality, loss of the normal pectoralis major shadow has been described as a reliable sign of rupture. Soft tissue shadowing is visible when a significant hematoma is present. Ultrasonography may be useful in confirming the site of rupture; MRI, if available, has the potential to demonstrate both the site and extent of muscle disruption.

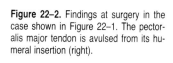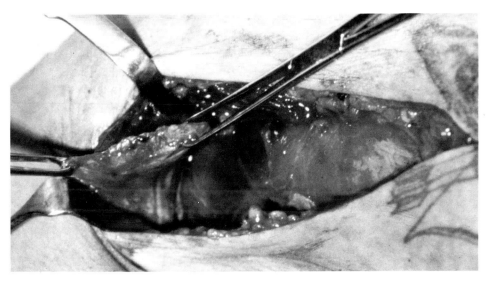

Figure 22–2. Findings at surgery in the case shown in Figure 22–1. The pectoralis major tendon is avulsed from its humeral insertion (right).

COMPLICATIONS

The most sinister complication of pectoralis major rupture is sepsis involving the associated hematoma. This has occurred in two reported cases,[61, 71] directly causing the death of one patient and leading to death by pneumonia of a second. Following a second injury to the pectoralis major muscle, pseudocyst formation occurring in a hematoma has been described by Ronchetti.[78] Associated neuromuscular injuries have been reported. Kawashima and associates[37] described a patient with a crush injury and total rupture of the pectoralis major at the musculotendinous junction with hypoesthesia of the C6–C8 and T1 dermatomes of the affected extremity. Several associated muscle injuries have also been described; these include rupture of the anteromedial portion of the adjacent deltoid, pectoralis minor rupture, and rotator cuff tears. Additional injuries in one patient included a fractured humerus and compound fractures of both forearm bones.

METHODS OF TREATMENT

Partial ruptures of the pectoralis major or lesions of the muscle belly respond to conservative treatment with initial icing and rest to control the hematoma. The early application of heat and ultrasound and a program of shoulder-mobilizing exercises, both passive and active assisted, help to restore shoulder function. Unresisted stretching exercises should be included early in the rehabilitation program, but resisted strengthening should await a six-week recovery with restoration of good shoulder mobility and settling of all pain.

Surgical Treatment

A complete rupture of the pectoralis major demands early surgical treatment in the active athlete. Results of late repair, although they may be satisfactory, are not as good as when primary repair is done.

Tendinous avulsion can be repaired by anatomical reattachment with heavy sutures through drill holes in the humeral cortex. When some tendon remains attached to the humerus, Orava and coworkers[64] have described an effective method of treatment by end-to-end repair of the tendons, reinforcing the repair with retention sutures into bone.

Musculotendinous junction tears can be sutured directly, but the shredding of tissue structure associated with muscle substance tears offers poor substance for repair and only imperfect results can be anticipated with this injury.

RESULTS OF TREATMENT

Park and Espiniella[67] in 1970 reviewed 31 patients reported in the literature. Surgical treatment produced an excellent result in 80 per cent of patients, with 10 per cent being rated good. This compared most favorably with the good results reported in only 58 per cent of patients treated nonoperatively. These authors stated that in the nonoperated group, varying degrees of weakness of adduction and internal rotation were present. However, over time the teres major, subscapularis, deltoid, and latissimus dorsi slowly take over the function of the pectoralis major. There are three cases reported of wrestlers returning to successful careers after nonoperative treatment. However, Gudmundsson[28] reports that normal power is rarely achieved in these instances. More recently, Zeman and colleagues[95] described nine athletes with ruptures of the pectoralis major. Surgical treatment was undertaken in four cases; all had excellent results. In the five patients treated nonoperatively, residual weakness was present in all; one professional boxer could not return to boxing, and two weightlifters had good results but were not entirely happy because of persistent weakness.

AUTHORS' PREFERRED TREATMENT

We use early surgical treatment for major avulsions at the musculotendinous junction. We treat ruptures of the muscle belly or partial lesions nonoperatively.

Rupture of the Deltoid

HISTORICAL REVIEW

The deltoid muscle is probably the single most important muscular structure in the shoulder girdle. Satisfactory function of the shoulder cannot be anticipated if it is irrevocably injured or its nerve supply compromised. Luckily, rupture of the deltoid muscle itself is a relatively uncommon clinical entity. First described by Clemens[13] in 1913 in a railway worker, reports in the literature have since been sparse. Davis[19] in 1919 reported one case in which the deltoid became detached following suppuration of its bony origin due to osteomyelitis of the clavicle. Gilcreest and Albi[27] described two further cases in 1939, but in the recent literature there is no report other than that of McEntire and coworkers[49] in 1972, describing a case associated with a rupture of the pectoralis major. Indeed, in the Mayo Clinic series of 1014 cases of musculotendinous rupture described by Anzel and colleagues,[2] no cases of deltoid rupture were seen.

ANATOMY

The deltoid is a multipennate muscle arising from the outer aspect of the anatomical "horseshoe" formed by the spine of the scapula, the acromion, and the outer end of the clavicle. It enfolds the shoulder and encloses the rotator cuff, inserting on the outer aspect of the humerus in the proximal one-third. Motor supply from the axillary or circumflex nerve reaches the muscle posteriorly on its undersurface.

MECHANISM

Minor strains of the deltoid are common in athletic activity, particularly in throwing sports. The anterior deltoid may be injured in the acceleration phase of throwing, when a forward body movement and a forcible contraction are simultaneously applied to an already stretched musculotendinous unit. In the follow-through phase at the end of forward motion of the arm, the posterior deltoid must restrain the shoulder and is vulnerable to injury.

Complete traumatic disruption of the deltoid, as the literature reviewed indicates, is extremely rare. Indeed, trauma to the deltoid most commonly seen in clinical practice is associated with misguided shoulder surgery. This is particularly true if the deltoid is detached from the acromion, resulting in a dehiscence. The posterior approach to the shoulder, releasing the deltoid from the spine of the scapula, is a major culprit in this regard.

In those instances in which traumatic rupture of the deltoid is incurred, it inevitably involves the application of a major external force to an already maximally contracted deltoid muscle.

The authors have recently reviewed one such case of a 62-year-old outdoor guide who had injured his right shoulder 10 years previously in a snowmobiling accident. After the machine rolled over him, notable swelling was defined at the deltoid insertion, with a palpable defect above.

CLINICAL PRESENTATION

Examination findings vary with the site of rupture. If the avulsion is from the origin, there is loss of the normal deltoid contour with weakness of abduction, flexion, or extension, depending upon the involved part. If the rotator cuff is also deficient, contraction of the remaining deltoid will cause the humeral head to protrude in the direction of the deltoid deficiency.

If the lesion is located near the deltoid insertion, a defect may be palpable, with an associated mass that becomes firmer upon contraction of the deltoid muscle.

METHODS OF TREATMENT

Minor strains and partial lesions of the deltoid muscle can be handled nonoperatively. Local icing in the acute phase followed by heat, mobilization of the shoulder, stretching, and gentle strengthening over the course of six weeks will usually restore the shoulder to full activity.

In the management of complete disruptions, there is no published experience to guide us. If such an injury is observed, consideration should be given to prompt surgical exploration in an effort to try to restore the structure anatomically. However, unless the injury is an avulsion from bone, the repair is likely to be weak. Midsubstance muscle injuries are difficult to suture effectively.

Delay in the repair with retraction and scarring makes the situation even more difficult. Davis[19] in 1919 first reported the management of a chronic defect of the anterior deltoid with a broad graft of fascia from the thigh. He recommended retaining a thick layer of subcutaneous fat to prevent adhesion formation between the rotator cuff and the fascial implant. Clearly, the late salvage of this injury is not satisfactory; if deltoid ruptures are to be dealt with satisfactorily, early identification and prompt surgical repair are mandatory.

Postoperative care following such surgery is vital. Abduction or flexion splinting to relieve the tension on the repair is maintained for six weeks or so before mobilization is commenced, and a strengthening program is not introduced for six to eight weeks following intervention.

AUTHORS' PREFERRED TREATMENT

We carry out early surgical treatment in those cases involving a complete disruption of one-third or more of the deltoid substance. Lesser degrees of tear and strains are treated nonoperatively. The problem of compromise of the deltoid origin by previous surgery is a difficult one. When an acromionectomy has been performed, reconstruction is not possible because the important anterolateral deltoid has lost its origin. With symptomatic failure of deltoid reattachment after acromioplasty, we consider re-exploration, mobilization of the superficial and deep aspects of the muscle, and repair back to the acromion. Postoperative protection is necessary to avoid active flexion and passive extension.

Rupture of the Triceps

HISTORICAL REVIEW

Partridge[69] in 1868 reported the first case of rupture of the triceps in a patient who fell partly on the roadway and partly on the sidewalk, striking the left arm just above and behind the elbow joint. He observed a 3/4-inch-long depression and a slight wound above and behind the elbow, in addition to tenderness over the triceps tendon. The arm was held extended and quiet for one week, following which passive motion commenced. Only eight more cases were reported over the next 100 years before Tarsney[88] added seven cases, clarifying the mechanism of injury and emphasizing the importance of the presence of avulsed bony fragments on the lateral radiograph in confirming the diagnosis. Although Tarsney described one patient with the combination of triceps rupture and fracture of the radial head, it was Levy and colleagues[44] who drew attention to this combination in 1978. In 1982[45] Levy and associates reported on 16 patients with triceps rupture, of whom 15 had associated radial head fractures and 1 a fracture of the capitellum.

ANATOMY

The triceps muscle consists of two aponeurotic laminae. The long head arising from the inferior glenoid neck and the lateral head from the humerus converge to form the superficial lamina, which commences at about the middle of the muscle and covers its lower half. The tendon inserts into the posterior part of the upper surface of the olecranon.

The medial head lies deep and arises from a broad origin on the humerus, inserting both directly into the olecranon and indirectly via the superficial lamina formed from the other two heads. A few fibers are inserted into the posterior capsule of the elbow joint to retract it during extension.

INCIDENCE AND MECHANISMS

Rupture of the triceps mechanism is a rare injury with only 43 cases reported in the literature. Patients with renal osteodystrophy are at greater risk of sustaining triceps rupture with bony avulsion.[23, 73] The condition may result from either indirect injury or a direct blow. Of the 39 cases in which the mechanism of injury is known, 29 (74 per cent) resulted from an indirect injury (the application of excessive tension to the muscle fibers), 7 (18 per cent) from a direct blow, and 3 (8 per cent) from a combination of both. The usual cause of injury is a fall onto the outstretched hand. This was the mechanism in 8 of 15 cases collected by Tarsney and in 13 of the 16 cases presented by Levy and coworkers in which the mechanism was known. One of the present authors (M.A.C.) has had personal experience of an indirect injury resulting from a vigorous fend in a rugby game. The resisted extension resulted in a combination of partial muscle and tendon rupture as well as bony avulsion, producing a complete disruption of the triceps mechanism.

Most direct injuries are a result of the elbow striking a fixed object, but crush injury is also described.[59] There appears to be no correlation between the mechanism of injury and the site of disruption of the triceps.

CLINICAL PRESENTATION

The patient gives a history of a direct blow or indirect injury, as described earlier. Particularly with an indirect injury, the patient may report a tearing sensation about the elbow. Pain, swelling, and weakness of elbow extension are commonly noted.

On examination a palpable defect is present, usually in the triceps tendon, and there is associated swelling and often bruising. The patient exhibits an inability to actively extend the elbow when the rupture is complete. When a fracture of the radial head has also occurred, tenderness and swelling are present over the fracture site and may dominate the clinical picture.[45]

X-RAY EVALUATION

Radiographs may be helpful in confirming triceps avulsion. In 6 of the 7 patients described by Tarsney and in 12 of 16 patients in Levy's series, avulsion fragments from the olecranon were present. X-rays are also important in excluding associated injuries. Radial head fracture is a common associated finding,[45] and fracture of the distal radius and ulna has also been reported.[42]

COMPLICATIONS

Levy and colleagues[45] emphasized the association of radial head fractures with triceps rupture, which was present in 15 of 16 of their patients. They therefore recommended that all patients with a radial head fracture be carefully assessed to exclude injury to the triceps tendon.

A most unusual complication described in 1987 by Brumbuck[10] involved avulsion of the origin of the lateral head of the triceps with an associated compartment syndrome. Partial ulnar nerve palsy following a direct blow that resulted in rupture of the triceps tendon has also been described.[1] A year later tenderness was still present over the ulnar nerve with hypoesthesia of the ulnar distribution; at surgery the nerve was found to be enclosed in a bed of adhesions. Ulnar nerve transposition was carried out.

METHODS OF TREATMENT

In complete rupture of the triceps tendon, experience with nonoperative treatment is limited. In 1962 Preston and Adicoff[73] described a patient with hyperparathyroidism who had suffered avulsion of the quadriceps tendons bilaterally and rupture of the triceps tendon with an avulsed bony fragment. The elbow was not immobilized, and in the 14 months following injury the patient was described as having little disability with ordinary activity. In a case described by Anderson and LeCocq[1] in which a 27-year-old woman had struck the triceps region against the gearshift of her car, the result was poor. At one year she still lacked 10 degrees of extension and was tender over the rupture site, and triceps strength was reduced to approximately one-half. Exploration revealed a completely ruptured tendon healed by scar in an elongated position. After scar excision and tendon shortening, she achieved an excellent result with nearly normal power. Sherman and coworkers[81] described a 24-year-old patient (a body builder) who was seen three months after injury. Resisted extension of the arm was markedly weak compared with the opposite side. Cybex testing revealed a 42 per cent extensor deficit at 60 degrees per second and a 74 per cent deficit at 180 degrees per second. After surgical repair at six months, normal function eventually was achieved. A patient described by Tarsney was originally treated in a plaster cast with the elbow flexed to 90 degrees. Although she regained some active extension initially, at four months increased weakness was noted; examination confirmed a palpable defect and loss of extension of the elbow. Delayed repair resulted in a return of full motion and power.

AUTHORS' PREFERRED TREATMENT

We prefer surgical treatment for both early and late injuries. Although there has been some variation in our method of repair, fixation via drill holes in the olecranon employing heavy suture material is effective. In one patient treated by the authors, the avulsed fragment was large enough to fix with Kirschner wires and a tension band wire, with supplementary sutures in the damaged tendon and muscle yielding sound fixation. The arm is immobilized in a cast at 30 degrees for a period of four weeks prior to mobilization.

Rupture of the Biceps

Lesions of the biceps tendon have been discussed in detail in Chapter 20. This section will focus on rupture of the biceps muscle.

HISTORICAL REVIEW

In documenting the history of biceps muscle rupture, we have had difficulty in confirming the site of the lesion. Reviewing the predominantly European literature, Gilcreest[26] noted that of the 81 cases of biceps rupture, only 15 had come to surgery. Difficulty in locating the site of rupture clinically is highlighted by the comments made in 1935 by Haldeman and Soto-Hall,[30] who noted that in recent tears of the biceps

The haematoma produced by a tear in the upper part of the tendon gravitates downward through the sheath to the region of the belly where it presents. The ecchymosis and tenderness suggest that the tear took place at the musculotendinous junction. This occurred in two cases in which we exposed the belly of the biceps muscle and then had to carry the incision upward to find the tear in the bicipital groove.

Many of the early cases of "muscle rupture" are likely to have been tears of the long head. Loos[47] in 1900 believed that 19.5 per cent of ruptures of the biceps were actually ruptures of the long head and 43.6 per cent occurred at the musculotendinous junction of the long head, while 15.1 per cent were total muscle ruptures and 21.8 per cent were partial muscle ruptures. In 1922 Gilcreest[25] stated, "According to most writers, about 66% are believed to occur in the muscle substance." Clearly these figures for muscle rupture are much too high; certainly, however, there are well-documented muscle ruptures in the earlier literature. Conwell[14] in 1937 described a 38-year-old man who sustained a traction injury to the limb while holding a drill handle. Operation revealed a complete rupture of both bellies of the biceps in the middle third, with the margins of the rupture being quite smooth, as if cut by a knife.

In 106 biceps ruptures in 100 patients, Gilcreest[26] diagnosed complete rupture of the entire muscle in 6, partial rupture in 1, complete rupture of the muscle of the long head in 3, and partial rupture in 5. There was 1 complete rupture of the muscle of the short head and 1 partial rupture.

In 1941 Tobin and associates[90] described ruptures of the biceps muscle occurring in parachutists. Heckman and Levine[34] in 1978 reported on 48 parachutists with ruptures of the biceps muscle, making this by far the largest series in the literature.

INCIDENCE AND MECHANISMS

Rupture of the biceps muscle is a rare injury. The lesion was overdiagnosed in the early literature for the reasons stated earlier, and the figures are therefore misleading. In the older literature, indirect injury from traction applied to a contracting biceps muscle is more common. The only recent reports in the literature involve injury in military parachutists.[34, 90] In the period from 1973 to 1975, Heckman and Levine encountered over 50 patients with closed transection of the biceps in a population of 40,000 paratroopers undertaking a total of over 100,000 parachute jumps each year.

The mechanism of injury is essentially the same for all parachutists. A 2-cm-wide woven nylon strap (the static line) is attached to the paratrooper's pack and the aircraft. The paratrooper jumps, and when a force of 6.33 kg per cm (80 pounds per square inch) is applied to the casing of the parachute it comes free, allowing the parachute to open. If the static line is incorrectly positioned in front of the arm, a severe force may be applied over the biceps, especially if the arm is simultaneously abducted after push-off.

CLINICAL PRESENTATION

The patient gives a history of direct or indirect injury, as described earlier. A tearing or popping sensation in the arm often accompanies indirect injury, followed by severe pain, swelling, and loss of strength. Gilcreest[26] states that the pain is more intense with muscle ruptures than with tendon ruptures and that a visible and palpable defect in the muscle may be present (Fig. 22–3), particularly if the patient is seen early, before a significant hematoma and swelling occur. He also states that the humerus may be felt beneath the skin in the defect, presumably with brachialis interposed. There is often extensive ecchymosis and pronounced bruising. Weakness is present, its severity depending on the extent of rupture. In the paratroopers described by Heckman and Levine, the skin always showed some degree of contusion or abrasion but was without laceration. These authors stated that although immediate, marked local hemorrhage and swelling occur, the defect may be difficult to appreciate immediately and the degree of the injury may be unrecognized. After the acute hematoma and swelling subside, however, the severity of the injury can more readily be appreciated.

X-RAY EVALUATION

In Heckman and Levine's series, radiographs at the time of injury were negative except in one patient with

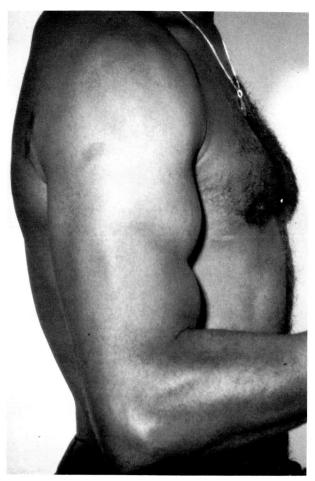

Figure 22–3. Biceps muscle rupture in a weightlifter.

an associated scapular neck fracture. There is no information in the literature regarding the use of ultrasonography or MRI in confirming the diagnosis and, particularly, the extent of injury, but they would be expected to be helpful.

COMPLICATIONS

Musculocutaneous nerve injury was common in Heckman and Levine's series. Although none of their patients showed alteration in sensation in the distribution of the lateral cutaneous nerve of the forearm, electromyographic studies were positive in 9 of 11 patients studied. One year later 2 of this group had normal electromyograms, 6 had signs of reestablishment of the nerve supply to the muscle, and 1 had persistent denervation. Two patients showed denervation of only one head of the biceps at three and four months after injury and were expected to recover. The authors concluded that there was frequently contusion of the musculocutaneous nerve but rarely permanent paralysis of the muscle.

The results of inadequately treated ruptures of the biceps muscle were well documented by Heckman and Levine. They evaluated 28 male paratroopers an average of 19 months after injury. In 25 there was weakness of the arm and fatigability, especially with activity requiring rapid, repeated elbow flexion. Seventeen complained of an unsightly cosmetic defect and 12 experienced pain, generally on using the muscle. The maximum force generated by elbow flexion at 90 degrees was measured with an ergometer as 53 per cent of that of controls.

METHODS OF TREATMENT

Heckman and Levine treated 20 patients whom they alternately allocated to one of two treatment regimens. Ten patients underwent acute surgical repair within 72 hours of injury. Through an anteromedial approach the muscle was explored. The typical lesion found in all cases was transection of the belly with an intact fascial envelope, with the space within the fascia being filled with blood. The hematoma was evacuated and the muscle belly reapproximated with double right-angled sutures of heavy catgut reinforced with a U-shaped flap of biceps fascia. The elbow was then immobilized in acute flexion for four weeks and at 90 degrees for an additional two weeks. The second group of 10 patients was treated by aspiration and splinting. It appeared to the authors that the intrafascial hematoma was the primary obstruction to closure of the muscle gap. Since it was seen at surgery that the hematoma could be aspirated with a 16-gauge needle and the muscle gap closed with acute elbow flexion, this treatment method was utilized. After aspiration the elbow was immobilized in a cast in acute flexion for six weeks; range-of-motion exercises were then begun.

At follow-up 8.8 months after surgery or 7.1 months after aspiration, the muscle power was virtually identical—76.5 per cent of normal and 77 per cent of normal, respectively. Both were superior to the 53 per cent of normal found in the original, untreated group. One patient in the surgical group developed a deep wound infection that required debridement, intravenous antibiotics, and secondary wound closure. In view of the equal strength of the two groups and the lack of complications with aspiration and splinting, this treatment was favored.

Delayed treatment gives only fair results. Heckman and Levine undertook repair in six patients at 4 to 18 months. The musculocutaneous nerve was intact in the base of the wound in all cases. Scar tissue was noted to be denser in those operated on later. At six months, three out of five showed improved power (an average of 42 per cent of normal power improving to 57 per cent) and the appearance was somewhat improved.

AUTHORS' PREFERRED TREATMENT

For patients seen acutely after biceps rupture, we prefer aspiration of the hematoma and immobilization of the elbow in acute flexion for six weeks. For subacute ruptures we favor open repair and immobilization in acute flexion for four weeks and flexion at 90 degrees for two weeks. When there is a significant delay before presentation, we base the decision to repair the muscle on the patient's occupation, functional deficit, and concern regarding cosmesis. The prognosis in such cases is guarded.

Rupture of the Serratus Anterior

Although traumatic winging of the scapula secondary to long thoracic nerve injury is not uncommon, there being several hundred cases reported in the English-language literature, rupture of the serratus anterior muscle is extremely uncommon. Fitchet[24] in 1930 was the first to report on injury to the serratus anterior muscle; he described five cases, although in none was the diagnosis confirmed surgically nor was electrodiagnostic equipment available to exclude injury to the long thoracic nerve. In 1940 Overpeck and Ghormley[65] reported on five additional cases of suspected serratus anterior muscle rupture. They believed that the severity of the pain was helpful in differentiating muscle rupture from long thoracic nerve palsy in that trauma to the muscle produced more severe pain than that seen with involvement of the nerve alone. Again, the cases were not confirmed surgically or electrodiagnostically.

Hayes and Zehr[32] in 1981 provided the first report of a surgically proven traumatic avulsion of the serratus anterior muscle. Their patient, a 25-year-old man who was driving an all-terrain vehicle that rolled over, sustained a mild cerebral contusion, a fractured jaw, and an injury to the right shoulder that resulted in a displaced fracture of the inferior angle of the scapula. The exact mechanism of injury was uncertain. He was treated in a sling, and at two weeks winging of the scapula was noted. The winging persisted; when he returned to work as a carpenter several months later he noted that the arm tired easily and was weak, particularly when he was working with the arm in front or overhead. He was also troubled by a grating sensation under the scapula. These symptoms persisted and at nine months he underwent exploration. The findings included rupture of both the rhomboideus major and serratus anterior muscles. The tendinous attachment of the serratus anterior to the separated inferior pole fragment remained intact. The inferior pole was excised, and both muscles were reattached to the freshened border of the scapula with No. 1 silk sutures. A Velpeau sling was used postoperatively and the shoulder protected for six weeks. Full strength was regained; there was no further winging of the scapula, and the patient returned to his former occupation. Hayes[31a] has subsequently treated a second patient who rolled a jeep over, sustaining a similar avulsion of the inferior pole of the scapula. He experienced pain and weakness in his work as a welder and was much improved following repair.

A second case of rupture of the serratus anterior was described by Meythaler and colleagues[58] in 1985 in a 64-year-old man with severe rheumatoid arthritis. His injury occurred with two episodes of rolling over in bed with the shoulder flexed and abducted. Winging of the scapula was evident clinically, along with marked infrascapular swelling and ecchymoses that extended along the lateral chest wall. Nerve conduction studies were normal in the long thoracic nerve, as was electromyography. Treatment was conservative, with rest followed by an intensive physiotherapy program; by 16 weeks the patient was independent in activities of daily living, but the winging persisted. In this case a number of predisposing factors existed. Gross restriction of glenohumeral joint movement resulted in increased stresses on the serratus anterior, which was already weakened by chronic prednisone therapy and Type II muscle atrophy associated with rheumatoid arthritis. Salicylate-induced coagulopathy may have contributed to the hematoma.

From the limited experience with disruption of the serratus anterior muscle reported in the literature, the authors advocate surgical repair in all but elderly and debilitated patients.

Rupture of the Coracobrachialis

Gilcreest and Albi in 1939[27] stated that they were unable to find any recorded case of rupture of the coracobrachialis in the literature. However, they reported a single case that was due to direct violence and at operation discovered a rupture of the belly of the muscle. The patient had experienced considerable impairment of function in the arm; he was reported as making a complete recovery postoperatively. A second case was described by Tobin and colleagues[90] in 1941 in a parachutist with a direct injury from his static line. No cases were included in a series of 1412 muscle ruptures reported by Anzel and coworkers[2] from the Mayo Clinic. This lesion appears to be extremely rare. Acute repair is recommended in young, active patients.

Rupture of the Subscapularis

Smith[83] in 1835 first reported an isolated tear of the subscapularis tendon in a cadaver. Speed[85] reported two patients in whom rupture of the subscapularis tendon had been diagnosed clinically but did not come to surgery. Gilcreest and Albi[27] reported one rupture found at operation, but no details of the site of rupture were available.

Partial rupture of the subscapularis in association with anterior dislocation of the glenohumeral joint is well documented.[21, 31, 60, 87] The part of the muscle that appears particularly vulnerable is the lower quarter, where the insertion may be directly from muscle into bone.[21, 87] Of 45 patients operated on for recurrent anterior dislocation, Symeonides reported 6 ruptures of the lower quarter of the subscapularis; in 24 patients there were partial ruptures of the muscle at various other points. Partial rupture of the subscapularis muscle has also been produced in cadavers from anterior dislocation of the shoulder.[21, 87] The presence of the muscle injury has been used as a rationale for immobilization in internal rotation following acute anterior dislocation of the shoulder.

Recently, McAuliffe and Dowd[48] reported a case of complete avulsion of the subscapularis insertion in a 54-year-old woman after a fall directly onto the shoulder. It was not possible to dislocate the shoulder under general anesthesia. Following reattachment at the fragment with nylon sutures, the patient regained full movement and returned to her normal activities in three months.

Conclusion

Muscle ruptures are not common, yet they can produce substantial disability after a direct or indirect injury to the shoulder or arm. Surgical repair is difficult because of the problem with suturing muscle tissue directly, but repair in the acute phase is to be commended whenever possible. Such repair can be further assisted by immobilization in a position that approximates the edges of the torn muscle. Careful protected exercise programs can then be initiated to further ensure optimal rehabilitation.

References

1. Anderson KJ, and Le Cocq JF: Rupture of the triceps tendon. J Bone Joint Surg 39A:444–446, 1957.
2. Anzel H, Covey KW, Weiner AD, et al: Disruption of muscles and tendons: an analysis of 1,014 cases. Surgery 45(3):406–414, 1959.
3. Bakalim G: Rupture of the pectoralis major muscle. A case report. Acta Orthop Scand 36:274–279, 1965.
4. Bayley I, Fisher K, Tsutsui H, and Matthews J: Functional biofeedback in the management of habitual shoulder instability. Proceedings of the 3rd International Conference on Surgery of the Shoulder, Fukuoka, Japan, Oct. 28–30, 1986.
5. Bennett BS: Triceps tendon ruptures. J Bone Joint Surg 44A:741–744, 1962.
6. Berson BL: Surgical repair of pectoralis major rupture in an athlete. Am J Sports Med 7(6):348–351, 1979.
7. Borchers E, and Iontscheff P: Die Subkutane Ruptur des grossen brustmuskels ein wenig bekanntes aber typishes Krankheitsbild. Zentralbl Chir 59:770–774, 1932.
8. Brickner WM, and Milch H: Ruptures of Muscles and Tendons. International Clinics Vol II Ser 38–7,97
9. Brownlee JJ: Rupture of the pectoralis major: a case report. Proceedings of the New Zealand Orthopaedic Association, Oct. 1987.
10. Brumback RJ: Compartment syndrome complicating avulsion of the origin of the triceps muscle. A case report. J Bone Joint Surg 69A:1445–1447, 1987.
11. Buck JE: Rupture of the sternal head of the pectoralis major: a personal description. J Bone Joint Surg 45B:224, 1963.
12. Butters AG: Traumatic rupture of the pectoralis major. Br Med J 2:652–653, 1941.
13. Clemens H: Traumatische Hemie des M. Deltoideus. Dsch Med Wochenschr 39:2197, 1913.
14. Conwell HL: Subcutaneous rupture of the biceps flexor cubiti; report of one case. J Bone Joint Surg 10:788–790, 1928.
15. Cougard P, Petitjean D, Hamonière G, and Ferry C: Rupture traumatique complète du muscle grand pectoral. Rev Chir Orthop 71:337–338, 1985.
16. Coughlin EJ, and Baker DM: Management of shoulder injuries in sport. Conn Med 29:723–727, 1965.
17. Cronkite AE: The tensile strength of human tendons. Anat Rec 64:173–186, 1936.
18. Danielsson L: Ruptur av.m. pectoralis major en brottningsskada. Nord Med 72:1089, 1964.
19. Davis CB: Plastic repair of the deltoid muscle. Surg Clin 3:287–289, 1919.
20. Delport HP, and Piper MS: Pectoralis major rupture in athletes. Arch Orthop Trauma Surg 100:135–137, 1982.
21. DePalma AF, Cooke AJ, and Prabhaker M: The role of the subscapularis in recurrent anterior dislocations of the shoulder. Clin Orthop 54:35, 1967.
22. Egan TM, and Hall H: Avulsion of the pectoralis major tendon in a weight lifter: repair using a barbed staple. Can J Surg 30:434, 1987.
23. Farrar EL, and Lippert FG: Avulsion of the triceps tendon. Clin Orthop 161:242, 1981.
24. Fitchet SM: Injury of the serratus magnus (anterior) muscle. N Engl J Med 303(17):818–823, 1930.
25. Gilcreest EL: Rupture of muscles and tendons, particularly subcutaneous rupture of biceps flexor cubiti. JAMA 84:1819–1822, 1922.
26. Gilcreest EL: The common syndrome of rupture, dislocation and elongation of the long head of the biceps brachii; analysis of 100 cases. Surg Gynecol Obstet 58:322–324, 1934.
27. Gilcreest EL, and Albi P: Unusual lesions of muscles and tendons of the shoulder girdle and upper arm. Surg Gynecol Obstet 68:903–917, 1939.
28. Gudmundsson B: A case of agenesis and a case of rupture of the pectoralis major muscle. Acta Orthop Scand 44:213–218, 1973.
29. Guerterbock P: Zerreissung der Sehn des M. triceps brachii. Arch Klin Chir 26:256–260, 1881.
30. Haldeman K, and Soto-Hall R: Injuries to muscles and tendons. JAMA 104:2319–2324, 1935.

31. Hauser FDW: Avulsion of the tendon of subscapularis muscle. J Bone Joint Surg 36A:139–141, 1954.

31a. Hayes JM: Personal communication, 1988.

32. Hayes JM, and Zehr DJ: Traumatic muscle avulsion causing winging of the scapula. J Bone Joint Surg 63A:495–497, 1981.

33. Hayes WM: Rupture of the pectoralis major muscle. Review of the literature and report of two cases. J Int Coll Surg 14:82–88, 1950.

34. Heckman JD, and Levine MI: Traumatic closed transection of the biceps brachii in the military parachutist. J Bone Joint Surg 60A:369–372, 1978.

35. Heimann W: Uber einige subkutane Muskel- und Sehnenverletzungen van den oberen Gliedmassen. Monatsschr Unfallh 15:266–279, 1908.

36. Jens J: The role of subscapularis muscle in recurring dislocation of the shoulder. J Bone Joint Surg 46B:780, 1964.

37. Kawashima M, Sato M, Torisu T, et al: Rupture of the pectoral major: report of 2 cases. Clin Orthop 109:115–119, June 1975.

38. Kingsley DM: Rupture of pectoralis major. Report of a case. J Bone Joint Surg 28:644–645, 1946.

39. Knaack WHL: Die subkutanen Verletzungen der Muskeln Veroffentl. Geb Mil Sanitatswesens 16:1–123, 1900.

40. Lage J de A: Ruptura do musculo grande pectoral. Rev Hosp Clin 6:37–40, 1951.

41. Law WB: Closed incomplete rupture of pectoralis major. Br Med J 2:499, 1954.

42. Lee MLH: Rupture of triceps tendon. Br Med J 2:197, 1960.

43. Letenneur M: Rupture sous-cutanée du muscle grand pectoral; guérison complète en quinze jours. Gaz de Hop 35:54, 1862.

44. Levy M, Fishel RE, and Stern GM: Triceps tendon avulsion with or without fracture of the radial head—a rare injury? J Trauma 18:677–679, 1978.

45. Levy M, Goldberg I, and Meir I: Fracture of the head of the radius with a tear or avulsion of the triceps tendon. J Bone Joint Surg 64B(1):70–72, 1982.

46. Lindenbaum BL: Delayed repair of a ruptured pectoralis major muscle. Clin Orthop 109:120–121, 1975.

47. Loos: Beitr Z Klin Chir 29:410, 1900.

48. McAuliffe TB, and Dowd GS: Avulsion of the subscapularis tendon: a case report. J Bone Joint Surg 69A:1454, 1987.

49. McEntire JE, Hess WE, and Coleman S: Rupture of the pectoralis major muscle. J Bone Joint Surg 43A:81–87, 1961.

50. MacKenzie DB: Avulsion of the insertion of the pectoralis major muscle. S Afr Med J July:147–148, 1981.

51. McKelvey D: Subcutaneous rupture of the pectoralis major muscle. Br Med J 2:611, 1928.

52. McMaster PF: Tendon and muscle ruptures. Clinical and experimental studies and locations of subcutaneous ruptures. J Bone Joint Surg 15:705–722, 1933.

53. Mandl F: Ruptur des Musculus pect. major. Wien Med Wochenschr 75:2192, 1925.

54. Malinovski I: Rare case of rupture of the pectoralis major at its attachment with process of the humerus. Voyenno Med J 153:136–138, 1885.

55. Manjarris J, Gershuni DH, and Moitoza J: Rupture of the pectoralis major tendon. J Trauma 25(8):810–811, 1985.

56. Marmor L, Bechtol CO, and Hall CB: Pectoralis major muscle function of sternal portion and mechanism of rupture of normal muscle: case reports. J Bone Joint Surg 43A:81–87, 1961.

57. Maydl K: Veber subcutane Muskel-urd Sehrerserrissungen, sowie Rissfracturer mit Berucksichligung der analogen, dirche directe Gewalt enstandenen und offerien verletzungen. Dtsch Z Chir 17:306–361, 1882; 18:35–139, 1883.

58. Meythaler JM, Reddy NM, and Mitz M: Serratus anterior disruption: a complication of rheumatoid arthritis. Arch Phys Med Rehabil 67:770–772, 1986.

59. Montgomery AH: Two cases of muscle injury. Surg Clin 4:871, 1920.

60. Moseley HF, and Overgaard B: The anterior capsular mechanism in recurrent anterior dislocation of the shoulder. J Bone Joint Surg 44B:913, 1962.

61. Moulonguet G: Rupture spontanée du grand pectoral chez un vieillard. Enorme hematome. Mort Bull Mem Soc Anat Paris 94:24–28, 1924.

62. Newmark H III, Olken SM, and Halls J: Ruptured triceps tendon diagnosed radiographically. Australas Radiol 29:60–63, 1985.

63. O'Donoghue DH: Injuries to muscle tendon unit. Am Surg 29:190–200, 1963.

64. Orava S, Sorasto A, Aalto K, and Kvist H: Total rupture of the pectoralis major muscle in athletes. Int J Sports Med 5:272–274, 1984.

65. Overpeck DO, and Ghormley RK: Paralysis of the serratus magnus muscle. JAMA 114(2):1994–1996, 1940.

66. Pantazopoulos T, Exarchov E, Stavrov Z, et al: Avulsion of the triceps tendon. J Trauma 15:827–829, 1975.

67. Park JY, and Espiniella JL: Rupture of pectoralis major muscle. A case report and review of literature. J Bone Joint Surg 52A:577–581, 1970.

68. Parkes M: Rupture of the pectoralis major muscle. Ind Med 12:226, 1943.

69. Partridge: A case of rupture of the triceps cubiti. Med Times Gaz 1:175–176, 1868.

70. Penhallow D: Report of a case of ruptured triceps due to direct violence. New York Med J 91:76–77, 1910.

71. Patissier P: Traite des Maladies des Artisans. Paris; 1822, pp 162–164.

72. Pirker H: Die Verletzungen durch Muskelzug. Ergebn d Chir u Orthop 25:553–634, 1934.

73. Preston FS, and Adicoff A: Hyperparathyroidism with avulsion of three major tendons. N Engl J Med 266:968–971, 1962.

74. Pulaski EJ, and Chandlee BH: Ruptures of the pectoralis major muscle. Surgery 10:309–312, 1941.

75. Pulaski EJ, and Martin GW: Rupture of the left pectoralis major muscle. Surgery 25:110–111, 1949.

76. Rédard P, cited by Deveny P: Contribution a l'étude des ruptures musculaires. Thesis no. 423:12, Paris, 1878.

77. Régeard A: Etude sur les ruptures musculaires. Thesis No. 182:51, Paris, 1880.

78. Ronchetti G: Rottura sottocutanea parziale del muscolo grand pettorale con formazione di pseudocistie ematica. Minerva Chir 14:22–28, 1959.

79. Schechter LR, and Gristina AG: Surgical repair of rupture of the pectoralis major muscle. JAMA 188:1009, 1964.

80. Searfoss R, Tripi J, and Bowers W: Triceps brachii rupture: case report. J Trauma 16:244–245, 1976.

81. Sherman OH, Snyder SJ, and Fox JM: Triceps avulsion in a professional body builder: a case report. Am J Sports Med 12(4):329, 1984.

82. Smart A: Rupture of pectoralis major. Guy's Hosp Gaz 2:61, 1873.

83. Smith JG: Pathological appearances of seven cases of injury of the shoulder joint with remarks. Am J Med Sci 16:219–224, 1835.

84. Solokoff L, and Hough AJ Jr: Pathology of rheumatoid arthritis and allied disorders. In McCarty DJ (ed): Arthritis and Allied Conditions: A Textbook of Rheumatology, 10th ed. Philadelphia; Lea & Febiger, 1985, pp 571–592.

85. Speed K: Personal communication to Gilcreest, 1939.

86. Stimson H: Traumatic rupture of the biceps brachii. Am J Surg 29(3):472–476, 1935.

87. Symeonides PP: The significance of the subscapularis muscle in the pathogenesis of recurrent anterior dislocation of the shoulder. J Bone Joint Surg 54B:476–483, 1972.

88. Tarsney FF: Rupture and avulsion of the triceps. Clin Orthop 83:177–183, 1972.

89. Tietjen R: Closed injuries of the pectoralis major muscle. J Trauma 20(3):262–264, 1980.

90. Tobin WJ, Cohen LJ, and Vandover JT: Parachute injuries. JAMA 117(16):1318–1321, 1941.

91. Urs ND, and Jani DM: Surgical repair of rupture of the pectoralis major muscle: a case report. J Trauma 16(9):749–750, 1976.

92. Von Eiselberg A: Cited by Mandl (reference 53).

93. Weinlechner J: Ueber subcutane Muskel-, Sehnen- und Knochenrisse. Wien Med Blatter 4:1561–1565, 1881.

94. Welsh RP, Macnab I, and Riley V: Biomechanical studies of rabbit tendon. Clin Orthop 81:171–177, 1971.

95. Zeman SC, Rosenfeld RT, and Lipscomb PR: Tears of the pectoralis major muscle. Am J Sports Med 7(6):343–347, 1979.

Tumors and Related Conditions

Ernest U. Conrad III, M.D.

The management of sarcomas is a broad and complex topic that represents less than 10 per cent of all orthopedic diagnoses.[1] This chapter stresses the initial assessment and evaluation because of the typical lengthy delay in diagnosis. The classification and staging of these lesions represents, in a broad sense, many of the improvements achieved in the last 10 to 15 years. A review of the salient radiographic and clinical features of the more common lesions is included without an in-depth discussion of any one particular lesion. The principles of biopsy and surgical resection, the definition and significance of surgical margins, and the classification of resections and reconstructions are all discussed. Most of the surgical reconstructive techniques (allografts, arthrodesis, and arthroplasty) presented have only short follow-up to date and should be considered accordingly.

Historical Review

The term "sarcoma" was used by Abernethy in the 19th century to describe tumors having a "firm and fleshy feel." Sarcoma refers to malignancies of mesenchymal, or connective tissue, origin. In that early period, sarcomas were lesions of the extremities, confused with osteomyelitis and other conditions. Even the most accomplished professors of surgery demonstrated little interest in the recognition of sarcomas as malignancies distinct from carcinomas, and consequently, there was little prior work involving their classification or treatment.

An exception to that rule was Samuel W. Gross (1837–1884), a well-known surgeon, pathologist, and anatomist at the Jefferson Medical College in Philadelphia, who authored one of the first works that attempted to deal with the classification of various sarcomas, their salient features, and indications for treatment and prognosis. Gross was one of the first in the world to identify sarcomas as a distinctly different group of tumors from carcinomas.[2] With the discovery and development of radiographs (1893), various lesions of bone were beginning to attract attention. Gross was one of the first to appropriately identify sarcomas as locally invasive, extremity tumors, with frequent metastases to the lungs and infrequently demonstrating lymphatic or hepatic metastases. These unusual lesions were associated with a history of trauma in half the cases and, according to Gross, required radical amputation or resection. In retrospect, his description of these first cases is remarkable for its accuracy.

The scientific and technical developments in radiology, surgery, and medicine in the early 20th century resulted in significant advances in orthopedics, reflected in improvements in the care of fractures, infections, and tumors. At that time, pathologists and surgeons such as John Ewing (New York), Ernest A. Codman (Boston), and James Bloodgood (Baltimore) became interested in various tumors of bone.[3] The treatment for sarcomas varied greatly over those early years, but the management of these unusual and difficult tumors gradually became more uniform as lesions were recognized histologically and radiographically as distinct entities. Surgical treatment also improved with the developments in pathology and radiology. Aggressive ablative surgery for sarcomas was first recommended by Gross in his classic article on sarcomas[2] and was followed by various reports in the early 20th century of various innovative surgical techniques.[4, 6] Linberg's classic article in 1928 regarding interscapulothoracic resections[5] for malignancies of the shoulder joint reported on aggressive surgery for skeletal tumors. Since those early reports, dramatic advances in imaging, chemotherapy, pathology, and surgical techniques have resulted in improved survival and allowed more limb-sparing surgery.

In the 20th century, Dallas B. Phemister (University

of Chicago, 1882–1951) was one of the first surgeons in North America to demonstrate a special interest in limb sparing or "limb salvage" surgery as we know it today.[7] Phemister reviewed the American College of Surgeons' records for osteosarcoma in 1938 and found that only 4 of 86 extremity cases (4.6 per cent) were treated with a limb-sparing resection.[7] Other reports of limb-sparing surgery at that time described variable results in terms of morbidity and mortality.[7-9] The popularity of "limb salvage" surgery reached its zenith in the past six to seven years, only to taper off to a more conservative approach, emphasizing the need for appropriate tumor resections and good functional results.

The specialty of musculoskeletal oncology has crystalized from various improvements in radiographic "staging" studies, chemotherapy, pathology, and surgery. One of the most significant developments has involved the evolution of a classification system for sarcomas of bone and soft tissue that allows the assessment of a patient's prognosis based on the stage of the tumor and the proposed treatment.[11, 12] It is one of the only systems that appropriately reflect a patient's prognosis based on the most significant determinants of that prognosis: a tumor's stage and its surgical and "adjuvant" treatment. It is a system that is useful for chemotherapists, surgeons, radiation therapists, radiologists, and pathologists in diagnosis and treatment and the assessment of treatment results.

Limb-sparing procedures, when properly executed, involve innovative reconstructive techniques to achieve an arthroplasty or arthrodesis associated with reasonable functional results. The indications for and assessment of these procedures in terms of functional results and tumor recurrence will be discussed briefly. Although the true worth of some of these procedures, in many instances, remains to be determined, the value of a classification system for sarcomas and the coordinated multidisciplinary treatment of musculoskeletal neoplasms is obvious. Sarcomas are unusual tumors requiring complex treatment. Their rarity and complexity has been a major reason for haphazard treatment in the past.

Anatomy

There are many anatomical considerations involved in the treatment of musculoskeletal tumors. In the shoulder girdle these considerations are amplified by the proximity of the brachial plexus and major vessels of the upper extremity to the scapula, humerus, and chest wall. The implications of these anatomical points involve many aspects of the treatment and prognosis of shoulder neoplasms.

While the evaluation of musculoskeletal tumors frequently refers to the various anatomical compartments of the region involved, the exact anatomy of the compartments about the shoulder remains poorly defined. The compartments of the shoulder include the deltoid compartment, the posterior scapular compartment (supraspinatus, infraspinatus, teres minor, and teres major), the subscapular compartments (subscapularis), the anterior pectoral compartment (pectoralis minor and major), the anterior humeral compartment (biceps and coracobrachialis), the lateral humeral compartment (brachialis), the posterior humeral compartment (medial, lateral, and long head of the triceps), and the intra-articular compartment of the glenohumeral joint.

Compartments seen at the level of the humeral head, proximal and middiaphysis, are seen in Figure 23–1. There has been little work on the true containment or integrity of these compartments, and their boundaries are theoretical. Although they are anatomically based, their actual potential for containment remains untested.

There are many anatomical clues that are helpful in making the initial diagnosis in patients presenting with an unknown musculoskeletal lesion. For instance, Ewing's sarcoma, in the majority of cases, occurs in the shaft or diaphysis of the humerus; it rarely occurs in the metaphysis of a long bone. On the other hand, osteogenic sarcoma rarely occurs in the shaft and usually occurs in the metaphysis. Similarly, whether a lesion is intra-articular or extra-articular is important for several reasons. Intra-articular tumors are unusual since most lesions have their epicenter in bone or in the soft tissues outside a joint. An intra-articular lesion is much more likely to represent a degenerative, traumatic, or other nontumor diagnosis. The fact that a tumor might involve a joint primarily or secondarily is of significance from the treatment point of view, because it requires a more complex, extra-articular resection. Secondary involvement of a joint by an intraosseous malignancy is usually a late phenomenon associated with a longer diagnostic delay or a more aggressive lesion and a worse prognosis[11, 15] (see Staging and Classification of Tumors).

Difficult locations for neoplasms in the shoulder girdle include those of the brachial plexus or lesions involving the axillary brachial vessels. Both the plexus and the axillary vessels are contained within their own sheaths that can eventually be penetrated or infiltrated by an aggressive lesion. Primary tumors of the brachial plexus (neurosarcomas) are usually manifested by a brachial plexus nerve deficit on clinical exam. Any patient who presents with distinct peripheral nerve symptoms associated with a shoulder mass should be assumed to have nerve involvement until demonstrated otherwise. A biopsy of that type of lesion is therefore very likely to involve that nerve and result in further nerve loss. Lesions involving the axillary or brachial vessels require magnetic resonance imaging (MRI) and arteriography in order to define the precise extent of involvement.

The shoulder girdle is unique in that it has one of the largest, most well-defined muscle compartments in the body in the deltoid muscle. To function normally,

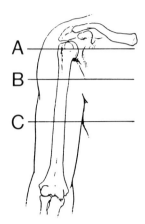

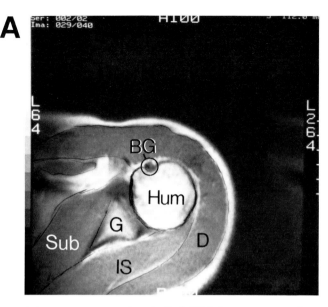

Transverse (axial) MRI image at the level of glenoid.

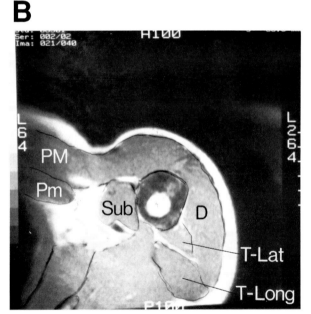

Transverse (axial) MRI image at the level of the proximal humerus.

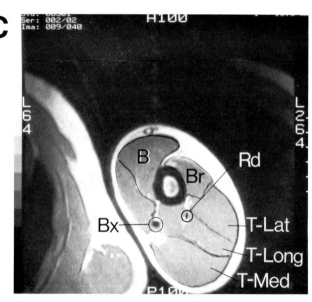

Transverse (axial) MRI image at the level of the mid-humerus.

D - Deltoid
Ax - Axillary vessels
TM - Teres Major
PM - Pectorals Major
CB - Coracobrachiallis
Md - Median Nerve
Hum - Humeral Head

Pm - Pectoralis Minor
BG - Bicipital groove
G - Glenoid
Sub - Subscapularis
B - Biceps brachii
Bx - Brachial vessels
IS - Infraspinatous

T-Lat - Triceps
      (lateral head)
T-Med - Triceps
      (mid-head)
T-Long - Triceps
      (long head)
Br - Brachiallis
Rd - Radial Nerve

Figure 23–1. Shoulder anatomy on axial MRI.

the shoulder is dependent on a well-innervated deltoid and rotator cuff in addition to adequate glenohumeral stability. The deltoid, like most muscle compartments, has anatomical subdivisions (acromial, clavicular, scapular), but grossly it is a well-defined muscle that is easily resectable, although very difficult to reconstruct functionally. Perhaps the most important anatomical consideration involved in the treatment of shoulder tumors is the anatomy of the axillary nerve and its relationship to the deltoid and placement of shoulder incisions, biopsies, etc. Injuries to the axillary nerve during tumor resections or biopsy may result in nearly total loss of deltoid function. Thus, the location of the axillary nerve at the time of biopsy and at the time of resection is of great significance. In general, the functional prognosis for tumors of the shoulder girdle is much better if the axillary nerve, deltoid, and rotator cuff are preserved. Whereas glenohumeral joint mechanics can be replaced by shoulder arthroplasty, reconstruction of the deltoid or rotator cuff is far more difficult.

Staging and Classification of Tumors

STAGING

The early classification system for musculoskeletal tumors was popularized by Lichtenstein according to basic histologic categories.[23] It was useful in identifying general trends in diagnosis and prognosis, but this descriptive histological system had limited significance for determining adjuvant treatment (chemotherapy, radiation therapy) and prognosis.

One of the greatest contributions to the improved treatment of sarcomas today has been the development of a staging system that assists with the selection of treatment, the assessment of prognosis, and the evaluation of results. Such a classification system was introduced by Enneking in 1980,[11] adopted by the Musculoskeletal Tumor Society, and subsequently accepted, with modifications, by the NIH Sarcoma Consensus Study Group as the staging system for all sarcomas.[12, 13] It represents a combined assessment of the histological, or "surgical grade" (G), the anatomical site of primary disease (T), and the presence or absence of metastases (M). Surgical grading is based on the histological assessment, identifying a lesion as benign (C_0), low-grade malignant (G_1), or high-grade malignant (G_2) (Tables 23–1 and 23–2).

The original concept of the staging system as devised by Enneking represented a departure from the staging system of the American Joint Committee for Cancer Staging and End-Results,[13] originally designed for the evaluation of various carcinomas. Enneking felt that system correlated poorly with the natural history of sarcomas. He described the salient features of sarcomas with reference to their distinction from carcinomas and the significance of those features regarding staging.[11–13]

Table 23–1. SURGICAL STAGING SYSTEM: BENIGN TUMORS

Stage	Grade	Site
1	Latent (G_0)	Intracapsular (T_0)
2	Active (G_0)	Intracapsular (T_0)
3	Aggressive (G_0)	Intracomparmental (T_1) or Extracompartmental (T_2)

From Enneking WF, Spanier SS, and Goodman MA: A system for the surgical staging of musculoskeletal sarcoma. Clin Orthop 153:105–120, 1980.

Most sarcomas, in contrast with carcinomas, were described as having a similar natural history, one of progressive local invasion and eventual hematogenous pulmonary metastasis. The surgical treatment of sarcomas of the extremities is significantly different from that of lesions of the head and neck, retroperitoneum, trunk, and abdomen. Appropriate surgery with or without radiation therapy remains the definitive treatment of the primary disease for most sarcomas. However, surgery must be combined with systemic chemotherapy to be curative. Chemotherapy or radiation therapy without surgery is rarely, if ever, curative for the primary lesion. It remains, however, an important adjuvant and palliative method of treatment.

The extent of disease in the Enneking system is defined by the "anatomical setting." Compartmentalization, or compartmental escape, is an important characteristic of sarcomas in contrast to previous classification systems and other tumors (carcinomas). It was postulated that the anatomical site (T) was the greatest factor in prognosis because it represented a composite of the following characteristics: anatomical site, rate of growth, and delay in diagnosis. The primary extent of disease is limited by the natural boundaries of the anatomical compartment in which the lesion is located. A lesion located in the anterior thigh is contained by the fascial envelope of the quadriceps compartment until progressive growth causes it to extend beyond the natural boundary. When that occurs, the patient has a worse prognosis and a higher risk of metastatic disease, reflecting a more aggressive tumor. Lesions that occur in poorly compartmentalized anatomical sites (groin, popliteal fossa, perivascular space) are, by the nature of that site, poorly compartmentalized and usually associated with a worse prognosis.

Table 23–2. SURGICAL STAGING SYSTEM: MALIGNANT BONE TUMORS

Stage	Grade	Site
IA	Low grade (G_1)	Intracompartmental (T_1)
IB	Low grade (G_1)	Extracompartmental (T_2)
IIA	High grade (G_2)	Intracompartmental (T_1)
IIB	High grade (G_2)	Extracompartmental (T_2)
III	Any grade (G_1 or G_2) with regional or distant mestastases (M_1)	any site (T_1 or T_2)

From Enneking WF, Spanier SS, and Goodman MA: A system for the surgical staging of musculoskeletal sarcoma. Clin Orthop 153:105–120, 1980.

The histological grading system for sarcomas in the Enneking system was simplified to a two-grade system, that of high-grade versus low-grade histology. Tumor grading should not be based on the histological type alone. The theory that some histological diagnoses always represent high-grade lesions and a worse prognosis, regardless of their histological grade, is not generally acceptable. No allowance for intermediate-grade histology was made since there was no intermediate surgical treatment. This system required the pathologist to classify all sarcomas as either high-grade or low-grade lesions, which contradicts most classical sarcoma grading systems that typically described high-, low-, and intermediate-grade histology. Grading remains a topic of controversy today, especially for soft tissue sarcomas, which do occur as intermediate-grade lesions in certain cases. The system has subsequently been modified to include intermediate-grade soft tissue tumors. The basic concept, however, remains a valid one, and intermediate-grade soft tissue tumors remain a treatment paradox regarding the indications for chemotherapy.

In the original Enneking staging system, the prognosis for a patient with regional lymph node involvement was believed to be as poor as that for the patient with pulmonary metastasis. Therefore, either lymph node metastasis or pulmonary metastasis was represented by Stage III disease.

The strength of the Enneking staging system is its simplicity. By emphasizing high-grade versus low-grade histology and limiting the number of tumor stages (IA, IB, IIA, IIB, III), this system is simple enough to be used by a wide group of specialists and to allow for a variety of treatments. The Enneking system employs a subtly but significantly different numbering system for benign and malignant disease. Benign disease is denoted as Grade 1, 2, or 3, depending on whether it is latent, active, or aggressive (see Table 23–1). A latent benign lesion does not show active growth. An active lesion shows active growth but is confined within the compartment defined by the surrounding natural boundaries. An aggressive lesion has the potential to penetrate or violate natural boundaries, such as cortical bone, periosteum, or fascial compartments, and remain locally aggressive without metastasizing. Theoretically, only malignant tumors (by definition) have the ability to metastasize: A contradiction in terms is presented by the ability of histologically "benign" giant cell tumors to "metastasize" to the lung in a small number of cases. Other aggressive benign tumors (chondroblastoma) have also demonstrated lung metastases in a small number of cases.

Malignant tumors are denoted as Stage I or II (see Table 23–2), depending on whether the histology is high grade or low grade, and as A or B, depending on whether the lesion is intracompartmental or extracompartmental. Thus, a IA lesion is malignant, low grade, and intracompartmental. A IIA lesion is high grade and intracompartmental, and IIB is high grade and extracompartmental (see Table 23–2). Grade III le-

sions are metastatic regardless of the grade or anatomical site of the lesion. The system is somewhat different for soft tissue.

The anatomical or surgical site classification (T) defines the primary lesion in relationship to its position in the anatomical compartment of origin. Tumors are described as encapsulated (T_0), intracompartmental (T_1), or extracompartmental (T_2). This designation is based on the Enneking compartmental theory, describing an anatomical compartment as a space or potential space defined by natural boundaries[11] (Table 23–3). Tumors contained within an anatomical compartment may violate the boundaries of the compartment with growth—usually a sign of an aggressive benign or malignant tumor. Active benign tumors are typically well encapsulated (T_0) and intracompartmental, while aggressive benign lesions may be poorly encapsulated but remain intracompartmental (T_1). Low-grade malignant lesions are typically intracompartmental (T_1), whereas extracompartmental lesions (T_2) usually represent high-grade malignancies. Extracompartmental tumors may extend from one compartment into another or from one compartment into a surrounding extrafascial plane, or they may arise within a poorly compartmentalized, extracompartmental space. Poorly compartmentalized anatomical spaces include perivascular areas such as the subsartorial space of the common femoral artery, the popliteal fossa, the antecubital fossa, or the midhand, midfoot, axilla, or groin (see Table 23–3).

The stage of the lesion and the surgical margin of the procedure are associated with a certain local recurrence rate as described in the work of Enneking (see section on Surgical Margin). These recurrence rates are based on an extensive retrospective review of the literature and reflect the risk of local recurrence following surgical resection without the use of adjuvant treatment. A benign aggressive (Stage 3) lesion treated

Table 23–3. SURGICAL SITES (T)

Intracompartmental	Extracompartmental
Intraosseous	Soft tissue extension
Intra-articular	Soft tissue extension
Superficial to deep fascia	Deep fascial extension
Parosseous	Intraosseous or extrafascial
Intrafacial compartments	Extrafascial planes or spaces
Ray of hand or foot	Mid- and hindfoot
Posterior calf	Popliteal space
Anterolateral leg	Groin–femoral triangle
Anterior thigh	Intrapelvic
Midthigh	Midhand
Posterior thigh	Antecubital fossae
Buttocks	Axilla
Volar forearm	Periclavicular
Dorsal forearm	Paraspinal
Anterior arm	Head and neck
Posterior arm	
Periscapular	

From Enneking WF, Spanier SS, and Goodman MA: A system for the surgical staging of musculoskeletal sarcoma. Clin Orthop 153:105–120, 1980.

with a wide margin has a recurrence rate of 10 per cent or less. This recurrence reflects surgical treatment alone and does not reflect the lower recurrence rate associated with surgery and adjuvant treatment, as is performed for most malignant conditions. High-grade malignant tumors (IIB), such as the typical osteosarcoma, require at least a wide surgical margin that includes a surrounding cuff of normal tissue in order to avoid a local recurrence.

After careful anatomical staging of the tumor, the appropriate surgical procedure can be predicted by considering the grade of the lesion and the extent of involvement at the primary site (stage). A patient's prognosis and risk for local recurrence can similarly be assessed by considering the grade of the tumor and the surgical margin achieved at the time of the surgical procedure. This "articulation" or correlation of the tumor "stage" and the "surgical margin" represents the first time that surgical details and staging specifics have been considered together in assessing and predicting the results of treatment for sarcomas.

Thorough initial evaluation and staging, before treatment, remain the crucial ingredients for a successful outcome. Without these initial studies and an adequate and accurate biopsy, a successful treatment plan is unlikely. A universally accepted staging classification system is important in order to direct patient care and to adequately assess clinical results regarding disease-free survival. This initial staging philosophy has remained one of the major contributions of the Enneking staging system.

The staging evaluation involves an assessment by various radiographic studies to determine the precise anatomical extent of primary disease, in addition to whether or not regional or distant metastases have occurred. Typical staging studies include plain radiographs, technetium bone scan, computed tomographic (CT) scans, MRI scans, and other studies that better define a lesion's location. A total body bone scan is the best study to assess the extent of the primary bone lesion and the possibility of metastatic disease.[15-17] CT scans are excellent for visualizing cortical geography and bony involvement at the primary site on a two-dimensional plane.[11] CT scanning of the lung is routinely carried out in most institutions to assess possible pulmonary metastasis, and it is a more sensitive method than plain radiographs.

MRI scans are indicated for evaluating soft tissue disease, intramedullary bony disease, and spinal or pelvic lesions.[18] The soft tissue or neurovascular margins are best assessed by the MRI scan because it is far more sensitive than the CT scan for evaluating soft tissue margins. MRI does image the peripheral inflammatory "reactive zone" with a bright signal that may or may not contain tumor. Similarly, the diagnostician may overread soft tissue margins when interpreting malignancies such as osteosarcoma and Ewing's sarcoma[18] because of the inability to distinguish inflammation from tumor on the MRI scan.

CLASSIFICATION OF TUMORS

Although the histological classification of tumors has some limitations in predicting prognosis and directing treatment, it does serve a purpose in identifying tumor types and their general tendencies. Knowing a tumor's histological type and the age of the patient is quite helpful in making a reliable tentative diagnosis in the majority of patients, especially when the x-ray appearance is added to that information. The most common lesions of bone, cartilage, and soft tissue will be described here in order to discuss their general histological, radiographic, and clinical characteristics.

Benign Osseous Lesions

Osteoid Osteoma

Benign osseous lesions of the shoulder are uncommon. Osteoid osteoma and osteoblastoma occur in the proximal humerus or scapula in 10 to 15 per cent of cases and, when they do occur, favor the proximal humerus or glenoid.[19, 20] Osteoid osteoma typically displays the classic symptom of night pain, relieved by salicylates. Radiographically, it is characterized by a large area of reactive bone surrounding a small lucent "nidus." On technetium bone scan, it has impressive increased activity, and the central nidus can be visualized as a distinct cortical hole on CT scanning or tomography. Histologically, this lucent nidus is a well-demarcated, small area of immature, very active osteoblastic tissue. Preoperative localization is an important strategy in order to avoid intraoperative difficulties in locating these lesions and thus in minimizing local recurrences.

Osteoblastoma

Some clinicians regard osteoblastoma as a larger version of osteoid osteoma ("giant osteoid osteoma") typified by a large lucent area of osteoblastic tissue surrounded by a thin sclerotic, reactive rim of bone.[20] Radiographically, osteoblastoma is typically seen as a lucent lesion that has expanded the overlying cortex into a thin rim. As with osteoid osteoma, osteoblastoma may be difficult to localize radiographically and requires careful preoperative imaging in order to avoid recurrences. Osteoblastoma, unlike osteoid osteoma, also occurs in an aggressive (Stage 3) form that is less well defined radiographically, has a high recurrence rate, and may have a histological appearance that is difficult to distinguish from low-grade osteosarcoma. Technetium bone scanning and CT scans are good imaging techniques for both of these lesions. Plain x-ray tomography remains an effective diagnostic tool for localizing many osteoid osteomas.

Myositis Ossificans

Myositis ossificans is a benign, reactive, bone-forming process occurring intramuscularly or in the "areolar tissues" (tendon, ligament, capsule, fascia) adjacent to bone. It may occur with or without a history of trauma and, in the latter instance, may be referred to as pseudomalignant myositis ossificans of soft parts.[14] The pseudomalignant form is typically seen as a symptomatic enlarging soft tissue mass that develops in the second decade of life, occurring in the shoulder in 15 per cent of cases. The typical radiographic appearance is a radio dense or osseous density in soft tissue that demonstrates a peripheral radiographic maturity or margination of the mass, separated from the adjacent cortical bone by a narrow zone of uninvolved soft tissue. This characteristic histological margination or zonation phenomenon (peripheral maturity) reflects the fact that the more active (immature) osteoblastic tissue is located centrally in the lesion. Most neoplasms, to the contrary, have their most active histology peripherally, not centrally. Isotope scans of myositis ossificans demonstrate a high uptake peripherally that may continue for 8 to 12 weeks or until spontaneous maturation occurs. Excision before that time is associated with a high recurrence rate.

In some patients, myositis ossificans may be confused with osteosarcoma, which does not demonstrate the same zonation or peripheral margination phenomenon, nor does it have the same radiographic characteristics. When there is confusion about the proper diagnosis, optimal management includes a complete radiographic evaluation and careful clinical observation rather than a hasty or premature excision or biopsy (which will be difficult to interpret).[44] The radiographic differential diagnosis for myositis ossificans includes extraosseous or parosteal osteosarcoma, synovial sarcoma, vascular lesions, and calcification of soft tissue secondary to necrosis or inflammation.

Malignant Osseous Lesions

Osteosarcoma

Osteosarcoma is the most common primary sarcoma of bone (excluding multiple myeloma). It represents the most common primary sarcoma occurring in the shoulder, followed by Ewing's sarcoma and chondrosarcoma. In the past, it has typically occurred in the adolescent age group, although a significant percentage of patients are young adults in their third decade of life.

Classic osteosarcoma is a high-grade, aggressive tumor that occurs in the metaphysis, typically as a Stage IIB lesion, usually demonstrated by an extraosseous soft tissue component by the time the diagnosis is made.[20–23] The typical patient presents with intrinsic bone pain at night that is frequently unrelated to activity. The average length of symptoms at presentation is three to six months, which reflects the subtle nature of the preliminary symptoms and the need for early recognition of intraosseous pain and night pain as warning symptoms.[29]

Approximately 10 to 15 per cent of all osteosarcomas occur in the proximal humerus, while 1 to 2 per cent

occur in the scapula or clavicle.[21–24] The typical radiograph for osteosarcoma has a sunburst or osteoblastic pattern, with penetration of the adjacent cortex (Fig. 23–2A). Osteosarcomas usually have increased activity on bone scan (Fig. 23–2B), and a soft tissue mass is seen on CT (Fig. 23–2C) and MRI (Fig. 23–2D). Arteriography is no longer the technique of choice for evaluating soft tissue involvement but may be obtained to evaluate major vessel involvement or for intra-arterial chemotherapy (Fig. 23–2E). Variants of osteosarcoma other than the classic type include telangiectatic (vascular) osteosarcoma,[28] secondary osteosarcoma (Paget's disease or radiation induced), and various low-grade lesions such as periosteal and parosteal osteosarcoma.[24–27] The basic histological criterion for the diagnosis of classic osteosarcoma includes a malignant stroma (spindle cells) producing tumor or immature, neoplastic osteoid.[21–23]

Benign Cartilaginous Lesions

Osteochondroma

The incidence of cartilaginous tumors in the shoulder is second only to those occurring about the pelvis.[29] Solitary osteochondroma or exostosis is the most common benign tumor of the shoulder; approximately one-fourth of all exostoses occur in the proximal humerus. Osteochondromas actually represent a developmental abnormality arising from the peripheral growth plate and are typically active, benign (Stage 2) lesions during skeletal growth. The plain radiograph is usually diagnostic in demonstrating a smooth "excrescence" of metaphyseal cancellous bone which is confluent and continuous with normal metaphyseal bone (Fig. 23–3). Exostoses may appear as pedunculated, stalk-like lesions or as flat, sessile lesions. Concern regarding a possible secondary chondrosarcoma may arise in adult patients who present with pain, an enlarging soft tissue mass, or intraosseous bony erosions. Evidence of a thickened cartilaginous cap (greater than 1 cm) on CT scan, in association with a soft tissue mass, pain, or radiographic evidence of possible malignant degeneration, suggests a secondary chondrosarcoma. The risk of a secondary chondrosarcoma arising out of an exostosis is approximately 1 per cent per lesion, although rates as high as 10 to 30 per cent have been referred to in the literature regarding secondary malignancy in patients with multiple hereditary exostoses.[29]

Exostoses are typically diagnosed in the skeletally immature. An enlarging or symptomatic exostosis should be considered with caution in the skeletally mature since parosteal osteosarcoma is an alternative diagnosis in that situation. The treatment for solitary exostosis involves an excision through the base of the lesion. In the sessile form, care should be taken to excise the cartilaginous cap in order to avoid recurrence. The most common complication of an exostosis is an iatrogenic or surgical injury to the adjacent growth plate or neurovascular structures at the time of excision. An adequate surgical exposure should be empha-

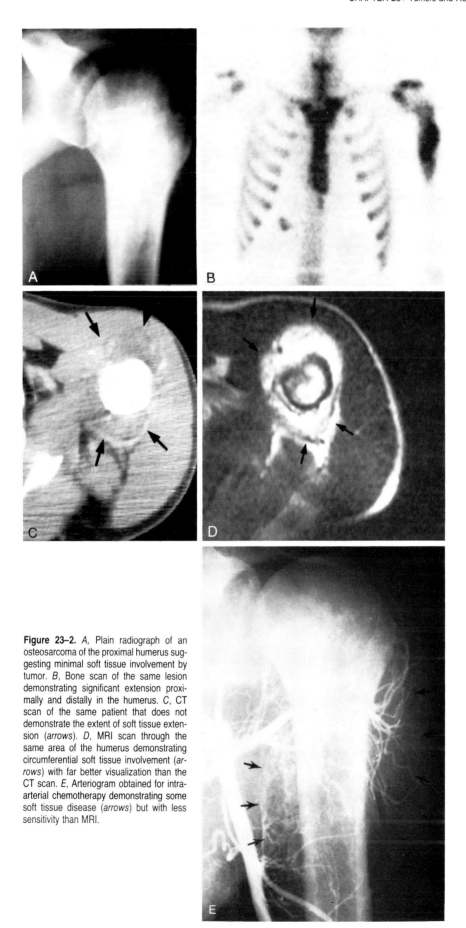

Figure 23–2. *A,* Plain radiograph of an osteosarcoma of the proximal humerus suggesting minimal soft tissue involvement by tumor. *B,* Bone scan of the same lesion demonstrating significant extension proximally and distally in the humerus. *C,* CT scan of the same patient that does not demonstrate the extent of soft tissue extension (*arrows*). *D,* MRI scan through the same area of the humerus demonstrating circumferential soft tissue involvement (*arrows*) with far better visualization than the CT scan. *E,* Arteriogram obtained for intra-arterial chemotherapy demonstrating some soft tissue disease (*arrows*) but with less sensitivity than MRI.

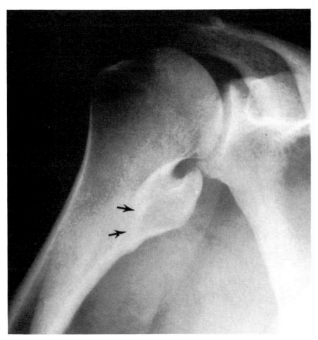

Figure 23–3. Osteochondroma of the proximal humerus demonstrating "confluence" of normal metaphyseal bone into the lesion (*arrows*).

sized, especially for proximal humeral and proximal femoral lesions, which are usually large and adjacent to the major neurovascular bundle of that extremity.

The diagnosis of secondary chondrosarcoma, arising out of an exostosis, is unusual and best made on the preoperative staging studies (thickened "cap" or enlarging soft tissue mass) and not by biopsy. Cartilage histology is very difficult to interpret, and thus, the diagnosis of a secondary malignancy is best made clinically and radiographically in most settings. The transition from benign to malignant is usually a protracted one involving relatively subtle histological changes.

Chondroblastoma

Chondroblastoma, or Codman's tumor, is an unusual benign, cartilaginous tumor that occurs in the proximal humeral epiphysis (25 per cent of cases) as a round or oval lesion containing fine calcifications surrounded by a reactive bony margin.[29–31] It occurs in the skeletally immature, and histologically it consists of aneurysmal tissue, "chicken wire" calcifications, and immature "paving stone" chondroblasts. Chondroblastoma occurs as an active, benign Stage 2 lesion, although it also has a more aggressive Stage 3 form. Treatment usually involves an extensive intralesional curettage that results in a large subchondral defect of the humeral head, requiring bone graft to prevent cartilaginous collapse. The radiographic appearance of this epiphyseal lesion is usually typical and involves adolescents or young adults. The differential diagnosis includes simple cyst, eosinophilic granuloma, osteomyelitis, or aneurysmal bone cyst.

Periosteal Chondroma

Periosteal chondroma is another benign cartilaginous lesion of the proximal humerus and is usually located just proximal to the deltoid insertion of the lateral humeral shaft. It typically presents as a minimally symptomatic or asymptomatic mass that is radiographically a sessile lesion with a distinct, well-defined margin of reactive cortex underlying the radiolucent cartilaginous mass.[32] Marginal excision results in a cortical defect of the humerus that may or may not require bone grafting. The differential diagnosis includes periosteal osteosarcoma, which does not have the well-defined underlying sclerotic cortex. Periosteal osteosarcoma is a more aggressive intracortical lesion that may extend into the medullary canal in a small percentage of cases.

Enchondroma

Solitary enchondroma is a benign, central cartilaginous lesion most commonly found in the small tubular bones of the hand but also occurring in the proximal humerus in 10 to 15 per cent of cases.[33, 34] As a benign lesion, enchondromas are asymptomatic and require no treatment. When they occur adjacent to a joint that is symptomatic for degenerative reasons, the clinical assessment of symptoms referable to the enchondroma is very difficult. This scenario is not uncommon, and it makes the initial evaluation of intraosseous cartilage tumors difficult, as intrinsic bone pain is an important symptom suggestive of a low-grade malignancy. Thus, the ability to distinguish intraosseous from intra-articular symptoms is a difficult but necessary challenge. The typical radiographic appearance of a benign enchondroma is that of a central lucent lesion with a well-defined bony margin and intrinsic calcifications. Figure 23–4 represents such a lesion in a 35-year-old female with rotator cuff symptoms and a heavily calcified benign cartilage lesion.

Malignant Cartilaginous Lesions

Chondrosarcoma

Chondrosarcoma may arise *de novo* as a primary chondrosarcoma, or it may arise out of a pre-existing benign cartilage lesion, which is then referred to as a secondary chondrosarcoma. Secondary chondrosarcoma occurs in young adults, accounts for approximately 25 per cent of all chondrosarcomas, and may be found in patients with a pre-existing enchondroma, osteochondroma, multiple enchondromatosis (Ollier's disease),[29, 35, 36] or multiple hereditary exostosis.[37] The radiographic evidence of a secondary, or low-grade, chondrosarcoma arising out of such a lesion includes enlarging radiolucent areas within the lesion or endosteal cortical erosions along the cortical margins (Fig. 23–5). Technetium bone scans are typically moderately "hot" for both enchondroma and low-grade chondrosarcoma and not helpful in distinguishing one from the

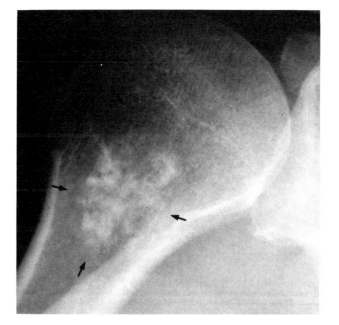

Figure 23–4. Plain radiograph of a 35-year-old woman with rotator cuff symptoms and an incidental benign enchondroma. There is no involvement or erosion of the endosteal cortical surface (*arrows*).

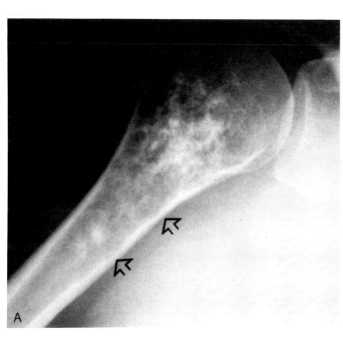

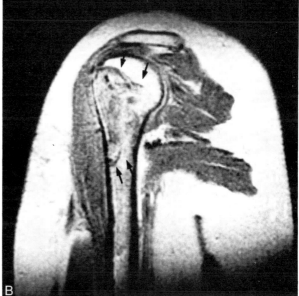

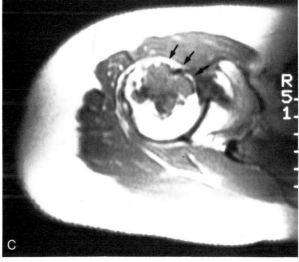

Figure 23–5. *A*, Plain radiograph of a 45-year-old woman with intrinsic intraosseous pain. There are distinct endosteal cortical erosions (*arrows*), suggesting a low-grade chondrosarcoma. *B*, Sagittal MRI scan of the proximal humerus demonstrating the extent of intraosseous involvement (*arrows*) by this low-grade chondrosarcoma. *C*, Axial (transverse) MRI scan through the humeral head demonstrating distinct bony erosions (*arrows*).

other. The microscopic evaluation of cartilage lesions is not diagnostic in a large percentage of cases. Histological characteristics suggestive of malignancy include cellularity, pleomorphism, and evidence of mitotic activity, such as double-nucleated lacunae. These are subtle findings, and the histological evidence for low-grade chondrosarcoma versus enchondroma is frequently incomplete and inconclusive.[34, 36] This confusion has led to the use of the term grade one-half chondrosarcoma to describe cartilage tumors that are histologically borderline between low-grade chondrosarcoma and benign enchondroma. The diagnosis of low-grade chondrosarcoma is best made radiographically with a biopsy at the time of definitive surgical treatment in order to confirm that it is a cartilaginous lesion. Low-grade, or secondary, chondrosarcomas are unique among intraosseous tumors in the difficulty in interpreting the light microscopic picture.

Primary chondrosarcoma is more commonly seen in the middle decades of life, and the incidence in the shoulder is second to that of the pelvis or hip joint.[38–43] These tumors typically present as intraosseous lesions with a poorly defined margin and faint intrinsic calcifications. Less commonly, a primary chondrosarcoma may arise from the surface of a bone or joint. Its clinical and radiographic appearance is very subtle, and a diagnostic delay of 6 to 12 months is not uncommon. Approximately two-thirds of primary chondrosarcomas are also low grade and may present as benign, encapsulated cartilage lesions. High-grade lesions are more invasive, have a higher metastatic rate, and usually occur in long-standing lesions as a "dedifferentiated" chondrosarcoma.[44–47]

Synovial Dysplasias

Cartilaginous loose bodies typically arise out of a proliferative synovium, in a reactive metaplastic process known as synovial chondromatosis (or osteochondromatosis).[48] It most commonly affects large joints (knee, elbow, shoulder, hip) in young adults and results in multiple small, cartilaginous, intra-articular loose bodies as the process matures. In the few cases where the nodules form a compact mass of cartilage, it may be confused with a low-grade, periarticular or juxta-articular chondrosarcoma. An intra-articular location favors the benign diagnosis of synovial chondromatosis; determining the intra-articular versus extra-articular location is sometimes one of the preoperative goals. In such cases, MRI or CT scans with or without arthrography might pinpoint the exact site of involvement. Synovial chondromatosis is typically a slowly progressive, degenerative disease that ultimately leads to joint destruction. It requires an aggressive total synovectomy to prevent persistence or recurrence, and in older patients with degenerative disease it is well treated with joint excision and replacement. A few cases in the literature associate malignant transformation with long-standing synovial chondromatosis which occurs over a prolonged period.[49]

Another disease associated with proliferating synovium is pigmented villonodular synovitis.[50] It is usually associated with a boggy, inflammatory synovitis, with or without bony erosions, in adolescents or young adults. It is histologically an aggressive synovial-histiocytic process that defies description as inflammatory or neoplastic. Treatment requires aggressive complete synovectomy for the diffuse form of the disease. Various forms of radiation therapy have been used in some centers with acceptable early clinical results.[51]

Miscellaneous Intraosseous Tumors

Simple Bone Cyst

Simple bone cysts, or unicameral bone cysts, occur most commonly in children between the ages of 4 and 12. Figure 23–6 demonstrates a simple cyst in the humerus of an eight-year-old. While the lesion appeared somewhat expansile, suggesting an aneurysmal bone cyst, the cortices remained intact, clear fluid was aspirated, and the cyst healed after the injection of intraosseous steroids. Simple bone cysts present as well-defined, central radiolucent lesions arising in the metaphysis adjacent to the physis (active) and, with maturation, migrate distally into the diaphysis (latent).

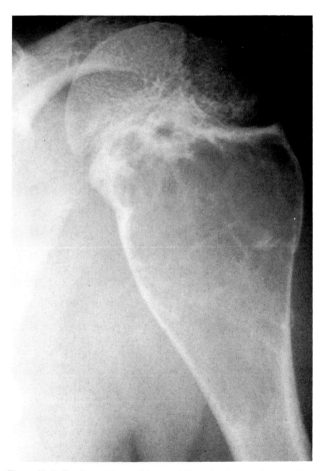

Figure 23–6. Simple cyst in an eight-year-old boy that is centrally located and juxtaepiphyseal (active).

They typically involve the proximal humerus (50 per cent), contain straw-colored fluid, and may be confused with an aneurysmal bone cyst (ABC).[52-57]

Pressure measurement of the cyst, aspiration, and intraosseous steroid injection is the treatment of choice and results in complete healing of the cystic area in approximately 50 per cent of cases and partial healing in 45 per cent. Approximately two-thirds of patients require multiple injections.[52] Complete repair following injection is most common in more inactive cysts with a lower pressure. Varying results in more recent reports have cast some doubt on the efficacy of steroid injections for simple bone cysts, especially when associated with a venogram at the time of dye injection into the lesion.[57] Recurrence or persistence of the cyst following surgical curettage and bone grafting occurs in approximately 30 per cent of cases. There is some diagnostic overlap between aneurysmal and simple cysts in children, as some simple cysts can have hemorrhagic fluid and yet not contain aneurysmal tissue.

Aneurysmal Bone Cyst

Aneurysmal bone cyst (ABC), nonossifying fibroma (NOF), and fibrous dysplasia are all benign lesions that also may occur in the shoulder. ABCs are not uncommon in the proximal humerus, but because of its widespread occurrence as a "secondary" lesion engrafted upon other tumors (simple cyst, giant cell tumor, chondroblastoma), the true incidence is unknown. The radiographic hallmark is that of a lucent, expansile. metaphyseal lesion. Treatment includes curettage and bone grafting,[58-59] which is associated with a recurrence rate of 20 to 30 per cent. Aneurysmal bone cysts can have an aggressive appearance and should have a careful biopsy prior to curettage in order to exclude the possibility of a telangiectatic osteosarcoma.

Fibrous Dysplasia

Fibrous dysplasia is a congenital dysplasia of bone that frequently surfaces as a painful lesion secondary to pathological fractures, microfracture, or the subtle, intrinsic, diaphyseal weakness resulting from pathological bone. The typical plain radiograph demonstrates a ground glass density with cortical thickening. Figure 23–7A and B are the plain radiograph and CT scan, respectively, of the humerus of a 20-year-old woman with severe polyostotic disease fibrous dysplasia. She had a history of chronic pseudarthroses (Fig. 23–7A) that had persisted despite bracing. When associated with symptoms or pathological fracture, diaphyseal involvement usually requires intramedullary fixation rather than bone grafting, as cancellous bone grafting is consistently "consumed" by the dysplastic process and is ineffective in resolving the weakened dysplasia process. Histologically, fibrous dysplasia demonstrates a furnace of dysplastic bone activity with a similar, impressive increased activity on the bone scan.[60-64]

Nonossifying Fibroma

Nonossifying fibroma (NOF) is a benign fibrous lesion that appears radiographically as an eccentric, well-defined, lucent lesion that has a scalloped border abutting the adjacent cortex (Fig. 23–8). It is more commonly found in the lower extremity than in the upper extremity. When the lesion is smaller than 2 cm, it may be referred to as a fibrous cortical defect. When larger than 3 cm or occupying more than half of the transverse diameter of the bone, these lesions are at risk for a pathological fracture. The majority of NOFs probably heal spontaneously and require no treatment. Treatment is reserved for those lesions with atypical radiographs (requiring biopsy) or for symptomatic or larger lesions (greater than 3 cm) that require treatment to prevent pathological fracture.[65]

Giant Cell Tumor

Giant cell tumor of bone is a common lesion in young adults that occurs primarily in the distal femur or proximal tibia (60 to 70 per cent) and also in the proximal humerus in 5 to 10 per cent of cases. It is a radiolucent, epiphyseal or metaphyseal tumor that most usually has a distinct bony margin and is frequently associated with extensive subchondral bone erosion. It is typically a Stage 2 active lesion (60 per cent of cases), but also shows up as a more aggressive, benign Stage 3 tumor in 20 per cent of cases. The treatment alternatives for giant cell tumor include curettage with or without local adjuvant treatment versus marginal resection. The local recurrence rate after curettage alone is 20 to 30 per cent for active lesions versus 5 to 10 per cent following marginal resection.[66-70] Local adjuvants used in conjunction with curettage include the application of phenol, bone cement (cementation), or liquid nitrogen freeze (cryotherapy). Histologically, "benign" giant cell tumor has demonstrated a potential for pulmonary metastasis in a very small percentage of cases.[70-78] The radiographic differential diagnosis in an adult includes aneurysmal bone cyst, metastatic adenocarcinoma, lymphoma, chondrosarcoma, and osteomyelitis.

Reticuloendothelial Tumors

Tumors of reticuloendothelial origin include a category of intraosseous lesions that arise from marrow stem cells and lesions of similar histology. They are also referred to as round cell or small blue cell tumors. This category of tumors includes diagnoses in the pediatric age group such as leukemia, lymphoma,[141] neuroblastoma, histiocytoses, rhabdomyosarcoma, Ewing's sarcoma, infection, and, in adults, multiple myeloma and metastatic adenocarcinoma.

Multiple Myeloma

Multiple myeloma is the most common primary malignancy of bone and typically occurs in the middle

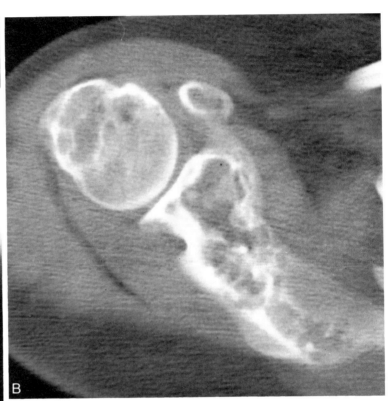

Figure 23–7. *A,* A 20-year-old woman with fibrous dysplasia of the humerus and a chronic pseudarthrosis (*arrow*) resistant to bracing. *B,* CT scan of the proximal humerus and scapula in the same patient demonstrating part of her extensive polyostotic disease, involving the humerus and scapula while sparing the glenohumeral joint.

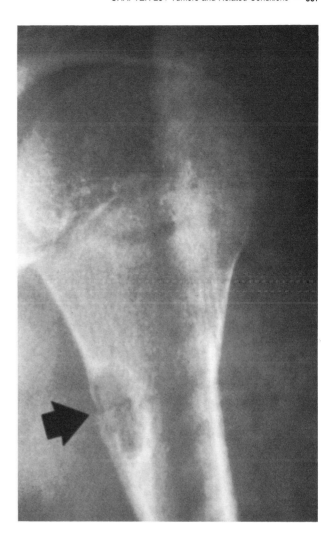

Figure 23–8. A small eccentric, juxtacortical, nonossifying fibroma that presented as a pathological fracture (*arrow*).

decades of life, involving the shoulder girdle in 5 to 10 per cent of cases.[79, 80] The most common site of involvement is in the axial skeleton, but a significant number of patients develop multiple distinct lesions in the extremities that may require surgical stabilization to prevent impending fracture if medical treatment has failed. In patients presenting initially with a solitary intraosseous myeloma or plasmacytoma of the shoulder, biopsy is indicated for diagnostic reasons. Elevated serum calcium levels, anemia, serum protein electrophoresis, or a distinctly cold bone scan may suggest the diagnosis of myeloma prior to biopsy in a patient with a solitary lesion or unknown diagnosis. The overall prognosis is poor; however, newer treatment involving aggressive chemotherapy and plasma cell antibodies offers hope for the future. Figure 23–9A is the plain radiograph of a 42-year-old man in apparent good health but experiencing shoulder pain. Coronal (Fig. 23–9B) and transverse (Fig. 23–9C) MRI scans demonstrate a suprascapular soft tissue lesion that extends anteriorly and posteriorly to the scapula. The preoperative diagnosis was a probable soft tissue sarcoma.

Open biopsy was diagnostic for multiple myeloma with extensive bony disease. The patient died suddenly one week after the biopsy, with an undocumented serum calcium level. All patients with the diagnosis of myeloma need to have careful documentation of their serum electrolytes.

Ewing's Sarcoma

The second most common intraosseous malignancy in adolescence is that of Ewing's sarcoma, an aggressive marrow cell tumor that appears as a permeative diaphyseal tumor which is poorly marginated and typically associated with a large, soft tissue mass.[81–82] Figure 23–10A demonstrates such a "permeative" lesion in the humeral diaphysis on a 16-year-old with a typically hot bone scan (Fig. 23–10B) and an associated soft tissue mass (Fig. 23–10C). Ewing's sarcoma today is primarily treated with aggressive chemotherapy and surgical resection or radiation therapy, depending on the size and location of the primary lesion.

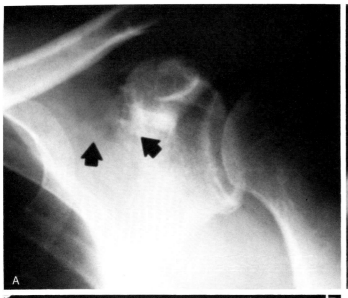

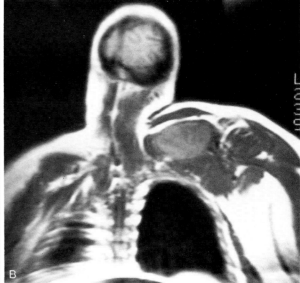

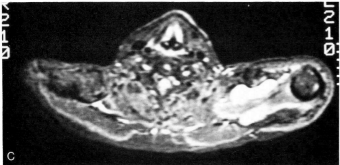

Figure 23–9. *A,* A 42-year-old man with left shoulder pain and a lytic scapular lesion (*arrows*). *B,* Coronal MRI view in the same patient demonstrates a suprascapular soft tissue mass. *C,* Axial MRI view in the same patient shows a lesion wrapped anteriorly and posteriorly over the scapula.

Miscellaneous Dysplasias

Gaucher's Disease

Gaucher's disease is an uncommon metabolic disorder of the reticuloendothelial system and glucocerebroside-glycolipid metabolism affecting the liver, spleen, and bone marrow.[83] The disease has an increased incidence in the Jewish population and occurs most commonly in the first three decades of life and without sexual preference. Patients typically experience pain secondary to bony involvement and marrow infiltration, which occurs most commonly in the femoral head, with a high degree of bilaterality. The disease in many ways represents a form of avascular necrosis of the femoral head. The humeral head is the second most common site of involvement, and radiographic changes include osteopenia, diaphyseal or medullary expansion, or cortical erosions. The differential diagnosis includes osteomyelitis in the acute setting and round cell tumors in the nonacute setting. Surgical treatment involves internal fixation for fracture prophylaxis, joint replacement for adults, when appropriate, and the appropriate management of pediatric femoral head necrosis in children.

Paget's Disease

Paget's disease (osteoporosis circumscripta, osteitis deformans) occurs after the fourth decade and has a slight preponderance in males.[84] Geographically, it appears to have a higher incidence in Great Britain, Europe, Australia, and the U.S.A., while relatively rare in India and most parts of Asia. Paget's disease occurs most commonly in the pelvis, skull, lumbosacral spine, femur, and humerus. It can occur in a polyostotic or a monostotic form usually manifested at the time of presentation. The typical radiographic picture shows cortical thickening and rarefaction, followed by pathological microfracture and diaphyseal bowing (Fig. 23–11A). The differential diagnosis in an adult includes metastatic adenocarcinoma, osteosarcoma, and osteomyelitis. Patients should be assessed by evaluating serum alkaline phosphatase and urinary hydroxyproline levels, total body bone scan, and CT scan or MRI.

Patients with Paget's disease undergoing orthopedic surgery should, in general, be pretreated. Paget's disease itself is best managed medically with diphosphonates or calcitonin. Sarcoma arising out of Paget's disease is associated with a history of progressive pain and a bony lytic lesion (Fig. 23–11B) associated with

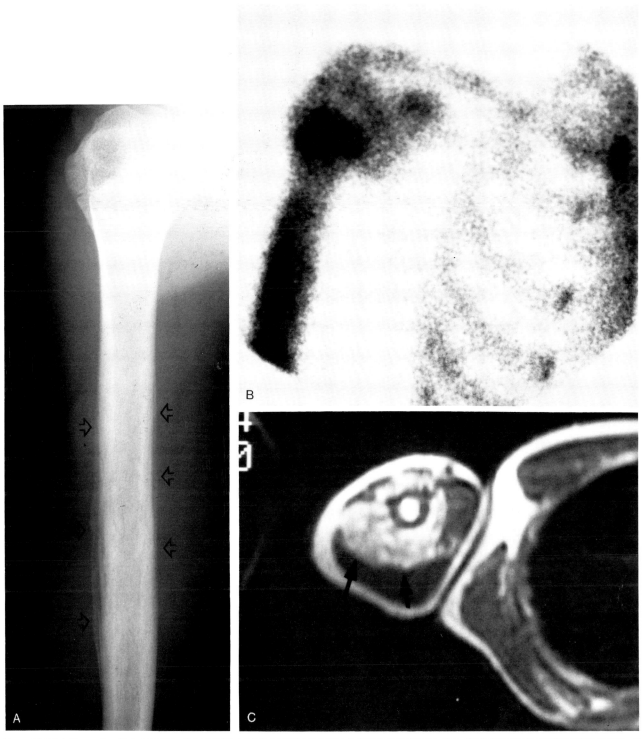

Figure 23–10. *A*, Permeative diaphyseal lesion demonstrating periosteal reaction in a 16-year-old boy (*arrowheads*). Open biopsy was consistent with Ewing's sarcoma. *B*, Bone scan of the same lesion demonstrates significant activity in the humerus. *C*, Axial MRI scan demonstrates a circumferential soft tissue mass (*arrow*) typical of Ewing's sarcoma.

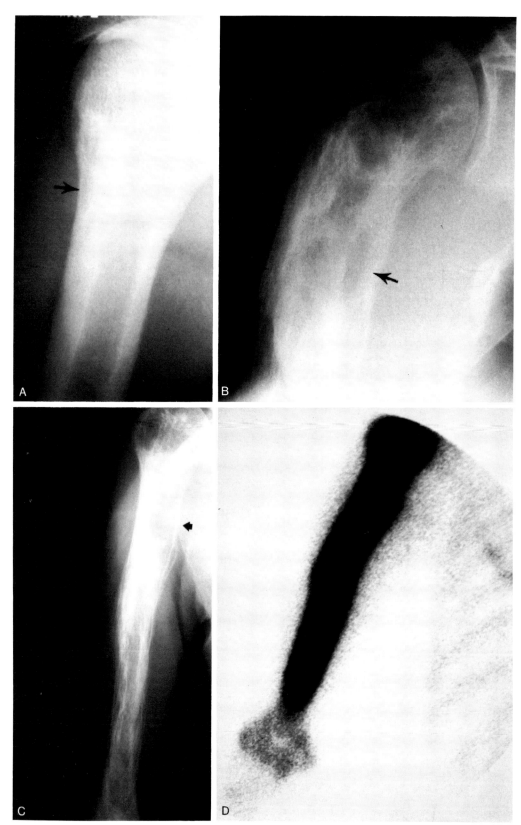

Figure 23–11. *A*, Early Paget's disease of the proximal humerus demonstrating cortical thickening and rarefaction (*arrows*). *B*, The same patient presented years later with shoulder pain and a lytic lesion of the humerus (*arrow*) consistent with a secondary osteosarcoma. *C*, Several months later this lytic process has become larger (*arrow*) and is associated with a large soft tissue mass (sarcoma). *D*, Bone scanning demonstrates intense humeral activity without distinguishing involvement by Paget's disease from sarcomatous changes.

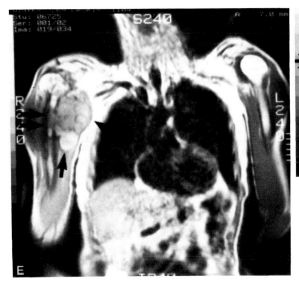
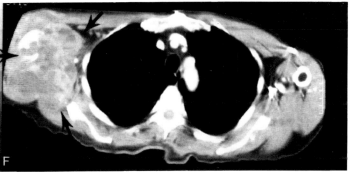

Figure 23–11 *Continued. E,* Coronal MRI shows a large soft tissue mass arising out of the proximal humerus (*double arrows*) and extending into the axilla. *F,* CT scan also demonstrates this secondary osteosarcoma with gross destruction of the proximal humerus (*arrows*).

a soft tissue mass. "Pagetoid sarcoma" is a rare variant of osteosarcoma and has been associated with a five-year mortality of 80 to 90 per cent.[85] Paget's sarcoma is best managed by a radical surgical margin because of the diffuse nature of the process of Paget's disease and the difficulty in assessing the extent of sarcomatous changes.

Figure 23–11*A* and *B* demonstrates the early and late radiographs of Paget's disease in the proximal humerus. The lytic lesion, combined with a history of increasing arm pain, serves notice of an early secondary osteosarcoma that showed up three months later (Fig. 23–11*C*) with a more impressive lytic lesion of the proximal humerus. Paget's disease affected the full humerus, and the bone scan (Fig. 23–11*D*) was of little help in demarcating bony margins or osseous involvement by this secondary, or Pagetoid, osteosarcoma.[23] MRI and CT scans again demonstrate the soft tissue and bony extent of disease (Fig. 23–11*E, F*) in the proximal humerus.

Benign Soft Tissue Tumors

Lipoma

Lipomas may occur intramuscularly or within normal fat planes of the axilla or the subscapular or other perivascular spaces. They frequently appear in the anterior deltoid as a large, soft, nontender, intramuscular mass.[86] A small number of lipomas may be tender or firm or have an equivocal history of a change in size. On an MRI or CT scan, a benign lipoma usually has a uniform, fatty consistency. Clinically, liposarcoma has a firmer, denser consistency than lipoma. If a lipoma feels very dense or firm clinically, it deserves an MRI scan for further evaluation. If the MRI scan demonstrates areas of distinctly different density, a biopsy should precede marginal excision to exclude the possibility of liposarcoma.

Hemangioma

Hemangiomas typically appear as "enlarging" intramuscular lesions in a child or young adult and are best visualized by MRI scan. If they are intimately involved with a major vessel, they should also be evaluated with an arteriogram. These lesions do not usually pose diagnostic or surgical problems, with the exception of large hemangiomas or hemangiomatosis of skeletal muscle. These are aggressive, congenital lesions that are frequently unresectable because of extensive neurovascular and soft tissue involvement.[87, 88] Many of these extensive lesions result in amputations for painful, dysvascular, or infected extremities. Most of these lesions are best diagnosed by open biopsy after an MRI scan, CT scan with contrast, or arteriography. Well-localized lesions are more easily resected than the more extensive congenital lesions. Embolization has had mixed results in halting the progression of disease.

Fibromatosis

Fibromatosis (desmoid) is a locally aggressive (Stage 2 or 3) lesion found in young children, teenagers, and young adults. These lesions have a firm consistency on clinical exam and may be associated with osseous erosions or invasion of a neurovascular bundle. Many of these lesions suffer a local recurrence because of inadequate preoperative staging, underestimation of their potential for local recurrence, and an inadequate surgical margin. The literature reveals considerable confusion and contradiction regarding the natural history of fibromatosis. Spontaneous regression as described in some publications is unusual except in some congenital forms, and the natural history for adolescent lesions is progressive growth and recurrence following marginal resections. These lesions rarely demonstrate pulmonary metastasis, and chemotherapy is not usually indicated for treatment.[89-92] The congenital form of the disease is referred to as a congenital fibrosarcoma primarily because of its very impressive histological cellularity. The adolescent version is best referred to as aggressive fibromatosis and behaves as an active aggressive lesion. Preoperative and postoperative MRI studies are mandatory in these patients in order to assess fully soft tissue involvement. Bone scans should also be carried out if there is any doubt about secondary bony involvement.

Soft Tissue Sarcomas

Soft tissue sarcomas occur in the upper extremity in approximately one-third of all cases. They are frequently misdiagnosed initially as a benign lesion and suffer a contaminated marginal resection before a definitive biopsy. Soft tissue sarcomas are characterized by four fairly typical clinical characteristics. They usually have a firm consistency, are deep to the superficial muscular fascia, are larger than 5 cm, and are nontender (Table 23-4). Adequate staging prior to biopsy is important for soft tissue sarcomas, just as it is for bony sarcomas (Fig. 23-12). Open biopsy is preferred in such lesions rather than needle biopsy so as to diagnose both the histological type and the histological grade of the lesion.

The most common soft tissue sarcoma in adults is malignant fibrous histiocytoma (MFH), which occurs most often in older adults (50 to 70 years).[93-95] Liposarcoma[96-98] typically occurs in the lower extremities in young adults as a large lesion with a histology ranging from low grade to high grade or pleomorphic. Synovial sarcoma[99] is a less common lesion associated with faint soft tissue calcifications, a juxta-articular location, and a high metastatic rate. Fibrosarcoma, rhabdomyosarcoma,[100] leiomyosarcoma, clear cell sarcoma, and epithelioid lesions are other, less common soft tissue malignancies.[101] Regardless of the tissue type, the grade of the lesion and the anatomical location of the primary tumor are the most significant factors determining prognosis and treatment. Soft tissue sarcomas of intermediate grade histology are problematic to treat because of a variable prognosis and response to chemotherapy. There has been some early experience with flow cytometry in identifying more active (aneuploid) tumors and may prove helpful in the future in subclassifying or grading intermediate grade tumors. Synovial sarcoma, epithelioid sarcoma, and rhabdomyosarcoma are characterized as soft tissue sarcomas with a high incidence (10 to 20 per cent) of

Table 23-4. SARCOMA: SIGNS AND SYMPTOMS

Bone	Soft Tissue
Bone pain	Firm mass
Night pain	Nontender mass
Pain (unrelated to joint motion)	Large (5 cm) or enlarging
Tender, soft tissue mass	Deep or subfascial

From Enneking WF, Spanier SS, and Goodman MA: A system for the surgical staging of musculoskeletal sarcoma. Clin Orthop 153:105–120, 1980.

regional lymph node metastasis and a poor prognosis,[102-109] but survival is generally recognized as being closely related to an individual tumor's histological grade.

Incidence of Neoplasms

Malignant tumors arising within the musculoskeletal system are rare and account for 0.5 to 0.7 per cent of all malignancies.[110] They are relatively more common in children, representing 6.5 per cent of all cancers in children. While there is little apparent sexual or racial predilection in the incidence of soft tissue sarcomas, osteosarcoma and Ewing's sarcoma have demonstrated a slight male preference (1.3 to 1.0).[111, 112] Approximately 4500 new cases of soft tissue sarcoma occur in the United States each year, with an incidence of 1.8 per 100,000, or approximately 18 cases per million. The number of new bone and cartilage or skeletal malignancies is similar. Various sources estimate 1000 to 2000 new cases of osteosarcoma occur annually in the United States.[110, 113, 114] The true incidence of most of these tumors remains somewhat speculative.

The most common tumor of the adult musculoskeletal system is metastatic adenocarcinoma, most commonly from the kidney, lung, breast, or prostate.[115] The most common primary malignancy of bone is multiple myeloma, a plasma cell malignancy usually diagnosed by the medical oncologist rather than the orthopedic surgeon.[116] Multiple myeloma has an incidence that is approximately twice that of osteosarcoma. Exclusive of multiple myeloma, the most common primary malignant tumor of bone is osteosarcoma. If both benign and malignant primary lesions of the musculoskeletal system are included, cartilaginous tumors are the most common primary lesion (benign and malignant) of the skeletal system.[111]

Age is a very important characteristic in the occurrence and distribution of tumors. The overall distribution of tumors by age in decades (Figs. 23-13 and 23-14) demonstrates the preponderance of benign tumors in the skeleton of the growing child; 58 per cent of all benign lesions occur in the second and third decades. Malignant tumors of the skeleton have a peak incidence in adolescents and middle-aged adults.[113-115] Osteosarcoma and Ewing's sarcoma are the most common malignant bone tumors in adolescents. In adults, osteosarcoma and chondrosarcoma occur with an incidence second to multiple myeloma and metastatic adenocarcinoma. Osteosarcoma represents approximately 40 per cent of all primary malignancies of bone, chondrosarcoma accounts for 20 per cent, and Ewing's sarcoma, 12.5 per cent.[113-115]

The incidence of tumors by anatomical location is best estimated by review of the works of Enneking[115] and Dahlin.[114] The overall incidence of primary sarcomas in the shoulder is approximately 15 per cent.[114, 115] Lesions of the shoulder are the third most common

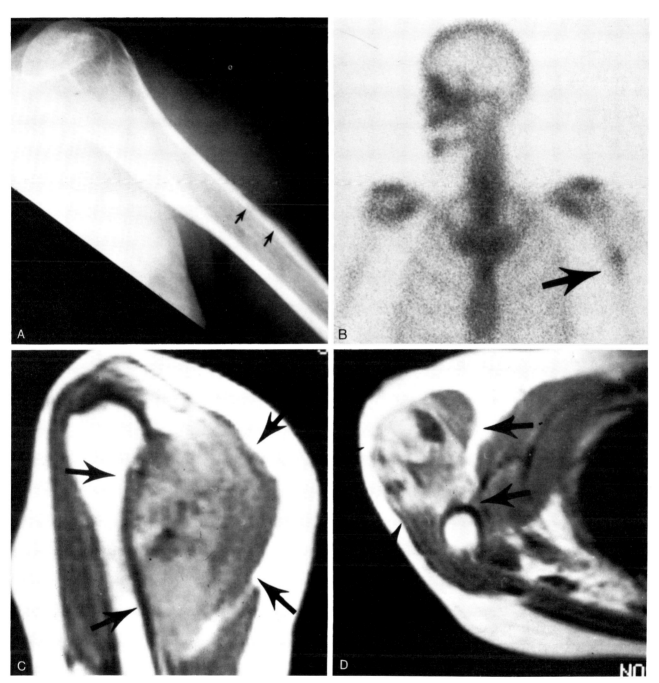

Figure 23–12. *A,* Plain radiograph in a 55-year-old woman with a large soft tissue sarcoma at the deltoid. Cortical irregularity at the deltoid insertion (*arrows*) is suggestive of bony invasion. *B,* The bone scan demonstrates distinct bony involvement at the deltoid tubercle with increased uptake (*arrow*). *C,* Sagittal MRI shows a large mass (*arrows*) abutting against the proximal humerus. *D,* Axial MRI also suggests posterior humeral cortical invasion by a large deltoid malignant fibrous histiocytoma (*arrows*).

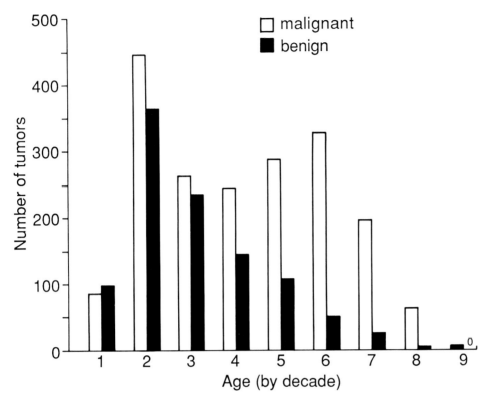

Figure 23–13. Distribution of musculo-skeletal tumors by age.

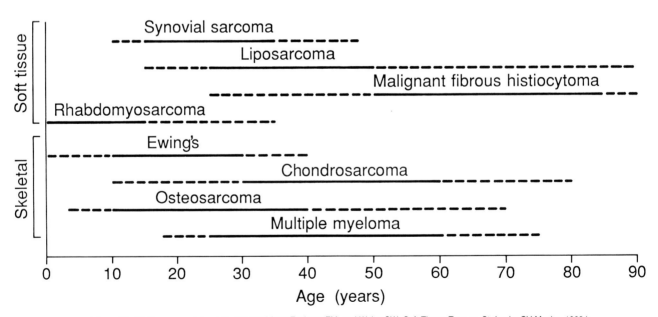

Figure 23–14. Sarcomas versus age. (Adapted from Enzinger FM, and Weiss SW: Soft Tissue Tumors. St. Louis: CV Mosby, 1983.)

overall site for sarcomas, behind the hip-pelvis (1) and the knee (distal femur and proximal tibia (2). In general, one-third of all sarcomas affect the upper extremity.[120] The majority of shoulder tumors occur in the proximal humerus (68.6 to 71.5 per cent) (Fig. 23–15). Tumors of the shoulder girdle occur in the clavicle (6 to 10 per cent of all cases) and in the scapula (18 to 24 per cent)[114, 115] to a much less common degree.

Clinical Presentation

Despite the refinement and developments in the field of musculoskeletal oncology, patients with musculo-skeletal malignancies, in general, experience a three- to six-month history of symptoms before an accurate diagnosis is made. The challenge for the general prac-titioner is to predict the diagnosis based on the initial history, physical exam, and plain radiographs. Most of these lesions have a subtle onset, and their initial diagnosis requires attention to certain details and an understanding of a few hallmark signs. The patient's

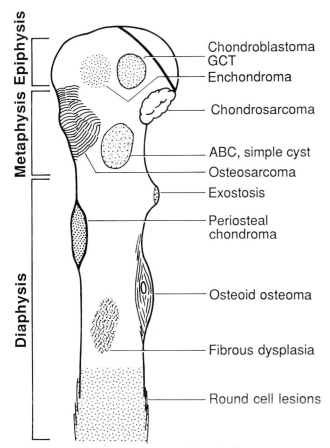

Figure 23–15. Common tumors of the proximal humerus.

Epiphysis
Metaphysis
Diaphysis

Chondroblastoma
GCT
Enchondroma

Chondrosarcoma

ABC, simple cyst
Osteosarcoma
Exostosis

Periosteal chondroma

Osteoid osteoma

Fibrous dysplasia

Round cell lesions

initial assessment remains the first and crucial step to a successful evaluation and treatment plan. In fact, in 70 to 80 per cent of cases it is possible to correctly diagnose and recognize most malignancies based on the initial history, physical exam, and plain radio-graphs.[115]

Patients with an intraosseous malignancy almost always complain of pain. The challenge to the physician is in distinguishing between the pain of malignancy and the other more common types of musculoskeletal pain secondary to degenerative joint disease, inflammatory joint disease, trauma, sepsis, and so forth. The hall-mark symptom of an intraosseous malignancy is that of night pain or pain at rest (see Table 23–4). Any patient who experiences a symptom of significant night pain should be very carefully assessed radiographically at the time of the first evaluation. Patients who expe-rience significant night pain should routinely have a technetium bone scan in addition to plain radiographs in order to evaluate their symptoms further. Some patients with inflammatory or degenerative joint dis-ease will complain of night pain, but in general, night pain as a prominent symptom is very suggestive of a possible tumor.

Other pertinent findings in the history that may be helpful include a strong family history for malignancy (adenocarcinoma or sarcoma) or a history of previous malignancy in the patient that may now be metastatic to the skeleton. Weight loss and general malaise may be significant symptoms for metastatic disease, and the physician should initiate a work-up to further evaluate the patient's general health. It is unusual, however, for a patient to have generalized symptoms or meta-static disease as the initial symptom of a sarcoma.

Musculoskeletal neoplasms present a clinical chal-lenge to the orthopedist in the determination of whether a patient has intraosseous pain or intra-artic-ular pain. This is not readily apparent in the early diagnosis of most intraosseous tumors. A careful phys-ical exam can sometimes elicit findings consistent with joint tenderness, impingement, or weakness, thus sug-gesting some sort of intra-articular process. It is un-usual for sarcomas to extend into a joint, and the presence of joint findings or symptoms is more consis-tent with trauma, degenerative disease, or some other nonneoplastic process. In general, intra-articular proc-esses are exacerbated by physical activities and joint motion (see section on physical examination). Simi-larly, some patients present with referred pain that may lead to the erroneous diagnosis of shoulder pain that has really originated from the cervical spine or hip pain that originates in the lumbar spine. The challenge of determining whether a particular patient's problem is intraosseous versus intra-articular requires a careful musculoskeletal evaluation which is usually best ac-complished by an orthopedist.

A careful orthopedic examination is important in evaluating all patients but is vital when evaluating the patient with difficult symptoms. Every adult patient being evaluated specifically for a possible neoplasm should have a careful general examination of the head and neck, cardiopulmonary status, abdomen, spine, breasts (women), prostate (men), and an examination for lymphadenopathy. This sort of general exam is most appropriate for adults who are more likely to have a metastatic adenocarcinoma. In addition to the specific exam evaluating patients for a possible neoplasm, all patients should have a complete general musculoskeletal exam evaluating for joint range of motion, strength, stability, and so forth. Regional adenopathy should be routinely checked on exam and will be found to be present with many tumors. It is usually an inflammtory phenomenon, reactive to the tumor. However, adenopathy involving lymph nodes greater than 1 cm should be evaluated further by MRI, and biopsy should be performed before definitive resection of the primary tumor.

Patients with an aggressive intraosseous malignancy usually have bony tenderness and a mass. The primary site may be deep and well covered by muscle and difficult to palpate. Usually, careful palpation will demonstrate the presence or absence of any soft tissue mass. However, low-grade intraosseous lesions may not involve the soft tissues. The ability to elicit joint findings is more suggestive of an intra-articular, a traumatic, an inflammatory, or a degenerative process. Thus, joint tenderness or stiffness can be a very helpful finding. Extension of an intraosseous malignancy medially toward the major neurovascular bundle, which is close to the humerus, may preclude limb-sparing surgery and is associated with a worse prognosis. The extent of involvement of the soft tissues on physical exam is an important finding to follow in addition to radiographic imaging. Clinical involvement of the soft tissues can be important information in directing the MRI scan and other studies. In general, the soft tissue mass produced by an intraosseous malignancy is relatively subtle as an early clinical finding and requires some attention on exam.

Soft tissue sarcomas most commonly have a history of a mass. Most soft tissue sarcomas, in contradistinction to intraosseous malignancies, are *not* painful. All soft tissue lesions should be carefully evaluated for the four characteristics of a soft tissue sarcoma: nontender mass, firm consistency, deep or subfascial location, and larger than 5 cm in size (see Table 23–4). There are exceptions to these characteristics, but as a general rule, they are very reliable guidelines in the initial evaluation of various soft tissue lesions. The most reliable finding of all is the consistency or density of the lesion. For instance, the most common soft tissue tumor in an adult is a lipoma, which may be large, deep in location, and nontender; however, its consistency will usually indicate whether it is malignant. Lipomas are typically very soft with the consistency of normal fat, while liposarcomas are usually firm. The ability to distinguish the consistency of a soft tissue mass can be a somewhat subtle but important finding.

Anything with a consistency more dense than normal fat should be evaluated carefully. Lipomas that feel firmer than normal fat or larger than 10 cm should be evaluated by MRI; intramuscular lesions that are firmer than normal muscle should also be evaluated by MRI. If a soft tissue mass is felt to be cystic, it is reasonable and advisable to attempt careful aspiration in the clinic in order to document whether that lesion contains fluid. Repeated or multiple aspirations are not advised and will only lead to contamination of a possible soft tissue sarcoma.

In summary, all patients with a possible musculoskeletal neoplasm (or an unknown diagnosis) should have a complete general examination and an orthopedic examination emphasizing the joints and the soft tissues. Always put your hand on the patient and consider the possibility of a mass when examining patients with a difficult problem. The size of any soft tissue mass should be carefully measured and recorded in the chart in order to give an objective finding for further follow-up. It is also helpful to take a photograph in the clinic for further objective documentation. The most common omission in the general physical examination is a failure to detect an obvious primary site of involvement for an adenocarcinoma (prostate, abdominal mass, prostatic mass). The most common mistake on the initial orthopedic exam is a failure to detect the true location of a lesion (referred pain) or to detect a soft tissue mass.

Routine clinical follow-up for a patient with a malignancy is important in order to detect progressive disease at an early stage. After the immediate postoperative evaluation, patients with sarcomas are generally followed every three to four months for two years, every six months for another two years, and every year thereafter. Frequent clinical follow-up is important in order to detect metastatic or recurrent disease at an early stage, thus enhancing further treatment. Frequent follow-up is also advisable in patients with undiagnosed skeletal pain. This is most appropriate in the adult who has significant joint symptoms and normal-appearing plain radiographs. If the plain radiographs are not consistent with the patient's symptoms, a total body technetium bone scan is well indicated in order to rule out a possible neoplasm. On the other hand, most patients who have a small (less than 5 cm) soft tissue mass can be followed without biopsy or MRI without significant danger of missing a possible malignancy. Similarly, intraosseous lesions that appear benign on plain x-rays or lesions that are picked up incidentally in the evaluation of a patient with intra-articular shoulder pathology can easily be followed if the plain radiographs are well demarcated and the lesions are obviously benign. If the initial plain radiographs are equivocal, a bone scan and CT or MRI are indicated to determine if the lesion is active and a biopsy needs to be done or if it can be followed clinically. Most low-grade, calcified or cartilaginous intraosseous lesions can be safely followed at 6-month intervals.

X-ray and Laboratory Evaluation

The orthopedist's interpretation of the initial plain radiographs is an important step in the early diagnosis of most musculoskeletal tumors. When dealing with intraosseous or skeletal lesions, the orthopedist should have a system for evaluating the initial plain radiographs and formulating the initial diagnosis. Every bony lesion has a characteristic location, margin, and density that typify it radiographically. These three radiographic characteristics are important in describing a lesion's growth rate and intrinsic density.[115] These concepts originated in a different format from that of Jaffee,[117] who first posed the questions "What is the lesion's density?" "What is it doing to bone?" "What is the bone doing to it?" and "What is its location?" in evaluating radiographs. This approach helps to focus attention on a lesion's growth rate, its degree of activity, and thus, its malignant potential. With these three characteristics in mind, the initial plain radiographs can be interpreted with the correct diagnosis in the majority of cases.

LOCATION

Where is the lesion located? Is it in the epiphysis, metaphysis, or diaphysis? Are there multiple metastatic sites or one primary site of involvement? For example, an aggressive metaphyseal tumor in an adolescent is very likely to be an osteosarcoma, whereas a diaphyseal lesion is much more likely to be a Ewing's sarcoma. Whether the lesion is central or eccentric with the bone also is important information. Nonossifying fibroma is almost always eccentric, while cartilaginous lesions (enchondroma) are usually centrally located.

MARGIN

The margin of the lesion on plain radiographs is the best reflection of that lesion's growth rate at the time of the initial evaluation. It refers to the margin or interface between the lesion and surrounding normal bone. If a tumor is slow growing, it will have a distinct or sclerotic margin that demonstrates the ability of the surrounding normal bone to react to it, thus marginating, or walling off, that lesion. A sclerotic or distinct peripheral bony margin indicates a slow-growing or benign lesion and is not usually seen with malignant or aggressive benign tumors. This type of margin reflects the ability of bone to respond to a slowly growing tumor. At the other end of the spectrum is the lesion that is not well marginated and does not have a sclerotic rim of reactive bone around it. This reflects a more rapidly growing tumor that enlarges at a rate that is faster than normal bone can react to it.

The best example of an aggressive lesion that infiltrates or percolates through bone is the permeative lesion of Ewing's sarcoma or any intramedullary round cell tumor or small blue cell tumor of bone. Round cell tumors occur more commonly in children, and the differential diagnosis includes lymphoma, leukemia, Ewing's sarcoma, rhabdomyosarcoma, neuroblastoma, histiocytoses, Wilms' tumor, or acute osteomyelitis. In contrast, the differential diagnosis for round cell tumors in adults includes metastatic carcinoma, Ewing's sarcoma, multiple myeloma, lymphoma, or osteomyelitis.

DENSITY

The intrinsic density of a lesion within bone or soft tissue is another piece of information that contributes to the initial diagnosis. Is the lesion making bone, cartilage (calcifications), fibrous dysplasia (ground glass density), or soft tissue (clear)? A truly cystic (or fluid-filled) lesion is most likely a benign or infectious lesion in bone or soft tissue, and this cystic nature may be determined clinically or demonstrated by the staging studies.

Thus, the complete assessment of the patient with a musculoskeletal lesion involves a careful evaluation of both the clinical and radiographic findings. The complex anatomy and frequency of referred pain make many diagnoses in the shoulder a challenge. A knowledge and an awareness of typical symptoms, physical findings, and radiographic clues for sarcomas are essential for successful treatment.

Appropriate initial radiographs for evaluating most patients include a well-exposed, properly positioned film. Accepting poor-quality radiographs can lead to disaster. It is essential that a well-exposed radiograph of the shoulder be obtained in all patients, especially those with persistent symptoms who may be failing conservative treatment for what is believed to be an intra-articular glenohumeral problem. There is no doubt that the best initial staging diagnostic study for evaluating a possible intraosseous malignancy is a technetium bone scan. The best staging study for a soft tissue lesion is an MRI scan. CT scans are routinely used for ruling out lung metastasis in addition to initial plain chest radiographs for all patients who have a probable soft tissue or bony malignancies.

The staging studies involved with assessing a high-grade intraosseous lesion, such as an osteosarcoma, include bone scan, MRI of the extremity, CT of the extremity, and CT of the lung. An MRI scan is indicated in order to assess the degree of soft tissue involvement and the neurovascular bundle margin before and after biopsy and induction chemotherapy. The CT scan of the extremity remains a good study to assess the degree of bony cortical involvement. A total body bone scan be carried out in all patients with musculoskeletal malignancies in order to assess the presence of distant bony metastases and to assess the extent of primary disease.

Possible tumor involvement of the neurovascular bundle and brachial plexus is best assessed by MRI, while arteriography is now reserved specifically for lesions located adjacent to a major vessel. Arteriography has also been used in the past to assess the extent of soft tissue involvement by sarcomas, but it has been more or less replaced at present by MRI scans. Other modalities for assessing the extent of soft tissue sarcomas have included gallium scans, which have generally been considered of inferior resolution quality when compared with MRI scans.

The assessment of possible chest wall involvement by shoulder lesions remains a difficult task. It is best assessed by CT, MRI, and bone scans. If there is rib uptake on the bone scan, bony chest wall involvement is obvious. It is somewhat unusual for proximal humeral malignancies to have chest wall involvement. However, soft tissue lesions that have extended from the brachial plexus, axilla, or scapula may well develop chest wall involvement.

LABORATORY

In general, laboratory studies for sarcomas are not of great assistance in making the initial diagnosis. The most common exception is the serum alkaline phosphatase, which is frequently elevated in osteosarcoma or in Paget's disease.[118] Serum acid phosphatase or prostatic specific antigen levels and a urinalysis (microscopic hematuria) are helpful in the evaluation of possible malignancies of the prostate or kidney.[119] A hematocrit, white blood cell count, and erythrocyte sedimentation rate (ESR) are well indicated in evaluating for possible sepsis, although both the white count and the sedimentation rate may be nonspecifically elevated with various tumors and the hematocrit may be nonspecifically low. Any patient who has plasmacytoma or multiple myeloma in his or her differential diagnosis should have serum calcium and serum electrolytes checked preoperatively in order to detect hypercalcemia. In addition, those patients should undergo a serum and urine protein electrophoresis study in order to evaluate their immunoglobin profile.[116]

Routine laboratory studies (liver enzymes, etc.) are checked in the routine follow-up of patients with a musculoskeletal malignancy; however, it is unusual for a sarcoma to metastasize to the liver, and thus liver enzymes are rarely elevated secondary to tumor. Elevated liver enzymes can occur for other reasons (hepatitis) and are included in routine follow-up blood work for that reason. It is useful to evaluate liver enzymes and complete blood counts in all sarcoma patients in order to assess a patient's general medical health.

Complications of Tumors

PATHOLOGICAL FRACTURES

One of the most significant complications of a musculoskeletal tumor is that of pathological fracture, the majority of which are secondary to metastatic adenocarcinoma. Approximately one-third of all diagnosed cases of breast, pulmonary, thyroid, renal, and prostatic carcinoma include skeletal metastases.[121–124] While the most common site for metastasis is the axial skeleton, approximately 25 per cent of all metastases are located in the shoulder girdle.

Surgery may be indicated to obtain a primary diagnosis by open biopsy or to achieve internal fixation for fracture prophylaxis. Patients with an established tumor diagnosis and lytic lesions representing bony metastases should, in general, be treated with chemotherapy and radiation therapy first, if the evidence indicates that that particular lesion is likely to respond to that treatment. Metastatic lesions that are generally considered to be resistant to radiation therapy or chemotherapy or those lesions that have failed similar previous treatment should be treated surgically (e.g., renal cell carcinoma). Surgical stabilization or internal fixation is indicated in any patient with an impending or completed pathological fracture who can tolerate a general anesthetic and has a life expectancy of at least one month. Coaptation splinting, as an alternative to surgery, does a relatively poor job of relieving fracture symptoms in the humerus because of persistent rotational instability. Figure 23–16 shows a pathological fracture of the proximal humerus in a 65-year-old patient with extensive metastatic disease. His pain was unrelieved with coaptation bracing, and he was treated surgically with methylmethacrylate and short Enders rods placed through the fracture site. His poor medical status and limited life expectancy (several months) dictated this more conservative surgical procedure rather than the usual treatment of hemiarthroplasty. Even patients with widespread metastatic disease can benefit greatly from a careful but aggressive approach to the management of pathological fractures versus impending fractures.

Intraosseous sarcomas that result in a pathological fracture represent less than 10 per cent of all sarcomas, and although they present a challenge, they are no longer considered an absolute indication for immediate amputation. Another problem seen is that of fractures occurring after a poorly designed biopsy, thus emphasizing the need for careful biopsy procedures. A particular problem with Ewing's sarcoma arises in patients who develop a recurrence in a diaphyseal lesion that has been previously irradiated. Such lesions should be stabilized prophylactically with an intramedullary rod to prevent possible fracture if there is any evidence of cortical involvement. Fractures through irradiated bone are unlikely to heal and should be internally fixed as

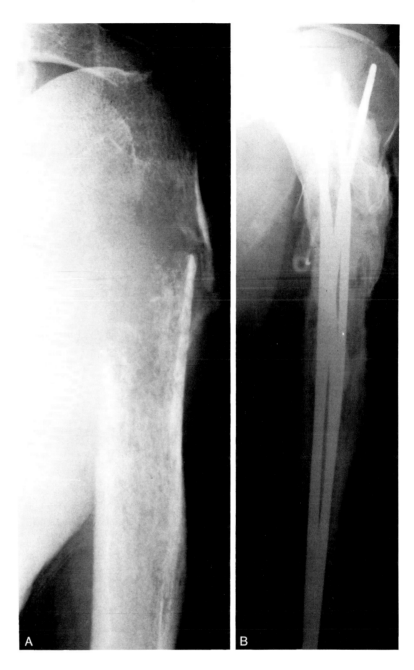

Figure 23–16. *A*, Metastatic adenocarcinoma of the lung in a 65-year-old man with extensive metastatic disease and a pathological fracture. *B*, A conservative surgical stabilization in this patient involved cementation and placement of a rod through the fracture site.

early as possible. Fibrous dysplasia represents another example of pathological bone that may require intramedullary fixation to prevent repeated fractures and progressive deformity. Intramedullary fixation is the method of choice because of its biomechanical superiority. Plating with screws is vastly inferior to intramedullary fixation of impending or completed pathological diaphyseal lesions.

Differential Diagnosis

The shoulder girdle is an area that presents a challenge to the diagnosis of many different conditions. Its close relationship with the cervical spine and brachial plexus can present a formidable challenge in distinguishing different anatomical lesions within a small anatomical space. The complexity of the soft tissue anatomy of the glenohumeral joint itself and the difficulty of making many common intra-articular diagnoses leave a significant margin for error, even for a skilled orthopedist. The confusion that may arise can delay the diagnosis for various musculoskeletal tumors for a significant period of time.

The differential diagnosis for various musculoskeletal lesions includes those lesions identified in Table 23–5. While the categories of trauma, tumor, infection, and inflammatory or degenerative disease include the diagnosis in the vast majority of cases, various dys-

Table 23–5. DIFFERENTIAL DIAGNOSIS OF
MUSCULOSKELETAL LESIONS

1. Trauma (subtle, bony, acute, or chronic)
2. Tumor (benign or malignant, primary or metastatic)
3. Infection (bacterial, viral, fungal, or venereal)
4. Inflammatory disease (rheumatoid arthritis, gouty arthropathy, collagen vascular disease, PVNS)
5. Degenerative disease (osteoarthritis)
6. Dysplasias (fibrous dysplasia, Paget's, disease, multiple hereditary exostoses, neurofibromatosis)
7. Hematological disorders (hemophilia, histiocytosis, myeloproliferative disorder)
8. Metabolic disorders (osteomalacia, rickets, hyperparathyroidism, renal osteodystrophy)

plastic, hematological or metabolic problems are important and require a more extensive evaluation. Certainly the process of separating out difficult problems starts with an accurate and thorough history and physical exam.

Trauma as the cause of lesions of the musculoskeletal system obviously often includes a history of an injury, but "incidental" trauma is also frequently associated with sarcomas, although no causal relationship has been demonstrated. Chronic injuries or stress fractures are often a more subtle and challenging diagnosis but are less common in the shoulder than in the lower extremity. Figure 23–17 demonstrates a degenerative condition of the sternoclavicular joint in an area that does not easily lend itself to imaging techniques; this degenerative lesion with an apparent soft tissue mass could be misinterpreted as a possible neoplasm of the proximal clavicle. An understanding of the pathology of the sternoclavicular joint is of great assistance in interpreting diagnostic studies of this area.

Infections are a common problem in healthy young children who suffer from acute hematogenous osteomyelitis or septic arthritis. In fact, the differential diagnosis for any lesion in a child should always include infection as a possible cause. Acute hematogenous osteomyelitis is an unusual problem in adults because adults usually develop osteomyelitis secondary to traumatic wounds, surgical complications, or chronic decubiti. Tuberculous or fungal infections are an even greater diagnostic and treatment challenge and a culture should be taken in all suspected infections. In general, tuberculous infections have an unimpressive amount of reactive bone on the radiographs and a chronic history. Whenever an infectious problem is being considered, a biopsy specimen should be sent in addition to abundant, appropriate cultures. The old adage "always biopsy an infection and culture a tumor" remains good advice as a general rule in the evaluation of any lesion. There are some necrotic soft tissue tumors that contain pus and strongly resemble a soft tissue abscess.

Inflammatory and degenerative disease is usually associated with typical findings on plain radiographs such as a joint space narrowing, subchrondal sclerosis, and cyst formation. Clinically, it can be very difficult to distinguish inflammatory or degenerative disease from a subtle neoplasm. The differential diagnosis can also be difficult in children, in whom pauciarticular juvenile rheumatoid arthritis in its initial presentation can be very difficult to distinguish from septic arthritis or other soft tissue tumors.

The most common dysplasias of bone masquerading as neoplasms include fibrous dysplasia in children and Paget's disease in adults. These are usually polyostotic

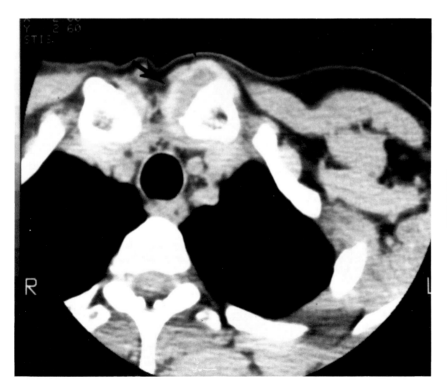

Figure 23–17. CT scan of the sternoclavicular joint in a patient with degenerative joint disease, an effusion and a soft tissue mass consisting of redundant synovium (*arrows*). This area is difficult to image and could be misinterpreted as a neoplasm.

"tumors" that actually represent dysplasias of bone. Fibrous dysplasia and Paget's disease can frequently be diagnosed by plain x-rays and bone scans, as can many of the polyostotic syndromes. Both fibrous dysplasia and Paget's disease may require intramedullary fixation in order to treat chronic, pathological painful, and weak long bones. Secondary malignancies are unusual and associated with increasing pain and obvious x-ray changes. Other dysplasias include multiple hereditary exostoses and enchondromatoses.

Hematological disorders (excluding myeloma) that may masquerade as tumors occur most commonly in children or young adults with the various histiocytoses, hemophilia, and other blood dyscrasias. The least aggressive form of histiocytosis is that of eosinophilic granuloma, which is truly the "great imitator" in children, as it can masquerade as a tumor. Eosinophilic granuloma occurs in the diaphysis and usually is seen as a solitary lesion in a healthy child. However, it may occur as multiple lesions, and when diagnosed in a young child (two years or younger), there is always the concern that this initial lesion may signal the presence of other lesions in the more severe form of the syndrome, such as Hand-Schüller-Christian disease (older children) or Letterer-Siwe disease (infants). Similarly, classic hemophilia or Factor 8 deficiency, although uncommon, may show up initially as a solitary knee effusion (septic knee). Therefore, it is important to obtain an accurate history, asking specifically about previous bleeding problems in other family members, in order to make the diagnosis.

Metabolic disorders in adults can also be difficult diagnoses to make. Adult patients with osteomalacia may present with a stress fracture, a hot bone scan, equivocal staging studies, and a risk factor in their history (renal disease, gastrointestinal malabsorption). Syndromes of renal osteodystrophy, osteomalacia, and osteoporosis are unlikely to show up as a problem of the upper extremity, but they remain an important part of any complete differential diagnosis. Patients with osteomalacia frequently appear with diffuse manifestations of their disease (vertebral fractures, osteopenia, etc.) and may require a full metabolic work-up: serum Ca, + PO_4, serum + urinary hydroxyproline, vitamin D, parathyroid hormone levels, bone scan, densitometry, and a tetracycline-labeled iliac crest biopsy.

Biopsy, Resections, Reconstructions, and the Management of Specific Lesions

THE BIOPSY

The management and treatment of any malignancy begins with a sound histological diagnosis. Although every institution has its own experiences and prejudices

regarding biopsy for sarcomas, open, or incisional, biopsy is regarded by most as the best method.[125] Incisional biopsy is an operative technique that involves incising a small wedge-shaped piece of tissue from the tumor for histological evaluation. Its primary advantage over a closed, or needle, biopsy is the acquisition of a larger, more adequate specimen, which is especially important in the face of challenging sarcoma diagnoses. However, open or incisional biopsies do carry a risk of tumor contamination from postoperative hemorrhage. It is important that the surgical principles of incisional biopsy be strictly observed in the shoulder, just as in any other anatomical site. A dissecting hematoma after any biopsy can easily contaminate otherwise normal tissue and expand the necessary margin for resection, or it can contaminate nearby major neurovascular structures such as the brachial plexus or brachial vessels and thus preclude the possibility of a limb salvage type of resection.

Mankin and colleagues, under the auspices of the Musculoskeletal Tumor Society,[126] carried out a retrospective comparison of 329 cases of sarcomas on which biopsies were performed in a referring (primary or secondary) hospital versus those done in a setting where there was experience with sarcomas. The study concluded that biopsy-related problems were three to five times more frequent in the outside referring hospital versus the treatment center. The referring hospitals without sarcoma experience had a higher incidence of major diagnostic errors, nonrepresentative biopsies, wound complications, treatment alterations, changes in results, and changes in final patient results. Last, the incidence of unnecessary amputations was 4.5 per cent of all the cases. This sort of study may be prejudiced in favor of the tertiary institutions by the fact that most patients were difficult cases that had been referred for treatment, but the study does emphasize a high complication rate for biopsies and the need for careful planning and execution. Higher complications and diagnostic errors do occur in less experienced centers, reflecting the complexity of the diagnosis and treatment of sarcomas. The best management for all patients with sarcomas is to have the biopsy carried out in an experienced center where the definitive treatment will be rendered.[127]

The best surgical approach for a biopsy of the proximal humerus has traditionally been through the anterior substance of the deltoid (Fig. 23–18). The deltopectoral groove should be avoided, as any hematoma after the biopsy might enter the groove and spread proximally into the axilla and lead to considerable proximal contamination. Approaching malignant lesions through the anterior deltoid requires resection of that portion of the deltoid with the definitive procedure but minimizes the risk of contamination; thus this is the traditional site for an incisional biopsy of the proximal humerus. Tumor contamination after the biopsy is a significant problem even in experienced hands and should observe the following principles of technique.[125]

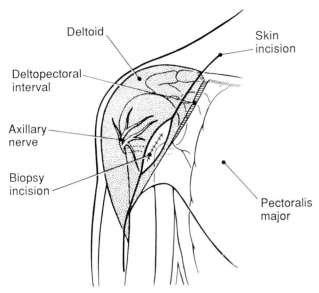

Figure 23–18. Biopsy of the proximal humerus.

Placement of the Incision

When biopsying lesions in the extremities, the surgeon should use a longitudinal (not transverse) incision, usually of 4 to 5 cm in length (see Fig. 23–18). The incision should be placed in the line of the proposed future definitive resection or placed such that it does not contaminate the lines of a possible future amputation. Around the scapula or clavicle, as in the pelvic girdle, an oblique or transverse incision is appropriate, but as a general rule, all extremity tumors should be biopsied through a longitudinal incision.

Contamination by Tumor Hematoma

If possible, always perform a biopsy of a tumor at its most superficial and accessible site. An incisional biopsy technique should involve as little soft tissue dissection as possible. A marginal, or excisional, biopsy should be reserved only for obviously benign lesions (e.g., lipoma) or for small (2 to 3 cm) lesions. Similarly, always biopsy the lesion away from a major neurovascular bundle or joint in order to avoid contaminating those structures and thus precluding a need for limb-sparing surgery. This precaution is especially important in the proximal humerus and shoulder because of the proximity of the brachial vessels and brachial plexus.

Before wound closure, strict hemostasis should be carefully accomplished. The use of a tourniquet is not possible in the shoulder and, even in areas where one is used, should be released before wound closure to achieve hemostasis. Very vascular malignant lesions (e.g., angiosarcoma, myeloma, hypernephroma, or Ewing's sarcoma) in the shoulder may prove to be a challenge regarding hemostasis. In those situations,

packing the wound with various coagulant materials in addition to a pressure dressing may prove helpful in enhancing hemostasis. The use of surgical drains or the practice of leaving the wound open following open biopsy is associated with a higher incidence of wound contamination or infection and is not an accepted method of management. After achieving hemostasis, the surgeon should meticulously close the biopsy wound and carefully close the deep and superficial layers to prevent late wound dehiscence. The skin is best closed with a subcuticular closure in order to minimize skin contamination and enable a smaller ellipse of skin to be excised with the main tumor specimen at the time of the definitive resection.

Adequacy of the Specimen

Prior to wakening the patient, it is essential to wait for the pathologist to confirm the adequacy of the specimen by frozen section under the microscope. Although it may not be possible to make a definitive diagnosis by frozen section in every case, it is possible to determine whether the specimen has diagnostic or lesional tissue and thus whether it is an adequate specimen. Bacterial and fungal cultures should be obtained routinely, in addition to sending tissue for special stains, electron microscopy, flow cytometry,[133] or immunohistochemistry. As a general rule, it is advisable to biopsy infections and culture tumors. If there is some doubt about the location of a biopsy site in the extremity, pelvis, or spine, an intraoperative radiograph with an appropriate marker should be taken before the biopsy. In many cases of osteogenic sarcoma, it is not necessary to biopsy the bone to obtain adequate tissue. A biopsy of a bony lesion can frequently be obtained from its soft tissue extension, thus avoiding fenestration of that bone and the complications of postoperative fracture and further contamination from osseous bleeding.

Open Versus Closed Biopsy

The alternatives to an incisional, or open, biopsy include a marginal, or excisional, biopsy or closed needle biopsy. In general, an excisional biopsy is not an accepted method for any lesion that may be malignant. It is an acceptable biopsy technique only when used to excise a small lesion (smaller than 3 cm) or to excise a lesion that is obviously benign (e.g., lipoma). The marginal excisional biopsy of a small lesion produces little more contamination than an incisional biopsy and thus is an adequate technique for that size lesion. Marginal excision of a tumor, however, is best indicated for benign lesions. Small (less than 5 cm) soft tissue sarcomas do exist in the upper extremity, and if there is concern or confusion about a lesion, a consultation with a specialist before the biopsy is the appropriate approach.[128]

Needle biopsy is an attractive method for use on

some tumors.[129–131] The disadvantage is the small size of the specimen and the difficulty of assessing whether a lesion is high grade or low grade.[132] Although needle biopsy techniques may give a reliable diagnosis regarding tissue type (MFH versus liposarcoma), they frequently do not give a reliable diagnosis regarding the grade of the lesion[125] (high, intermediate, or low grade). Thus, in determining contemporary treatments that require the knowledge of high-grade versus low-grade histology, a needle biopsy is frequently an inadequate way to achieve a definitive histological diagnosis with soft tissue sarcomas. The attraction of a needle biopsy is that it avoids the operative setting and is achievable in the clinic, giving a quick diagnosis that may be useful in initiating preoperative chemotherapy if a lesion is obviously high grade. The disadvantage remains that of sampling error, which has been reported in approximately 25 per cent of cases.[125] Needle biopsy is the preferred method for biopsying osteosarcoma when the radiographs are typical and only a tissue diagnosis (malignant stroma or osteoid) is required. It has the advantage of a small bony fenestration, minimizing both the potential for postbiopsy hemorrhage and the risk of pathological fracture. The best indications for a needle biopsy include the following:

1. **To achieve a "tissue" diagnosis** (i.e., metastasis, recurrence, or confirming an otherwise classic presentation). Needle biopsy as a general rule is not a reliable method for assessing the histological grade of a lesion.

2. **For cystic lesions or abscesses**. Cystic lesions are usually not malignancies, and in children, a needle biopsy is a good way to quickly rule out possible infections. It is the preferred method of diagnosing and treating many cystic lesions. If purulent drainage is not obvious, beware of soft tissue sarcomas with central necrosis; a definitive open biopsy should accompany any surgical drainage procedure.

3. **Vertebral or pelvic tumors**. Needle biopsy is an appropriate technique for vertebral and pelvic lesions, thus avoiding a more extensive open biopsy. Most of these lesions are biopsied with CT guidance in the radiology department.

The instruments required for needle biopsy are not complex. Needle biopsy for soft tissue sarcomas typically involves the use of a trocar cutting needle that delivers a small strip of tissue. Larger trephine or bone marrow needles (3 to 5 mm in diameter) are used for bony lesions. The skinny needle technique for soft tissue tumors uses a 22-gauge needle for a cytological smear; this smear requires interpretation by an experienced cytopathologist.

Immediately proceeding with the definitive resection following an open biopsy is a treatment alternative that offers the advantage of minimizing the risk of postbiopsy hematoma and contamination. It requires appropriate intraoperative precautions, such as a change in gowns, gloves, instruments, and the operative drapes, between the biopsy and the definitive resection. The issue of whether or not it is prudent to proceed with a definitive surgical resection immediately following the frozen section histological diagnosis depends on the lesion involved and the confidence level of the pathologist giving the diagnosis. This course of action requires careful planning and a confident, well-informed pathologist at the time of the frozen section biopsy. It is not a reasonable alternative for patients who are candidates for preoperative adjuvant therapy or when the differential diagnosis includes radiosensitive tumors, such as lymphoma, which are not treated with resection. When there is doubt regarding whether a lesion is malignant or benign, high grade or low grade, treatment should be delayed until a definitive diagnosis is reached.

Biopsies are a challenging aspect of sarcoma management, reflecting both the rarity and the complexity of diagnosing and treating these lesions. Although the biopsy appears to be a technically small operative procedure, it represents a significant hurdle to the achievement of an appropriate and successful treatment plan. The complexities of the diagnosis of most sarcomas require that this significant, initial step in the treatment be carried out in a center experienced in the management of sarcomas.[127]

SURGICAL RESECTIONS ABOUT THE SHOULDER GIRDLE

The Surgical Margin

Appropriate surgery remains the definitive treatment for most sarcomas at their primary site. The surgical treatment is best described by separately defining the tumor resection part of the procedure and the reconstructive part of the procedure. These two aspects of any surgical procedure for a tumor are potentially conflicting in their objectives, and great care should be taken to ensure that the resection is not minimized or compromised to facilitate the reconstructive part of the procedure and thus enhance function. The resection must take precedence over the reconstruction to accomplish a cure. It is imperative that these two procedures remain separate in principle. In some institutions, different surgeons carry out these two parts of the procedure in order to achieve that goal.

When discussing the probable success of a procedure in terms of local tumor control, the resection procedure is best defined by the surgical margin achieved. The surgical margin describes the efficacy of the procedure in terms of possible future tumor recurrence.[115] Assessing and describing the surgical margin requires a cooperative effort by both the surgeon and the pathologist, who must immediately review the surgical specimen. The four fundamental types of margins are intracapsular, marginal, wide, and radical (Table 23–6 and Fig. 23–19).

An *intracapsular*, or *intralesional*, surgical margin describes an inadequate margin resulting from a resection that violates the tumor's pseudocapsule and runs

LIMB SALVAGE RESECTION

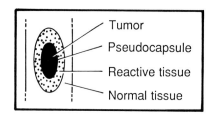

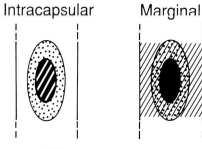

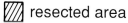

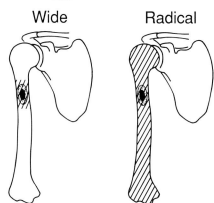

Figure 23–19. Surgical margins.

AMPUTATION

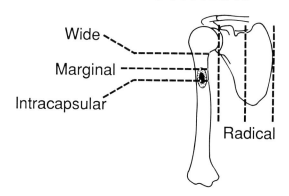

Table 23–6. SURGICAL MARGINS

Surgical Margin	Surgical Procedure	Result
Intralesional	Piecemeal debulking or curettage	Leaves macroscopic tumor
Marginal	Excision of tumor and pseudocapsule through reactive zone	Leves microscopic tumor
Wide	Excision of tumor, pseudocapsule, reactive zone, and a cuff of normal tissue	Risk of leaving microscopic tumor
Radical	Extracompartmental procedure removes tumor, pseudocapsule, reactive zone, and entire compartment	Minimal risk of residual microscopic tumor

From Enneking WF, Spanier SS, and Goodman MA: A system for the surgical staging of musculoskeletal sarcoma. Clin Orthop *153*:105–120, 1980.

through the tumor, leaving gross residual tumor. It involves a partial and incomplete excision of tumor. In general, debulking procedures such as this are grossly inadequate and not indicated for any tumor.

A *marginal* surgical margin (see Fig. 23–19) involves a plane of dissection through the reactive zone located between tumor and normal tissue. The reactive zone refers to areolar tissue surrounding the tumor that is compressed and inflamed by tumor invasion and enlargement. Although it is located outside a tumor's pseudocapsule, it potentially contains foci of microscopic tumor, and thus a dissection through this plane is associated with a high recurrence rate, especially when dealing with high-grade malignant tumors. This reactive or inflammatory zone usually demonstrates a significant decrease in activity with appropriate chemotherapy.

A *wide* margin (see Fig. 23–19) involves a surgical procedure that excises the tumor, its pseudocapsule, the surrounding reactive zone, and a cuff of normal tissue. The dissection remains outside the zone of reactive tissue, and thus the tumor specimen contains a cuff of normal tissue around its entire circumference. There are no specifications or requirements for the thickness of this cuff of normal tissue. According to this system, however, it is generally felt that a wide margin extends at least one to two cm.

A *radical* margin (see Fig. 23–19) involves an en bloc excision of tumor, its pseudocapsule, reactive zone, and the entire compartment within which it is contained.

A malignant intraosseous tumor of the proximal humerus treated with a radical surgical margin requires an excision of the entire humerus. A similar lesion of the deltoid treated with a radical surgical margin would involve a procedure that includes a total excision of the deltoid compartment from origin to insertion. The surgical margin is defined by its worst or closest margin. If a specimen has primarily a wide margin but is marginal in one aspect, it is described as marginal and not as a wide margin. Each particular surgical margin may be achieved by local resection or by amputation

(see Fig. 23–19). Determination of the surgical margin is the critical step that allows the surgeon to integrate the surgical treatment with the staging system and thereby outline treatment and assess clinical results. By assessing the surgical margin and the stage of the lesion, a prediction of local recurrence can be made based on past experience (Table 23–7).

Limb Salvage Surgery

The surgical treatment of high-grade sarcomas of bone may involve amputation or limb salvage. In the skeletally immature with significant remaining growth potential, amputation is preferable to resection, although expandable prostheses are also available. These are metallic arthroplasties that have an extendable screw mechanism that can be lengthened at intervals to allow for skeletal growth. Limb salvage surgery is a reasonable alternative to amputation when a wide surgical margin is achievable and when enough soft tissue is preserved to allow a reasonably good functional result. In most cases, the functional criteria for limb-sparing surgery are stricter than the criteria for tumor control. Sufficient functional muscle mass is required to obtain a reasonable functional result and to avoid wound complications.[207]

Limb salvage, or limb-sparing, resections of the shoulder girdle are generally indicated for neoplasms that have no major neurovascular involvement and have enough remaining bone stock proximally and distally to allow a reasonable reconstruction. In addition, adequate soft tissue coverage and deltoid function is required in order to avoid wound complications and achieve sufficient functional results.[134–140]

Patients with soft tissue sarcomas or bony sarcomas of the proximal humerus with considerable soft tissue extension are challenging limb salvage candidates. The brachial neurovascular structures and glenohumeral joint are not infrequently involved by tumor, and careful preoperative staging is essential before deciding on a surgical plan or attempting limb salvage procedures. High-grade malignant tumors of the proximal humerus typically present as extracompartmental lesions (IIB) and require a wide surgical resection to achieve a cure. Patients who undergo marginal resections for high-grade malignancies are at risk for local recurrences in the majority of cases, no matter how

Table 23–7. RECURRENCE RATE BY SURGICAL MARGIN VERSUS STAGE

Surgical Margin	Benign			Malignant			
	1	2	3	IA	IB	IIA	IIB
Intracapsular	0%	30%	50%	90%	90%	100%	100%
Marginal	0%	0%	50%	70%	70%	90%	90%
Wide	0%	0%	10%	10%	30%	50%	70%
Radical	0%	0%	0%	0%	0%	10%	20%

Adapted by permission from Enneking WF: Musculoskeletal Tumor Surgery. New York: Churchill-Livingstone, 1983, p 99.

efficacious their adjuvant chemotherapy. Thus, a typical IIB osteosarcoma of the proximal humerus requires a wide surgical margin for an adequate margin. Determining appropriate surgical candidates and the feasibility of a wide surgical margin preoperatively is accomplished by the preoperative staging studies. Most osteosarcomas show up as IIB lesions with soft tissue involvement by the tumor. The amount of soft tissue involvement and the proximity of the medial neurovascular bundle present a preoperative challenge to determining candidates for limb salvage. Another preoperative challenge for high-grade sarcomas involves the assessment of the extent of bony disease and whether disease extends into the glenohumeral joint. If the joint is involved, an extracapsular or extra-articular resection is indicated with resection of the glenoid *en bloc* with the capsule of the glenohumeral joint and the remainder of the proximal humerus. Preoperative tasks include assessing distant, metastatic disease and determining the extent of bony and soft tissue margins with the planned resection.[135]

The primary site of a tumor to some extent predicts certain resection and reconstruction tendencies. High-grade sarcomas of the proximal humerus are likely to have a close relationship to the medial neurovascular bundle (brachial plexus or brachial artery or vein) axillary nerve, deltoid, or the glenohumeral joint. Chest wall involvement with these tumors is less common and usually occurs as a late finding after involvement of the medial neurovascular structures. Obviously, the best limb salvage candidates are those with primary bone tumors with minimal extraosseous extension. Soft tissue sarcomas of the shoulder region are easily resected when located in the deltoid, but deltoid resection precludes arthroplasty as a reasonable alternative because of the subsequent loss of active abduction. The following classification system is useful for describing these different resections and the various reconstructive principles (Fig. 23–20).

Type 1—Short Proximal Humeral Resection

Type 1 resections, short proximal humeral resections, are proximal to the deltoid insertion of the humerus (Fig. 23–20). These resections are intra-articular; that is, the bony resection includes the humeral head and the proximal plane of resection goes through the glenohumeral joint. These resections may or may not involve an *en bloc* resection of the abductor mechanism. The abductor mechanism refers to the rotator cuff, deltoid muscle, and its (axillary) innervation. The sacrifice of any part of this composite results in significantly weakened abduction and a significant change in the expectation of postoperative function (see various reconstructive procedures). Axillary nerve injury or resection is a common consideration because of its strategic location at the inferior and posterior humeral neck.

The deltoid muscle inserts into the humerus at approximately 10 to 14 cm from the articular surface of the proximal humeral head. Removing the deltoid insertion from the humerus involves a reconstructive procedure with greater complications and longer rehabilitation than a procedure without detachment of the deltoid insertion. Thus, bony resections distal to the deltoid insertion are associated with more complications or more limited functional results. If the deltoid and rotator cuff with their respective innervations are preserved, good active abduction can be achieved postoperatively and a better functional result can be expected following the reconstruction. Sacrifice of the rotator cuff, the deltoid, its innervation, or vascular supply leads to a significant reduction in potential shoulder abduction. There is a great difference between resections of the proximal humerus that include the deltoid muscle, axillary nerve, or rotator cuff and those that do not. Proximal humeral resections including a part of the abductor mechanism are referred to in this classification system as Type 1B humeral resections (see Fig. 23–20). Resections of the humerous that do not sacrifice a part of the abductor mechanism are referred to as 1A resections. This subclassification of A (preservation or an active abductor mechanism) and B (resection or sacrifice of a part of the abductor mechanism) is also used to classify the other resection types as described.

Type 2   Long Proximal Humeral Resections

Type 2 resections (see Fig. 23–20) refer to proximal humeral resections where the distal osteotomy is made distal to the deltoid insertion. This type usually includes proximal humeral resections longer than 12 cm. They are referred to as 2A or 2B, depending on whether or not they spare or include (respectively) the abductor mechanism with the resection. Type 1 or Type 2 resections of the proximal humerus may be reconstructed with an arthroplasty or an arthrodesis, depending on whether or not the potential for active abduction remains following the resection. Type 2, or long humeral resections, have a longer rehabilitative period and a greater overall incidence of complications or more limited functional results because of the long bony reconstruction and the need for reattachment of the deltoid.

Type 3—Glenohumeral Resections

Type 3 resections of the proximal humerus extend to the glenoid side of the glenohumeral joint in an extra-articular or extracapsular fashion (see Fig. 23–20). The proximal bony resection is through the base of the glenoid or scapular neck. If enough bone stock remains in the glenoid area, an arthroplasty or an arthrodesis may be achieved, depending on the competency of the abductor mechanism. Without a good abductor mechanism, an arthrodesis is preferable, but adequate bone stock must exist in the lateral scapula, either at the acromion or at the remaining scapular neck or glenoid area. Type 3 resections are typically

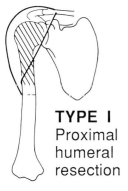

TYPE I
Proximal
humeral
resection

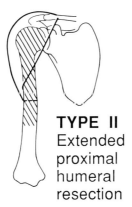

TYPE II
Extended
proximal
humeral
resection

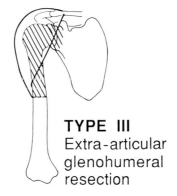

TYPE III
Extra-articular
glenohumeral
resection

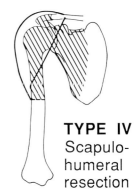

TYPE IV
Scapulo-
humeral
resection

Scapular Resections

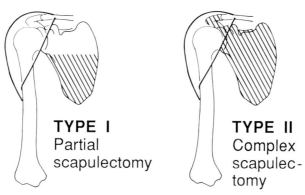

TYPE I
Partial
scapulectomy

TYPE II
Complex
scapulec-
tomy

A. Deltoid preserved
B. Deltoid resected

Figure 23–20. Classification of shoulder resections.

carried out for a high-grade malignancy of the proximal humerus or humeral head with intra-articular invasion, as can occur with osteosarcoma or chondrosarcoma.

Type 4—Scapulohumeral Resections

Type 4 resections refer to scapulohumeral resections of the proximal humerus and scapula (see Fig. 23–20), including the classic Tikhoff-Linberg procedure that involves a full scapular resection with a resection of the humeral head.[145–148] An extended Tikhoff-Linberg resection refers to a full scapular resection with a lengthy proximal humeral resection. The resection may or may not include a portion of the deltoid or abductor mechanism (A or B). Modifications of the original Tikhoff-Linberg involve a subtotal scapular resection *en bloc* with an extra-articular resection of the proximal humerus. These large resections are typically carried out for high-grade lesions of the proximal humerus with glenohumeral joint involvement. One criterion for a Tikhoff-Linberg procedure, as with any limb-sparing surgery, is a lack of involvement of the neurovascular structures (brachial artery, vein, and brachial plexus). It involves a large scapular resection that usually is left without reconstruction.

Scapulohumeral resections are an example of a limb-sparing procedure that results in very limited postoperative function. They are accepted well by the patient when the functional limitations are fully discussed before surgery. Postoperatively, patients typically have varying degrees of proximal humeral stability and a well-innervated, functional hand and elbow. Elbow motion depends on the degree of postoperative humeral stability. In this setting, where the surgical alternative is an amputation, many patients are satisfied with this limited degree of function. Patients frequently prefer to retain the extremity even with limited functional expectations. When the patient is well informed preoperatively and a functional hand persists postoperatively, the patient's subjective evaluations are quite good despite limited functional results.[145–148]

Types 1 and 2—Scapular Resections

Scapular resections may be classified as partial Type 1 or complex Type 2 resections, depending on whether they include the glenoid (complex) or not (partial) (see Fig. 23–20). Partial resections of the scapula are associated with relatively high functional results postoperatively, compared with the more restricted functional performance following complex or complete resections of the scapula.[142–144] This classification system does not include other, less common resections about the shoulder such as various partial or intercalary resections of the humerus that may or may not involve reconstruction. These resections are associated with excellent function postoperatively when there is preservation of the surrounding neurovascular structures and the abductor mechanism. Partial resections of the humerus may be undertaken for less aggressive benign lesions, such as periosteal chondroma or chondroblastoma. Generally, these partial resections lead to superior functional results. Partial resections of the scapula and clavicle also are unusual and may be undertaken for malignant or benign lesions.[184, 185]

RECONSTRUCTIVE PROCEDURES OF THE SHOULDER

There are three basic choices for reconstruction following limb-sparing resections of the shoulder: arthroplasty, arthrodesis, or a flail shoulder (Fig. 23–21). A flail shoulder is defined as a shoulder that lacks functional motor power and stability. It is functionally inferior to arthroplasty or arthrodesis but superior to a painful arthroplasty or arthrodesis. The flail shoulder, such as the shoulder that results following a Tikhoff-Linberg procedure, constitutes an acceptable result for the patient who has undergone a large scapulohumeral resection for an aggressive tumor and who is satisfied with limited shoulder and elbow function. Elbow motion is limited by instability of the proximal humerus and thus stabilization of the proximal humerus significantly enhances function of both the elbow and the hand. Multiple techniques have been attempted in the past to stabilize the remaining humerus to the chest wall. The original technique of using an intramedullary rod sutured to a proximal rib was discontinued because of migration of the rod into the wound flaps.[144] In addition, suspension of the midhumerus to the remaining clavicle to achieve some degree of stability has also been carried out. The best method of stabilization involves reattachment of any remaining proximal musculature to the proximal humerus. Although a flail shoulder is not functionally attractive, it does allow a generous tumor resection and is usually associated with a predictable relief of pain. It remains a viable alternative following large resections and for the complications of a painful, infected, or failed arthroplasty or arthrodesis. However, in the true sense of the word, a flail joint is unstable, and an attempt should be made to limit instability by soft tissue reconstruction whenever possible.[145–149]

The choice of arthroplasty versus arthrodesis following shoulder resections should be considered carefully with the patient before surgery. A patient's personality, vocation, lifestyle, and handedness all affect the decision, and all these factors should be taken into account. In general, an arthroplasty requires active abduction and glenohumeral stability, both of which require a competent, functional abductor mechanism. What constitutes a functionally competent abductor mechanism is a source of some debate. The abductor mechanism has three basic anatomical components: the deltoid muscle, the rotator cuff muscles (supraspinatus, infraspinatus, and teres minor), and their respective blood supply (circumflex and suprascapular vessels) and innervation (axillary and suprascapular nerves). Resections or injuries to the axillary nerve after resection or biopsy of the humerus are not uncommon, and the loss

Arthroplasty

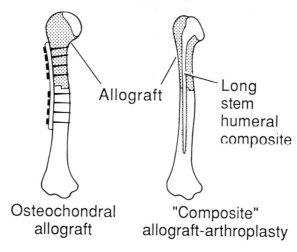

Allograft

Long
stem
humeral
composite

Osteochondral
allograft

"Composite"
allograft-arthroplasty

Figure 23–21. Reconstruction alternatives.

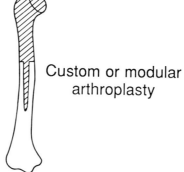

Custom or modular
arthroplasty

Arthrodesis

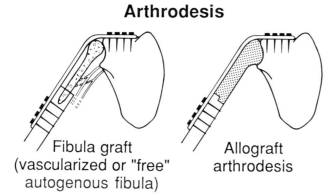

Fibula graft
(vascularized or "free"
autogenous fibula)

Allograft
arthrodesis

of deltoid function has significant functional conse-quences. A well-innervated deltoid is the minimum requirement for a functional, stable arthroplasty. Loss of rotator cuff function has, in the past, required a constrained or semiconstrained arthroplasty, which is associated with greater complications, and may have served as an indication for an arthrodesis.[150] Newer reconstructive procedures have achieved functional ar-throplasties using various unconstrained prostheses with oversized humeral components instead of con-strained glenohumeral designs.[151] These techniques and others have improved results significantly over the previous high failure rates in earlier series (50 per cent), but they lack long-term follow-up.[152–155]

Currently, the techniques of arthroplasty employ metallic, ceramic, or osteochondral allograft im-plants.[155–164] The increasing use of allograft transplan-tation[165, 167] has had two major effects on the reconstruc-tion of humeral resections. First, it has increased the length of the proximal humerus that can be recon-structed, thus expanding the indications for limb sal-vage procedures. Previously, resections were limited to those that could be reconstructed by an autogenous fibular graft or a custom long-stem humeral compo-nent. It is now possible to replace resections within 8 cm of the distal humerus. Second, allograft reconstruc-tions may be a more reasonable reconstructive alter-native in younger patients because of their potential as a biological structure. An allograft reconstruction of-fers the advantages of enhanced soft tissue attachment to the graft, bony union to the remaining humerus, and the potential for the transplantation of viable cartilage. The relative complications of an allograft versus a prosthetic reconstruction have not yet been demonstrated to be significantly different.

Arthroplasty reconstructions following tumor resec-tions involve the choice of an allograft,[155] a metallic[169] or ceramic[159, 160, 170–171] prosthesis, or the combination of an allograft and a prosthesis, referred to as a composite reconstruction[168] (Fig. 23–22). This compos-ite reconstruction involves an allograft that is fixed with a long-stem humeral component through the graft and cemented into the remaining humeral bone stock. It can be cemented or press fit into the allograft or the remaining humerus. With this type of reconstruction, reattachment of the deltoid or rotator cuff to the allograft represents a distinct advantage compared with reattachment to metallic prostheses. Thus, there is the potential for enhanced stability, strength, motion, and function. However, the preliminary results for trans-planted allograft rotator cuff and other allograft liga-ments show a high failure rate.[152]

The greatest challenge following a proximal humeral hemiarthroplasty reconstruction with an allograft is in the reconstruction of the surrounding soft tissues. Great care has to be taken in reconstructing the glenohumeral joint capsule, the rotator cuff, and the deltoid insertion at the time of transplantation. The processes of bony ingrowth and remodeling, soft tissue attachment, graft fixation, revascularization, and car-

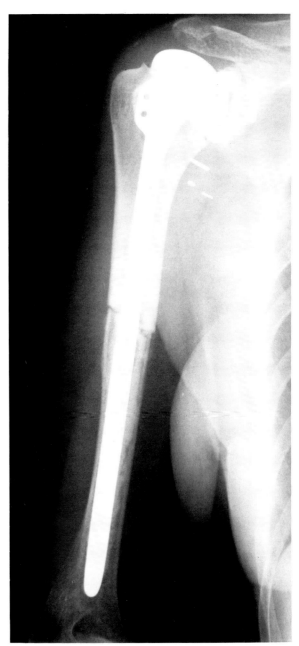

Figure 23–22. "Composite" reconstruction of the proximal humerus.

tilage survival remain areas of active research and clinical investigation. Graft fractures, infection, rejec-tion, and instability remain serious potential compli-cations that occur in 20 to 30 per cent of all pa-tients.[165–167]

The reconstructive alternative to allograft transplan-tation lies with a custom prosthetic implant of accept-able metals or ceramics.[155–164, 168–171] Prosthetic implants offer the advantage of strength and custom fit and are an excellent alternative, especially in older patients. To date, the functional results of arthroplasties in the proximal humerus are excellent for both composite reconstructions and metallic implants.[168–171] As yet, no studies have described comparative differences in function, infection, and revision surgery for these procedures. Newer modular prosthetic designs provide the attractive alternative of a readily available implant that can be customized to the resection defect intraoperatively without delay. These are newer designs with little clinical follow-up, but they appear to have significant application in reconstructing the humerus after tumor resections.[168]

When the deltoid muscle is sacrificed by resection, the best reconstructive choice is an arthrodesis. As a technique, arthrodesis has changed significantly. An arthrodesis following tumor resection may be achieved with various bone graft materials including free or vascularized autogenous fibular grafts or allograft transplantation.[173-177] Resections of 5 to 6 cm or less may use autogenous cancellous grafts from the iliac crest, with or without some shortening of the humerus itself.[177-180] The remaining humerus should be buttressed against the acromion and may or may not be offset from the glenoid with autogenous grafts. Resections of the humerus up to 20 cm in length may be reconstructed with a vascularized autogenous fibular graft. Free (nonvascularized) autogenous fibular grafts may be used for defects less than 12 cm.[172] Nonvascularized fibular grafts longer than 12 cm are associated with a high incidence of graft fractures.[179]

Frozen allograft is a reasonable alternative graft material for shoulder arthrodesis. However, its use has been reported in several series with short follow-up, and there may be some potential problems with the increased risk of nonunion or loss of fixation following nonunion.[220] The use of postoperative radiation therapy or chemotherapy has deleterious effects on the bony union of any reconstruction. Patients with high-grade lesions needing arthrodesis are immediately at even higher risk for nonunion and fracture if they receive postoperative radiation therapy. Most surgeons consider postoperative radiation therapy a contraindication to an allograft arthrodesis.

Internal fixation of an arthrodesis is best achieved with the use of a long-angled custom plate that enables patients to avoid prolonged postoperative immobilization and has enhanced fixation and positioning of the fusion. Such long-angled plates are required for long humeral resections, while shorter, more conventional plates may be used for shorter humeral resections.[175] Newer implants to enhance fixation of the proximal humerus to the scapula are currently being evaluated clinically.

The use of a long-angled plate with adequate purchase of the scapula and remaining humerus has improved postoperative function by avoiding immobilization with a postoperative shoulder spica cast. Proper positioning of the plate on the scapular spine, acromion, and lateral border of the humerus is crucial to achieve proper positioning of the arm and adequate postoperative function. Intraoperative positioning remains a demanding part of the procedure and significantly affects the rotational position of the arm by its

orientation proximally and distally. When such a plate is used, at least eight cortices are required for adequate distal humeral fixation. Likewise, the scapular fixation requires four to five good scapula screws to prevent failure of fixation proximally. Careful positioning of the plate at the acromion is necessary in order to avoid prominence and wound complication. Spica cast immobilization is not required postoperatively if adequate fixation is achieved, as it is in most cases.[175] Postoperatively, patients may use a sling with a soft bolster under the elbow. They begin exercises to improve rhomboid and periscapular strength six weeks after surgery and may carefully begin abduction exercises at eight weeks.[175]

The greatest functional disadvantage in an arthrodesis is the restriction of rotation inherent in the procedure. Most patients are happy with the functional results and obtain adequate abduction (70 to 80 degrees) postoperatively. Limited abduction after arthrodesis usually reflects prolonged immobilization, poor rehabilitation, or a persistent or painful nonunion. The abduction that does occur after arthrodesis is at the scapulothoracic interval and is powered by the rhomboids and other scapular muscles. Patients who are not candidates for an arthroplasty are frequently good candidates for an arthrodesis, as their alternative reconstructive choice is usually a flail shoulder.[173-176]

Scapular resections are unusual procedures that may involve partial or complex resections.[142-144, 182-185] Complex scapular resections in this classification system (see Fig. 23–18) involve a portion of the glenoid. There is some experience with the prosthetic replacement of the scapula following total scapulectomy.[181] Reconstruction with a scapular prosthesis requires humeral head replacement to articulate with the prosthetic glenoid. According to the most recent report of this procedure, the ideal indication for such a prosthesis is a partial scapulectomy.[181] Eckhard[181] reports a series of eight patients treated with endoprosthetic replacement of the scapula for various malignant or benign aggressive lesions. The follow-up on these patients was limited (20 months mean follow-up), and 50 per cent achieved acceptable (good to excellent) functional results. As yet, scapular prosthetic replacement remains a somewhat experimental procedure for which only early, short-term clinical results have been reported. The best indication for such a prosthesis is a partial scapulectomy for shoulders that can be reconstructed in other ways. It remains an attractive area for further development in the patient who has had a complete scapulectomy.

MANAGEMENT OF SPECIFIC LESIONS

Aggressive Benign Bone Tumors

The surgical treatment of active or aggressive bone tumors presents a greater challenge when the tumor occurs adjacent to significant structures such as a major nerve or vessel, a joint or joint surface, or active growth plate. Aggressive benign lesions of bone presenting with significant subchondral bone loss frequently present the greatest challenge in preserving a functional joint.

Aggressive and active benign tumors are typified in the adult by benign giant cell tumor of bone, which occurs in the proximal humerus in 15 to 20 per cent of cases. The treatment choice for such a lesion includes resection versus intralesional curettage. The latter is usually associated with the use of a local adjuvant to enhance the opportunity to kill the tumor. Various local adjuvants that have been used in the recent past include the application of liquid nitrogen (cryosurgery) or phenol (phenolization), the placement of methylmethacrylate (cementation), and various forms of cauterization. Wide surgical resection offers the lowest risk of tumor recurrence but, to some extent, diminishes joint function. For that reason, the slightly less effective intralesional procedures are preferred when associated with a relatively low rate of recurrence tumor (10 per cent). Experience with curettage and cryosurgery has demonstrated a lower recurrence rate (less than 10 per cent) compared with other forms of local adjuvant treatment and may represent the preferred intralesional treatment.[70, 78]

Surgical resection is more effective at controlling tumor and is the preferred method for more aggressive or recurrent lesions. Reconstructions following humeral head resection usually involve an allograft or a custom or modular arthroplasty. Thus, a larger resection that enhances tumor control requires a larger, more complicated reconstruction.

Aggressive benign soft tissue tumors are best exemplified by aggressive fibromatosis in young adults and are lesions which also require a wide surgical margin to minimize the risk of recurrence. Lesions that are juxtaposed to a major neurovascular structure may be treated with a marginal surgical margin in addition to radiation therapy. Radiation therapy appears to be efficacious in minimizing the recurrence rate following marginal resections, despite controversy to the contrary.

Low-Grade Malignancies of Bone

Chondrosarcoma

Chrondrosarcoma represents the most common low-grade malignancy of bone. It occurs frequently in the proximal humerus and presents a clinical challenge in interpreting the source of pain (intra-articular versus extra-articular) and early radiographic signs of malignancy. The definitive treatment for low-grade chondrosarcoma is appropriate surgery. Chemotherapy and radiotherapy have no added benefit in the treatment of an intermediate- or low-grade intraosseous lesion such as chondrosarcoma. Patients who develop a local recurrence after surgery can also be treated surgically for the local recurrence, but if multiple occurrences appear, restaging and adjuvant therapy should be considered.

The appropriate surgical treatment for a low-grade intraosseous chondrosarcoma that is well contained within the cortices of the proximal humerus is either an intralesional curettage with cryosurgery or wide surgical resection. In general, the functional results of an intralesional procedure will be superior to that of a resection and reconstruction. Control of tumor is better with resection than with any intralesional procedure, and thus there are trade-offs between tumor control and functional results. Many chondrosarcomas that are intraosseous in the proximal humerus are low grade in nature and may be treated with curettage alone. A significant proportion of those patients will develop a local recurrence over 5 to 10 years; thus curettage should include some type of adjuvant treatment in order to optimize tumor control.

The resection of a chondrosarcoma involving the glenohumeral joint necessitates an extra-articular resection of the shoulder. This is a more difficult procedure, requiring a total shoulder arthroplasty. The risk of a contaminated surgical margin is higher with this procedure; however, the alternative tumor procedure is either an inadequate, contaminated resection or a forequarter amputation.

Intermediate- or high-grade chondrosarcomas are less common and require a wide surgical margin and appropriate arthroplasty reconstruction. These higher-grade malignancies cannot be reasonably treated using intralesional procedures with or without local adjuvant because of an increased risk of local recurrence and metastatic disease. Results of chemotherapy for high-grade chondrosarcoma are quite limited, but chemotherapy is nonetheless indicated.

High-Grade Malignancies of Bone

Osteosarcoma

High-grade malignant lesions of bone, such as osteosarcoma, are best treated with preoperative (induction) chemotherapy, reassessment of the response to chemotherapy (restaging), surgical resection or amputation, and postoperative chemotherapy.[186–189] Postoperative chemotherapy is tailored or adjusted, depending on the degree of necrosis in the surgical tumor specimen. This type of treatment was first developed in the Sloan Kettering T10 methotrexate protocol and has become the standard treatment for osteosarcoma in many centers.[187–188, 207] Controlled studies specifically evaluating the true significance of preoperative chemotherapy, the significance of the histological response to that preoperative therapy, and the effect of postoperative tailoring of chemotherapy remain to be evaluated.[189] We do not know how much of a histological response to chemotherapy is required to improve survival. We do not know which tumor types respond to which drugs. We do not know which drug combinations are more efficacious (cisplatinum versus methotrexate).

We do not know if the intra-arterial administration of chemotherapy has a greater tumor effect and so forth. There are proponents for many of these theories but very few well-controlled studies.[189]

Adequate evidence does exist to demonstrate improved survival with the addition of chemotherapy to surgery.[190] There has been little experience with radiation therapy in the primary treatment of osteosarcoma, and such therapy does not have a significant role in the curative treatment of osteosarcoma in most centers today. Although there has been a significant increase in survival with more aggressive chemotherapy, many of the significant studies have yet to be carried out.[191–194] In addition, the protocols for managing metastatic pulmonary disease remain to be written. Although it is apparent that pulmonary resection aids survival, its integration with chemotherapy has been poorly defined.[195–200]

Ewing's Sarcoma

The treatment of Ewing's sarcoma today is somewhat similar to the treatment of osteosarcoma in that preoperative induction chemotherapy is delivered after a histological diagnosis is obtained with an appropriate biopsy.[200–205] Placement of the biopsy is very important in Ewing's sarcoma because of the high risk of pathological fracture following radiation therapy. Although the treatment of Ewing's sarcoma 10 years ago involved the combination of chemotherapy and radiation therapy, several studies documenting a high local recurrence rate, especially with large tumors (more than 10 cm), have led to a greater emphasis on surgical treatment of the disease.[202] Thus, lesions that are surgically resectable, especially when larger than 8 to 10 cm, are frequently treated with preoperative chemotherapy, restaging, and surgical resection. A wide surgical margin should be the goal of surgical resection. If a marginal surgical resection results, postoperative radiation therapy is indicated. Patients with Ewing's sarcoma typically present with a large soft tissue mass that usually demonstrates an impressive shrinkage with reasonable response to chemotherapy.[201–202] Patients who do not demonstrate this shrinkage of the inflammatory border of the soft tissue part of Ewing's sarcoma probably have lesions that are not responding well to chemotherapy and should be reassessed very carefully, both pre- and postoperatively. The total treatment protocol for Ewing's sarcoma usually involves approximately 12 months of treatment (chemotherapy).

Amputation may be indicated for treatment of young patients with Ewing's sarcoma with significant growth potential remaining if they present with a lesion in the lower extremity. The alternative is to treat that patient with chemotherapy and radiation therapy, which will usually result in physeal arrest and a discrepancy in leg length. There is significant experience with morbidity following the radiation treatment of lower extremity lesions in young children with Ewing's sarcoma.[203–206]

In addition, these patients represent one of the highest risks for secondary sarcomas, such as osteosarcoma, arising from their radiation field. In the upper extremity, Ewing's sarcoma not infrequently occurs in the proximal humerus, and a surgical resection of the humerus should be considered for all large lesions (8 to 10 cm or more) in children older than 12 years.

Soft Tissue Sarcomas

Soft tissue sarcomas may present as high-grade, low-grade, or intermediate-grade neoplasms. Low-grade and intermediate-grade soft tissue sarcomas with adequate surgical margins are best treated with a surgical resection and postoperative radiation therapy. Worrisome surgical margins may serve as an indication for preoperative radiation therapy. High-grade soft tissue sarcomas have been treated in the past with preoperative radiation therapy followed by surgical resection and chemotherapy. Local recurrence has not been a significant problem (<10 per cent), while pulmonary metastases have (10 to 30 per cent). The institution of preoperative radiation therapy usually delays surgical resection by approximately seven to eight weeks. Chemotherapy in that setting is given postoperatively and is usually not possible until 2 to 3 weeks after resection or 10 to 12 weeks after the institution of treatment. Because of this delay in chemotherapy and the real problems of pulmonary metastases, chemotherapy may be given preoperatively in order to assess the histological response and treat systemic disease. Postoperative therapy is adjusted according to the histological response and is given two to three weeks after surgery. Radiation therapy is indicated for marginal surgical margins and is integrated with postoperative chemotherapy.

Author's Preferred Methods of Treatment

BIOPSY

The biopsy of musculoskeletal tumors will always represent the initial and probably one of the most important steps in the evaluation and treatment of these challenging lesions. The biopsy site should always be placed in the line of a possible future resection and should not be executed before an adequate clinical evaluation and diagnostic radiographic staging studies have been completed. When the staging studies and the clinical presentation of the patient are suggestive of a particular lesion, a needle biopsy is an excellent method. A fairly reliable, tentative diagnosis can be made after staging studies have been completed. This can then be easily confirmed with a needle biopsy. Thus, most classic osteosarcomas have a fairly typical x-ray and can be easily diagnosed with a needle biopsy. However, when a lesion's diagnosis is still uncertain, even after initial staging studies, an open biopsy provides the best diagnosis. In that situation, the more generous the biopsy specimen, the easier the diagnosis. Providing enough of a biopsy specimen without contaminating an extremity remains a challenge even for the experienced oncology surgeon. In general, the biopsy should be executed by the surgeon who will carry out the definitive resection.

SURGICAL CHOICES

In terms of treatment choices, there are three different categories of lesions which remain a challenge in today's setting: aggressive benign lesions, such as giant cell tumor; low-grade malignant lesions, such as chondrosarcoma; and high-grade malignant lesions, such as osteosarcoma or Ewing's sarcoma.

Giant cell tumor, in many instances, is a difficult lesion to treat because it is locally aggressive and destructive to the adjacent joint. It is a difficult tumor to grade histologically and radiographically, and the specific indications for various surgical treatments are nebulous. In the vast majority of cases, a bony resection is the optimal treatment for tumor control. However, curettage supplemented with liquid nitrogen freezing (cryosurgery) may be a better method of treatment in terms of preserving function and controlling tumor. Aggressive recurrent lesions will not be resolved with curettage alone and require curettage with liquid nitrogen freezing or a wide surgical resection. The experience with curettage and liquid nitrogen has been good regarding tumor control and function of the extremity.[70, 78] It requires very careful intraoperative monitoring of the patient for both embolic precautions and protection of the soft tissues and neurovascular structures. It should be carried out only by someone experienced in the technique and is best combined with a subchondral bone graft and internal fixation or cementation of the remaining bony defect. Patients should be advised of the risks and benefits of cryosurgery versus wide resection in the treatment of a giant cell tumor. In many clinical settings, either procedure is a reasonable alternative.

Low-grade malignancies are typified by low-grade chondrosarcomas, which are difficult lesions to define histologically. Microscopically, a low-grade chondrosarcoma is defined by increased cellularity, binucleated lacunae, and microscopic bony resorption, in addition to the clinical radiographic picture of endosteal cortical resorption and bony destruction. Most of these low-grade lesions are located at the metaphyseal-diaphyseal junction in intramedullary or cancellous bone. In general, biopsy and surgical treatment are indicated only in the symptomatic patient (intraosseous pain). When there is doubt about the diagnosis, the patient is far better off being followed carefully with repeat x-rays every 3 to 6 months and a repeat CT scan or MRI scan. Low-grade chondrosarcomas of the extremities (secondary chondrosarcoma) are a very low-grade malignancy in the typical case, with very little threat of pulmonary metastasis. They can be comfortably followed clinically with little or no risk to the patient. Biopsy of such a low-grade cartilaginous lesion is frequently difficult to interpret and may result in an equivocal histological diagnosis regarding the malignant grade or potential. Thus, the diagnosis of benign versus low-grade malignant is best made in the clinical setting rather than in the pathology department. This is a rare exception to the general rule of relying on the histological evaluation of all musculoskeletal lesions in order to define their true nature.

The treatment of a low-grade malignancy (chondrosarcoma) is similar to that of an aggressive benign lesion (giant cell tumor). Curettage alone will be associated with a very high (70 to 80 per cent) recurrence rate for low-grade malignancies, although that recurrence may take 5 to 10 years to show up. Thus, curettage alone is really, in the strict sense of the word, an inadequate form of treatment. Lesions that have failed to respond to previous curettage should be treated with a resection in order to minimize multiple recurrences and wider contamination. For patients willing to take the risk of recurrence (10 per cent), in an attempt to maximize function, curettage with freezing (cryosurgery) is indicated.

HIGH-GRADE TUMORS AND PREOPERATIVE CHEMOTHERAPY

High-grade malignancies in the shoulder have a distribution similar to those in other sites, with the most common lesions being osteosarcoma and Ewing's sarcoma. Most patients with a high-grade malignancy of bone or soft tissue are best treated with chemotherapy before surgical resection in order to minimize local recurrence and to attempt to evaluate tumor response. The Sloan Kettering T10 protocol of preoperative chemotherapy was the first to use methotrexate-based therapy in high dosages (combination of methotrexate, cisplatinum, and adriamycin) given before surgical resection and then tailored postoperatively according to the histological response of the tumor specimen. It has been effective in significantly improving the five-year survival for osteosarcoma in several different clinical studies. Five-year survival went from 25 to 30 per cent previously to a current rate of approximately 50 to 60 per cent. Other improvements in treatment (radiology, pathology, surgery) have also contributed to this improved survival rate. The chemotherapy protocols are complex and demand a multidisciplinary setting with real communication between the chemotherapist and the surgeon. Preoperative chemotherapy is also used for Ewing's sarcoma, that is, preoperative chemotherapy followed by surgery and then maintenance chemotherapy. When a patient with Ewing's sarcoma appears to have a lesion that will have a close or marginal surgical margin, the alternative treatment choice for that patient is chemotherapy and radiation therapy without surgery or chemotherapy with preoperative radiation therapy and surgical resection. The pendulum has more or less swung away from radiation therapy and toward surgical resection for Ewing's sarcoma because of higher recurrence rates following radiation therapy of the primary site alone. Ewing's sarcomas smaller than 8 to 10 cm may be reasonably treated with chemotherapy and radiation therapy in some settings. However, lesions larger than 8 to 10 cm require surgical resection and chemotherapy with or without radiation therapy as the definitive treatment of their primary disease. There are many experienced musculoskeletal tumor surgeons who believe that radiation therapy has no role at all in the treatment of Ewing's sarcoma, especially in the young child with a juxtaepiphyseal lesion that should be treated with an amputation in order to maximize survival. The dilemma of when to use radiation therapy for Ewing's sarcoma persists; however, higher local recurrence rates and greater morbidity in young patients have resulted in little enthusiasm for radiation therapy as the treatment for primary disease, especially in the skeletally immature.

Soft tissue sarcomas are also best treated with preoperative chemotherapy, surgery, and further postoperative chemotherapy. The benefit of preoperative chemotherapy for soft tissue sarcomas is the early systemic treatment of a systemic disease, the minimization of local recurrences, and the opportunity to evaluate the tumor specimen for response to chemotherapy. The majority of patients who present with a soft tissue sarcoma have microscopic circulating tumor cells in their blood stream. A delay in the institution of systemic chemotherapy may represent a deleterious delay in systemic treatment. This explains a significant pulmonary metastasis rate despite adequate local control with any treatment. Protocols that call for radiation therapy before surgical resection and chemotherapy for soft tissue sarcomas usually result in a six-week delay in the institution of chemotherapy and systemic treatment. At the University of Washington, we have therefore elected to give preoperative chemotherapy to all high-grade soft tissue sarcomas followed by restaging and surgical resection after three cycles of chemotherapy. If the surgical margin is marginal, patients also receive postoperative radiation therapy interposed with their postoperative chemotherapy. There are other similar protocols elsewhere that have replaced preoperative radiation therapy with preoperative chemotherapy.

Much has been written and proclaimed about limb-sparing procedures. In fact it is relatively easy to carry out a limb-sparing procedure in the current context of preoperative chemotherapy and to have adequate local control without recurrence at the primary tumor site. It is a much greater challenge, however, to carry out limb-sparing procedures and have a good or excellent functional result following that procedure. Thus, soft tissue involvement may be more important than bone and joint involvement. A good functional result requires well-innervated muscle, adequate soft tissues, and a stable joint. If the soft tissues, strength, or stability of the reconstruction are inadequate, the emotional and financial investment in limb-sparing surgery is probably not warranted. Appropriately carried out, limb-sparing procedures do not increase a patient's risk for local recurrence or diminish the chances for survival.[207] These procedures should, however, be very carefully planned and coordinated in the treatment of all patients. Surgical complications need to be limited enough to enable the resumption of chemotherapy within two to three weeks after surgery.

Because of the emotional effect of losing an extremity, most patients are naturally drawn to the idea of limb salvage surgery. The responsibility of outlining the true risks and benefits of such a procedure rests with the surgeon, who will transmit his or her own prejudices. The gold standard for comparison is an amputation, and all rehabilitation time should be compared with the limited recovery time of an upper or lower extremity amputation (six months). These comparisons and differences should be well thought out beforehand so that a clear picture can be presented to the patient. In the final analysis, tumor control should be emphasized, and any attempt at limb salvage should stress stabilization and mobilization in order to maximize functional results. These are challenging problems that require challenging treatments, and only experience and a carefully coordinated team approach will meet that challenge.

All of these treatment protocols are logistically complex and demand a close relationship between the chemotherapist, surgical oncologist, and radiation therapist. The specialized treatment of these patients also requires a clinical nurse specialist to serve as a clinical coordinator and a source of continuity for patients. It is very difficult to treat sarcoma patients only occasionally and do it well.

References

1. Orthopaedic Practice in the U.S. 1986–1987. American Academy of Orthopaedic Surgeons, Department of Professional Affairs, Chicago, 1987.
2. Gross SW: Sarcoma of the long bones: based upon a study of one hundred and sixty-five cases. Am Med *18*:17–57, 1879.
3. Lichtenstein L: Preface to the First Edition. General Remarks, Classification of Primary Tumors of Bone. *In* Bone Tumors. St. Louis: CV Mosby, 1959, pp 6–34.
4. Lexer E: Die Gesamte Widerherstellungs Chirurgie. Leipzig: Barth, 1931.
5. Linberg BF: Interscapulothoracic resection for malignant tumors of the shoulder joint region. J Bone Joint Surg *10*:344, 1928.
6. Hardin CA: Interscapulothoracic amputations for sarcomas of the upper extremity. Surgery *49*:355, 1961.
7. Phemister DB: Conservative surgery in the treatment of bone tumors. Surg Gynecol Obstet *70*:355, 1940.
8. Albee FH: The treatment of primary malignant changes of bone by radical resection and bone graft replacement. JAMA *107*:1693, 1936.
9. Eiselsberg A: Zur Heilung Groesserer. Defects der Tibia Durch Gestielte Haut-Periost-KnochenLappen. Arch Klin Chir *55*:435, 1897.

10. Klapp R: Ueber Einen Fall Ausgedehnter Knochev-transplantation. Deutsche Ztschr Chir 54:576, 1900.

11. Enneking WF, Spanier SS, and Goodman MA: A system for the surgical staging of musculoskeletal sarcoma. Clin Orthop 153:106, 1980.

12. Proceedings of NIH Consensus Development Conference on Limb-Sparing Treatment of Adult Soft Tissue Sarcomas and Osteosarcoma. U.S. Dept. of Health and Human Services, Public Health Services, NIH Cancer Treatment Symposia, Vol. 3, 1985.

13. American Joint Committee for Cancer Staging and End-Results Reporting: Manual for Staging of Cancer. Chicago: AJC, 1977.

14. Ogilvie-Harris DJ, Hans CB, and Fornasier VL: Pseudomalignant myositis ossificans: heterotopic new bone formation without a history of trauma. J Bone Joint Surg 62-A:1274–1283, 1980.

15. Simon MA and Hecht JD: Invasion of joints by primary bone sarcomas in adults. Cancer 50:1649–1655, 1982.

16. Simon MA and Bos GD: Epiphyseal extension of metaphyseal osteosarcoma in skeletally immature individuals. J Bone Joint Surg 62-A:195–204, 1980.

17. Hudson TM, Schakel M, Springfield DS, et al: The comparative value of bone scintigraphy and computed tomography in determining bone involvement by soft-tissue sarcomas. J Bone Joint Surg 66-A:1400–1407, 1984.

18. Sundaram M, McGuire MH, Herbold DR, et al: Magnetic resonance imaging in planning limb-salvage surgery for primary malignant tumors of bone. J Bone Joint Surg 68-A:809–819, 1986.

19. Huvos AG: Osteoid osteoma. In Bone Tumors: Diagnosis, Treatment and Prognosis. Philadelphia: WB Saunders, 1979, pp 8–46.

20. Enneking WF: Osseous lesions originating in bone. In Musculoskeletal Tumor Surgery. New York: Churchill-Livingstone, 1983, pp 1021–1123.

21. Huvos AG: Osteogenic sarcoma. In Huvos AG (ed): Bone Tumors. Philadelphia: WB Saunders, 1979, pp 47–93.

22. Dahlin DC: Bone tumors: general aspects and data on 6,221 cases. Osteosarcoma, 3rd ed., Chapter 17. Springfield, IL: Charles C Thomas, 1978, pp 156–185.

23. Lichtenstein L: Bone Tumors, 4th ed. St. Louis: CV Mosby, 1972.

24. Enneking WF, Springfield DS, and Gross M: The surgical treatment of parosteal osteosarcoma in long bones. J Bone Joint Surg 67A:125–135, 1985.

25. Unni KK, Dahlin DC, Beabout JW, and Ivins JC: Parosteal osteogenic sarcoma. Cancer 37:2466–2475, 1976.

26. Unni KK, Dahlin DC, and Beabout JW: Periosteal osteogenic sarcoma. Cancer 37:2467–2485, 1976.

27. Unni KK, Dahlin DC, McLeod RA, et al: Interosseous well-differentiated osteosarcoma. Cancer 40:1337–1347, 1977.

28. Matsuno T, Unni KK, McLeod RA, and Dahlin DC: Telangiectatic osteosarcoma. Cancer 38:2538–2547, 1976.

29. Enneking WF: Cartilaginous lesions in bone. In Musculoskeletal Tumor Surgery. New York: Churchill-Livingstone, 1983, pp 875–997.

29. Lane JM, Hurson B, Boland PJ, and Glasser DB: Osteogenic sarcoma, ten most common bone and joint tumors. Clin Orthop 204:93–110, 1986.

30. Huvos AG: Chondroblastoma. In Bone Tumors: Diagnosis, Treatment and Prognosis. Philadelphia: WB Saunders, 1979.

31. Dahlin DC and Ivins JC: Benign chondroblastoma: a study of 125 cases. Cancer 30:401–413, 1972.

32. Enneking WF: Periosteal chondroma. In Musculoskeletal Tumor Surgery. New York: Churchill-Livingstone 1983, pp 913–919.

33. Huvos AG: Osteochondroma and enchondromas. In Bone Tumors: Diagnosis, Treatment and Prognosis, Philadelphia: WB Saunders, 1979, pp 139–170.

34. Enneking WF: Enchondroma. In Musculoskeletal Tumor Surgery. New York: Churchill-Livingstone, 1983, pp 878–892.

35. Shapiro F: Ollier's disease: an assessment of angular deformity, shortening, and pathological fracture in twenty-one patients. J Bone Joint Surg 64A:95–103, 1982.

36. Kreicbergs A, Boquist L, Borssen B, and Larsson SE: Prognostic factors in chondrosarcoma: a comparative study of cellular DNA content and clinicopathologic features. Cancer 50:577–583, 1982.

37. Garrison RC, Unni KK, McLeod RA, et al: Chondrosarcoma arising in osteochondroma. Cancer 49:1890–1897, 1982.

38. Enneking WF: Primary chondrosarcoma. In Musculoskeletal Tumor Surgery. New York: Churchill-Livingstone, 1983, pp 945–964.

39. Gitellis S, Bertoni F, Chieti PP, et al: Chondrosarcoma of bone. J Bone Joint Surg 63A:1248–1256, 1981.

40. Mankin HJ, Cantley KD, Lipielo L, et al: The biology of human chondrosarcoma. I. Description of the cases, grading, and biochemical analyses. J Bone Joint Surg 62:160–176, 1980.

41. Bjornsson J, Unni KK, Dahlin DC, et al.: Clear cell chondrosarcoma of bone: observations in 47 cases. Am J Surg Pathol 8:223–230, 1984.

42. Pritchard DJ, Lunke RJ, Taylor WF, et al: Chondrosarcoma: a clinicopathologic and statistical analysis. Cancer 45:149–157, 1980.

43. Huvos AG, Rosen G, Dabska M, and Marcove RC: Mesenchymal chondrosarcoma: a clinicopathologic analysis of 35 patients with emphasis on treatment. Cancer 51:1230–1237, 1983.

44. Dahlin DC and Beabout JW: Dedifferentiation of low-grade chondrosarcomas. Cancer 28:461–466, 1971.

45. Marcove RC, Mike V, Hutter RVP, et al: Chondrosarcoma of the pelvis and upper end of femur. J Bone Joint Surg 54:561–572, 1972.

46. Frassica FJ, Unni KK, Beabout JW, and Sim FH: Differentiated chondrosarcoma. A report of the clinicopathological features and treatment of 78 cases. J Bone Joint Surg 68A:1197, 1986.

47. Capanna R, Bertoni F, Bettelli G, et al: Dedifferentiated chondrosarcoma. J Bone Joint Surg 70A:60–69, 1988.

48. Milgram JW: Synovial osteochondromatosis. J Bone Joint Surg 59A:792–901, 1977.

49. Mullins F, Berard CW, and Eisenberg SH: Chondrosarcoma following synovial chondromatosis. Cancer 18:1180, 1965.

50. Rao A, Srinvasa V, and Vincent J: Pigmented villonodular synovitis (giant-cell tumor of the tendon sheath and synovial membrane). A review of eighty-one cases. J Bone Joint Surg 66A:76–94, 1984.

51. Sledge CB, Atcher RW, Shoetkeoff S, et al: Intra-articular radiation synovectomy. Clin Orthop 182:37–40, 1984.

52. Scaglietti O, Marchetti PG, and Bartolozzi P: The effects of methylprednisolone acetate in the treatment of bone cysts. Results of three years follow-up. J Bone Joint Surg 61:200–204, 1970.

53. Neer CS, Francis KC, Kiernan HA, et al: Current concepts in the treatment of solitary unicameral bone cysts. Clin Orthop 97:40–51, 1973.

54. Malawer MM, McKay DW, Markle B, et al: Analysis of 40 consecutive cases of unicameral bone cysts treated by high pressure renograffin injection and intracavitary methylprednisolone acetate: prognostic factors and hemodynamic evaluation. 52nd Annual Meeting, American Academy of Orthopaedic Surgeons, Las Vegas, Nevada, 1985.

55. Oppenheimer WL, and Galleno H: Operative treatment versus steroid injection in the management of unicameral bone cysts. J Pediatr Orthop 4:1–7, 1984.

56. Enneking WF: Simple cyst. In Musculoskeletal Tumor Surgery. New York: Churchill-Livingstone, 1983, pp 1494–1513.

57. Griffith M, Betz RR, Mardjetko S, et al: Review of treatment of unicameral bone cysts. Presented at American Association of Orthopaedic Surgeons, Annual Meeting, Atlanta, Georgia Feb. 8, 1988.

58. Beisecker JL, Marcove RC, Huvos AG, and Moke V: Aneurysmal bone cysts: a clinicopathologic study of 66 cases. Cancer 26:615, 1970.

59. Enneking WF: Aneurysmal bone cysts. In Musculoskeletal Tumor Surgery. New York: Churchill-Livingstone, 1983, pp 1513–1530.

60. Harris WH, Dudley HR, Jr, and Barry RJ: The natural history

of fibrous dysplasia. An orthopaedic, pathological and roentgenographic study. J Bone Joint Surg *44A*:207–233, 1962.

61. Henry A: Monostotic fibrous dysplasia. J Bone Joint Surg *51B*(2):300–306, 1969.

62. Jaffe HL: Fibrous dysplasia. *In* Tumors and Tumorous Conditions of the Bones and Joint. Philadelphia: Lea & Febiger, 1958, pp 117–142.

63. Lichtenstein L: Polyostotic fibrous dysplasia. Arch Surg *36*:874–898, 1938.

64. Stewart MJ, Gilmer WS, and Edmonson AS: Fibrous dysplasia of bone. J Bone Joint Surg *44B*(1):302–318, 1962.

65. Arata MA, Peterson HA, and Dahlin DC: Pathologic fractures through non-ossifying fibromas. J Bone Joint Surg *63A*:980–988, 1981.

66. Goldenberg RR, Campbell CJ, and Bonfiglio M: Giant-cell tumor of bone: an analysis of two hundred and eighteen cases. J Bone Joint Surg *52A*:619–663, 1970.

67. Dahlin DC, Cupps RE, and Johnson EW, Jr.: Giant cell tumor: a study of 195 cases. Cancer *25*:1061–1070. 1970.

68. Campanacci M, Baldini N, Boriani S, and Sudanese A: Giant-cell tumor of bone. J Bone Joint Surg *69A*:106–114, 1987.

69. McDonald DJ, Sim FH, McLeod RA, and Dahlin DC: Giant-cell tumor of bone. J Bone Joint Surg *68A*:235–242, 1986.

70. Conrad EU III, Enneking WF, and Springfield DS: Giant cell tumor treated with curettage and cementation. *In* Limb Salvage in Musculoskeletal Oncology. New York: Churchill Livingstone, 1987, p 626.

71. Persson BM, and Wouters HW: Curettage and acrylic cementation in surgery of giant cell tumors of bone. Clin Orthop *120*:125–133, 1976.

72. Persson BM, Ekelund L, Lovdahl R, and Gunterberg B: Favourable results of acrylic cementation for giant cell tumors. Acta Orthop Scand *55*:209–214, 1984.

73. Linder L: Reaction of bone to the acute chemical trauma of bone cement. J Bone Joint Surg *59A*:82, 1977.

74. Marcove RC: A 17-year review of cryosurgery in the treatment of bone tumors. Clin Orthop *163*:231–233, 1982.

75. Marcove RC, Lyden JP, Huvos AC, and Bullough PB: Giant cell tumor treated by cryosurgery. A report of twenty-five cases. J Bone Joint Surg *55*:1633–1644, 1973.

76. Marcove RC, Stovell P, Huvos AC, et al: The use of cryosurgery in the treatment of low and medium grade chondrosarcoma: a preliminary report. Clin Orthop *122*:147–156, 1977.

77. Marcove RC, Weis LD, Vaghaiwall MR, et al.: Cryosurgery in the treatment of giant cell tumors of bone. A report of 52 consecutive cases. Cancer *41*:957–969, 1978.

78. Malawer MM, Dunham WK, Zaleski T, and Zielinski CJ: Cryosurgery in the management of benign (aggressive) and low grade malignant tumors of bone: analysis of 40 consecutive cases. Presented at the meeting of the American Academy of Orthopedic Surgeons (AAOS), New Orleans, February 1986.

79. Goodman MA: Plasma cell tumors. Clin Orthop *204*:87–92, 1986.

80. Durie BGM, and Salmon SE: A clinical staging system for multiple myeloma. Correlation of measured myeloma cell mass with presenting clinical features, response to treatment and survival. Cancer *36*:842–854, 1975.

81. Enneking WF: Ewing's sarcoma. *In* Musculoskeletal Tumor Surgery. New York: Churchill-Livingstone, 1983, pp 1345–1380.

82. Bacci G, Picci P, Gherlinzoni F, et al: Localized Ewing's sarcoma of bone: ten years' experience at the Istituto Ortopedico Rizzoli in 124 cases treated with multimodal therapy. Eur J Cancer Clin Oncol *21*:163–173, 1985.

83. Goldblatt J, Sacks S, and Beighton P: The orthopaedic aspects of Gaucher disease. Clin Orthop *137*:208, 1978.

84. Kanis JA, and Gray RE: Long term follow-up observations on treatment in Paget's disease of bone. Clin Orthop *217*:99–125, 1987.

85. Price CHG, and Golde W: Paget's sarcoma of bone. A study of eighty cases. J Bone Joint Surg *51B*:205–224, 1969.

86. Enneking WF: Lipoma. *In* Musculoskeletal Tumor Surgery. New York: Churchill-Livingstone, 1983, pp 1225–1240.

87. Enneking WF: Vascular lesions. *In* Musculoskeletal Tumor Surgery. New York: Churchill-Livingstone, 1983, pp 1175–1190.

88. Allen PW, and Enzinger FM: Hemangioma of skeletal muscle. Cancer *29*:8, 1972.

89. Enneking WF: Fibromatosis. *In* Musculoskeletal Tumor Surgery. New York: Churchill-Livingstone, 1983, pp 760–773.

90. McKenzie DH: The fibromatoses: a clinicopathologic concept. Br Med J *4*:777, 1972.

91. Enzinger FM, and Weiss SW: Fibromatoses. *In* Soft Tissue Tumors. St. Louis: CV Mosby, 1983, p 45.

92. Rock MG, Pritchard DJ, Reiman HM, et al.: Extra-abdominal desmoid tumors. J Bone Joint Surg *66A*:1369–1374, 1984.

93. Enzinger FM, and Weiss SW: Malignant fibrohistiocytic tumors. *In* Soft Tissue Tumors. St. Louis: CV Mosby, 1983, p 166.

94. Capanna R, Bertoni F, Bacchini P, et al: Malignant fibrous histiocytoma of bone: the experience at the Rizzoli Institute: report of 90 cases. Cancer *54*:177–187, 1984.

95. Weiss SW, and Enzinger FM: Malignant fibrous histiocytoma: an analysis of 200 cases. Cancer *41*:2250–2266, 1978.

96. Enzinger FM, and Weiss SW: Liposarcoma. *In* Soft Tissue Tumors. St. Louis: CV Mosby, 1983, p 242.

97. Reszel PA, Soule EH, and Coventry MB: Liposarcomas of the extremities and limb girdles. A study of 222 cases. J Bone Joint Surg *48A*:229, 1966.

98. Shiu MH, Castro EB, Hajdu SI, and Fortner JG: Results of surgical and radiation therapy in the treatment of liposarcoma arising in an extremity. AJR *123*:577, 1975.

99. Wright PH, Sim FH, Soule EH, and Taylor WF: Synovial sarcoma. J Bone Joint Surg *64A*(1):112–122, 1982.

100. Maurer HM, Moon T, Donaldson M, et al: The intergroup rhabdomyosarcoma study. Cancer *40*:2015, 1977.

101. Enzinger FM, and Weiss SW: Rhabdomyosarcoma. *In* Soft Tissue Tumors. St. Louis: CV Mosby, 1983, p 338.

102. Simon MA, Spanier SS, and Enneking WF: The management of soft tissue tumors of the extremities. J Bone Joint Surg *60*:317, 1976.

103. Enneking WF, Spanier SS, and Malawer MM: The effect of the anatomic setting on the results of surgical procedures for soft parts sarcoma of the thigh. Cancer *47*:1005–1022, 1981.

104. Rydholm A: Management of patients with soft-tissue tumors: strategy developed at a regional oncology center. Acta Orthop Scand [Suppl.] *203*:3–76, 1983.

105. Eilber FR, Eckhardt J, and Morton DL: Advances in the treatment of sarcomas of the extremity: current status of limb salvage. Cancer *54*:2695–2701, 1984.

106. Rosenberg SA, Kent H, Cost J, et al: Prospective randomized evaluation of the role of limb sparing surgery, radiation therapy, and adjuvant chemoimmunotherapy in the treatment of adult soft tissue sarcomas. Surgery *84*:62–69, 1978.

107. Suit HD, Proppe KH; Mankin HJ, et al: Preoperative radiation therapy for sarcoma of soft tissue. Cancer *47*:2267–2274, 1981.

108. Rosenberg SA, Suit FD, and Baker LH: Sarcomas of soft tissue. *In* DeVita VT, Hellman S, and Rosenberg SA (eds): Cancer. Principles and Practice of Oncology, 2d ed. Philadelphia: JB Lippincott, 1985, pp 1243–1293.

109. Lindberg RD, Martin RG, Romsdahl MM, and Barkley HT, Jr.: Conservative surgery and postoperative radiotherapy in 300 adults with soft-tissue sarcomas. Cancer *47*:2391–2397, 1981.

110. Cancer Patient Survival. Report No. 5, U.S. Dept. of Health, Education and Welfare. Publication No. (NIH) 77-992, 1976.

111. Dahlin DC: Bone Tumors: General Aspects and Data on 6,221 Cases, 3rd ed. Springfield, IL: Charles C Thomas, 1978, pp 3–17.

112. Huvos AG: Bone Tumors: Diagnosis, Treatment and Prognosis. Philadelphia: WB Saunders, 1979.

113. Rubin P: Clinical Oncology, 6th ed. American Cancer Society, 1983.

114. Dahlin DC: Bone Tumors: General Aspects and Data on 6,221 Cases, 3rd ed. Springfield, IL: Charles C Thomas, 1978, pp 156–175.

115. Enneking WF: Musculoskeletal Tumor Surgery. New York: Churchill-Livingstone, 1983, pp 1–60.

116. Goodman MA: Plasma cell tumors. Clin Orthop 204:87–92, 1986.

117. Jaffe HL: Tumors and Tumorous Conditions of the Bone and Joints. Philadelphia: WB Saunders, 1979.

118. Levine AM, and Rosenberg SA: Alkaline phosphatase levels in osteosarcoma tissue as related to prognosis. Cancer 44:2291–2293, 1979.

119. Paulson DF, Perez CA, and Anderson T: Cancer of the kidney and ureter. In DeVita VT, Hellman S, and Rosenberg SA (ed): Cancer: Principles and Practice of Oncology, 2nd ed. Philadelphia: JB Lippincott, 1985, pp 895–905.

120. Rosenberg SA, Suit FD, and Baker LH: Sarcoma of soft tissue. In DeVita VT, Hellman S, and Rosenberg SA (eds): Cancer: Principles and Practice of Oncology, 2nd ed. Philadelphia: JB Lippincott, 1985, pp 1243–1293.

121. Harrington KD: Metastatic disease of the spine. Curr Conc Rev 68A:1110–1115, 1986.

122. Berrettoni BA, and Carter JR: Mechanisms of cancer metastasis to bone. Curr Conc Rev 68A:308–312, 1986.

123. Weiss L, and Gilbert HA: Bone Metastases. Boston: GK Hall, 1981.

124. Fidler IJ, and Hart IR: Biological diversity in metastatic neoplasms: origins and implications. Science 217:998–1003, 1982.

125. Simon MA: Biopsy of musculoskeletal tumors. J Bone Joint Surg 64A:1253–1257, 1982.

126. Mankin HJ, Lange TA, and Spanier SS: The hazards of biopsy in patients with malignant primary bone and soft-tissue tumors. J Bone Joint Surg 64A:1121–1127, 1982.

127. Enneking WF: The issue of the biopsy. Editorial. J Bone Joint Surg 644:1119–1120, 1982.

128. Enneking WF: Biopsy. In Musculoskeletal Tumor Surgery. New York: Churchill-Livingstone, 1983, pp 185–201.

129. DeSantos LA, Murray SA, and Ayaler AG: The value of percutaneous needle biopsy in the management of primary bone tumors. Cancer 43:735–744, 1979.

130. Moore TM, Meyers MH, Patzakis MJ, et al.: Closed biopsy of musculoskeletal lesions. J Bone Joint Surg 61:375–380, 1979.

131. Schajowicz F, and Derquie JC: Puncture biopsy in lesions of the locomotor system: review and results in 4050 cases, including 941 vertebral punctures. Cancer 21:5331–5487, 1968.

132. Broders AC: The microscopic grading of cancer. In Pack GT, and Arrel IM (eds): Treatment of Cancer and Allied Diseases. New York: PB Hoeber, 1964.

133. Mankin HJ, Connor JF, Schiller AL, et al: Grading of bone tumors by analysis of nuclear DNA content using flow cytometry. J Bone Joint Surg 67A:404–413, 1985.

134. Enneking WF: Functional evaluation of reconstruction after tumor resection. Proceedings of the Second International Workshop on the Design and Application of Tumor Prostheses for Bone and Joint Reconstruction, Vienna, 1983.

135. National Institutes of Health, Consensus Development Panel: Limb-sparing treatment of adult soft-tissue sarcomas and osteosarcomas. JAMA 254:1791–1794, 1985.

136. Eilber FR, Morton DL, Eckardt JJ, et al: Limb salvage for skeletal and soft tissue sarcomas. Cancer 53:2579, 1984.

137. Enneking WF: Modified system for functional evaluation of surgical management of musculoskeletal tumors from limb salvage. In Enneking WF (ed): Musculoskeletal Oncology. New York: Churchill-Livingstone, 1987.

138. Lugli T: The facts of an exceptional intervention and the prosthetic method. Clin Orthop 133:215–218, 1978.

139. Albee FH: The treatment of primary malignant changes of bone by radical resection and bone graft replacement. JAMA 107:1693, 1936.

140. Phemister DB: Conservative bone surgery in the treatment of bone tumors. Surg Gynecol Obstet 70:355, 1940.

141. Sweet D, Mass DP, Simon MA, and Shapiro CM: Histiocytic lymphoma of bone: current strategy for orthopaedic surgeons. J Bone Joint Surg 63A:79–84, 1981.

142. Turnbull A, Blumencranz P, and Fortner J: Scapulectomy for soft tissue sarcoma. Can J Surg 21:37, 1981.

143. Marhade G, Monastryrski J, and Steuner B: Scapulectomy for malignant tumors, function and shoulder strength in five patients. Acta Orthop Scand 56:332, 1985.

144. Burwell HN: Resection of the shoulder with humeral suspension for sarcoma involving the scapula. J Bone Joint Surg 47B:300, 1965.

145. Pack GT, McNeer G, and Coley BL: Interscapulo-thoracic amputation for malignant tumors of the upper extremity. Surg Gynecol Obstet 74:161, 1942.

146. Linberg BF: Interscapulothoracic resection for malignant tumors of the shoulder joint region. J Bone Joint Surg 10:344, 1928.

147. Marcove RC, Lewis MM, and Huvos AG: En bloc upper humeral-interscapular resection: the Tikhoff-Linberg procedure. Clin Orthop 124:219–228, 1977.

148. Malawer MM, Sugarbaker PH, et al: The Tikhoff-Linberg procedure and its modifications. In Atlas of Extremity Sarcoma. Philadelphia: JB Lippincott, 1984, pp 205–226.

149. Francis KC, and Worcester JN Jr.: Radical resection for tumors of the shoulder with preservation of a functional extremity. J Bone Joint Surg 44A:1423–1429, 1962.

150. Post M, Haskell SS, and Jablon M: Total shoulder replacement with a constrained prosthesis. J Bone Joint Surg 62A:327–335, 1980.

151. Matsen FA III: Personal communication, January 1988.

152. Gore DR, Murray MP, Sepic MS, and Gardner GM: Shoulder-muscle strength and range of motion following surgical repair of full-thickness rotator-cuff tears. J Bone Joint Surg 68A:266, 1986.

153. Barrett WP, Franklin JL, Jackins SE, et al: Total shoulder arthroplasty. J Bone Joint Surg 69A:865–872, 1987.

154. Neer CS, Watson KC, and Stanton FJ: Recent experience in total shoulder replacement. J Bone Joint Surg 64A:319–337, 1982.

155. Poppen NK, and Walker PS: Forces at the glenohumeral joint in abduction. Clin Orthop 135:165–170, 1978.

156. Burrows HJ, Wilson JN, and Scales JT: Excision of tumors of humerus and femur, with restoration by internal prostheses. J Bone Joint Surg 57B:140, 1975.

157. Salzer M, Zweymueller K, Locke H, et al: Further experimental and clinical experience with aluminum oxide endoprothesis. J Biomed Mater Res 10:847, 1976.

158. Imbriglia JE, Negr CS, and Dick HM: Resection of the proximal one half of the humerus in a child for chondrosarcoma. J Bone Joint Surg 60A:262, 1978.

159. Salzer M, et al: A bioceramic endoprosthesis for the replacement of the proximal humerus. Arch Orthop Trauma Surg 93:169, 1979.

160. Sim FH, Chao EYS, Prichard DJ, and Salzer M: Replacement of the proximal humerus with a ceramic prosthesis: a preliminary report. Clin Orthop 146:161, 1980.

161. Koelbel R, Rohlmann A, and Bergmann G: Biomechanical considerations in the design of a semi-constrained total shoulder replacement. In Bayley I, and Kessel L (eds): Shoulder Surgery. Berlin: Springer-Verlag, 1982.

162. Rock MG, Sim FH, and Chao EYS: Limb salvage procedures for primary bone tumors of the shoulder. In Bateman JE and Welsh RP (eds): Surgery of the shoulder. Philadelphia: BC Decker, 1984.

163. Gebhart MJ, Lane JM, McCormack RR, and Glasser D: Limb salvage in bone sarcomas—Memorial Hospital experience. Orthopaedics 8:262, 1985.

164. Wilson PD, and Lance EM: Surgical reconstruction of the skeleton following segmental resection for bone tumors. J Bone Joint Surg 47A:1629, 1965.

165. Parrish FF: Treatment of bone tumors by total excision and replacement with massive autologous and homologous grafts. J Bone Joint Surg 48A:968–990, 1966.

166. Mankin HJ, Doppelt SH, Sullivan TR, and Tomford WW: Osteoarticular and intercalary allograft transplantation in the

management of malignant tumors of bone cancer. *50*:613–630, 1982.

167. Mankin HJ, Fogelson FS, Thrasher AA, et al: Massive resection and allograft transplantation in the treatment of malignant bone tumors. N Engl J Med *294*:1247–1255, 1976.

168. Rock M: Intercalary allograft and custom Neer prothesis after en block resection of the proximal humerus. *In* Enneking WF (ed): Limb Salvage in Musculoskeletal Oncology. (Bristol-Myers/Zimmer Orthopaedic Symposium.) New York: Churchill-Livingstone, 1987, p 586.

169. Bos G, Sim FH, Pritchard DJ, et al: Prosthetic proximal humeral replacement: the Mayo Clinic experience. *In* Enneking WF (ed): Limb Salvage in Musculoskeletal Oncology. (Bristol-Myers/Zimmer Orthopaedic Symposium.) New York: Churchill-Livingstone, 1987, p 61.

170. Sekera J, Ramach W, Pongracz N, et al: Experience with ceramic and metal implants for the proximal humerus in cases of malignant bone tumor. *In* Enneking WF (ed): Limb Salvage in Musculoskeletal Oncology (Bristol-Myers/Zimmer Orthopaedic Symposium.) New York: Churchill-Livingstone, 1987, p 211.

171. Shibata: Reconstruction of skeletal defects after the Tikhoff-Linberg procedure using aluminum ceramic endoprosthesis and stabilization of the shoulder. *In* Enneking WF (ed): Limb Salvage in Musculoskeletal Oncology (Bristol-Myers/Zimmer Orthopaedic Symposium.) New York: Churchill-Livingstone, 1987, p 553.

172. Schauffler RM: Transplant of the upper extremity of the fibula to replace the upper extremity of the humerus. J Bone Joint Surg *8*:723, 1926.

173. Rowe CR: Re-evaluation of the position of the arm in arthrodesis of the shoulder in the adult. J Bone Joint Surg *56A*:913, 1974.

174. Cofield R: Glenohumeral anthrodesis. J Bone Joint Surg *61A*:673, 1979.

175. Conrad EU, and Enneking WF: Shoulder arthrodesis following tumor resection. Presented to AAOS, February 1986.

176. Gebhardt MC, McGuire MH, and Mankin HJ: Resection and allograft arthrodesis for malignant bone tumors of the extremity. *In* Enneking WF (ed): Lung Salvage in Musculoskeletal Oncology. New York: Churchill-Livingstone, 1987.

177. Weiland AJ, Daniel RK, and Riley CH: Application of the free vascularized bone graft in the treatment of malignant or aggressive bone tumors. Johns Hopkins Med J *140*:85, 1977.

178. Burchardt H, Jones H, Glowczewskie F, et al: Freeze dried allogenic segmental cortical bone grafts in dogs. J Bone Joint Surg *60A*:1081–1090, 1978.

179. Burchardt H, Busbee GA III, and Enneking WF: Repair of experimental autologous grafts or cortical bone. J Bone Joint Surg *57A*:814–819, 1975.

180. Smith WS, and Struhl S: Replantation of an autoclaved autogenous segment of bone for treatment of chondrosarcoma. Long-term follow-up. J Bone Joint Surg *70A*:70, 1988.

181. Eckardt JJ, Eilber FR, Jinnah RH, and Mirra JM: Endoprosthetic replacement of the scapula, including the shoulder joint, for malignant tumors: a preliminary report. *In* Enneking WF (ed): Limb Salvage in Musculoskeletal Oncology. New York: Churchill-Livingstone, 1987, pp 542–553.

182. DeNancrede CBG: The end results after total excision of the scapula. Ann Surg *50*:1, 1909.

183. Ryerson EW: Excision of the scapula: report of a case with excellent functional result. JAMA *113*:1958, 1939.

184. Papaioannou AN, and Francis KD: Scapulectomy for the treatment of primary malignant tumors of the scapula. Clin Orthop *41*:125, 1965.

185. Samilson RL, Morris JM, and Thompson RW: Tumors of the scapula: a review of the literature and an analysis of 31 cases. Clin Orthop *58*:105, 1968.

186. Simon MA: Current concepts review. Causes of increased survival of patients with osteosarcoma: current controversies. J Bone Joint Surg *66A*:306–310, 1984.

187. Rosen G, Caparros B, Huvos AC, et al: Preoperative chemo-

therapy for osteogenic sarcoma: selection of postoperative adjuvant chemotherapy based upon the response of the primary tumor to preoperative chemotherapy. Cancer *49*:1221–1230, 1982.

188. Rosen G: Neoadjuvant chemotherapy for osteogenic sarcoma. A model for treatment of malignant neoplasm. *In* Recent Results in Cancer Research, Vol 103. Berlin: Springer-Verlag, 1986, pp 48–157.

189. Goorin AM, Abelson HT, and Freil E III: Osteosarcoma: fifteen years later. N Engl J Med *313*:1637–1643, 1985.

190. Bleyer WA, Haas JE, Feigl P et al: Improved 3-year disease-free survival in osteogenic sarcoma: efficacy of adjunctive chemotherapy. J Bone Joint Surg *64B*:233–238, 1982.

191. Campanacci M, Bacci G, Bertoni F, et al: The treatment of osteosarcoma of the extremities: twenty years' experience at the Istituto Ortepedico Rizzoli. Cancer *48*:1569–1581, 1981.

192. Jaffe N, Prudich J, Knapp J, et al: Treatment of primary osteosarcoma with intra-arterial and intravenous high-dose methotrexate. J Clin Oncol *1*:428–431, 1983.

193. Murray JA, Jessup K, Romsdahl M, et al: Limb salvage surgery in osteosarcoma: early experience at M.D. Anderson Hospital. Proceedings of NIH Consensus Development Conference on Limb-Sparing Treatment of Adult Soft Tissue Sarcomas and Osteosarcoma. U.S. Dept. of Health and Human Services. Public Health Services. NIH Cancer Treatment Symposia, Vol. 3, 1985.

194. Winkler K, Beron G, Kotz R, et al: Neoadjuvant chemotherapy for osteogenic sarcoma: results of a cooperative German/Austrian study. J Clin Oncol *2*:617–624, 1984.

195. Martini N, Huvos AG, Mike V, et al: Multiple pulmonary resections in the treatment of osteogenic sarcoma. Ann Thorac Surg *12*:271–280, 1971.

196. Schaller RT, Jr, Haas J, Schaller J, et al: Improved survival in children with osteosarcoma following resection of pulmonary metastases. J Pediatr Surg *17*:546–550, 1982.

197. Giritsky AS, Etcubanas E, and Mark JBD: Pulmonary resection in children with metastatic osteosarcoma. J Thorac Cardiovasc Surg *75*:354–362, 1978.

198. Burgers JMV, Breur K, van Dobbenburgh OA, et al: Role of metastatectomy without chemotherapy in the management of osteosarcoma in children. Cancer *45*:1664–1668, 1980.

199. Rosenberg SA, Fyle MW, Conkle D, et al: The treatment of osteosarcoma. II. Aggressive resection of pulmonary metastases. Cancer Treat Rep *63*:753–762, 1979.

200. Goorin AM, Deloney MJ, Lack EE, et al: Prognostic significance of complete surgical resection of pulmonary metastases in patients with osteogenic sarcoma: analysis of 32 cases. J Clin Oncol *2*:425–430, 1984.

201. Thomas PRM, Perez CA, Neff JR, et al: The management of Ewing's sarcoma: role of radiotherapy in local tumor control. Cancer Treat Rep *68*:703–710, 1984.

202. Rosen G, Caparros B, Nirenberg A, et al: Ewing's sarcoma. Ten-year experience with adjuvant chemotherapy. Cancer *47*:2204–2213, 1981.

203. Wilkins RM, Pritchard DJ, Burgert EO, and Unni KK: Ewing's sarcoma of bone—experience with 140 patients. Cancer *58*(11):2551–2555, 1986.

204. Springfield DS, and Pagliarulo C: Fractures of long bones previously treated for Ewing's sarcoma. J Bone Joint Surg *67A*:477–481, 1985.

205. Miser J, Kinsella T, Tsokos M, et al: High response rate of recurrent childhood tumors to etoposide (VP16), ifosfamide (IFOS0, and mesna (MES) uroprotection. Proc Soc Clin Oncol *5*:209, 1986.

206. Lewis RJ, Marcove RC, and Rosen G: Ewing's sarcoma: functional effects of radiation therapy. J Bone Joint Surg *59A*:325–331, 1977.

207. Simon MA, Aschliman MA, Thomas N, and Mankin HJ: Limb-salvage treatment versus amputation for osteosarcoma of the distal end of the femur. J Bone Joint Surg *68A*:1331–1337, 1986.

Sepsis of the Shoulder: Molecular Mechanisms and Pathogenesis

Anthony G. Gristina, M.D.
Gordon Kammire, M.D.
Anna Voytek, M.D.
Lawrence X. Webb, M.D.

General principles in the pathogenesis of shoulder sepsis are similar to those pertaining to all intra-articular infections. There are three fundamental pathways for infection to enter a joint: (1) spontaneous hematogenous seeding via the synovial blood supply, (2) contiguous spread from adjacent metaphyseal osteomyelitis via the intra-articular portion of the metaphysis, and (3) penetration of the joint by trauma, therapy, or surgery.

Susceptibility to infection is determined by the adequacy of the host defenses. Spontaneous bacteremia, trauma, and surgery are common opportunities for infection. Shoulder infection is uncommon, however, because of normal defense mechanisms, the use of antibiotic prophylaxis, and a good local blood supply.

Certain patient groups with immune system depression or aberrations are at increased risk for infection. Patients with rheumatoid disease manifest a spontaneous and somewhat cryptic sepsis in joints.[57, 69] Diabetics, infants, children, the aged, patients with vascular disease, drug abusers, and HIV patients are at increased risk to specific organisms, as are patients with hematological dyscrasia and neoplastic disease. Joint infection requires a threshold inoculum of bacteria and is facilitated by damaged tissue, foreign body substrata, the acellularity of cartilage surfaces, and the presence of receptors. Total joint arthroplasty is at potential risk because of the presence of metallic and polymeric biomaterials and the decreased phagocytic ability of macrophages in the presence of methylmethacrylate. Biomaterials and adjacent damaged tissues and substrata are readily colonized by bacteria in a polysaccharide biofilm which is resistant to macrophage attack and antibiotic penetration.[37, 47, 50, 56] With antibiotic prophylaxis, published infection rates of total joint arthroplasty are low—1 to 5 per cent, depending on device and location.[24, 26, 52, 90, 124] However, once infected, biomaterials and damaged tissues are exceedingly resistant to treatment.

Clinical infection in tissue- and biomaterial-related disease in normal or immunosuppressed patients involves the maturation of an inoculum of known pathogens (for example, Staphylococcus aureus or Pseudomonas aeruginosa) or the transformation of nonpathogens (S. epidermidis) to a septic focus of adhesive, "slime-producing," virulent organisms. This transformation occurs in the presence of, and is potentiated by, the surface of biomaterials[46, 47, 49, 50, 56, 122] or damaged tissue[87] and is also particularly virulent on acellular, susceptible, and defenseless cartilage matrix surfaces.[129]

History

Experiences in shoulder infection have paralleled those of other large joints, although with less frequency. The work of outstanding scientists, such as Louis Pasteur (1822–1895), Joseph Lister (1827–1912), and Robert Koch (1843–1910), in the last quarter of the 19th century, ushered in the modern age of bacteriology and an early understanding of intra-articular sepsis. Koch's experiments with culture media at the Berlin Institute for Infectious Disease verified the role of the tubercle bacillus in musculoskeletal infection. In 1893, J. E. Péan attempted to reconstruct the tuberculous shoulder of a 30-year-old man using a prosthetic replacement made of platinum and rubber.

The latter part of the 19th century also saw the development of the concept of antisepsis. Lister maintained that sepsis was the main obstacle to significant advances in surgery. He documented a dramatic drop in cases of empyema, erysipelas, hospital gangrene, and surgical infection through the use of antiseptic techniques. Although the popularization of antiseptic technique in the surgical theater greatly reduced the rate of complication owing to infection, it was not until the 1930s that specific antimicrobial therapy was discovered. In 1935, a German bacteriologist, Gerhard Domagk, discovered that sulfonamides protected mice against fatal doses of hemolytic staphylococci. Sulfonamides were soon employed for infections in patients with excellent results.

Although the history of bacteriology and subsequent antiseptic techniques in surgery and the development of antibiotics are well documented, very little of the early literature relates specifically to infections about the shoulder. In Codman's book, *The Shoulder*, published in 1934, infection of the shoulder and, in particular, osteomyelitis of the proximal humerus were considered very rare lesions.[23] Codman cited a report by King and Holmes in 1927 in which a review of 450 consecutive symptomatic shoulders evaluated at the Massachusetts General Hospital revealed 5 cases of tuberculosis of the shoulder, 1 luetic infection of the shoulder, 3 unspecified shoulder infections, and 2 cases of osteomyelitis of the proximal humerus. The rarity of tubercular lesions of the shoulder was documented through the results of four large series of tuberculosis involving the musculoskeletal system (Townsend, 21 of 3244 cases; Whitman, 38 of 1833 cases; Young, 7 of 5680 cases; Billroth, 14 of 1900 cases). As microbial culturing and identification techniques developed in the early 20th century, streptococcal and staphylococcal species were more frequently identified as the causative agents in shoulder infection.

Septic Anatomy of the Shoulder

A review of shoulder anatomy reveals specific structural relationships that are intimately linked to the pathogenesis of joint sepsis and osteomyelitis. The circulation of the proximal humerus and periarticular structures (particularly the synovium) and the intricate system of bursae about the shoulder are critical factors.

Classically, diverse, age-dependent presentations of hematogenous osteomyelitis and septic arthritis of the shoulder (and other large joints such as the hip and knee) have been attributed to the vascular development about the growth plate and epiphysis. The most detailed studies of the vascular development in this area have been done on the proximal femur but are analogous to the same development about the proximal humerus. Experimental work by Trueta[126] demonstrated that, before eight months of age, there are direct vascular communications across the growth plate between the nutrient artery system and the epiphyseal ossicle. This observation was felt to account for the frequency of infection involving the epiphyseal ossicle and subsequent joint sepsis in infants. At some point between 8 months and 18 months of age (an average of 1 year), the growth plate forms a complete barrier to direct vascular communication between the metaphysis and epiphysis. The last vestiges of the nutrient artery turn down acutely at the growth plate and reach sinusoidal veins. At this point the blood flow "slows down," creating an ideal medium for the proliferation of pathogenic bacteria.[127] In addition, there is evidence that the afferent tracts of the metaphyseal vessels have no or insufficient phagocytizing properties.[120]

In the adult shoulder, the intra-articular extent of the metaphysis is located in the inferior sulcus and is intracapsular for approximately 10 to 12 mm.[22] Infection of the proximal metaphysis, once established, may gain access to the shoulder joint via the haversian and Volkmann canals at the nonperiosteal zone (Fig. 24–1). With obliteration of the growth plate at skeletal maturity, anastomoses of the metaphyseal and epiphyseal circulation are again established.

In his study of the vascular development of the proximal femur, Chung did not find evidence of direct communications between the metaphyseal and epiphyseal circulation across the growth plate in any age group.[20] Chung's work demonstrated a persistent extraosseous anastomosis between metaphyseal and epiphyseal circulation on the surface of the perichondral ring. He found no evidence of vessels penetrating the growth plate in the infant population and attributed apparent changes in the arterial supply with age to enlargement of the neck and ossification center.

Branches of the suprascapular artery and the circumflex scapular branch of the subscapular artery from the scapular side of the shoulder anastomose with the anterior and posterior humeral circumflex arteries from the humeral side of the shoulder. This anastomotic system supplies the proximal humerus by forming an extra-articular and extracapsular arterial ring. Vessels from this ring traverse the capsule and form an intra-articular synovial ring. This fine anastomosis of vessels in the synovial membrane is located at the junction of the synovium and the articular cartilage over an area that has been termed the transition zone.[109] This subsynovial ring of vessels was first described by William Hunter in 1743 and named the *circulus articuli vasculosus*.[63] At the transitional zone, synovial cells become flattened over this periarticular vascular fringe. Fine arterioles at this boundary acutely loop back toward

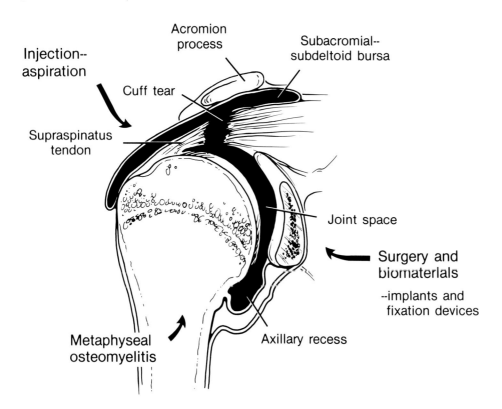

Figure 24–1. Routes of infection for intra-articular sepsis.

the periphery. Again, blood flow at this level may be slowed and provides a site for the establishment of an inoculum of pathogenic organisms. Rather than hemodynamic changes, however, it is more probable that receptor-specific, microbe-to-cell surface interactions potentiate the infectious process.

Another consideration in the septic anatomy of the shoulder is the communication between the joint space and capsule and the system of bursae about the shoulder. Anteriorly, there is direct communication between the capsule and the subscapular bursa located just below the coracoid process. Posteriorly, the capsule communicates with the infraspinatus bursa. A third opening in the capsule occurs at the point at which the tendon of the long head of the biceps enters the shoulder. From the transverse humeral ligament to its entry into the shoulder capsule, the tendon of the long head of the biceps is enveloped in folds of synovium. Intentional or inadvertent injection of the subscapular bursa, the infraspinatus bursa, or the tendon of the long head of the biceps provides the potential for intra-articular bacterial inoculation. Injection of the subdeltoid or subacromial bursa in the presence of rotator cuff tear (degenerative or traumatic) provides another potential setting for bacterial contamination of the joint.

MICROANATOMY AND CELL BIOLOGY

The articular cavity is unique because the surface of hyaline cartilage, although noncrystalline, is essentially acellular and is composed of horizontally arranged collagen fibers in proteoglycan macromolecules. The boundaries of joint cavities are composed of a richly vascularized cellular synovial tissue. Recent studies indicate that collagen fibers and the glycoprotein matrix, rather than the synovium, are the target substrata for microbial adhesion and colonization.[118, 129]

Synovial cells are somewhat phagocytic and appear to combat infection as part of the inflammatory response. Microscopic examination of infected joints in a rabbit animal model indicated predominant colonization of cartilaginous, rather than synovial, surfaces.[129] Receptors for collagen have been identified on the cell surfaces of certain strains of *S. aureus*.[118] The infrequent occurrence of bacteria on synovial tissue may reflect innate resistance of synovial cells to colonization, the lack of appropriate synovial ligands, or functional host defense mechanisms at a synovial level.[10]

The synovial intima is composed of several layers of cells designated types A and B.[14] A cells are predominant and have phagocytic qualities. B cells have pinocytic characteristics. The subintimal vascularized layer contains fibroadipose tissue, lymphatic vessels, and nerves.[109]

Ultrastructural studies of the synovial subintimal vessels reveal that gaps between endothelial cells are bridged by a fine membrane.[109] There is no epithelial tissue in the synovial lining and, therefore, no structural barrier (basement membrane) to prevent the spread of infection from synovial blood vessels to the joint.

The synovial lining in the transition zone is rarely more than three or four cell layers thick, which places the synovial blood vessels in a superficial position and makes them susceptible to damage from relatively minor trauma.

Intra-articular hemorrhage caused by trauma, coupled with transient bacteremias, may be implicated as a factor in the pathogenesis of joint sepsis. Random hematogenous seeding allows bacterial penetration of synovial vessels, producing an effusion consisting primarily of neutrophils which release cartilage-destroying lysosomal enzymes.[14] Staphylococci also release enzymes and toxins that destroy tissue matrix and cells.

Articular (hyaline) cartilage varies from 2 to 4 mm in thickness in the large joints of adults. This avascular, aneural tissue is composed of a relatively small number of cells and chondrocytes and an abundant extracellular matrix. The extracellular matrix contains collagen and a ground substance composed of carbohydrate and noncollagenous protein and has a high water content. The chondrocytes are responsible for the synthesis and degradation of matrix components and are therefore ultimately responsible for the biomechanical and biological properties of articular cartilage.

Collagen produced by the chondrocytes accounts for more than one-half of the dry weight of adult articular cartilage (Type II). Individual collagen fibers, with a characteristic periodicity of 640 Å, vary from 300 Å to 800 Å in diameter, depending on their distance from the articular surface.[109]

The principal component of the ground substance produced by chondrocytes is a protein polysaccharide complex called proteoglycan. The central organizing molecule of proteoglycan is hyaluronic acid. Numerous glycosaminoglycans (mainly chondroitin sulfate and keratin sulfate) are covalently bound from this central strand. Glycosaminoglycans carry considerable negative charge. The highly ordered array of electronegativity on the proteoglycan molecule interacts with large numbers of water molecules (small electric dipole). Approximately 75 per cent of the wet weight of articular cartilage is water, the majority of which is structured by the electrostatic forces of the proteoglycan molecule.[109]

The structure of articular cartilage varies relative to its distance from the free surface. For purposes of description, the tissue has been subdivided into zones that run parallel to the articular surface. Electron microscopy of the free surface reveals a dense network of collagen fibers (40 Å to 120 Å in diameter) which

is arranged tangentially to the load-bearing surface and at approximately right angles to each other. This dense, mat-like arrangement, the *lamina obscurans*, is approximately 3μ thick. No cells have been identified in this layer.[109, 128]

Zone 1 contains large bundles of collagen fibers that are approximately 340 Å thick and lie parallel to the joint surface and at right angles to each other (Fig. 24–2).[109, 128] This zone, the *lamina splendins*, has little or no intervening ground substance and contains the highest density of collagen. Chondrocytes in Zone 1 are ellipsoid in shape and are oriented parallel to the articular surface. They show little electron microscopic evidence of metabolic activity.

In Zone 2, the collagen consists of individual, randomly oriented fibers of varying diameters. The chondrocytes in Zone 2 tend to be more spherical and larger than those of Zone 1, with abundant mitochondria and extensive endoplasmic reticulum, suggesting greater metabolic activity. The proteoglycan-to-collagen ratio in Zone 2 is much higher than that near the surface.

In Zone 3, the collagen fibers are thicker, often in the range of 1400 Å, and tend to form a more orderly meshwork which lies radial to the articular surface. The chondrocytes in Zone 3 are larger and tend to be arranged in columns, often appearing in groups of two to eight cells. The cells are noted to have enlarged Golgi complexes, many mitochondria, and an extensively developed endoplasmic reticulum, indicating a high degree of metabolic activity.

Bone is a composite structure incorporating calcium hydroxyapatite crystals in a collagen matrix grossly similar to synthetic composites or to partially crystalline polymers. Devitalized bone provides a passive substratum for bacterial colonization and the ultimate incorporation of its proteinaceous and mineral constituents as bacterial metabolites.[49, 51, 120]

Classification

Intra-articular sepsis may be classified in order of pathogenesis and frequency as (1) direct hematogenous, (2) secondary to contiguous spread from osteomyelitis, or (3) secondary to trauma or surgery (Table 24–1). Most joint infections are caused by hematoge-

Table 24–1. CLASSIFICATION OF OSTEOMYELITIS AND INTRA-ARTICULAR SEPSIS

Hematogenous
Contiguous Spread
   Osteomyelitis
   Soft tissue sepsis
   Vascular insufficiency
Direct Inoculation
   Trauma ⎫
   Surgery ⎭ with or without foreign body or biomaterials

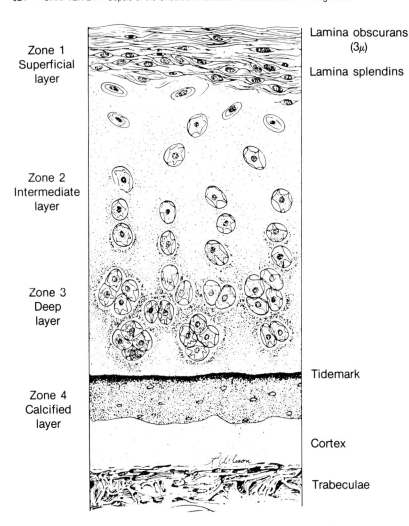

Figure 24–2. The zones of adult articular cartilage. (Modified with permission from Turek SL: Orthopaedics: Principles and Their Application. Philadelphia: JB Lippincott, 1977.)

nous spread, although direct contamination is not uncommon with trauma.

Osteomyelitis of the humerus may spread intra-articularly, depending on the age of the patient, the type of infecting organism, and the severity of infection. Osteomyelitis of the clavicle or scapula is uncommon, although it does occur after surgery and internal fixation, from retained shrapnel fragments, or in heroin addicts.[12, 39, 74, 79, 119, 138]

Hematogenous osteomyelitis, although common in children,[85] is uncommon in adults until the sixth decade or later and is usually associated with a compromised immune system. Direct spread from wounds or foreign bodies, including total joint and internal fixation devices, is the most common etiology for shoulder sepsis in adults.

Incidence and Pathogenic Mechanisms of Septic Arthritis and Osteomyelitis

SURFACES AS SUBSTRATA FOR BACTERIAL COLONIZATION

The pathogenesis of bone and joint infections is related, in part, to preferential adhesive colonization of inert substrata whose surfaces are not integrated with healthy tissues composed of living cells and intact extracellular polymers such as the articular surface of joints or damaged bone (Fig. 24–3).[11, 51, 58, 112, 121, 135]

Almost all natural biological surfaces are lined by a cellular epithelium or endothelium. Exceptions are intra-articular cartilage and the surface of teeth. Mature enamel is the only human tissue that is totally acellular; it is primarily composed of inorganic hydroxyapatite crystals (96 per cent by weight), with a small amount of water (3 per cent) and organic matrix (less than 1 per cent).[5] Proteins in the organic matrix are distributed between the hydroxyapatite crystals, forming a framework that strengthens the enamel by decreasing its tendency to fracture or separate. These proteins are unique among mineralized tissue because they are not a fibrous collagen protein like that found in bone, dentin, and cementum or in cartilage but are similar to the keratin family of proteins.[5]

Cartilage and enamel are readily colonized by bacteria because they lack the protection by natural desquamation or by intact extracapsular polysaccharides that is provided by an active cellular layer. Their acellular surfaces are similar to many of those in nature for which bacteria have developed colonizing mechanisms. Certain strains of *S. aureus* adhere to specific

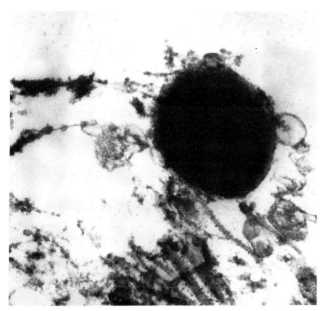

Figure 24–3. Electromicrograph of rabbit articular cartilage illustrating direct bacteria-to-collagen fiber contact. (Reproduced from Voytek A, Gristina AG, Barth E, et al: Staphylococcal adhesion to collagen in intra-articular sepsis. Biomaterials 9:107–110, 1988, by permission of the publishers, Butterworth & Co, Ltd, © 1988.)

sites on collagen fibrils, a process that is mediated by specific surface receptor proteins. Dissimilarities in surface structure are probably responsible for the specificity of bacterial species colonization of these surfaces.

Enamel is mostly crystalline and inorganic, and cartilage is organic and noncrystalline. Enamel contains no collagen, while collagen is ubiquitous in cartilage and bone. *S. aureus* is the natural colonizer of cartilage but not of enamel because it contains collagen receptors.[60, 61, 123] The specificity of colonization is also modulated in part by lectins and the host-derived synovial fluid, blood, and serum, conditioning films of protein, and polysaccharide macromolecules.

The colonization of teeth by *Streptococcus mutans* and other organisms is a natural polymicrobial process and may be symbiotic or slowly destructive; for joint cartilage, bacterial colonization is unnatural and rapidly destructive.[38] The acellular cartilage matrix and inanimate biomaterial surfaces offer no resistance to colonization by *S. aureus* and *S. epidermidis*, respectively. The observed invasion and gradual destruction of the cartilage over time supports clinical observations of the course of untreated septic arthritis (Fig. 24–4).[60, 86, 115, 116] Several strains of *S. aureus* produce collagenase, which, along with host-originated inflammatory products, is probably the main cause of progressive cartilage destruction.[82, 86, 109] The acellular cartilaginous surfaces of joints are particularly vulnerable to sepsis because they allow direct exposure to bacteria from open trauma, surgical procedures, or hematogenous spread. This mechanism parallels previous observations on the mechanism of osteomyelitis, which suggest that the adhesion of bacteria to dead bone or naked cartilage (surfaces not protected by living cells) via recep-

tors and extracellular polysaccharides is a factor in pathogenesis.[49, 51, 117]

INTRA-ARTICULAR SEPSIS

The articular cavity is a natural dead space, becoming a major closed abscess and media bath for bacteria. In this avascular and acellular space, host defense mechanisms are at a disadvantage. Synovial cells are not actively antibacterial, although they are somewhat phagocytic. White blood cells must be delivered to the area and lack a surface for active locomotion. Under such conditions it is expected that phagocytic action is impaired, especially against encapsulated organisms.

Spontaneous intra-articular sepsis of the shoulder is derived from random hematogenous bacterial seeding. Synovial vasculature is abundant, and the vessels lack a limiting basement membrane. Bacteremia, especially by *Neisseria gonorrhoeae*, increases the risk of intra-articular spread. Contiguous spread from adjacent and intracapsular metaphyseal osteomyelitis also occurs. Surgery, arthroscopy, total joint replacement, aspirations, and steroid injections also can result in direct inoculation of bacteria into the intra-articular space. The presence of foreign bodies from trauma or after surgery (stainless steel, chrome cobalt alloys, ultra–high molecular weight polyethylene, and methylmethacrylate) increases the possibility of infection by providing a foreign body nidus for colonization, allowing antibiotic-resistant, slime-enclosed colonization to occur.[47, 49, 51] The presence of a foreign body also lowers the size of the inoculant required for sepsis and perturbs host defense mechanisms.

Septic arthritis of the shoulder complex most frequently involves the glenohumeral joint. The acromioclavicular and sternoclavicular joints are occasionally infected in specific patient groups or after steroid

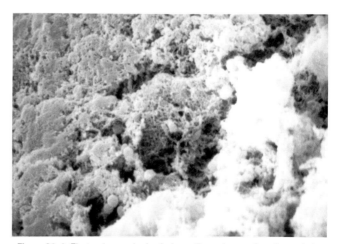

Figure 24–4. Electromicrograph of articular cartilage at seven days demonstrates destructive changes occurring beneath matrix-enclosed cocci. (Reproduced from Voytek A, Gristina AG, Barth E, et al: Staphylococcal adhesion to collagen in intra-articular sepsis. Biomaterials 9:107–110, 1988, by permission of the publishers, Butterworth & Co, Ltd, © 1988.)

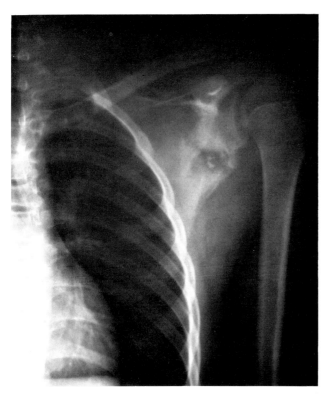

Figure 24–5. Staphylococcal osteomyelitis of the scapula secondary to closed trauma and hematological seeding with abscess formation. The shoulder joint is not involved. (From the Department of Radiology, Wake Forest University Medical Center, Winston-Salem, NC.)

injections in arthritis. Direct contamination from open wounds is also possible. Sternoclavicular sepsis is more common in drug addicts and usually involves gram-negative organisms, specifically *P. aeruginosa*. *S. aureus*, *Escherichia coli*, *Brucella*, and *N. gonorrhoeae* have also been reported.[89]

Septic arthritis of the shoulder represents up to 14 per cent of all septic arthritis cases.[81] In earlier studies, the incidence was 3.4 per cent.[72] A more elderly population, increased trauma, and the common use of

articular and periarticular steroids may be factors in this epidemiology (Fig. 24–5). The primary causal organism of shoulder sepsis also appears to have changed from pneumococcal to staphylococcal (*S. aureus*). The shift in causal organisms involved in intra-articular sepsis is probably a result of antibiotic use and increased diagnostic accuracy. Sepsis in immuno-compromised patients may be polyarticular as well as polymicrobial. Ten per cent of septic arthritis involves more than one joint and is likely in children. Viral infections commonly involve more than one joint.

OSTEOMYELITIS

Hematogenous osteomyelitis accounts for 80 to 90 per cent of osteomyelitis in children. Contiguous os-teomyelitis is more common in adults, secondary to surgery and direct inoculation. Over 50 years of age, contiguous osteomyelitis and disease related to vascular insufficiency are predominant.

Osteomyelitis in children is usually caused by one organism and by mixed organisms (*S. aureus*, gram-negative, and anaerobic bacteria) in adults.

Of the bones of the shoulder, the humerus is most frequently involved in osteomyelitis. The clavicle is occasionally involved in drug addicts by hematogenous spread. The scapula is rarely involved; usually infection occurs by direct inoculation or contiguous spread (Table 24–2).

Microbial Adhesion and Intra-articular Sepsis

An understanding of microbial adhesion is required for complete clinical and therapeutic insights in joint sepsis. Studies of bacteria in marine ecosystems indicate that they tend to adhere in colonies to surfaces or

Table 24–2. FREQUENCY OF JOINT INVOLVEMENT IN INFECTIOUS ARTHRITIS[a] (PERCENT)

	Bacterial (Suppurative)		Mycobacterial[b]	Viral
	Children[b]	Adults[c]		
Knee	41	48	24	60
Hip	23	24	20	4
Ankle	14	7	12	30
Elbow	12	11	8	20
Wrist	4	7	20	55
Shoulder	4	15	4	5
Interphalangeal and metacarpal	1.4	1	12	75
Sternoclavicular	0.4	8	0	0
Sacroiliac	0.4	2	0	0

Reprinted with permission from Mandell L, Douglas KG Jr, and Bennett JE (eds): Principles and Practice of Infectious Diseases, 2nd ed. New York: John Wiley & Sons, 1985, p. 698.
[a]More than one joint may be involved, so percentage exceeds 100%.
[b]Compiled from Nelson and Koontz[91] and Jackson and Nelson.[64]
[c]Compiled from Kelly and colleagues,[71] Argen and colleagues,[3] and Gifford and associates.[39]
[d]Compiled from Smith and Sanford[114] and Medical Staff Conference.[83]

substrata. The number of bacteria that can exist in a given environment is directly related to stress and nutrient supply.[62, 137] Since surface attachment, rather than a floating or suspension population, is a favored survival strategy, it is the state of the major portion of bacterial biomasses in most natural environments[62, 102] and is a common mode of microbial life in man.

Bacterial attachment to surfaces is influenced by proteinaceous bacterial receptors and by an extracapsular exopolysaccharide substance within which bacteria aggregate and multiply.[25, 32] Once bacteria have developed a biofilm-enclosed, adhesive mode of growth, they become more resistant to biocides,[102] antiseptics,[80] antibiotics,[44] antagonistic environmental factors.[25, 62] and host defense systems.[7, 45, 108] Free-floating, nonadhesive bacteria or microbes that lack a well-developed outer layer or exopolysaccharide are more susceptible to host-clearing mechanisms[7, 108] and to lower concentrations of antibacterial agents.[44]

Gibbons and van Houte[38] first described the significance of this adhesive phenomenon in the formation of dental plaque. In diseases such as gonococcal urethritis,[134] cystic fibrosis,[136] and endocarditis, bacterial colonization and propagation occurs along endothelial and epithelial surfaces. The association between bacterial growth on biomaterial surfaces and infection was

first described in 1963,[48] with the adhesive colonization of biomaterials first being reported in 1979.[50]

Microbial adhesion and associated phenomena also explain the foreign body effect, an increased susceptibility to infection experienced in the presence of a foreign body. Infections centered on foreign bodies are resistant to host defenses and treatment and tend to persist until the infecting locus is removed.[51] Foreign bodies include implanted biomaterials, fixation materials, prosthetic monitoring and delivery devices, traumatically acquired penetrating debris and bone fragments,[46] and compromised tissues.[46, 47, 51]

MOLECULAR AND ATOMIC MECHANISMS IN ADHESION

Initial bacterial attachment or adhesion depends on the long range physical forces characteristic of the bacterium, the fluid interface, and the substratum. Specific irreversible adhesion, which occurs after initial attachment, is based on time-dependent adhesin-receptor interactions and on extracapsular polysaccharide synthesis.[33, 38, 66, 122]

Biomaterial surfaces present sites for environmental interactions derived from their atomic structures (Fig. 24–6).[125] Metallic alloys have a thin (100 Å to 200 Å) ox-

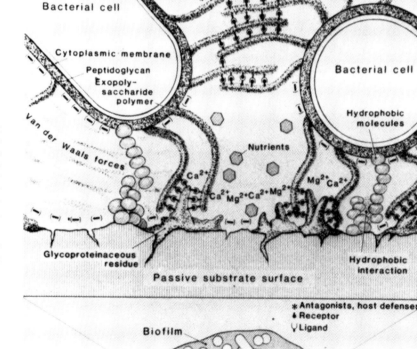

Figure 24–6. Mechanism of bacterial adherence. At specific distances the initial repelling forces between like charges on the surfaces of bacteria and substrate are overcome by attracting Van der Waals forces, and there are hydrophobic interactions between molecules. Under appropriate conditions extensive development of exopolysaccharide polymers occurs, allowing ligand-receptor interaction and proteinacious binding of the bacteria to the substrate. (Reproduced with permission from Gristina AG, Oga M, Webb LX, and Hobgood CD: Adherent bacterial colonization in the pathogenesis of osteomyelitis. Science 228:990–993, 1985. Copyright 1985, American Association for the Advancement of Science.)

ide layer that is the true biological interface.[1, 68] The surfaces of polymers and metals are modified by texture, manufacturing processes, trace chemicals, and debris, and by host-derived ionic, polysaccharide and glycoproteinaceous constituents (conditioning films). The finite surface structure of conditioning film in a human host has not been defined for any biomaterials but is specific for each individual biomaterial, type of tissue cell, and local host environment.[1, 6, 26]

Biomaterial surfaces may also act as catalytic hot spots for molecular and cellular activities.[1, 49, 68, 76] Tissue cells and matrix macromolecules also provide substrata for bacterial colonization. Bacteria have developed adhesins or receptors that interact with tissue cell surface structures (Fig. 24–7). Intermediary macromolecules or lectins may also play a role. Cells (endothelial) are more susceptible to bacterial colonization when their extramembranous outer polysaccharide glycocalyx has been traumatized or damaged by toxins.

Subsequent to or concomitant with initial attachment, fimbrial adhesins (*E. coli*) and substratum receptors may interact, as in bacteria-to-tissue cell pathogenesis or for the glycoproteinaceous conditioning films that immediately coat implants.[6, 19] The production and composition of the extracellular polysaccharide polymer, which tends to act like a glue, is a pivotal factor.[18, 137] The bacterial extracapsular exopolysaccharides may bind to surfaces or to surface absorbates and may act to consolidate microbial and polymicrobial environments.[105]

After colony maturation, cells on the periphery of the expanding biomass may separate or disaggregate and disperse, a process that is moderated by colony size, nutrient conditions, and hemodynamic or mechanical shear forces; in natural environments disaggregation is a survival strategy. In humans, however, it is involved in the pathogenesis of septic emboli. Disaggregation (dispersion) and its parameters may explain the phenomena of intermittent or short-term "bacterial showers" or disseminated bacterial emboli.

Bacterial Pathogens

The following organisms are involved in septic arthritis and osteomyelitis of the shoulder and are listed in order of frequency.[70]

Bacteria: *S. aureus, S. epidermidis, Streptococcus Group B, E. coli, P. aeruginosa, Haemophilus influenzae Type B, Neisseria gonorrhoeae, Mycobacterium tuberculosis*, and *Salmonella* and *Pneumococcus* species.

Fungi: *Actinomyces, Blastomyces, Coccidioides, Candida albicans*, and *Sporothrix schenckii*.

H. influenzae Type B is most frequently isolated in children under two years of age and is rarely found

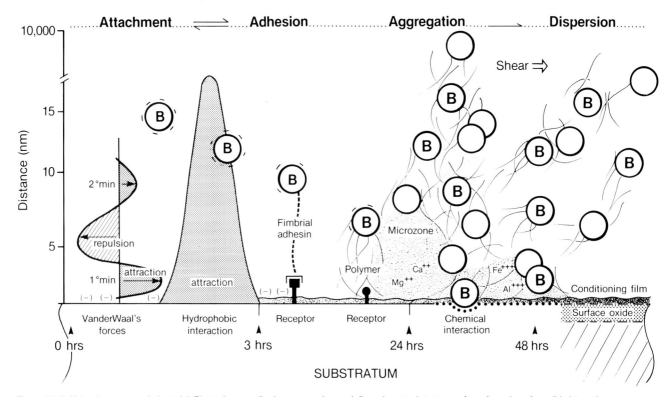

Figure 24–7. Molecular sequence in bacterial (B) attachment, adhesion, aggregation, and dispersion at substratum surface. A number of possible interactions may occur, depending on the specificities of the bacteria or substratum system (graphics, nutrients, contaminants, macromolecules, species, and materials). (Reproduced with permission from Gristina AG: Biomaterial-centered infection: microbial adhesion versus tissue integration. Science 237:1558–1595, 1987. Copyright 1987, American Association for the Advancement of Science.)

after age five. Group B *Streptococcus*, gram-negative bacilli, and *S. aureus* are common infecting organisms in the neonatal period. *S. aureus* is most common in adults; *N. gonorrhoeae* is common in adults under age 30.[35] Beta-hemolytic *streptococci* are the most common streptococci in adults and children; however, Group B is more common in neonates and diabetics. Hematogenous septic arthritis in infants is primarily streptococcal, whereas hospital-acquired infections are primarily staphylococcal but may also feature *Candida* and gram-negative organisms, especially in infants.[107]

Gram-negative bacilli are found in approximately 15 per cent of joints, especially in association with urinary tract infections or debilitating disease. *E. coli*, *P. aeruginosa*, and other gram-negative bacilli have been isolated more frequently in the last decade, along with Group A streptococci and an occasional appearance by Group B and G streptococci. Pneumococcal arthritis is now unusual.

M. tuberculosis involves the knee, hip, ankle, and wrist more frequently than the shoulder. *M. marinum* is found in marine environments.

Coccidioides immitis involves the knee more frequently than the shoulder. *Blastomyces* usually spreads from osteomyelitis to the intra-articular space. *Candida albicans* may spread via the hematogenous route in debilitated patients or directly from steroid injections.

S. aureus is often the major pathogen in biometal, bone and joint, and soft tissue infections and is the most common pathogen isolated in osteomyelitis when damaged bone or cartilage acts as a substratum.[21, 49, 51] The predominance of *S. aureus* in adult intra-articular sepsis[17, 98] may be explained by its ubiquity as a tissue pathogen seeded from remote sites, its natural invasiveness and toxins, and its receptors for collagen, fibronectin, fibrinogen, and laminin. *S. epidermidis* is most frequently involved when the biomaterial surface is a polymer or when a polymer is a component of a complex device (extended-wear contact lenses,[112] vascular prostheses,[135] an artificial heart,[56] and total joint prostheses[49]).

Studies of chronic adult osteomyelitis have revealed polymicrobial infections in more than two-thirds of cases.[15, 21, 51] The most common pathogens isolated included *S. aureus* and *S. epidermidis* and *Pseudomonas*, *Enterococcus*, *Streptococcus*, *Bacillus*, and *Proteus* species. Polymicrobial infections, therefore, appear to be an important feature of substratum-induced infections, are probably present more often than is realized, and should be regarded as a poor prognostic sign for total joint revision surgery.[53] Polymicrobial infection is a feature of chronic intra-articular sepsis and sinus formation and may be a feature of HIV infection with suppression of host defense mechanisms.[53, 54]

In summary, *S. aureus* is the most common organism in septic infections and is usually spread via hematogenous seeding. *S. epidermidis* is the principal organism in biomaterial-related infections, especially those centered on polymers. Mixed (polymicrobial), gram-neg-

ative, and anaerobic infections are probably more common than past studies have indicated and are frequently associated with open wounds and sinus tracts.

Clinical Presentation

SYMPTOMS AND SIGNS

Pain, loss of motion, and effusion are early signs of infection.[17] Shoulder effusion is difficult to detect and often missed. Motion is painful and the arm is adducted. X-rays may show a widened glenohumeral joint space and later signs of osteomyelitis (Fig. 24–8). Systemic signs include fever, leukocytosis, and sedimentation rate changes. The symptoms of immunosuppressed and rheumatoid patients may be muted.

The sternoclavicular joint may be involved and should be suspected in unilateral enlargement without trauma in patients under 50. Gonococcal and staphylococcal infections have been reported.[89] Intravenous drug addicts are susceptible to infection by gram-negative organisms, especially *P. aeruginosa* and *Serratia marcescens*. The acromioclavicular joint is rarely involved in sepsis but may be contaminated by steroid injections.

TOTAL SHOULDER REPLACEMENT

Sepsis after total joint replacement of the shoulder is rare (<0.5 per cent) because of antibiotics, excellent blood supply, and the axial gradient or proximal location of the shoulder. Symptoms of infection include pain, loss of motion, and subluxation. Pain relief is so

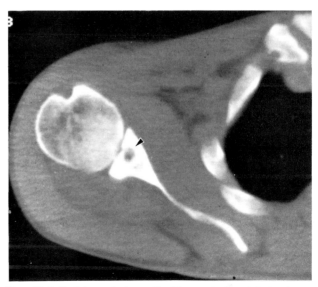

Figure 24–8. Staphylococcal osteomyelitis of the scapula. *Arrow* indicates abscess secondary to infection caused by intra-articular steroid injection. (Courtesy of Mark Warburton, M.D., High Point, NC.)

universal after total shoulder replacement that infection should be suspected if pain, radiographic joint distention, and later, a widening around the cement, especially about the humerus, are present.

RHEUMATOID ARTHRITIS

Patients with chronic rheumatoid arthritis are susceptible to spontaneous septic arthritis.[57, 69] Because the active destructive process of the rheumatoid arthritis masks the septic condition, detection of infection is often delayed. The onset of septic arthritis should be suspected when the clinical course of the rheumatoid patient worsens acutely, especially if the disease is long term. When infection is present, the patient experiences a sudden aggravation of pain and swelling and increased temperature in the joint. Sudden chills may also occur. The physician should stress to chronic rheumatoid patients (and to himself or herself) that a sudden exacerbation of symptoms warrants investigation.

If septic arthritis is suspected, the synovial fluid should be examined. The following findings indicate septic arthritis: the leukocyte count is usually more than 50,000 cells; the glucose level tends to be low (however, this is not a reliable indication of sepsis); and more than 75 per cent of the cells are polymorphonuclear. These findings are beyond the range compatible with uncomplicated rheumatoid arthritis.[133]

DIFFERENTIAL DIAGNOSIS

Aspiration of the joint is essential; however, it is often possible to diagnose septic arthritis from the external appearance of the joint. Roentgenograms are not very useful in early diagnosis because septic arthritis does not significantly alter the bone destruction owing to rheumatoid arthritis and because bone and joint radiographic changes are delayed.

Other acute arthritic disorders may imitate or mask sepsis, including gout, pseudogout, rheumatic fever, juvenile rheumatoid arthritis, and the oligoarthritic syndromes. Trauma and tumors may cause adjacent joint effusions and must be considered.

Laboratory and X-ray Evaluation

Culturing and analysis of synovial fluid is critical for diagnosis. Aspiration of the joint should always be performed when sepsis is suspected. X-ray control is indicated if the approach is difficult or about total joints. The injection of saline or simultaneous arthrogram of the glenohumeral joint may be helpful in certain cases. When cultures are negative and diagnosis is difficult, arthroscopic biopsy can be useful. In expert hands, frozen sections and touch preparations may be helpful at surgery but tend to give only an indication of pyogenic versus granulomatous or traumatic lesions. A synovial biopsy and culture for acid-fast organisms and fungi should be performed in patients with chronic monarticular arthritis, especially those with tenosynovitis. The leading infectious cause of chronic monarticular arthritis is atypical mycobacteria, such as *M. kansasii*, followed closely by *Sporothrix schenckii*. *M. tuberculosis* is rare today.[9, 113, 119] Viral infection must be considered when bacteria cannot be identified. Serological tests are required, using acute and convalescent sera, since viruses cannot be cultured from joint fluid.

SYNOVIAL FLUID ANALYSIS

In bacterial infections aspiration may yield 10 ml or more of fluid. Synovial joint fluid is usually opaque or brownish, turbid, and thick but may be serosanguineous in 15 per cent of cases with poor mucin clot. Proteins are elevated, primarily because of an elevated white blood cell count (usually greater than 50,000, frequently as great as 100,000, and primarily composed of neutrophils).[133] One-half of adults and a lower percentage of children will have a joint fluid glucose level of 40 mg less than serum glucose drawn at the same time.[64, 111, 132] These findings are more common later in infection. Polymorpholeukocytes are dominant (90 per cent). Counts over 100,000 per mm³ are typical of staphylococcal and acute bacterial infection. Monocytes are more predominant in mycobacterial infections. Rheumatoid, rheumatic, and crystalline joint diseases also elevate leukocytes, but the presence of these diseases does not exclude concomitant sepsis. Crystal examination is needed to rule out gout or pseudogout.

Gram stains are positive about 50 per cent of the time, but false positives do occur.[131] Methylene blue–stained smears are more sensitive.[113] Positive joint cultures occur in 90 per cent of established bacterial septic arthritis cases and 75 per cent of patients with tubercular arthritis.[131] Blood cultures should also be obtained and are positive in approximately 50 per cent of patients with acute infection. Depending on the type of systemic disease and organism, distant sites such as gastrointestinal, genitourinary, respiratory, and central nervous systems should also be cultured.[113] Some prosthesis-centered infections are difficult to detect unless tissues are biopsied and vortexed and homogenates are prepared for culture (Table 24–3).

Culture specimens should be taken for gram-positive, gram-negative, aerobic, and anaerobic bacteria, mycobacteria, and fungi. In approximately two-thirds of cases, the causative organism may be identified by Gram staining. Laboratory technique and media selection should be based on the type of antibiotic given to the patient and the special nutrient requirements of suspected bacteria. Use of blood agar is routine; chocolate agar is the best medium for culturing *Neisseria*

Table 24–3. SYNOVIAL FLUID FINDINGS IN ACUTE PYOGENIC ARTHRITIS

| | | Inflammatory Fluids | |
Joint Fluid Examination	Noninflammatory Fluids	*Noninfectious*	*Infectious*
Color	Colorless, pale yellow	Yellow to white	Yellow
Turbidity	Clear, slightly turbid	Turbid	Turbid, purulent
Viscosity	Not reduced	Reduced	Reduced
Mucin clot	Tight clot	Friable	Friable
Cell count (per mm³)	200–1000	3000–>10,000	10,000–>100,000
Predominant cell type	Mononuclear	PMN*	PMN*
Synovial fluid/blood glucose ratio	0.8–1.0	0.5–0.8	<0.5
Lactic acid	Same as plasma	Higher than plasma	Often very high
Gram stain for organism	None	None	Positive†
Culture	Negative	Negative	Positive†

Reprinted with permission from Schmid FR: Principles of diagnosis and treatment of bone and joint infections. In McCarty DJ (ed): Arthritis and Allied Conditions. A Textbook of Rheumatology. Philadelphia: Lea & Febiger, 1985, p. 1638.
*PMN = polymorphonuclear leukocyte.
†In some cases, especially in gonococcal infection, no organisms may be demonstrated.

and *Haemophilus* species. Thayer-Martin media may be used to isolate gonococcal organisms, but since it contains vancomycin and colistin methanesulfonate, *Haemophilus* species or other mixed flora will not grow on it.[106] Sabouraud's medium is specific for fungi. An egg-glycerol-potato and synthetic agar combination is used to culture mycobacteria.[106] Centrifugation is recommended for detection of mycobacteria (which are less frequently present) if sufficient fluid can be obtained. The magnitude of anaerobic septic arthritis has been underestimated in the past.[30]

RADIOGRAPHIC, ULTRASOUND, CT, MRI, AND ISOTOPE TECHNIQUES

X-rays and computed tomography (CT) of the septic shoulder may indicate changes ranging from widening to subluxation and from bone destruction to new bone formation (Figs. 24–9 to 24–11).[130] Arthrography may be useful for identifying rotator cuff tears,[4] which are present in many patients with septic arthritis. Ultra-

sonography is useful in assisting aspiration and in assessing the infected shoulder joint.[42] Positive technetium bone scanning has been reported in 75 to 100 per cent of septic arthritis cases, but technetium, gallium, and indium scans are not consistent.[36, 84, 139] Schmidt found that technetium bone scans performed on children with septic arthritis were frequently negative.[107] Indium scans may be more accurate indicators of sepsis, but conclusive data are lacking. Indium scintigraphy for osteomyelitis should be preceded by a positive technetium scan. If an indium scan is negative, infection is unlikely. A positive indium scan increases the specificity of diagnosis. Indium uptake should be evaluated against the normal reticuloendothelial background.[139]

CT is useful in identifying small early lytic lesions caused by osteomyelitis that might be obscured in ordinary x-rays. Diagnosis of sternoclavicular joint sepsis and clavicular osteomyelitis infections may be improved using CT because it overcomes the tissue overlap problem that occurs with ordinary x-rays; however, CT does not offer much advantage in imaging the humerus.

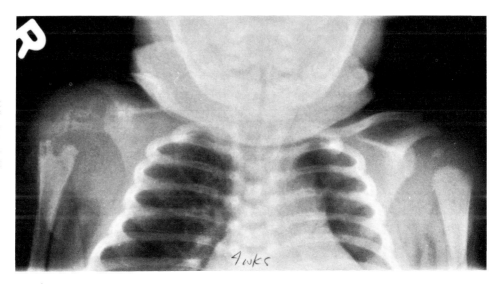

Figure 24–9. Septic arthritis of the right shoulder with destruction and widening of the proximal humerus. Also note healing of a right clavicle fracture. Organism: beta-hemolytic streptococci. (From the Department of Radiology, Wake Forest University Medical Center, Winston-Salem, NC.)

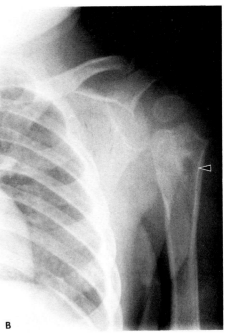

B

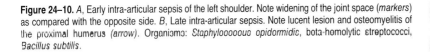

Figure 24–10. *A,* Early intra-articular sepsis of the left shoulder. Note widening of the joint space *(markers)* as compared with the opposite side. *B,* Late intra-articular sepsis. Note lucent lesion and osteomyelitis of the proximal humerus *(arrow).* Organisms: *Staphyloooooooouo opidormidic,* bota-homolytic streptococci, *Bacillus subtilis.*

In chronic osteomyelitis, large areas of abnormal or low signals with magnetic resonance imaging (MRI) may indicate an area of possible sequestration and hyperemia, especially along sinus tracts.[27] Capsular distention of articular cartilage and fluid-filled spaces are clearly visible on MRI, as are damaged surfaces, loose bodies, and avascular regions. MRI has not been used extensively for the detection of intra-articular sepsis or osteomyelitis. However, it will probably be

quite sensitive in early detection and specific for the localization and identification of sequestra.[31, 59, 104]

Complications

Inadequately treated intra-articular sepsis or osteomyelitis may result in recurrent infection, contiguous spread, bacteremia, distant septic emboli, anemia, septic shock, and death. Delayed diagnosis with adequate treatment may result in joint surface destruction, contractures, subluxation, arthritis, and growth aberrations (Fig. 24–12).[97] Inflammation, bacterial products, and lysosomal enzymes break down cartilage.[73] Within weeks, bacterial antigens stimulate destructive inflammation that may persist after the infection is treated. Bacterial endotoxins are chemotactic and bacterial proteolytic enzymes further destroy surfaces. Increased intra-articular pressure also causes ischemia. Thrombotic events are also stimulated by burgeoning infection, further destroying the joint and adjacent bone. Long-term complications of chronic osteomyelitis include amyloidosis, nephrotic syndromes, and epidermal carcinoma.

Treatment

A retrospective study of a 10-year period at the Bowman Gray School of Medicine revealed 17 septic shoulders in 16 patients.[124] Patients with gonococcal infections were excluded from the study. The patients' ages ranged from 26 days to 72 years (average age, 33 years). The causative organism was *S. aureus* in five

Figure 24–11. Cystic lesions in the humeral head consistent with tuberculosis sicca in a 19-year-old woman. (Reproduced with permission from DePalma AF (ed): Surgery of the Shoulder, 3rd ed. Philadelphia: JB Lippincott, 1983.)

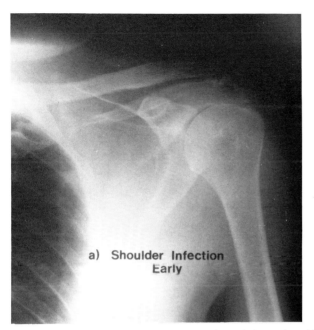 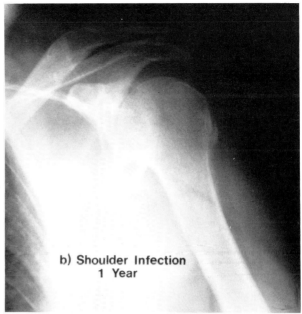

Figure 24-12. Hematogenous osteomyelitis secondary to intra-articular sepsis. *a*, Minimal lucency of proximal humerus at two weeks after probable onset of infection. *b*, After arthrotomy, antibiotic treatment, and resolution of infection, x-ray reveals periosteal new bone formation and joint contracture. Organism: *Staphylococcus aureus*.

patients, Group B *Streptococcus* in two patients, *Pneumococcus* in three, multiple organisms in one patient, *Proteus* in one patient, and *Haemophilus* in one patient. Three patients had obvious clinical infection with negative cultures owing to treatment, technique, and timing.

Ten septic shoulder patients (treated by different physicians) underwent arthrotomy; one was treated by arthrocentesis; and another was treated initially with aspirations, but later an arthrotomy was performed for osteomyelitis of the glenoid. Total joints were involved in two patients. Both infections were delayed and due to seeding from distant sites; one was associated with repeated local trauma. One total joint infection was resolved by removal of the component and resulted in a nonpainful pseudarthrosis. A second patient had chronic drainage and a markedly decreased range of motion, even after debridement.

One patient treated with aspirations and intravenous antibiotics expired owing to septic shock. Five patients developed chronic drainage or osteomyelitis. Underlying shoulder pathology significantly delayed diagnosis and treatment of shoulder sepsis in four patients.

All patients received intravenous antibiotics, and the duration of treatment ranged from seven days to four weeks. All patients received at least a total of three weeks of antibiotic therapy, including oral and intravenous administration. All children had complete resolution and excellent function at several months follow-up. Complete resolution of symptoms occurred with the treatment provided in 9 of the 16 patients. We suggest early active motion and therapy as tolerated.

Predisposing factors included rheumatoid arthritis, previous surgery, steroid injections, trauma, burns,

and septic emboli from distant infections. CT scans were positive 60 per cent of the time.

Intra-articular sepsis should be treated swiftly.[116] Variables that influence the selection of treatment methods include the duration of infection, host immune status, the types of infecting organisms, and the presence of foreign bodies or adjacent osteomyelitis. The most critical factors in treatment are the infecting organism and the presence of a foreign body.

Most clinicians agree that systemic antibiotic therapy should begin immediately following the diagnosis of septic arthritis, but there is less agreement on subsequent therapy. In internal medicine, repeated needle aspiration is recommended as a primary treatment;[71, 132] however, orthopedic surgeons and the authors believe that immediate arthrotomy is the treatment of choice, especially for the shoulder.[67, 100]

In general, the literature suggests that treatment of septic arthritis with repeated needle aspiration and appropriate intravenous antibiotics may be adequate except for the hip. However, conclusive studies of initial surgical drainage versus needle aspiration are lacking. A retrospective study comparing 55 infected joints treated by needle aspiration with 18 joints treated surgically concluded that 60 per cent of surgically treated patients had sequelae, whereas 80 per cent of medically treated patients recovered completely.[41] The authors question these data. Most orthopedic surgeons believe that the anatomy of the shoulder and the nature of shoulder sepsis demand surgical treatment. Septic arthritis that does not respond to medical management in seven days should be surgically drained. Sternoarticular infections in drug abusers usually involve bone and joint. For these

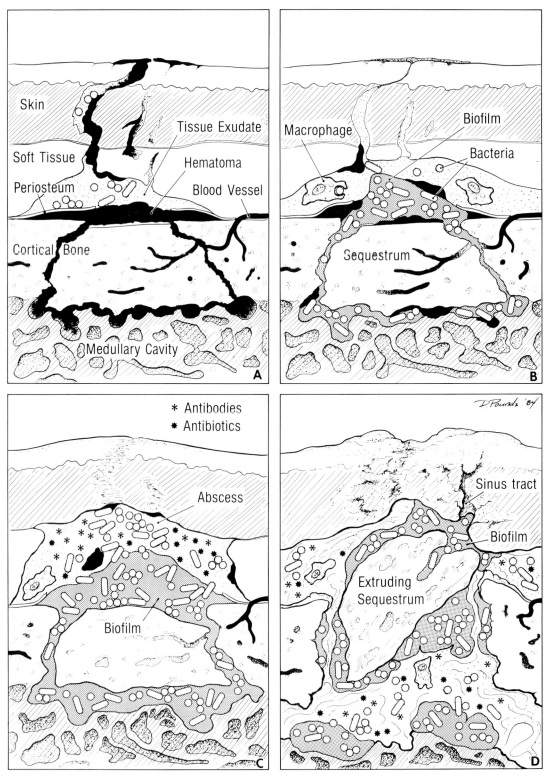

Figure 24–13. The sequence of pathogenesis in osteomyelitis. *A,* Initial trauma produces soft tissue destruction and bone fragmentation, as well as wound contamination by bacteria. In closed wounds, contamination may occur by hematogenous seeding. *B,* As the infection progresses, bacterial colonization occurs within a protective exopolysaccharide biofilm. The biofilm is particularly abundant on the devitalized bone fragment, which acts as a passive substratum for colonization. *C,* Host defenses are mobilized against the infection but are unable to penetrate or be effective in the presence of the biofilm. *D,* Progressive inflammation and abscess formation eventually result in the development of a sinus tract and, in some cases, ultimate extrusion of the sequestrum that is the focus of the resistant infection. (Reproduced with permission from Gristina AG, Barth E, and Webb LX: Microbial adhesion and the pathogenesis of biomaterial-centered infections. *In* Gustilo RB, Gruninger RP, and Tsukayama DT (eds): Orthopaedic Infection. Diagnosis and Treatment. Philadelphia: WB Saunders, 1989, pp 3–25.)

patients, needle aspiration has not been useful in establishing the diagnosis. However, surgical drainage has been useful in providing the pathogen. It also allows debridement of necrotic bone and permits drainage of abscesses, which are often present.[8, 101, 120]

Osteomyelitis of the proximal metaphysis may either precede or be secondary to septic arthritis of the glenohumeral joint (Fig. 24–13). Therefore, drilling of the metaphysis has been recommended for pediatric septic glenohumeral arthritis to rule out osteomyelitis and to allow adequate decompression of the bone. Diagnosed osteomyelitis should be surgically treated.

Immobilization is usually recommended for septic arthritis. However, Salter's study of septic arthritis in a rabbit model indicated that the use of continuous passive motion was superior to immobilization or to intermittent active motion.[103] Possible explanations for these results include prevention of bacterial adhesion, enhanced diffusion of nutrients, improved clearance of lysosomal enzymes and debris from the infected joints, and stimulation of chondrocytes to synthesize the various components of the matrix.

The majority of children do well following treatment for septic shoulder arthritis. In a study of nine children with glenohumeral arthritis, Schmidt suggested surgical treatment with exploration of the biceps tendon sheath.[107] Growth center damage is possible. The prognosis for adults with septic arthritis of the shoulder is poor, but shoulders treated within four weeks or less of the onset of symptoms may do well. Poor results are associated with delayed diagnosis, virulent (gram-negative) infecting organisms, persistent pain, drainage, osteomyelitis, and destruction of the joint.

Gonococcal septic arthritis may be polyarticular.[40] Fever is low grade, usually below 102° F. Articular and periarticular structures are swollen, stiff, and painful, followed by desquamation of skin over the joints. During septicemia, macular and occasionally vesicular rash occurs in one-third of patients but is also caused by *Neisseria meningitidis*, *Haemophilus*, and *Streptobacillus*.[16, 110] Organisms are not common in joint fluid and, therefore, are not isolated in most cases. The general picture of gonococcal septic arthritis is less acute than staphylococcal infection. Gonococcal arthritis responds well to systemic antibiotic therapy and needle aspiration; however, in refractory cases, the authors have used arthrocentesis.

Antimicrobial agents used to treat joint infections generally achieve levels intra-articularly equal to or greater than serum levels except for erythromycin and gentamicin (Table 24–4). Intra-articular antibiotics are generally not advocated and may cause sterile abscesses. The authors do, however, use bacitracin in irrigating solutions at surgery. Rarely, carefully monitored intra-articular aminoglycosides may be indicated. In osteomyelitis, antibiotic penetration into bone is unreliable.[95] Clindamycin achieves higher bone levels than cephalothin or methicillin.[94] When healthy bone in children is being treated, absent sequestration, delivery of antibiotics to the infected site is likely. The

Table 24–4. EMPIRIC ANTIBIOTIC THERAPY FOR BONE (B) AND JOINT (J) INFECTIONS

Age	Clinical Status	Site	Antibiotic	Likely Pathogens
≤3 months	normal host	B; J	Nafcillin + aminoglycoside[1] + ampicillin	Enteric gram-negative bacilli, *Staphylococcus aureus* (*S. aureus*), group B streptococci
3 mos. to 6 yrs	normal host	B; J	Cefuroxime	*S. aureus*, *Haemophilus influenzae*
6 to 10 yrs	normal host	J	Nafcillin	*S. aureus*
>6 to 59 yrs	normal host	B	Nafcillin	*S. aureus*
>10 to 59 yrs	normal host	J	Nafcillin, penicillin G	*S. aureus*, *Neisseria gonorrhoeae*
≥60 yrs	UTI	B; J	Nafcillin + aminoglycoside[1] + ampicillin	*S. aureus*, enteric gram-negative bacilli, Enterococci
All ages	sickle cell anemia	B; J	Nafcillin + TMP-SMX[2]	*S. aureus*, Salmonella species
All ages	bite wound	B; J	Cefoxitin	*Pasteurella multocida* (animals), *S. aureus*, anaerobes, *Eikenella corrodens* (human)
All ages	immunocompromised[3]	B; J	Ceftriaxone + aminoglycoside[1]	*S. aureus*, gram-negative bacilli
All ages	IV drug abuse	B; J	Nafcillin + aminoglycoside[1] + anti-pseudomonal penicillin[2]	*S. aureus*, *Pseudomonas aeruginosa*
All ages	trauma	B; J	Nafcillin + aminoglycoside[1] + anti-pseudomonal penicillin[2]	*S. aureus*, gram-negative bacilli
All ages	foreign body—early, acute	B; J	Vancomycin + ceftriaxone or TMP-SMX[2]	*S. aureus*, *Staphylococcus epidermidis*, gram-negative bacilli, streptococcal species
All ages	foreign body—late, chronic	B; J	Await culture results	Variable
Adult	decubitus ulcer, diabetic foot ulcer	B	Cefoxitin	Anaerobe; streptococci, gram-negative bacilli

Reprinted with permission from Luskin RL, and Kabins SA: Antimicrobial therapy in orthopaedic patients. *In* Post M (ed): The Shoulder. Surgical and Nonsurgical Management, 2nd ed. Philadelphia: Lea & Febiger, 1988, p 117.

[1]Tobramycin, gentamicin, amikacin, netilmicin

[2]Trimethoprim-sulfamethoxazole

[3]Neutropenic, diabetic, systemic lupus erythematosus, alcoholic or chronic debilitating illness

[4]Ticarcillin, piperacillin, carbenicillin, azlocillin

opposite situation exists in adults, the aged, vascularly compromised patients, and patients with chronic osteomyelitis, sequestration, and sinus formation. Animal studies have suggested that antibiotic combinations (for example, oxacillin and aminoglycosides) may be more effective in osteomyelitis.[95] The new quinolone group of antibiotics under evaluation for treatment of bone and joint infections may be useful because of their broad spectrum of activity against staphylococci, *Pseudomonas* species, and gram-negative bacteria.[28] These agents achieve excellent local levels in living and dead bone. The emergence of mutant strains may occur but can be reduced by intelligent use of quinolones in combination with other antibiotics.

Staphylococci may persist after nafcillin therapy owing to selection of cell wall–deficient organisms, requiring the use of an antistaphylococcal such as clindamycin.[2] Intravenous therapy is generally continued for more than three weeks in septic arthritis and more than four to six weeks in osteomyelitis and is monitored by systemic signs, white blood count, and sedimentation rates.[96, 113] Serum levels greater than or equal to 1:8, MIC, and MBC are suggested.[77] Oral antibiotics may be used after intravenous therapy as required.[77, 94]

Surgical debridement is the *sine qua non* of treatment for septic arthritis and osteomyelitis of the shoulder. The logic is as follows: (1) toxic products, damaged tissue, and foreign bodies must be removed to prevent damage and to treat infection effectively; and (2) laboratory studies have shown that the MIC and MBC levels needed to treat surface-adherent bacterial populations are 10 to 100 times higher than those for suspension populations.[55, 65, 75, 97] These findings suggest that it is possible to clear a bacteremia or bacteria suspended in synovial fluid but very difficult to sterilize an infected cartilaginous joint surface or sequestrum covered with debris without administering toxic levels of antibiotics.

Antibiotic impregnated beads (gentamicin or tobramycin) may be indicated in certain cases of osteomyelitis and articular sepsis.[13, 34, 43] We suggest their removal at 6 to 12 weeks. Studies suggest that eventually, these methylmethacrylate surfaces may provide a substratum for resistant organisms.[135a] Closed suction and irrigation may be used for short periods (less than three days) if necessary in special cases in septic joints, provided the system does not allow retrograde contamination. However, the literature does not indicate a definite advantage with this treatment, and it is seldom required in *de novo* joint sepsis since adequate antibiotic levels can be achieved systemically.

Open wounds involving joints are by definition contaminated, even though bacteria are not always detected. Type 3 open fractures, especially those involving joints, have a very high rate of infection, as do tibia wounds. There are indications that these should be treated with a combination of cefazolin and gentamicin.[95] Topical or local antibiotics may be used in the future for damaged tissue or chronic infections in certain population groups because these infections require higher antibiotic levels than can be achieved via the bloodstream. A biodegradable, resorbable, antibiotic-loaded substrate placed in a surgically debrided musculoskeletal site may be even more effective than methylmethacrylate beads.

PROPHYLAXIS

Antibiotic prophylaxis is effective because bacteria are cleared before they establish slime-shielded, surface-adherent, rapidly growing populations at sites deep within bone or on biomaterials. The authors suggest using antibiotic prophylaxis, such as cefazolin, 2 gm intravenously at anesthesia and repeated at four hours.[93] The use of prophylactic antibiotics is suggested for all implant surgery, including both prosthetic and internal fixation of fractures, and trauma. Antibiotics may be varied, depending on the special conditions of each case and patient.[95] Treatment for 48 hours in clean cases is believed sufficient. Clean air, laminar flow, and ultraviolet light are also effective based on local cost/benefit ratios.

Authors' Preferred Methods of Treatment

The shoulder joint is capacious and anatomically complicated. For this reason, open surgical drainage rather than aspiration or arthroscopic drainage is indicated. We use an anterior deltopectoral approach. The deltoid and coracoid are not detached. Infected surfaces are debrided of adhesins, clots, and debris. Surgical lavage with antibiotics is an appropriate technique. In most cases, the wound may be loosely closed and a large hemovac inserted for 24 hours to remove postsurgical accumulations. In cases of chronic sepsis or infection by gram-negative organisms, the wound is left open. Adequate intra-articular concentrations of antibiotics can be achieved by intravenous and intramuscular administration.[92] The duration of antibiotic treatment varies, depending on the host and organism; three weeks of intravenous therapy followed by three weeks of oral treatment is a reasonable base. Patient response is the key to duration of treatment.

Infection occurs in less than 1 per cent of cases after total joint arthroplasty of the shoulder.[52, 90] Parallels in hip surgery indicate that early infection may be treated with irrigation and debridement if it is largely due to an infected hematoma. This is rarely the case, however, and removal of components is usually required. All damaged tissue and methylmethacrylate should be removed if possible. The prognosis for revision total joint arthroplasty after infection is poor.[88] A fusion may be performed. Our studies indicate that patients have surprisingly good function one year after removal of components without fusion. Thus resection, rather than fusion, is our standard salvage method for failed, infected shoulders and elbows.

In summary, intra-articular shoulder sepsis is becoming increasingly frequent in adults. Shoulder anatomy is unique in that bursae communicating with the joint provide a pathway for bacteria for which cartilage is the target substratum. Successful treatment depends on immune system response, the type of infecting organism, and early surgical debridement.

References

1. Albrektsson T: The response of bone to titanium implants. CRC Crit Rev Biocompat 1:53–84, 1985.
2. Antibiotics for osteomyelitis. Lancet 1:153–154, 1975.
3. Argen RJ, Wilson DH, Jr., and Wood P: Suppurative arthritis. Arch Intern Med 117:661–666, 1966.
4. Armbuster G, Slivka J, Resnick D, et al: Extraarticular manifestations of septic arthritis of the glenohumeral joint. AJR 129:667–672, 1977.
5. Avery JK (ed): Oral Development and Histology. Baltimore: Williams & Wilkins, 1987.
6. Baier RE, Meyer AE, Natiella JR, et al: Surface properties determine bioadhesive outcomes: methods and results. J Biomed Mater Res 18:337–355, 1984.
7. Baltimore RS, and Mitchell M: Immunologic investigations of mucoid strains of Pseudomonas aeruginosa: comparison of susceptibility to opsonic antibody in mucoid and nonmucoid strains. J Infect Dis 141:238–247, 1980.
8. Bayer AS, Chow AW, Louie JS, et al: Gram-negative bacillary septic arthritis: clinical, radiologic, therapeutic, and prognostic features. Semin Arthritis Rheum 7:123–132, 1977.
9. Berney S, Goldstein M, and Bishko F: Clinical and diagnostic features of tuberculous arthritis. Am J Med 53:36–42, 1972.
10. Bhawan J, Das Tandon H, and Roy S: Ultrastructure of synovial membrane in pyogenic arthritis. Arch Pathol 96:155–160, 1973.
11. Birinyi LK, Douville C, Lewis SA, et al: Increased resistance to bacteremic graft infection after endothelial cell seeding. J Vasc Surg 5:193–197, 1987.
12. Broadwater JR, and Stair JM: Sternoclavicular osteomyelitis: coverage with a pectoralis major muscle flap. Surg Rounds Orthop 2(9):47–50, 1988.
13. Buccholz HW, and Gartmann HD: Infektionsprophylaxe und operative Behandlung der schleichenden tiefen Infektion bei der totalen Endoprothese. Chirurg 43:446–452, 1972.
14. Bullough PG, and Vigorita VJ: Atlas of Orthopaedic Pathology. Baltimore: University Park Press, 1984, p 94.
15. Burch KK, Fine G, Quinn EL, and Eisses JF: Cryptococcus neoformans as a cause of lytic bone lesions. JAMA 231:1057–1059, 1975.
16. Cabot RC (ed): Case records of the Massachusetts General Hospital. An obscure general infection. Boston Med Surg J 197:1140–1142, 1927.
17. Calhoun J, Cantrell J, and Mader J: Septic shoulders. Paper #28. The Society of American Shoulder and Elbow Surgeons, 4th Open Meeting, Atlanta, Georgia, February 7, 1988.
18. Calleja GB, Atkinson B, Garrod DR, et al: Aggregation. Group report. In Marshall KC (ed): Microbial Adhesion and Aggregation. Berlin: Springer-Verlag, 1984, pp 303–321.
19. Christensen GD, Simpson WA, and Beachey EH: Adhesion of bacteria to animal tissues: complex mechanisms. In Savage DC, and Fletcher M (eds): Bacterial Adhesion, Mechanisms and Physiological Significance. New York: Plenum Press, 1985, pp 279–305.
20. Chung SMK: The arterial supply of the developing proximal end of the human femur. J Bone Joint Surg 58A:961–970, 1976.
21. Cierny G, Couch L, and Mader J: Adjunctive local antibiotics in the management of contaminated orthopaedic wounds. In

22. Final Program. American Academy of Orthopaedic Surgeons, 53rd Annual Meeting, New Orleans, Louisiana, 1986, p 86.
22. Clemente C (ed): Gray's Anatomy of the Human Body, 5th ed. Philadelphia: Lea & Febiger, 1985.
23. Codman EA: The Shoulder. Rupture of the Supraspinatus Tendon and Other Lesions in or About the Subacromial Bursa, 2nd ed. Malabar, FL: Robert E. Kreiger, 1984.
24. Cofield RH: Total shoulder arthroplasty with the Neer prosthesis. J Bone Joint Surg 66A:899–906, 1984.
25. Costerton JW, Geesey GG, and Cheng K-J: How bacteria stick. Sci Am 238:86–95, 1978.
26. Dankert J, Hogt AH, and Feijen J: Biomedical polymers: bacterial adhesion, colonization, and infection. CRC Crit Rev Biocompat 2:219–301, 1986.
27. David R, Barron BJ, and Madewell JE: Osteomyelitis, acute and chronic. Radiol Clin North Am 25:1171–1201, 1987.
28. Desplaces N, and Acar JF: New quinolones in the treatment of joint and bone infections. Rev Infect Dis 10(Suppl. 1):S179–S183, 1988.
29. DePalma AF (ed): Surgery of the Shoulder, 3rd ed. Philadelphia: JB Lippincott Co., 1983.
30. Fitzgerald RH, Rosenblatt JE, Tenney JH, and Bourgault A-M: Anaerobic septic arthritis. Clin Orthop 164:141–148, 1982.
31. Fletcher BD, Scoles PV, and Nelson AD: Osteomyelitis in children: detection by magnetic resonance. Radiology 150:57–60, 1984.
32. Fletcher M: Adherence of marine micro-organisms to smooth surfaces. In Beachy EH (ed): Bacterial Adherence. Receptors and Recognition, series B, vol. 6. London: Chapman & Hall, 1980, pp 347–374.
33. Fletcher M: Effect of solid surfaces on the activity of attached bacteria. In Savage DC, and Fletcher M (eds): Bacterial Adhesion: Mechanisms and Physiological Significance. New York: Plenum Press, 1985, pp 339–362.
34. Flick AB, Herbert JC, Goodell J, and Kristiansen T: Noncommercial fabrication of antibiotic-impregnated polymethylmethacrylate beads. Technical note. Clin Orthop 223:282–286, 1987.
35. Gelberman RH, Menon J, Austerlitz S, and Weisman MH: Pyogenic arthritis of the shoulder in adults. J Bone Joint Surg 62A:550–553, 1980.
36. Gentry LO: Osteomyelitis: options for diagnosis and management. J Antimicrob Chemother 21:[Suppl]:115–128, 1988.
37. Gibbons RJ, and Van Houte J: Dental caries. Annu Rev Med 26:121–136, 1975.
38. Gibbons RJ, and Van Houte J: Bacterial adherence and the formation of dental plaques. In Beachey EH (ed): Bacterial Adherence: Receptors and Recognition, Series B, vol 6. London: Chapman & Hall, 1980, pp 63–104.
39. Gifford DB, Patzakis M, Ivler D, and Swezey RL: Septic arthritis due to Pseudomonas in heroin addicts. J Bone Joint Surg 57-A:631–635, 1975.
40. Goldenberg DL: Gonococcal arthritis. In McCarty DJ (ed): Arthritis and Allied Conditions. A Textbook of Rheumatology, 10th ed. Philadelphia: Lea & Febiger, 1985, pp 1651–1661.
41. Goldenberg DL, and Reed JI: Bacterial arthritis. N Engl J Med 312:764–771, 1985.
42. Gompels BM, and Darlington LG: Septic arthritis in rheumatoid disease causing bilateral shoulder dislocation: diagnosis and treatment assisted by grey scale ultrasonography. Ann Rheum Dis 40:609–611, 1981.
43. Goodell JA, Flick AB, Hebert JC, and Howe JG: Preparation and release characteristics of tobramycin-impregnated polymethylmethacrylate beads. Am J Hosp Pharm 43:1454–1460, 1986.
44. Govan JRW, and Fyfe JAM: Mucoid Pseudomonas aeruginosa and cystic fibrosis: resistance of the mucoid form to carbenicillin, flucloxacillin and tobramycin and the isolation of mucoid variants in vitro. J Antimicrob Chemother 4:233–240, 1978.
45. Govan JRW: Mucoid strains of Pseudomonas aeruginosa: the influence of culture medium on the stability of mucus production. J Med Microbiol 8:513–522, 1975.
46. Gristina AG, and Costerton JW: Bacteria-laden biofilms: a hazard to orthopedic prostheses. Infect Surg 3:655–662, 1984.

47. Gristina AG, and Costerton JW: Bacterial adherence to biomaterials and tissue. The significance of its role in clinical sepsis. J Bone Joint Surg 67A:264–273, 1985.

48. Gristina AG, and Rovere GD: An in vitro study of the effects of metals used in internal fixation on bacterial growth and dissemination. J Bone Joint Surg 45A:1104, 1963.

49. Gristina AG, Hobgood CD, and Barth E: Biomaterial specificity, molecular mechanisms and clinical relevance of S. epidermidis and S. aureus infections in surgery. In Pulverer G, Quie PG, and Peters G (eds): Pathogenesis and Clinical Significance of Coagulase-negative Staphylococci. Stuttgart: Fischer Verlag, 1987, pp 143–157.

50. Gristina AG, Kolkin J, Leake E, et al: Bacteria and their relationship to biomaterials. First World Biomaterials Conference, Final Programme Book of Abstracts, p 2.39. Vienna, European Society for Biomaterials, 1980.

51. Gristina AG, Oga M, Webb LX, and Hobgood CD: Adherent bacterial colonization in the pathogenesis of osteomyelitis. Science 228:990–993, 1985.

52. Gristina AG, Romano RL, Kammire GC, and Webb LX: Total shoulder replacement. Orthop Clin North Am 18:445–453, 1987.

53. Gristina AG, Webb LX, and Barth E: Microbial adhesion, biomaterials, and man. In Coombs R, and Fitzgerald R (eds): Infection in the Orthopaedic Patient. London: Butterworths Press, 1989, pp 30–42.

54. Gristina AG, Barth E, and Myrvik Q: Materials, microbes and man. The problem of infection associated with implantable devices. In Williams DF (ed): Current Perspectives on Implantable Devices. London: JAI Press, in press.

55. Gristina AG, Hobgood CD, Webb LX, and Myrvik QN: Adhesive colonization of biomaterials and antibiotic resistance. Biomaterials 8:423–426, 1987.

56. Gristina AG: Biomaterial-centered infection: microbial adhesion versus tissue integration. Science 237:1558–1595, 1987.

57. Gristina AG, Rovere GD, and Shoji H: Spontaneous septic arthritis complicating rheumatoid arthritis. J Bone Joint Surg 56A:1180–1184, 1974.

58. Hamill RJ, Vann JM, and Proctor RA: Phagocytosis of Staphylococcus aureus by cultured bovine aortic endothelial cells: model for postadherence events in endovascular infections. Infect Immun 54:833–836, 1986.

59. Hendrix RW, and Fisher MR: Imaging of septic arthritis. Clin Rheum Dis 12:459–487, 1986.

60. Holderbaum D, Spech T, Ehrhart L et al: Collagen binding in clinical isolates of Staphylococcus aureus. J Clin Microbiol 25:2258–2261, 1987.

61. Holderbaum D, Hall GS, and Ehrhart LA: Collagen binding to Staphylococcus aureus. Infect Immun 54:359–364, 1986.

62. Hoppe HG: Attachment of bacteria. Advantage or disadvantage for survival in the aquatic environment. In Marshall KC (ed): Microbial Adhesion and Aggregation. New York: Springer-Verlag, 1984 pp 283–301.

63. Hunter W: Of the structures and diseases of articulating cartilage. Philos Trans R Soc Lond 42:514–521, 1743.

64. Jackson MA, and Nelson JD: Etiology and medical management of acute suppurative bone and joint infections in pediatric patients. J Pediatr Orthop 2:313, 1982.

65. Jennings R, Myrvik Q, Naylor P, et al: Comparative in vitro activity of LY146032 against biomaterial-adherent Staphylococcus epidermidis. In Abstracts of the Annual Meeting of the American Society for Microbiology, p 18, Washington, D.C., 1988.

66. Jones GW, and Isaacson RE: Proteinaceous bacterial adhesins and their receptors. CRC Crit Rev Microbiol 10:229–260, 1984.

67. Karten I: Septic arthritis complicating rheumatoid arthritis. Ann Intern Med 70:1147–1151, 1969.

68. Kasemo B, and Lausmaa J: Surface science aspects on inorganic biomaterials. CRC Crit Rev Biocompat 2:335–380, 1986.

69. Kellgren JH, Ball J, Fairbrother RW, and Barnes KL: Suppurative arthritis complicating rheumatoid arthritis. Br Med J 1:1193–1200, 1958.

70. Kelly PJ, and Fitzgerald RH Jr.: Bacterial arthritis. In Braude AI, Davis CE, and Fierer J (eds): Infectious Diseases and Medical Microbiology, 2nd ed. Philadelphia: WB Saunders, 1986, pp 1468–1472.

71. Kelly PJ, Martin WJ, and Coventry MD: Bacterial (suppurative) arthritis in the adult. J Bone Joint Surg 52A:1595–1602, 1970.

72. Kelly PJ, Conventry MB, and Martin WJ: Bacterial arthritis of the shoulder. Mayo Clin Proc 40:695–699, 1965.

73. Klein RS: Joint infection, with consideration of underlying disease and sources of bacteremia in hematogenous infection. Clin Geriatr Med 4:375–394, 1988.

74. Krespi YP, Monsell EM, and Sisson GA: Osteomyelitis of the clavicle. Ann Otol Rhinol Laryngol 92:525–527, 1983.

75. Ladd TI, Schmiel D, Nickel JC, and Costerton JW: Rapid method for detection of adherent bacteria on Foley urinary catheters. J Clin Microbiol 21:1004–1006, 1985.

76. Lehninger AL: Principles of Biochemistry. New York: Worth Publishers, 1982.

77. Luskin RL, and Kabins SA: Antimicrobial therapy in orthopaedic patients. In Post M (ed): The Shoulder. Surgical and Nonsurgical Management, 2nd ed. Philadelphia: Lea & Febiger, 1988, pp 108–138.

78. Mandell GL, Douglas RG Jr., and Bennett JE (eds): Principles and Practice of Infectious Diseases, 2nd ed. New York: John Wiley & Sons, 1985.

79. Manny J, Haruzi I, and Yosipovitch Z: Osteomyelitis of the clavicle following subclavian vein catheterization. Arch Surg 106:342–343, 1973.

80. Marrie TJ, and Costerton JW: Prolonged survival of Serratia marcescens in chlorhexidine. Appl Environ Microbiol 42:1093–1102, 1981.

81. Master R, Weisman MH, Armbuster TG, et al: Septic arthritis of the glenohumeral joint. Unique clinical and radiographic features and a favorable outcome. Arthritis Rheum 10:1500–1506, 1977.

82. McCarty DJ (ed). Arthritis and Allied Conditions. A Textbook of Rheumatology, 10th ed. Philadelphia: Lea & Febiger, 1985.

83. Medical Staff Conference: Arthritis caused by viruses. California Med 119(3):38–44, 1973.

84. Merkel KD, Brown ML, DeWanjee MK, and Fitzgerald RH: Comparison of indium-labeled leukocyte imaging with sequential technetium-gallium scanning in the diagnosis of low-grade musculoskeletal sepsis. J Bone Joint Surg 67A:465–476, 1985.

85. Morrey BF, and Bianco AJ: Hematogenous osteomyelitis of the clavicle in children. Clin Orthop 125:24–28, 1977.

86. Morrissy RT: Bone and joint sepsis in children. In American Academy of Orthopaedic Surgeons Instructional Course Lectures. 55th Annual Meeting of the American Academy of Orthopedic Surgeons, Atlanta, Georga, February 4–9, 1988.

87. Neihart RE, Fried JS, and Hodges GR: Coagulase-negative staphylococci. Southern Med J 81:491–500, 1988.

88. Neer CS, and Kirby RM: Revision of humeral head and total shoulder arthroplasties. Clin Orthop 170:189–195, 1982.

89. Neer CS, and Rockwood CA Jr.: Fractures and dislocations of the shoulder. In Rockwood CA, and Green DP (eds): Fractures in Adults, Vol. 1. Philadelphia: J. B. Lippincott Company, 1984, pp 675–721.

90. Neer CS, Watson KC, and Stanton FJ: Recent experience in total shoulder replacement. J Bone Joint Surg 64A:319–337, 1982.

91. Nelson JD, and Koontz WC: Septic arthritis in infants and children: a review of 117 cases. Pediatrics 38:966–971, 1966.

92. Nelson JD: Antibiotic concentrations in septic joint effusions. N Engl J Med 284:349–353, 1971.

93. Neu HC: Cephalosporin antibiotics as applied in surgery of bones and joints. Clin Orthop 190:50–64, 1984.

94. Norden CW: Osteomyelitis. In Mandell G, Gordon D, and Bennett J (eds): Principles and Practice of Infectious Diseases, 2nd ed. New York: John Wiley & Sons, 1985, pp 704–711.

95. Norden C: Experimental osteomyelitis IV. Therapeutic trials with rifampin alone and in combination with gentamicin, sisomicin, and cephalothin. J Infect Dis 132:493–499, 1975.

96. Norden CW: A critical review of antibiotic prophylaxis in orthopedic surgery. Rev Infect Dis 5:928–932, 1983.

97. O'Meara PM, and Bartal E: Septic arthritis: process, etiology,

treatment outcome. A literature review. Orthopedics *11*:623–628, 1988.

98. Patzakis MJ, Wilkins M, and Moore TM: Use of antibiotics in open tibial fractures. Clin Orthop *178*:31–35, 1983.

99. Post M: The Shoulder: Surgical and Nonsurgical Management. Philadelphia: Lea & Febiger, 1988.

100. Rimoin DL, and Wennberg JE: Acute septic arthritis complicating chronic rheumatoid arthritis. JAMA *196*:617–621, 1966.

101. Roca RP, and Yoshikawa TT: Primary skeletal infections in heroin users: a clinical characterization, diagnosis and therapy. Clin Orthop *144*:238–248, 1979.

102. Ruseska I, Robbins J, and Costerton JW: Biocide testing against corrosion-causing oil-field bacteria helps control plugging. Oil Gas J *10*:253–264, 1982.

103. Salter RB, Bell RS, and Keeley FW: The protective effect of continuous passive motion in living articular cartilage in acute septic arthritis: an experimental investigation in the rabbit. Clin Orthop *159*:223–247, 1981.

104. Sartoris DJ, and Resnick D: Magnetic resonance imaging of septic arthritis. Infect Surg January:12–14, 1988.

105. Savage DC, and Fletcher M (eds): Bacterial Adhesion: Mechanisms and Physiological Significance. New York: Plenum Press, 1985.

106. Schmid FR: Principles of diagnosis and treatment of bone and joint infections. *In* McCarty DJ (ed): Arthritis and Allied Conditions. A Textbook of Rheumatology. Philadelphia: Lea & Febiger, 1985, pp 1627–1650.

107. Schmidt D, Mubarak S, and Gelberman R: Septic shoulders in children. J Pediatr Orthop *1*:67–72, 1981.

108. Schwarzmann S, and Boring JR III: Antiphagocytic effect of slime from a mucoid strain of *Pseudomonas aeruginosa*. Infect Immun *3*:762–767, 1971.

109. Scott JT (ed): Copeman's Textbook of the Rheumatic Diseases, 6th ed., Vol. 1. New York: Churchill Livingstone, 1986.

110. Sharp JT: Gonococcal arthritis. *In* McCarty DJ (ed): Arthritis and Allied Conditions. A Textbook of Rheumatology, 9th ed. Philadelphia: Lea & Febiger, 1979, pp 1353–1362.

111. Sharp JT, Lidsky MD, Duffey J, and Duncan MW: Infectious arthritis. Arch Intern Med *139*:1125–1130, 1979.

112. Slusher MM, Myrvik QN, Lewis JC, and Gristina AG: Extended-wear lenses, biofilm, and bacterial adhesion. Arch Ophthalmol *105*:110–115, 1987.

113. Smith JW: Infectious arthritis. *In* Mandell GL, Douglas RG Jr., and Bennett JE (eds): Principles and Practice of Infectious Diseases. New York: John Wiley & Sons, 1985, pp 697–704.

114. Smith JW, and Sanford JP: Viral arthritis. Ann Intern Med *67*:651–659, 1967.

115. Smith RL, and Schurman DJ: Comparison of cartilage destruction between infectious and adjuvant arthritis. J Orthop Res *1*:136–143, 1983.

116. Smith RL, Schurman DJ, Kajiyama G, et al: The effect of antibiotics on the destruction of cartilage in experimental infectious arthritis. J Bone Joint Surg *69A*:1063–1068, 1987.

117. Speers DJ, and Nade SML: Ultrastructural studies of adherence of *Staphylococcus aureus* in experimental acute haematogenous osteomyelitis. Infect Immun *49*:443–446, 1985.

118. Speziale P, Raucci G, Visai L, et al: Binding of collagen to *Staphylococcus aureus* Cowan 1. J Bacteriol *167*:77–81, 1986.

119. Srivastava KK, Garg LD, and Kochhar VL: Tuberculous osteomyelitis of the clavicle. Acta Orthop Scand *45*:668–672, 1974.

120. Steigbigel NH: Diagnosis and management of septic arthritis. *In* Remington JS, and Swartz MN (eds): Current Clinical Topics in Infectious Diseases. New York: McGraw-Hill Book Company, 1983, pp 1–29.

121. Stern GA, and Lubniewski A: The interaction between *Pseudomonas aeruginosa* and the corneal epithelium. Arch Ophthalmol *103*:1221–1225, 1985.

122. Sugarman B, and Young EJ (eds): Infections Associated with Prosthetic Devices. Boca Raton, FL: CRC Press, 1984.

123. Switalski LM, Ryden C, Rubin K, et al: Binding of fibronectin to *Staphylococcus* strains. Infect Immun *42*:628–633, 1983.

124. Toby EB, Webb LX, Voytek A, and Gristina AG: Septic arthritis of the shoulder. Orthop Trans *11*:230, 1987.

125. Tromp RM, Hamers RJ, and Demuth JE: Quantum states and atomic structure of silicon surfaces. Science *234*:304–309, 1986.

126. Trueta J: The normal vascular anatomy of the human femoral head during growth. J Bone Joint Surg *39B*:358–394, 1957.

127. Trueta J: The three types of acute hematogenous osteomyelitis. A clinical and vascular study. J Bone Joint Surg *41B*:671–680, 1959.

128. Turek SL: Orthopaedics. Principles and Their Application. Philadelphia: JB Lippincott, 1977.

129. Voytek A, Gristina G, Barth E, et al: Staphylococcal adhesion to collagen in intra-articular sepsis. Biomaterials *9*:107–110, 1988.

130. Waldvogel FA, Medoff G, and Swartz MN: Osteomyelitis. Clinical Features, Therapeutic Consideration, and Unusual Aspects. Springfield, IL: Charles C Thomas, 1971.

131. Wallace R, and Cohen AS: Tuberculous arthritis. A report of two cases with review of biopsy and synovial fluid findings. Am J Med *61*:277–282, 1976.

132. Ward JR, and Atcheson SG: Infectious arthritis. Med Clin North Am *61*(2):313–329, 1977.

133. Ward J, Cohen AS, and Bauer W: The diagnosis and therapy of acute suppurative arthritis. Arthritis Rheum *3*:522–535, 1960.

134. Watt PJ, and Ward ME: Adherence of *Neisseria gonorrhoeae* and other *Neisseria* species to mammalian cells. *In* Beachey EH (ed): Bacterial Adherence. Receptors and Recognition, series B, vol 6. London: Chapman & Hall, 1980, pp 251–288.

135. Webb LX, Myers RT, Cordell AR, et al: Inhibition of bacterial adhesion by antibacterial surface pretreatment of vascular prostheses. J Vasc Surg *4*:16–21, 1986.

135a. Webb LX, Naylor P, and Gristina AG: Unpublished data.

136. Woods DE, Bass JA, Johanson WG Jr., and Straus DC: Role of adherence in the pathogenesis of *Pseudomonas aeruginosa* lung infection in cystic fibrosis patients. Infect Immun *30*:694–699, 1980.

137. Wrangstadh M, Conway PL, and Kjelleberg S: The production and release of an extracellular polysaccharide during starvation of a marine *Pseudomonas* sp. and the effect thereof on adhesion. Arch Microbiol *145*:220–227, 1986.

138. Wray TM, Bryant RE, and Killen DA: Sternal osteomyelitis and costochondritis after median sternotomy. J Thorac Cardiovasc Surg *65*:227–233, 1973.

139. Wukich DK, Abreu SH, Callaghan JJ, et al: Diagnosis of infection by preoperative scintigraphy with indium-labeled white blood cells. J Bone Joint Surg *69A*:1353–1360, 1987.

Amputations and Prosthetic Replacement

Robert L. Romano, M.D.
Ernest M. Burgess, M.D.

Amputations about the shoulder joint are infrequent. Although exact figures are not available, it is estimated that less than 5 per cent of all major amputations occur at this level. Cross-sectional anatomy at the shoulder is complex. The standard techniques presented in this chapter are generally accepted as being based on well-established anatomical, surgical, and prosthetic considerations. Since many of these amputations are for complicated neoplasms and severe trauma, considerable surgical ingenuity is often required. The nature of the pathological process requiring the amputation will direct the surgeon to emphasize plastic and reconstructive surgical principles to best utilize available tissues and permit uncomplicated healing.

Types of Amputations

Amputations at the shoulder can be separated into two categories:

1. Those that ablate the extremity—through the proximal humerus or by disarticulation of the glenohumeral joint, forequarter amputation, or revision of congenital amputations.

2. Those that preserve the distal extremity—scapulectomy, claviculectomy, and shoulder resection (Tikhor-Linberg).

Amputations through the proximal humerus above the level of the axillary fold are treated as shoulder disarticulations. Function and prosthetic rehabilitation are comparable. The real advantage of retaining the head of the humerus is cosmetic; shoulder disarticulation leaves an unsightly concavity at the glenoid fossa with sharp prominence of the acromion process, whereas the retained head of the humerus presents a more natural appearance with a rounded shoulder contour. Wearing of clothes is thus facilitated.

Disarticulation of the shoulder joint, when carried out through relatively normal anatomy or when an adequate amount of remaining soft tissue is available, becomes essentially a plastic reconstructive exercise. Pliable scars, mobile soft tissues, and appropriate muscle and tendon management will be described (see the section on Technique).

Forequarter amputation, often described as interscapulothoracic amputation, is the surgical removal of the upper extremity in the interval between the scapula and the thoracic wall. A short medial portion of the clavicle is usually retained. This amputation is a deforming procedure since the lateral neck structures slope directly onto the chest wall. It is possible, however, to recontour body form by modern cosmetic surface restoration to achieve a reasonable degree of appearance, using light, state-of-the-art materials, so that under clothing the unsightly trunk appearance is considerably improved.

Amputations that preserve the distal extremity are rarely done except in certain cases of tumor but may occasionally be indicated for the residual effects of chronic infection or radiation damage and, in particular, for the patient who refuses ablation of the limb. Preservation of the neurovascular supply to the distal extremity is, of course, a necessity. The patient will have a degree of hand and elbow function but will be severely limited in overall function of the limb owing to inability to appropriately position the arm, and—depending on the nature of the partial shoulder resection—the hand. The hand can function only at the side as the extremity dangles without stability. Orthotic support may assist in hand placement. The interscapulothoracic resection was suggested by Tikhor, the Russian surgeon; however, the procedure was first done by Linberg. This unusual block resection of the shoulder area was developed for the patient who refused a more radical procedure for certain tumors or for instances when the tumor did not involve the neurovascular bundle and the distal extremity could be preserved. It involves resection of the scapula, most of the clavicle, and the head, neck, and a portion of the proximal shaft of the humerus, as well as involved soft tissues. The distal limb, the vascular supply, and the brachial plexus are preserved.

Scapulectomy alone may be done for primary bone tumors. The technique was first described by Syme in 1864. Its indications are rare since the malignancy is ordinarily not confined to the scapula itself. Adequate function without prosthetic assistance is expected, although the limb will be left weakened.

Claviculectomy is also rarely used for neoplastic disease localized to the clavicle. This procedure yields a good functional result with satisfactory cosmesis, range of motion, and reasonable (though diminished) strength in shoulder abduction, flexion, and adduction.

Precipitating Factors

The necessity for shoulder amputation results primarily from trauma and neoplasm. This has been the case in past centuries and remains mostly true today. The great increase in amputations of the lower limb for peripheral vascular disease is not reflected at the shoulder level; rarely does ischemia result in such amputations. Fulminating infections, particularly in Third World countries, may justify shoulder amputation as a life-saving, staged procedure. An occasional congenital limb defect with phocomelia will require revision amputation. This circumstance seldom occurs, however, since even the presence of small residual fingers, including a partial hand or limb at shoulder level, may be useful in prosthetic rehabilitation. Function, not cosmesis, is the overriding consideration in such circumstances. A concentrated experience in congenital anomalies was acquired from the thalidomide disaster in England and northern Europe. Quite commonly, afflicted children were born with flipper-like, rudimentary upper limbs extending out from shoulder level; the condition was often bilateral. Management of this severe functional loss stimulated remarkable improvements in prosthetic design and terminal device control for shoulder-level ablation.

Trauma, which is by far the major cause of amputations through the shoulder area, often follows well-defined patterns. Physicians staffing major trauma centers are accustomed to occasionally seeing the worker whose arm has been caught in moving machinery and avulsed at the shoulder joint. A portion of the chest wall soft tissues is often torn away, leaving a large, ragged wound. The injury can be life threatening. Road accidents, often involving motorcycles, result in the person being thrown from the vehicle and dragged along with the arm often engaged, then torn from the body. Similarly, individuals unrestrained by seat belts are thrown from cars or trucks; their limbs are caught in the door, the steering wheel, or another part of the vehicle's machinery and severed from the body. Since these accidents are severe, multiple associated injuries are often sustained, complicating treatment of the shoulder avulsion. When these injuries are accompanied by burns, reconstruction of the amputation site is particularly challenging.

Specific Procedures

AMPUTATION THROUGH THE SURGICAL NECK AND SHAFT OF THE HUMERUS

Exposure is obtained through the lateral aspect of the shoulder area. The patient is placed supine on the operating table with support beneath the shoulder, allowing access to the entire shoulder area. The arm is draped free. The incision begins anteriorly at the level of the coracoid process. It is carried distally, following the anterior border of the deltoid muscle, to cross the lateral proximal humerus just below the level of the deltoid insertion. It continues along the posterior border of the deltoid muscle to the level of the axillary fold, then transversely across the axilla to connect with the anterior arm (Fig. 25–1). Care should be taken to leave an adequate amount of skin, particularly in the axilla. Skin closure can be compromised when the flap is short and tight medially.

The next step is to identify, ligate and divide the cephalic vein in the deltopectoral groove. The interval between the deltoid and pectoralis major muscles is developed and the deltoid muscle retracted laterally and upward. The pectoralis major muscle is now divided at its humeral insertion and reflected medially. The pectoralis minor and coracobrachialis muscles can then be identified, with the neurovascular bundle exposed in the interval between them. The axillary artery and vein and adjacent tributaries are identified, isolated, doubly ligated, and divided.

The median ulnar, radial, and musculocutaneous nerves are then isolated individually, drawn gently down into the wound, ligated circumferentially, and sectioned with a knife distal to the ligatures. They will then retract comfortably under the pectoralis minor muscle.

The deltoid muscle is sectioned at its insertion and further retracted proximally with the lateral skin flap. The insertions of the teres major and latissimus dorsi muscles are then identified at the bicipital groove, and the muscles are sectioned near their insertions. The long and short heads of the biceps, the triceps, and the coracobrachialis are then divided approximately 3/4 inch distal to the planned level of bone section.

With the proximal humerus thus isolated, it is divided at the desired level with a small-tooth, recipro-

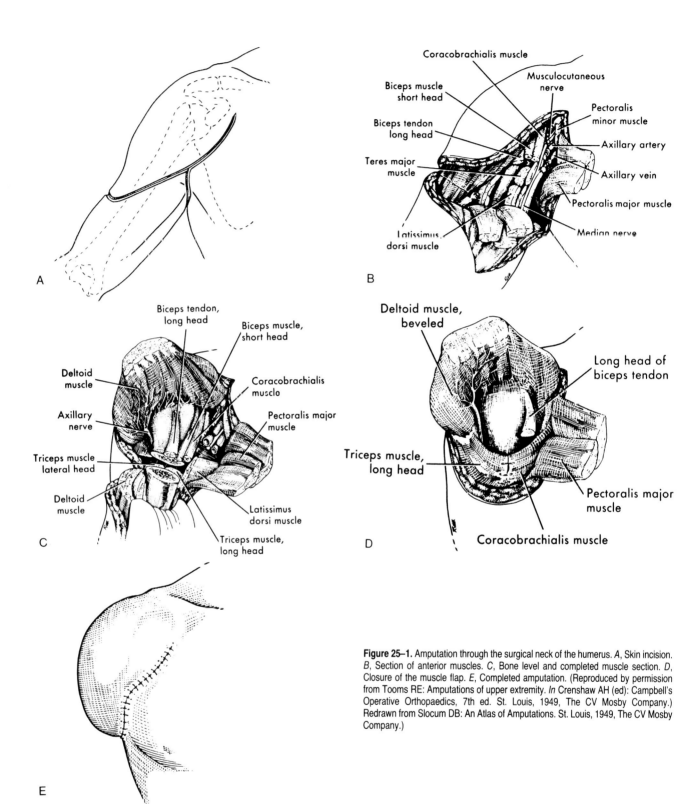

Figure 25–1. Amputation through the surgical neck of the humerus. *A*, Skin incision. *B*, Section of anterior muscles. *C*, Bone level and completed muscle section. *D*, Closure of the muscle flap. *E*, Completed amputation. (Reproduced by permission from Tooms RE: Amputations of upper extremity. *In* Crenshaw AH (ed): Campbell's Operative Orthopaedics, 7th ed. St. Louis, 1949, The CV Mosby Company.) Redrawn from Slocum DB: An Atlas of Amputations. St. Louis, 1949, The CV Mosby Company.)

cating power saw. Sharp, bony margins are rounded smooth and the wound is thoroughly irrigated.

The limb is then removed. Closure is accomplished by drawing the long head of the triceps, together with both heads of the biceps and the coracobrachialis, over the cut end of the humerus and swinging the pectoralis major muscle laterally, suturing it to the end of the bone without tension.

The deltoid muscle and skin flaps are tailored to an accurate closure, using interrupted sutures or skin clips. The wound is drained either by through-and-through drainage or by suction drainage, or both. Supportive compression dressings are applied to assist in eliminating postsurgical dead space. Dressings are changed in 48 hours, and the drains are removed. Compressive soft dressings are continued until the wound is stable.

DISARTICULATION OF THE SHOULDER

Shoulder disarticulation has been referred to in many military medical writings over the centuries. Baron Dominique Jean Larrey, military surgeon to Napoleon for 16 years, described and illustrated his technique, which established the standard of the day. Baron Larrey was a skilled anatomist and an expert surgical technician; it has been said that he amputated more limbs than any surgeon before or since. He described performing 200 thigh amputations in one 24-hour period while accompanying Napoleon during the battle of Borodino. (A modified illustration of his shoulder disarticulation technique is shown in Figure 25–2.)

The patient is positioned supine with support under the affected shoulder, allowing complete access to the shoulder and shoulder girdle area. The incision begins anteriorly at the coracoid process and continues along the anterior border of the deltoid muscle, then is carried transversely across the proximal lateral humerus at the level of the deltoid muscle insertion (Fig. 25–3A). It is then continued superiorly along the posterior border of the muscle to end at the posterior axillary fold, where the two ends of the incision are joined with a second incision passing across the axilla. The cephalic vein is identified in the deltopectoral groove and ligated. The deltoid and pectoralis major muscles are separated anteriorly. The deltoid is then retracted laterally; the pectoralis major is divided at its humeral insertion and reflected medially.

The interval between the coracobrachialis and the short head of the biceps is opened to expose the neurovascular bundle (Fig. 25–3B). The axillary artery and vein are doubly ligated independently of each

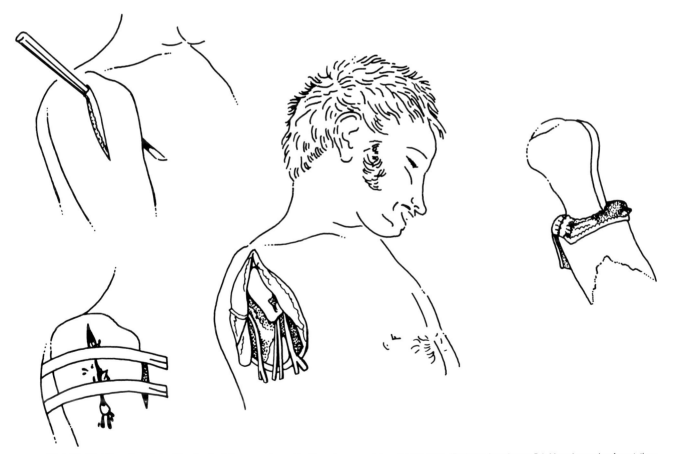

Figure 25–2. Modified illustration of shoulder disarticulation as performed by Baron Larrey and described in 1797. (Redrawn from Larrey DJ: Memoire sur les Amputations des Membres a La Suite des Coups de Feu Etaye de Plusieurs Observations. Paris: Du Pont, 1797.)

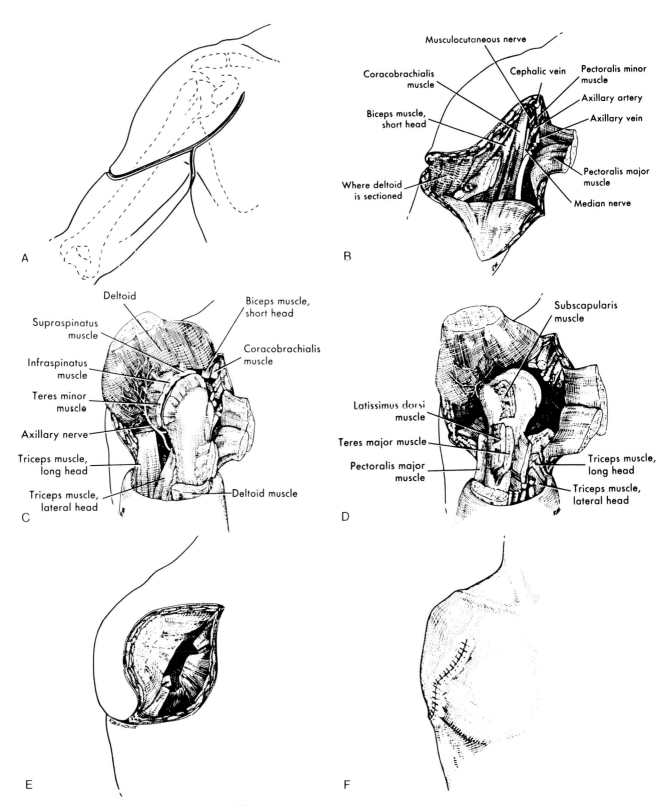

Figure 25–3. Disarticulation of the shoulder. *A*, Incision. *B*, Exposure and section of the neurovascular bundle. *C*, Reflection of the deltoid; the arm is placed in internal rotation; section of the supraspinatus, infraspinatus, and teres minor tendons and of the posterior capsule; section of the coracobrachialis and biceps at the coracoid. *D*, Arm placed in external rotation; subscapularis and anterior capsule section. *E*, Suture of muscles in the glenoid cavity. *F*, Completed amputation. (Reproduced by permission from Tooms RE: Amputations of upper extremity. *In* Crenshaw AH (ed): Campbell's Operative Orthopaedics, 7th ed. St. Louis, 1987, The CV Mosby Company. Redrawn from Slocum DB: An Atlas of Amputations. St. Louis, 1949, The CV Mosby Company.)

other and then sectioned. The thoracoacromial artery, just proximal to the pectoralis minor muscle, is identified, ligated, and divided. The vessels then retract superiorly under the pectoralis minor muscle. The median, ulnar, musculocutaneous, and radial nerves can then be identified, drawn gently distally into the wound, ligated with a circumferential suture, and sectioned under mild tension. They then retract beneath the pectoralis minor muscle.

The coracobrachialis and short head of the biceps are then sectioned near their insertions on the coracoid process (Fig. 25–3C). The deltoid muscle is freed from its insertion on the humerus and reflected superiorly to expose the capsule of the shoulder joint. The teres major and latissimus dorsi muscles are divided at their insertions and the arm is placed in internal rotation to expose the short external rotator muscles, the posterior aspect of the shoulder joint, and the adjacent fascia. All of these structures are divided.

The arm is then rotated into full external rotation, and the anterior aspect of the joint capsule, the remaining shoulder capsule, and the subscapularis muscle are sectioned (Fig. 25–3D). The triceps muscle is divided near its insertion, and the limb is severed from the trunk by dividing the inferior capsule of the shoulder joint. The cut ends of all muscles are reflected into the glenoid cavity and sutured there to help fill the hollow left by the removal of the humeral head (Fig. 25–3E).

The deltoid muscle flap is then brought down inferiorly to permit suturing just below the glenoid (Fig. 25–3F). The closure is accomplished without tension using optimal wound closure technique. Drains, either suction or through-and-through or both, are inserted and closure is carried out in layers. Compression dressings are applied to assist in eliminating any residual dead space. Scar adhesions about the site of surgery can be painful and can complicate both cosmetic and functional prosthetic fit. Drains are ordinarily removed in 48 hours, and the effective compression dressings are reapplied.

FOREQUARTER AMPUTATION

This radical procedure involves the surgical removal of the entire upper limb in the interval between the scapula and the thoracic wall. Its primary indication is the presence of malignant tumors about the shoulder girdle. Since such tumors often invade the regional lymph nodes and chest wall, the operation is considered essentially a life-saving salvage procedure. The surgery may control intractable pain for a time, although in present neoplastic management pain is best handled by a variety of medical techniques. Open ulceration and infection can further require careful planning to obtain skin and soft tissue coverage.

Most forequarter amputations performed today in Western countries are carried out by surgical services specializing in neoplastic diseases. The management of

connective tissue malignant tumors of the limbs has been changing dramatically over the past decade and continues to change. In those few cases in which forequarter amputation seems to be indicated, the management team should consist of oncologists, plastic and reconstructive surgeons, and orthopedic or general surgeons. The surgery itself—except in unusual circumstances of trauma or tumor—is not complicated when carried out with the standard accepted techniques that have been used successfully for most of this century. Occasionally, staged procedures and skin or composite grafts are required to achieve wound closure.

Anterior Approach

The incision begins at a point 4 cm lateral to the sternoclavicular articulation at a point corresponding to the lateral border of the sternocleidomastoid muscle insertion (Fig. 25–4A). It follows the entire anterior aspect of the clavicle and passes over the top of the shoulder to the spine of the scapula. At this point, the arm is flexed over the chest to rotate the scapula forward and outward so that its bony contour is outlined in greater relief. The posterior aspect of the upper incision then proceeds down over the spine to its vertical border, which it follows distally to the angle of the scapula. The lower portion of the ellipse starts in the middle third of the clavicle and passes downward in the groove between the deltoid and pectoral muscles to the anterior axillary fold. The arm is abducted and the incision is continued across the axilla at the level of the junction of the skin of the arm with the axillary skin. As the incision passes the posterior axillary fold, it continues medially across the back to join the upper incision at the angle of the scapula. The head is bent toward the normal side so that the sternocleidomastoid muscle may be better outlined, and the pectoralis major muscle is severed from its clavicular insertion; the dissection starts at the lateral border of the insertion and proceeds close to bone to the lateral border of the sternocleidomastoid muscle. The pectoralis major muscle is then reflected downward and medially. If further exposure is needed, the humeral insertion of the pectoralis major may be divided. The upper border of the clavicle is exposed by sectioning the superficial layer of the deep fascia along the upper border of the clavicle as far medially as the sternocleidomastoid muscle. Further dissection beneath the clavicle is carried out by means of the finger or a blunt curved dissector. The external jugular vein, which emerges just above the clavicle at the lateral border of the sternocleidomastoid, may be sectioned and ligated if it is in the way.

The clavicle is now divided by a Gigli or reciprocating power saw at the lateral border of the sternocleidomastoid muscle. It is not desirable to section the clavicle more medially because of the danger of injuring the veins that hug its medial inch. The clavicle is sectioned at or near the acromioclavicular joint, and the freed portion is removed (Fig. 25–4B). If the

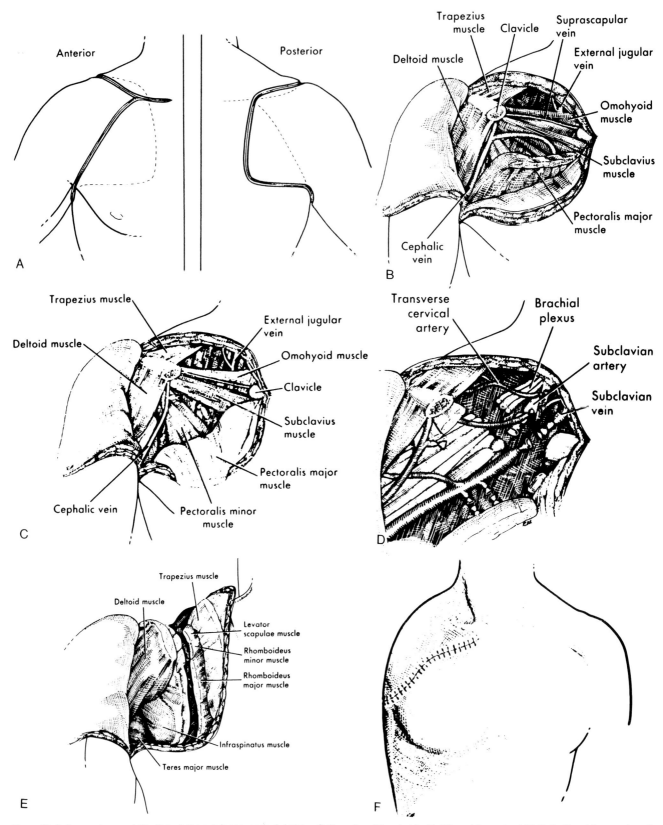

Figure 25–4. Forequarter amputation through the anterior approach. *A,* Incision. *B,* Resection of the clavicle. *C,* Lifting of the pectoral lid. *D,* Section of the vessels and nerves after incision through the axillary fascia, the insertion of the pectoralis minor, the costocoracoid membrane, and the subclavius. *E,* Section of supporting muscles of the scapula. *F,* Completed amputation. (Reproduced by permission from Tooms RE: Amputations of upper extremity. *In* Crenshaw AH (ed): Campbell's Operative Orthopaedics, 7th ed. St. Louis, 1987, The CV Mosby Company. Redrawn from Slocum DB: An Atlas of Amputations. St. Louis, 1949, The CV Mosby Company.)

humeral insertion of the pectoralis major muscle has not already been sectioned, this is done. This whole muscle may then be reflected downward, and the entire shoulder girdle may be retracted outward and downward so that the axillary and subclavian region is in full view. The axillary fascia is sectioned, the pectoralis minor is severed from its coracoid insertion, and the costocoracoid membrane that lies between the pectoralis minor and the subclavius is divided (Fig. 25–4D). The second layer of deep fascia up to the level of the omohyoid muscle, the periosteum at the back of the clavicle, and the subclavius are divided to complete the exposure of the neurovascular bundle. The subclavian artery is isolated, sectioned, and doubly ligated. The blood in the extremity is emptied into the general circulation by elevation; the subclavian vein is then clamped, cut, and doubly ligated. The brachial plexus is identified and each trunk carefully ligated circumferentially. The nerves are sectioned one by one at the cranial end of the incision and allowed to retract. The latissimus dorsi muscle and all remaining soft tissues binding the shoulder girdle to the anterior chest wall are sectioned, and the limb falls freely backward.

Section of the Posterior Muscles

The arm is placed across the chest and held with gentle downward traction. The posterior incision is deepened through the fascia, and the skin is retracted medially. The remaining muscles fixing the shoulder girdle to the scapula are divided as they are encountered from above downward. The muscles holding the scapula to the thorax are divided (Fig. 25–4E). The incision starts at the insertion of the trapezius to the clavicle and acromion and is carried downward along the upper border of the spine of the scapula. After sectioning, each muscle is retracted medially. The muscles along the superior angle of the vertebral border of the scapula—the omohyoid, levator scapulae, rhomboideus major and minor, and serratus anterior—are sectioned by placing double clamps near their insertions and cutting between the clamps from above downward. The extremity is removed and hemostasis is controlled with meticulous care.

Closure

Careful inspection is made to ensure that all malignant tissue has been removed. If the pectoralis major has not, of necessity, been removed, it should be sutured to the trapezius muscle. Closure is accomplished in layers, with all remaining muscular structures grouped over the lateral chest wall to afford as much padding as possible. The skin flaps are brought together and tailored to form an accurate approximation. The wound is closed with interrupted sutures (Fig. 25–4F), and adequate drainage is accomplished. Dry dressings are applied, and a snug pressure dressing is placed over the lateral chest wall. The drains are removed in 48 to 72 hours, and the sutures are removed between the 10th and 14th days.

Posterior Approach

Littlewood, in 1922, described a technique of forequarter amputation requiring two incisions and approaching the shoulder area from the posterior aspect (Fig. 25–5). This posterior approach is considered technically easier. We have used the conventional (Berger) anterior approach for cases under our care over the years but recognize the advantages of the two-incision technique, especially in atypical cases.

The patient is positioned on the uninvolved side near the edge of the operating table (Fig. 25–5). Two incisions are required—one posterior (cervicoscapular) and one anterior (pectoroaxillary). The posterior incision is made first. Beginning at the medial end of the clavicle, it extends laterally for the entire length of the bone, carries over the acromion process to the posterior axillary fold, continues along the axillary border of the scapula to a point inferior to the scapular angle, and finally curves medially to end 2 inches from the midline of the back. From the scapular muscles an entire full-thickness flap of skin and subcutaneous tissue is elevated medially to a point just medial to the vertebral border of the scapula.

Next, the trapezius and latissimus dorsi muscles are identified and divided parallel with the scapula. The same is done to the levator scapulae, the rhomboideus major and minor, and the scapular attachments of the serratus anterior and the omohyoid. As the dissection progresses, vessels are ligated as necessary, especially the branches of the transverse cervical and transverse scapular arteries. The soft tissues are then freed from the clavicle and the bone is divided at its medial end. The subclavius muscle is also divided.

The extremity is then allowed to fall anteriorly, thus placing the subclavian vessels and brachial plexus under tension and making their identification easier. The cords of the plexus are clamped close to the spine, and the subclavian artery and vein are clamped, doubly ligated, and divided.

The anterior incision is then begun at the middle of the clavicle. It curves inferiorly just lateral to but parallel with the deltopectoral groove, extends across the anterior axillary fold, and finally carries inferiorly and posteriorly to join the posterior axillary incision at the lower third of the axillary border of the scapula. As the final step in the operation, the pectoralis major and minor muscles are divided and the limb is removed. The skin flaps are trimmed to allow a snug closure and their edges sutured with interrupted sutures of nonabsorbable material. Effective through-and-through and suction drains are inserted to eliminate fluid accumulation. Firm chest wall pressure dressings are required. Drains can be removed after 48 hours.

Surgical variations, based on the nature and extent of the pathological process, may indicate the need for

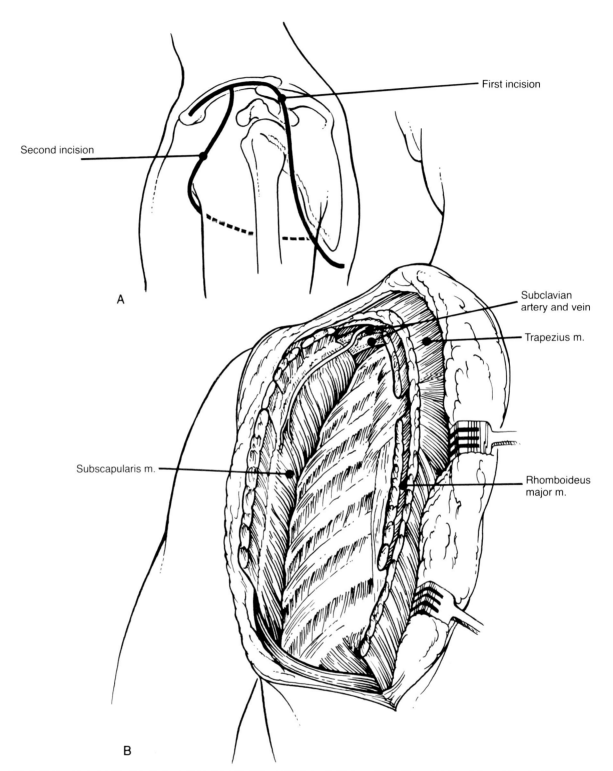

Figure 25–5. Forequarter amputation through the posterior approach (Littlewood technique). (Redrawn from Littlewood H: Amputations at the shoulder and at the hip. Br Med J 1:381, 1922.)

regional lymph node resection and for soft tissue removal at the chest wall when the tumor has extended into these structures. Skin grafts, including composite tissues, may be necessary to obtain primary or secondary closure.

INTERSCAPULOTHORACIC RESECTION

Intercalary shoulder resection (the Tikhor-Linberg technique) achieves a massive removal of the musculoskeletal elements of the shoulder girdle, including the scapula, the lateral three-fourths of the clavicle, and a portion of the proximal humerus, with extensive removal of all adjacent muscles. The neurovascular structures supplying the arm and hand are preserved. Excessive skin is often left following this radical resection. The remaining connecting soft tissues across the former shoulder joint consist only of the axillary vessels and the brachial plexus, together with the axillary skin. Closure of the soft tissues, including the skin, is individualized according to the nature of the malignancy for which the surgery is performed. It is necessary to stabilize the proximal humerus to the remaining medial stump of the clavicle and/or the chest wall in order to prevent excessive drooping and telescoping of the arm.

This operation is rarely used in surgical practice today. A patient's refusal to allow formal amputation can, however, justify its use. The author's experience is limited to two patients (both male), one with chondrosarcoma of the shoulder girdle and one with reticulum sarcoma. The latter patient achieved a 5-year survival and, in fact, is alive and well 12 years following the surgery; he has retained a quite remarkable degree of function of the elbow, forearm, and hand. An avid tennis player, he manages a competitive game as a bimanual athlete.

The operation is carried out with the patient in the full lateral position and lying on the uninvolved side. The entire upper extremity, chest, and neck are prepared and draped so that the arm, shoulder, and shoulder girdle are free for manipulation and positioning. The incision resembles a tennis racquet—the "handle" extends from the medial third of the clavicle laterally, while the anterior limb extends downward along the deltopectoral groove to the midpoint of the medial edge of the biceps, proceeds distally for 7 to 8 cm, then curves upward to cross the lateral surface of the arm at or just below the middeltoid level (Fig. 25–6). From this point the posterior limb of the "racquet" curves from the middeltoid area downward and medially toward the inferior angle of the scapula, where it again curves upward to join the original clavicular incision near the acromioclavicular joint.

Deeper dissection can be carried out from either an anterior or a posterior approach. We have utilized a combination of both approaches in our cases. In effect, this dissection combines the classical anterior technique of forequarter amputation with the posterior approach (Littlewood) technique of this surgery. The brachial plexus is preserved, as are major vessels. It is necessary to ligate the transverse cervical, suprascapular, circumflex scapular, circumflex humeral, and thoracoacromial arteries. With the scapulothoracic muscles detached and the deltoid, biceps, and triceps sectioned, the humerus can be transected at or below the surgical neck at the level of election. The biceps, triceps, and deltoid muscles are attached to the thoracic wall, and the trapezius suspends the arm as firmly as possible without compromising neurovascular integrity. The wound is drained both by suction and through-and-through drains, which are removed in 48 hours. Soft compression dressings and a Velpeau-like sling support are used postoperatively.

The skin and soft tissue resection is modified to accommodate removal of the neoplasm. The arm should be supported until sufficient scarring has occurred at the operative site to provide some stability. No attempt is made to regain a semblance of shoulder function. Rehabilitation concentrates on the neck and trunk muscles and on the arm distal to the site of amputation of the humerus. An adequate degree of hand, wrist, forearm, and elbow function can be achieved. Cosmesis is also surprisingly good, considering the massive tissue resection. The defect in the shoulder girdle and shoulder contour can be concealed with a light, modern prosthetic cosmetic restoration, using currently available materials—particularly the urethanes—that provide a more normal appearance of the shoulder area under clothing.

SCAPULECTOMY

Syme in 1864 described excision of the scapula for primary bone tumors. The operation is used for isolated neoplasms of the scapula, a condition rarely seen. Neglected, slow-growing osteocartilaginous tumors arising in the scapula may cause functional compromise sufficient to warrant excision of the scapula, which usually is accompanied by adjuvant chemotherapy and radiation. A general description of the operative technique is presented here in the realization that there literally is no standard operative approach. When the tumor has extended beyond the confines of the bone, the surgery may require excision of lymph nodes in the complicated chains surrounding the shoulder girdle. Scapulectomy following biopsy should include wide resection of the biopsy site, including skin and deep tissues.

The operation is carried out with the patient in the prone position, supported under the affected shoulder. The arm is draped free to allow movement of the humerus and scapula as the dissection proceeds. Regardless of the nature and type of the incision, adequate access to the entire superior border of the scapula is mandatory.

The classical incision begins laterally at the tip of the acromion and extends posteriorly directly below the acromion spine to its midportion, then gently

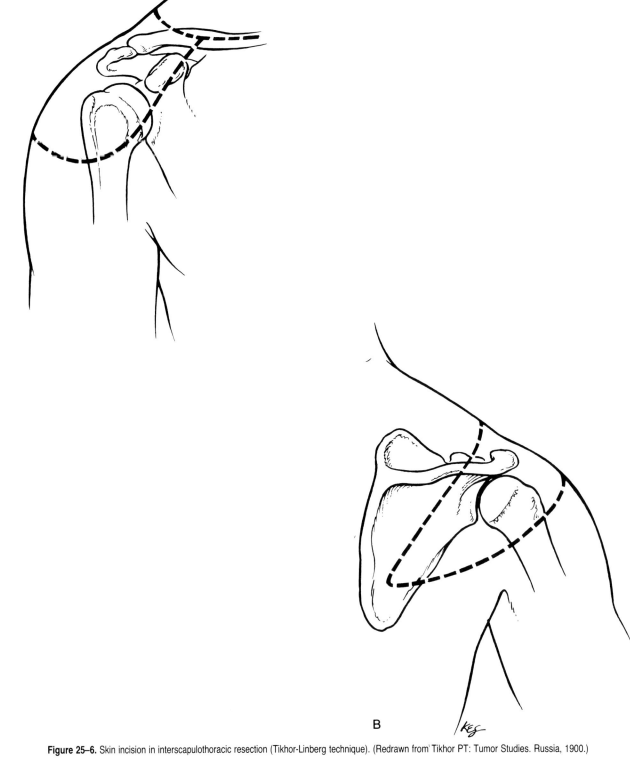

Figure 25–6. Skin incision in interscapulothoracic resection (Tikhor-Linberg technique). (Redrawn from Tikhor PT: Tumor Studies. Russia, 1900.)

curves distally across the body of the scapula to its inferior angle (Fig. 25–7). The nature of the pathological process will determine the management of muscles and, specifically, those muscles that should be resected. Detaching the latissimus dorsi from the inferior angle allows the scapula to be tilted upward and outward, thereby affording free access to the subscapular space.

The vertebral border of the scapula is then freed and the remaining insertions of the inferior and middle trapezius are detached from the spine of the scapula, exposing the rhomboids for division. The superior trapezius is divided from the scapular spine, the acromion, and the distal clavicle. The levator scapulae is sectioned. The superficial cervical and descending scapular vessels are identified and ligated. The suprascapular vessels and nerves are exposed; as the scapula is lifted further laterally from the thorax, the brachial plexus and axillary vessels come into view. It is important to remove the supraspinatus and infraspinatus and the serratus anterior along with the scapula itself. The nature and extent of the pathological process will dictate whether it is possible to preserve the acromion and the continuity of the superior trapezius–deltoid suspensory system.

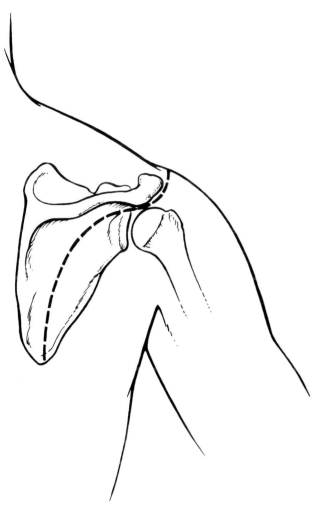

Figure 25–7. Skin incision in scapulectomy.

The axillary border of the scapula is then approached with transection of the deltoid from the spine of the scapula and from the acromion. The teres major and long head of the triceps muscles are transected, the subscapular artery is identified, and ligated, and the underlying axillary and radial nerves are carefully preserved. The disarticulation of the acromioclavicular joint and detachment of the coracoclavicular ligaments or division of the clavicle just medial to the coracoclavicular ligaments allows the scapula to be further freed from the chest. The pectoralis minor, coracobrachialis, and short head of the biceps muscles can then be detached from the coracoid process and the rotator cuff transected by external and internal rotation of the humerus. It may be appropriate to modify the level of section of the rotator cuff so that after removal of the scapula, the distal cuff can be sutured about the distal clavicle to suspend and stabilize the humerus and to preserve a more cosmetic shoulder outline. The wound is closed in layers over adequate drainage systems. Compression dressings are applied, and the arm is supported in a Velpeau-type dressing.

Variations of the scapulectomy technique are the rule rather than the exception. Even with modern imaging systems, it may not be possible to identify the extent of the tumor until surgery. In general, oncologists prefer other nonoperative and surgical means of treatment of neoplasms involving the scapula. Similarly, scapulectomy to control intractable pain caused by tumor can be unsuccessful. Finally, metastatic malignancy involving the scapula is not an indication for scapulectomy; nonsurgical management is considered the treatment of choice.

CLAVICULECTOMY

En bloc resection of the clavicle has been recommended for localized malignancy. It is rarely indicated. To a large degree, the specific surgical technique will depend on the type and location of the neoplasm. The surgical approach is over the anterior aspect of the entire length of the clavicle, extending from the sternoclavicular joint to the acromioclavicular joint (Fig. 25–8). Biopsy sites, if present, are widely excised. Dissection is carried down to the deltoid insertion, which is divided from the clavicle, leaving an intact proximal muscular cuff. The conoid and trapezoid ligaments are divided near their clavicular attachment and the sternocleidomastoid muscle is carefully sectioned, avoiding injury to the external jugular vein. The omohyoid muscle is retracted and the pectoralis major incised. The clavicle is then elevated, leaving the subclavicular muscle attached to the clavicle. The sternoclavicular capsule, sternohyoid muscle insertion, and costoclavicular ligament are all excised. Immediately adjacent vascular structures are carefully protected, and the branches of the transverse cervical artery are ligated. The clavicle is then removed.

Closure in layers, eliminating dead spaces, is carried

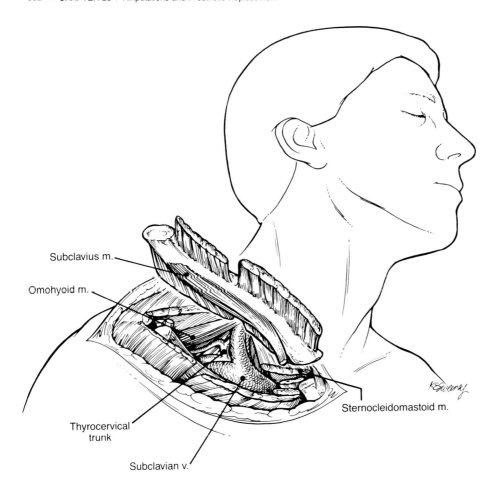

Subclavius m.

Omohyoid m.

Thyrocervical trunk

Subclavian v.

Sternocleidomastoid m.

Figure 25–8. Claviculectomy. (Redrawn from Lewis MM, Ballet FL, Kroll PG, and Bloom N: En bloc clavicular resection, operative procedure and postoperative testing of function. Clin Orthop *193*:214, 1985.)

out over drainage. Compression dressings and a sling are applied, with drains being removed in 24 to 48 hours. The shoulder and arm are mobilized as early as is consistent with wound healing.

Technical variations, based on the site and nature of the tumor, individualize the surgery to such a degree that each case must be planned surgically as a specific technical challenge. Reported series usually include only three or four cases. We have not had occasion to perform this resection-amputation.

Prosthetic Rehabilitation

Shoulder-area amputations present the most difficult challenge for functional restoration by external prosthetic replacement. Many unilateral amputees reject a functional prosthesis, preferring a light, cosmetic substitute or merely an empty sleeve. The remaining limb, whether initially dominant or not, rapidly accommodates to permit most basic activities associated with ordinary, normal life. Bilateral shoulder amputations create just the opposite functional demand. The handicap is so severe that prostheses, even though uncomfortable, heavy, and functionally crude compared with the normal limbs, provide sufficient critically needed

function to justify the training, discomfort, and inconvenience associated with their use.

Children born with amelia of both upper limbs rapidly learn to use their legs and feet to substitute. Remarkable skill can be achieved. Lower limb joints, particularly the hips, ankles, and feet, develop abnormally large ranges of movement to facilitate a wide range of foot placement. The intrinsic muscles of the feet as well as the tarsal joints respond by adaptation to perform many grasp, hook, and pinch functions ordinarily not present in feet. This adaptive substitution continues up through the amputee's adult life. Although fitted with cosmetic or functional upper limb prostheses, the individual usually discards the artificial limbs in the home and work setting, using them only for social purposes.

Lower limb substitution following bilateral shoulder-level amputation in the adult, and in particular in the elderly, does not elicit a similar lower limb functional response. Some substitution can occur, although under most circumstances such a severely disabled individual requires constant attendant help.

TYPES OF PROSTHESES

Prostheses for shoulder-level amputees are of three types: (1) body powered, (2) externally powered, and

(3) cosmetic. The amputee is often best served by a combination of body powering and external powering with interchangeable terminal devices, including a cosmetic hand. The simplest artificial substitute is nonfunctional, a strictly cosmetic device (Fig. 25–9). Modern designs are light, usually fabricated of urethanes or similar synthetics, with light internal or external frame rigidity (where necessary) supplied by graphite, light metals, or semirigid thermoplastics. The shoulder cup of the prosthesis is contoured to correspond with the opposite shoulder shape. Light shoulder strap suspension stabilizes the limb and prevents it from slipping off. The elbow is simple and nonfunctional and permits stable positioning at various angles by the opposite limb. The hand can be individually constructed to match the remaining hand. The psychological advantage of a cosmetic prosthesis often plays a very important and integral part in physical rehabilitation.

These cosmetic limbs can be quite elegant and expensive. They are obtained through regular prosthetic sources with the services of a cosmetic restoration artist, who is responsible for the shape, texture, and surface detail, including color. Most major population centers in the United States, Canada, and Europe can provide these services. Contact with these skilled professionals is made in cooperation with conventional professional prosthetists.

This passive cosmetic replacement is not entirely without function. The hand can assist in stabilizing objects on a table or workbench. In general, the active

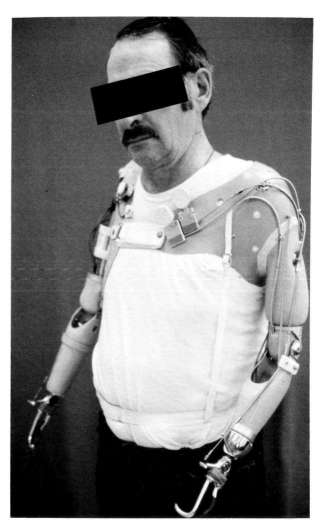

Figure 25–10. Cable-operated left arm with a positive-locking cable-operated elbow, positive-locking wrist rotation unit, positive-locking wrist flexion unit, and cable-operated split hook. The elbow lock is controlled by a tether to a waist belt. The locks of the two wrist components are controlled by the two nudge controls on the anterior panel of the socket. (Courtesy of Dudley S. Childress, Ph.D., Prosthetics Research Laboratory, Northwestern University and the Orthotics and Prosthetics Clinical Services Department, Rehabilitation Institute of Chicago.)

unilateral amputee will use a cosmetic prosthesis only for special social occasions and not in the course of daily work and living activities.

Body-Powered Functional Prostheses

A substitute limb that can perform useful functions poses a difficult engineering challenge. It requires articulation at the elbow and should permit a degree of positioning of the terminal device (wrist/hand) (Fig. 25–10). Some degree of shoulder abduction and elbow rotation is also required if positioning of the hand or hook is to operate within a significant range of usefulness. Suspending the limb and attaching it sufficiently to the body to provide stability dictates the use of a large shoulder cap, usually made of semiflexible materials, and additional straps around the trunk and across the opposite shoulder. Activation of the hand

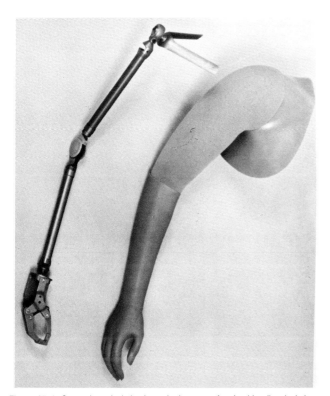

Figure 25–9. Cosmetic endoskeletal prosthetic system for shoulder disarticulation. (Courtesy of Otto Bock Orthopedic Industry, Minneapolis, MN.)

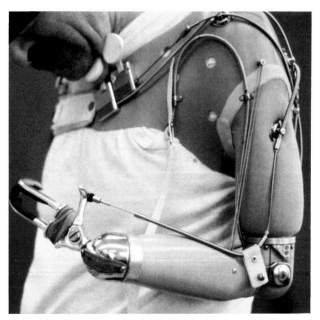

Figure 25–11. The patient releasing the lock of the wrist flexion unit. (Courtesy of Dudley S. Childress, Ph.D., Prosthetics Research Laboratory, Northwestern University and the Orthotics and Prosthetics Clinical Services Department, Rehabilitation Institute of Chicago.)

or hook is accomplished by opposite shoulder movement using a shoulder loop attached to cabling, either light, housed metal or nylon. The prosthesis can be either prepositioned and then locked or, in the case of the elbow, cable controlled (Fig. 25–11).

For years prosthetic engineers have attempted to simplify this prosthesis. Attempting to duplicate, even to a small degree, the unbelievably complex motor and sensory function of the upper limb frustrates such engineering attempts. As a result, even with present technology the body-powered limbs are rather crude, uncomfortable, and severely limited in function. More often, such limbs are designed for a special purpose, such as working at a bench or desk. When the zone of functional activity of the terminal device is confined to a relatively small area, it is more feasible to accommodate design, thus making the prosthesis more acceptable (Figs. 25–12 to 25–15).

Externally Powered Prostheses

For the reasons just outlined, prosthetic engineers have turned to external power sources. Following the thalidomide experience, which produced a significant

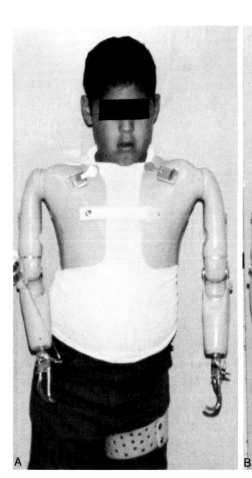
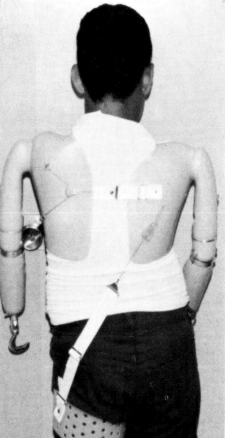

Figure 25–12. Body-powered prosthesis for bilateral phocomelia. (Courtesy of Alpha Orthopedic Appliance Co, Los Angeles, CA.)

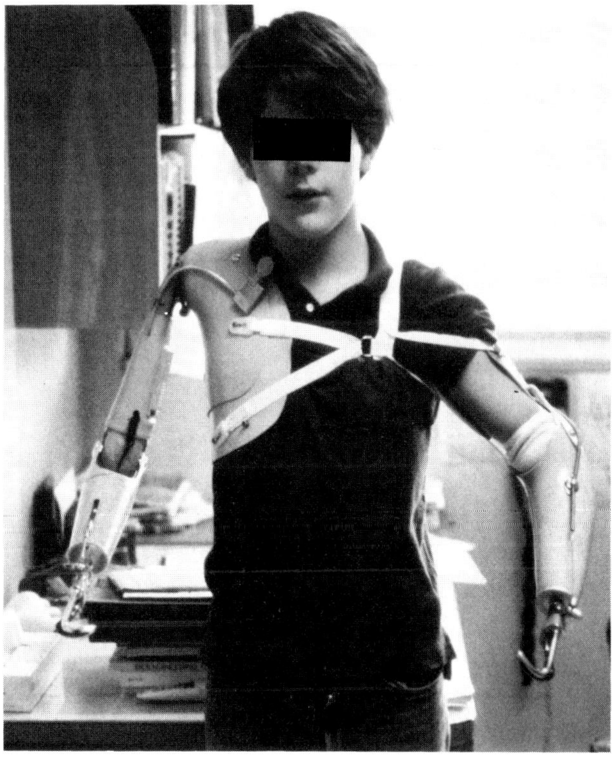

Figure 25–13. Prosthetic management for bilateral upper limb amputation. Right shoulder disarticulation and left below-elbow prostheses. (Courtesy of Eric Baron, C.P.O., University of California, Child Amputee Prosthetics Project, Los Angeles, CA.)

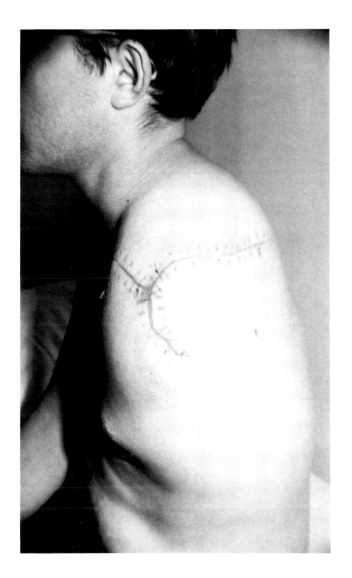

Figure 25–14. Forequarter amputee ready for prosthetic fitting.

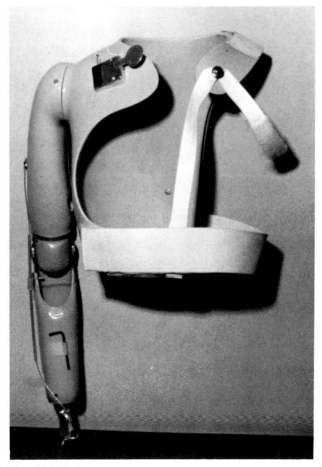

Figure 25–15. Body-powered forequarter amputation prosthesis. (Courtesy of Alpha Orthopedic Appliance Co, Los Angeles, CA.)

number of bilateral shoulder disarticulations, prosthetic engineers sought to activate prosthetic substitutes by using compressed gas and/or electricity. Although useful under certain circumstances, the compressed-gas systems have been discarded for lighter, more responsive electrical power systems. Currents generated by body muscles activate the prosthesis. A number of such prosthetic systems have been developed worldwide. The current state of electronic technology has allowed considerable ingenuity in myoelectric control. With amputations about the shoulder, it is practical to seek elbow and terminal-device control only. The elbow can be positioned through electrical means (Fig. 25–16). It can then be stabilized in the locked position and the terminal device operated through signals (Fig. 25–17). Hybrid limbs are most commonly worn, i.e., partially body powered and partially powered by electricity. In the author's opinion, the prosthesis developed at the University of Utah (the Utah Arm) represents the current state of the art for this approach (Fig. 25–18). The elbow of this device can be controlled electrically and the terminal device by body power (Fig. 25–19). This combination has been particularly successful in the young, vigorous

amputee. Even with the lightest materials, weight is a limiting factor.

To be successful, functional prostheses require a high degree of motivation on the part of the user. With one remaining functional upper limb, most daily acts of living can be carried out by the normal arm with increasing skill as training proceeds. Even after being fitted with a state-of-the-art prosthesis, users tend to gradually discard it as they find themselves increasingly functional with the opposite normal limb. The cosmetic substitute then becomes the limb of choice.

SPECIAL CONSIDERATIONS

Postural Abnormalities

Normally, the weight of the arm and the muscle activity associated with shoulder/arm function keep the shoulders appropriately level. Unilateral hypertrophy of an upper limb, including the shoulder girdle, occurs in certain occupations and is also seen in some sports. Some people are born with a degree of asymmetry of shoulder level. These are relatively minor postural abnormalities and do not require special clothing.

When the arm is removed and the clavicle and scapula remain, the shoulder girdle elevators are unopposed by the weight of the arm and by those muscles passing across the shoulder that tend to depress the shoulder and arm. The consequence of this imbalance is an upward elevation described as "hiking" of the shoulder girdle. This "high shoulder" tends to accentuate the cosmetic loss, even when the individual is wearing a cosmetic shoulder filler and/or a cosmetic limb. Abnormal shoulder elevation can be countered by corrective exercises beginning as soon as they are tolerated following the amputation. The wearing of a prosthesis with its dependent weight also diminishes shoulder "hike." In most circumstances the shoulder girdle elevation is inevitable; however, its degree can be minimized by appropriate physical measures.

Removal of the entire upper limb in the growing skeleton routinely results in a sharp scoliosis of the dorsal spine at the mid and upper dorsal levels. Muscular imbalance is considered to be the cause of the deformity. It may be seen to a slighter degree in the adult but is primarily confined to the growing skeleton. The combined postural deformity of upper dorsal spine scoliosis and elevation of the shoulder girdle produces asymmetry of the head and neck on the trunk, with the head appearing to be placed asymmetrically as the person stands.

In general, there is no corrective splinting or orthotic device that successfully counteracts the postural changes associated with shoulder-level amputation. Neck and shoulder-girdle exercises offer the most effective prophylaxis and treatment. The postural deficits are particularly evident with forequarter amputation. Soft, light polyurethane cosmetic restoration, either as part of a cosmetic prosthesis or separately

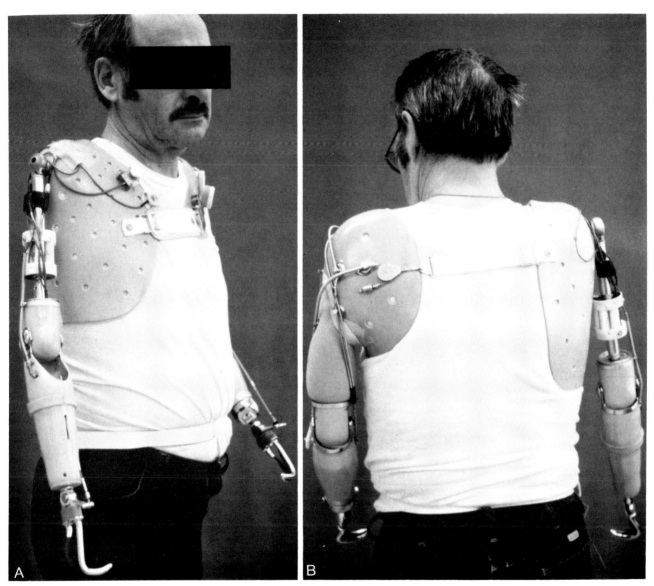

Figure 25–16. Patient with a right shoulder disarticulation electrically powered prosthesis. The powered components are the Hosmer electric elbow and the NY/Hosmer Prehension Actuator. Both components are controlled by chin-actuated push switches near the anterosuperior border of the socket. The shoulder, turntable, and forearm rotation joints are all manually positioned friction joints. The crepe band around the forearm provides surface friction for rotation against objects. (Courtesy of Dudley S. Childress, Ph.D., Prosthetics Research Laboratory, Northwestern University and the Orthotics and Prosthetics Clinical Services Department, Rehabilitation Institute of Chicago.)

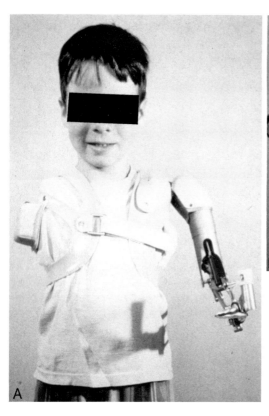

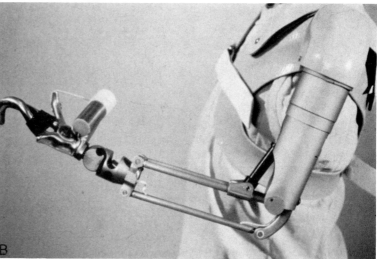

Figure 25–17. *A*, Child provided with a noncommercial prosthesis—the NU/Michigan Feeder Arm—with parallelogram linkage in forearm (kinematic coupling of elbow and wrist). *B*, The prehensor is the electrically powered Michigan Hook. (Courtesy of Dudley S. Childress, Ph.D., Prosthetics Research Laboratory, Northwestern University and the Orthotics and Prosthetics Clinical Services Department, Rehabilitation Institute of Chicago.)

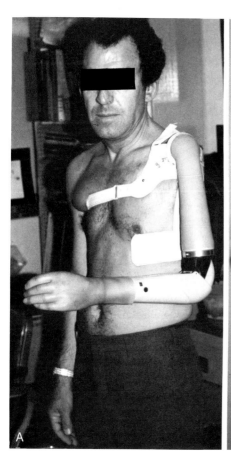

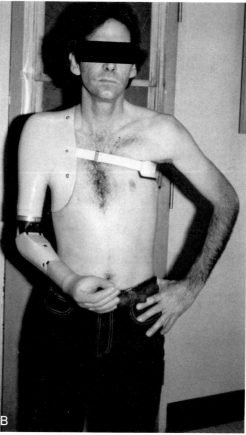

Figure 25–18. Myoelectrical prostheses for proximal humerus/shoulder disarticulation amputations (Utah Arm). (Courtesy of Eric Baron, C.P.O., University of California, Child Amputee Prosthetics Project, Los Angeles, CA.)

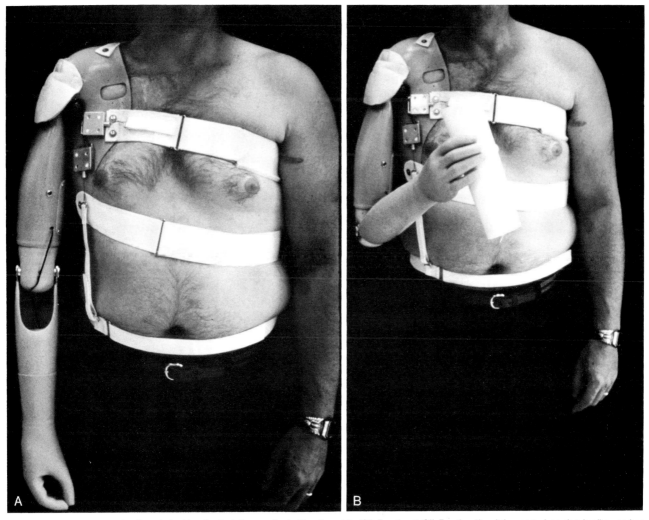

Figure 25–19. Switch-activated unilateral shoulder disarticulation prosthesis. Two four-state (Off–Function 1–Off–Function 2) switches control an electric elbow and an electric hand. Both switches are attached to the exterior of the anterior panel of the socket. The switch for the elbow is connected to a waist belt so that elevation of the shoulder moves the switch through its four states. The switch for the hand is connected to the chest strap and is operated by chest expansion. (Courtesy of Dudley S. Childress, Ph.D., Prosthetics Research Laboratory, Northwestern University and the Orthotics and Prosthetics Clinical Services Department, Rehabilitation Institute of Chicago.)

used with the empty sleeve, will counter to some degree the unsightly upper body contour.

Pain

Long-term, regional, and phantom pain sensations are encountered in a high percentage of shoulder-level amputations. This is particularly true with limb loss caused by trauma. Avulsion of the arm can cause severe traction trauma to nerve trunks and nerve roots up to their spinal origin. Painful neoplasms requiring shoulder-area amputation tend to "carry over" established pain patterns following ablation.

There is no direct surgical relief for these pain phenomena, either at the time of amputation or subsequently. Careful, meticulous isolation and ligation of nerve trunks followed by sharp knife sectioning below the level of ligature has proved to be the most effective method of handling nerves at the time of surgery. The

sectioned nerves should retract well under remaining muscles and are thus protected by soft tissues. Nerve cautery and injecting the nerve ends with a long-acting local anesthetic or with tissue-destroying chemicals such as phenol or absolute alcohol have been ineffective. The ligated nerve will form a neuroma, but if encapsulated by the nonabsorbable suture it does not tend to grow out in tentacle-like fashion to adhere to adjacent structures.

When pain remains a serious problem the best management is nonsurgical. Central neural surgery, particularly, is to be avoided. High nerve division and/or tractotomy are almost routinely unsuccessful and, in fact, may aggravate the pain patterns. Local physical measures including massage, cold, exercise, neuromuscular stimulation by external electrical currents, acupuncture, and regional sympathectomy may under given circumstances have a place in therapy when the pain is intractable. A technique that has gained some acceptance and success is the incorporation of transcutaneous electrical nerve stimulators (TENS) in a shoulder-cap type prosthesis, which is worn by the amputee at night and even during the day with the battery pack attached to the belt or inside a pocket. We have used this TENS system with moderate success. Psychological support can be beneficial, particularly when personality problems seem to accentuate the occurrence of pain. The individual needs patience and reassurance that the discomfort will improve over time, especially when a supportive social environment is present.

References

1. Abbott LC, and Lucas DB: The function of the clavicle; its surgical significance. Ann Surg 140:583–599, 1954.
2. Bauman PK: Resection of the upper extremity in the region of the shoulder joint. Khirurg Arkh Velyaminova 30:145–149, 1914.
3. Berger P. Amputation du membre superieur dans la contiguite du tronc (des articulation de l'omoplate). Bull Mem Soc Nat Chir 9:656, 1883.
4. Blumenfeld I, Schortz RH, Levy M, and Lepley JB: Fabricating a shoulder somatoprosthesis. J Prosthet Dent 45(5):542–544, 1981.
5. Bogacki W, and Spyt T: Interscapular-thoracic amputation of the arm. Nowotwory 30(30):261–264, 1980.
6. Burgess EM: Sites of amputation election according to modern practice. Clin Orthop 37:17–22, 1964.
7. Burton DS, and Nagel DA: Surgical treatment of malignant soft-tissue tumors of the extremities in the adult. Clin Orthop 84:144–148, 1972.
8. Copland SM: Total resection of the clavicle. Am J Surg 72:280, 1946.
9. DeNancrede CBG: End-results of total excision of the scapula for sarcoma. Ann Surg 50:1–22, 1909.
10. DePalma AF: Scapulectomy and a method of preserving normal configuration of the shoulder. Clin Orthop 4:217–224, 1954.
11. Fanous N, Didolkar MS, Holyoke ED, and Elias EG: Evaluation of forequarter amputation in malignant diseases. Surg Gynecol Obstet 142(3):381–384, 1976.
12. Grimes OF, and Bell HG: Shoulder girdle amputation. Surg Gynecol Obstet 91:201, 1950.
13. Guerra A, Capanna R, Biagini R, et al: Extra-articular resection of the shoulder (Tikhoff-Linberg). Ital J Orthop Traumatol 11(2):151–157, 1985.
14. Haggart GE: The technique of interscapulothoracic amputation. Lahey Clin Bull 2:16, 1940.
15. Hall CB, and Bechtol CO: Modern amputation technique in the upper extremity. J Bone Joint Surg 45A:1717, 1963.
16. Hardin CA: Interscapulothoracic amputations for sarcomas of the upper extremity. Surgery 49:355, 1961.
17. Harty M, and Joyce JJ: Surgical approaches to the shoulder. Orthop Clin North Am 6(2):553–564, 1975.
18. Hau T: The surgical practice of Dominique Jean Larrey. Surg Gynecol Obstet 154:89, 1982.
19. Herberts P: Myoelectric signals in control of prostheses. Studies on arm amputees and normal individuals. Acta Orthop Scand (Suppl) 124:1+, 1969.
20. Janecki CJ, and Nelson CL: En bloc resection of the shoulder girdle: technique and indications. J Bone Joint Surg 54A:1754–1758, 1972.
21. Knaggs RL: Mr. Littlewood's method of performing the interscapulothoracic amputation (Letter to the editor). Lancet 1:1298, 1910.
22. Kochhar CL, and Strivastava LK: Anatomical and functional considerations in total claviculectomy. Clin Orthop 118:199, 1976.
23. Larrey DJ: Memoire sur les Amputations des Membres a La Suite des Coups de Feu Etaye de Plusieurs Observations. Paris: Du Pont, 1797.
24. Levinthal DH, and Grossman A: Interscapulothoracic amputations for malignant tumors of the shoulder region. Surg Gynecol Obstet 69:234, 1939.
25. Lewis MM, Ballet FL, Kroll PG, and Bloom N: En bloc clavicular resection, operative procedure and postoperative testing of function. Clin Orthop 193:214, 1985.
26. Littlewood H: Amputations at the shoulder and at the hip. Br Med J 1:381, 1922.
27. Luiberg BE: Interscapulothoracic resection for malignant tumors of the shoulder joint region. J Bone Joint Surg 10:344–349, 1928.
28. Mansour KA, and Powell RW: Modified technique for radical transmediastinal forequarter amputation and chest wall resection. J Thorac Cardiovasc Surg 76(3):358–363, 1978.
29. Marcove RC: Neoplasms of the shoulder girdle. Orthop Clin North Am 6(2):541–552, 1975.
30. McLaughlin J: Solitary myeloma of the clavicle with long survival after total excision: report of a case. J Bone Joint Surg 55B:357, 1973.
31. McLaurin CA, Sauter WF, Dolan DM, and Harmann GR: Fabrication procedures for the open-shoulder above-elbow socket. Artif Limbs 13(2):46–54, 1969.
32. Moseley HF: The Forequarter Amputation. Edinburgh: E. and S. Livingstone, 1957, p 49.
33. Nadler SH, and Phelan JT: A technique of interscapulo-thoracic amputation. Surg Gynecol Obstet 122:359, 1966.
34. Neff G: Prosthetic principles in bilateral shoulder disarticulation or bilateral amelia. Prosthet Orthot 2(3):143–147, 1978.
35. Oible JH: Napoleon's Surgeon. London: William Heinemann Medical Books, 1970.
36. Pack GT: Major exarticulations for malignant neoplasms of the extremities: interscapulothoracic amputation, hip joint disarticulations and interilioabdominal amputation: a report of end results in 228 cases. J Bone Joint Surg 38A:249, 1956.
37. Pack GT, and Baldwin JC: The Tikhor-Linberg resection of shoulder girdle. Surgery 38:753–757, 1955.
38. Pack GT, and Crampton RS: The Tikhor-Linberg resection of the shoulder girdle: indications for its substitution for interscapulothoracic amputation, recent data on end-results of the forequarter amputation. Clin Orthop 19:148, 1961.
39. Pack GT, Ehrlich HE, and Gentil F: Radical amputations of the extremities in the treatment of cancer. Surg Gynecol Obstet 84:1105–1116, 1947.
40. Pack GT, McNeer G, and Coley BL: Interscapulo-thoracic amputations for malignant tumors of the upper extremity: a report of thirty-one consecutive cases. Surg Gynecol Obstet 74:161, 1942.
41. Roth JA, Sugarbaker PH, and Baker AR: Radical forequarter amputation with chest wall resection. Ann Thorac Surg 37(5):432–437, 1984.
42. Salzer M, and Knahr K: Resection of malignant bone tumors. Recent Results Cancer Res 54:239–256, 1976.
43. Sauter WF: Prostheses for the child amputee. Orthop Clin North Am 3(2):483–494, 1972.
44. Slocum DB: Atlas of Amputations. St. Louis: CV Mosby, 1949.
45. Spar I: Total claviculectomy for pathological fractures. Clin Orthop 129:236, 1977.
46. Sperling P, and Rloding H: Interthoracoscapular amputation (forequarter amputation). Zentralbl Chir 106(5):340–343, 1981.
47. Syme J: Excision of the Scapula. Edinburgh: Edmonton and Douglas, 1864.
48. Tikhor PT: Tumor Studies (monograph). Russia, 1900.
49. Tooms RE: Amputation surgery in the upper extremity. Orthop Clin North Am 3(2):383–395, 1972.
50. Trishkin VA, Saakian AM, Stoliarov VI, and Kochnev VA: Interscapulothoracic amputation in treating malignant tumors of the upper extremity and shoulder girdle. Vestn Khir 124(1):75–78, 1980.
51. Turnbull A, Blumencranz P, and Fortner J: Scapulectomy for soft tissue sarcoma. Can J Surg 24(1):37–38, 1981.
52. Zancolli E, Mitre HJ, Bick M, et al: Interscapulo-cleidothoracic disarticulation. Indications and technic. Prensa Med Argent 52(16):1122–1126, 1965.

The Shoulder in Sports

Frank W. Jobe, M.D.
James E. Tibone, M.D.
Christopher M. Jobe, M.D.
Ronald S. Kvitne, M.D.

The goals of physicians treating athletes have changed over the centuries, depending on the expectations of the athlete, the technology available, and the state of medical knowledge. The earliest recorded team physician was Galen, who cared for the Pergamum gladiators. He made valuable contributions to the field of shoulder surgery in the second century A.D. and was the first to recognize that there is a conflict between stability and freedom of movement. He also recognized labral detachment and glenoid fractures as part of the pathology of dislocation. However, his knowledge of biomechanics was insufficient to recognize the high magnitude of forces across the joint.

The early goals in sports medicine were limited to prevention of the recurrence of injury. In the case of dislocation, preventing recurrence rather than post-treatment performance was the hallmark of success. Today, such goals are too limited. We now have the technology to study performance and correlate many kinds of pathology with errors in athletic technique. Satisfactory post-treatment performance is an essential characteristic of sports medicine.

Much of the anatomy and biomechanics of the shoulder is presented in other chapters of this text. This chapter addresses the particular anatomy and kinesiology of the shoulder specific to sports participation. An accurate picture of performance in an elite athlete is invaluable in understanding the pathology found in these patients.

The rotator cuff, the static stabilizers, and the other scapular muscles work as a triumvirate, the interaction of which optimizes the delicate balance between stability and function. In the laboratory, as shoulder function borders on instability at the glenohumeral joint, muscle activity becomes aberrant in an attempt to stabilize the glenohumeral joint by fixing the scapula. The rotator cuff muscles attempt to substitute for the inadequate stabilizers and scapular rotators. If the instability persists or worsens, muscle spasm occurs, creating a second source of pain and abnormal kinematics. These secondary adjustments to increase stability will impose an elevated muscle load that leads to early muscle fatigue. This fatigue, in turn, contributes to suboptimal kinetics. Instability, muscle spasm, fatigue—each potentiates the other two and a downward spiral ensues.

Instability, in particular, then may be the key unlocking that compartment of Pandora's box wherein lies shoulder pathology in the athlete. We cannot prevent shoulder problems if we cannot control minor instability early in the pathological sequence. Control requires early recognition. The drive for anatomical stability can lead the shoulder to asynchronous muscle firing, sometimes into impingement and beyond, to frank tears of the rotator cuff.

Biomechanics of the Throwing Shoulder

The forces generated and the energies used in athletics are much larger than those that could ever be generated by the shoulder musculature alone.[37, 38] The exercises used in postsurgical and post-traumatic recovery are actually a form of "rest" compared with the kinesiological tasks performed during athletics.

The biomechanics of the athletic shoulder differ quantitatively rather than qualitatively from the biomechanics of the shoulder in the activities of daily living. The focus is on the higher energies involved in athletic motion. Such a focus is essential to understand the mechanism of acute trauma and the need for conditioning prior to athletic performance. We will describe the mechanism of chronic overuse and discuss the need for conditioning and proper coaching technique. Knowing these forces will allow us to understand how the performance of an exercise program as part of a rehabilitation scheme can still be considered a form of rest for a high-performance athlete.

Beginning the section with a discussion of the baseball throw is appropriate for two reasons. First, it is the most studied athletic activity involving the shoulder and therefore offers the largest quantity of and, probably, the best documented data.* Second, with minor modifications, the same type of activity also occurs in a number of other athletic activities such as throwing a football or a javelin, as well as in racquet sports.[37]

The central thesis of throwing biomechanics can be outlined as follows: The thrower uses his or her own body weight and large muscles to generate kinetic energy, which is guided across the shoulder in the direction of the thrown object. After the object is released, the retained energy within the throwing arm is released by reversing this process, whereby the energy is dissipated by the larger muscles of the lower limb and back. In general, pathology occurs in one of two ways: (1) improper mechanics generating the necessary throwing speed requires more shoulder muscle force to propel the object, leading to fatigue; and (2) improper dissipation of this energy results in the retention of unwanted energy within the soft tissues about the shoulder, resulting in tissue damage.

An exercise used by pitching coaches demonstrates the use of the entire body. First, sit in a chair and throw a ball as far as possible. Next, stand and throw. The ball will go at least twice as far. The muscles of the shoulder alone cannot generate sufficient energy to produce such a throw nor can they dissipate the energy after the throw is completed. Therefore, inju-

*See references 3–5, 12, 23, 25, 28, 29, 47.

ries are likely to occur when shoulder muscles are asked to generate or dissipate energies beyond their capacity.

The throwing motion generates high speed in the thrown object in the same fashion that a skater increases his or her rate of spin, by following the law of conservation of rotational energy. Rotational energy is the product of $1/2\ IW^2$. W is the rate of rotation, I is the moment of inertia, dependent upon the mass of an object and its distance from the axis of rotation. Given a constant rotational energy, decreasing I increases W. The skater cannot suddenly lose weight, so he brings the arms in tight to bring his mass closer to the center of rotation.

A thrower uses the same principle. By utilizing the whole body to generate momentum and by then transferring momentum to smaller and smaller portions of the body, the rate of rotation will be maximized. The phases of throwing were defined by surgeons focusing on the shoulder; these names reflect shoulder activity during each phase (Fig. 26–1). For the purposes of the following discussion, let us assume that the pitcher is two meters tall and weighs 100 kg. The first phase of throwing—*wind-up*—consists of the thrower picking up his contralateral lower limb. In mechanical terms, he is raising his center of gravity to the highest point possible. Different throwers will use different styles depending on the exact situation in the game, but the end result is roughly the same in terms of how much potential energy he is producing. The next phase begins when the hand with the ball leaves the glove and ends when the contralateral foot touches the ground. The pitcher begins moving his upper limb toward a position where it can best accept energy transfer. The most important mechanical event during this *early cocking* phase is taking place below the arm. The pitcher falls

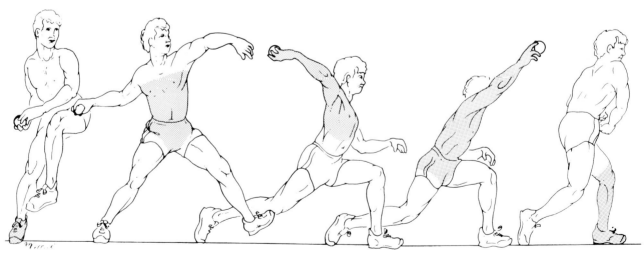

Figure 26–1. The five phases of pitching a baseball (from left to right): wind-up, early cocking, late cocking, acceleration, and follow-through. Wind-up or preparation: preliminary activity dominated by flexion of the upper extremity, with both hands holding the ball. Early cocking: a period of abduction and external rotation of the shoulder that begins as the ball is released from the nondominant hand. Late cocking: contact of the forward foot with the ground divides this stage from early cocking. Late cocking continues until maximum external rotation at the shoulder is attained. Acceleration: starts with the posture of maximum abduction and external rotation at the shoulder and continues until release of the ball, as the ball leaves the fingers. Follow-through: the final interval of motion as the arm flexes and internally rotates across the chest and is thus decelerated. (Reproduced with permission from Glousman RE, Jobe FW, Tibone JE, et al: Dynamic EMG analysis of the throwing shoulder with glenohumeral instability. J Bone Joint Surg *70A*:220–226, 1988.)

toward the catcher, creating an angular motion rotating around an axis at the level of the foot. If his center of gravity lowers by 0.3 meters, the pitcher loses approximately 300 joules of potential energy. If we assume that all of the energy added by the force of the pitcher's muscles exactly counterbalances the energy lost in performing the action, we have an idea of how much kinetic energy is set in motion: 300 joules. The next phase is *late cocking*. At the shoulder, abduction and external rotation are taken to maximum or supramaximum; as before, the important mechanical action is not at the shoulder. The kinetic energy is transferred to the forward rotating torso. Since only the upper body is moving, the total mass contributing to the angular moment of inertia is cut in half. In addition, that mass is more tightly configured around the new axis of rotation, leading to a further decrease in the angular moment of inertia. Again, assuming that muscles make up for any energy lost in inefficiency (the second law of thermodynamics), the conservation of angular kinetic energy leads to an increase in the rate of rotation. As the torso faces the catcher in midrotation, it slows, isolating the kinetic energy in the upper limb.

Since the upper limb is a mere fraction of the total body mass, it experiences a quantum leap in the rate of rotation. This phase is called *acceleration* and takes place both at the shoulder and at the elbow. The phase ends with the release of the ball and the loss of some of the kinetic energy to the ball. A 90-mile-per-hour pitch departs with about 88.2 joules of energy, leaving 212 joules behind, mostly in the throwing arm.

The problem occurs with the need to dissipate this remaining energy without allowing it to injure body tissue. The *follow-through* phase is a continuation of the throwing motion. Its sequence is exactly reversed from that occurring prior to ball release, although the direction remains the same. The muscles now fire eccentrically, dissipating the remaining energy as the heat of the chemical reaction between actin and myosin. The primary strategy of follow-through is to return the angular kinetic energy to a slower-moving object, i.e., to the entire body as it rotates over the contralateral foot. In the first phase of follow-through, the arm continues in horizontal flexion and internal rotation as it was during acceleration. The muscles now act to decelerate the arm. The torso begins to rotate forward as in late cocking. This accomplishes two things: (1) it decreases the relative motion at the glenohumeral and scapulothoracic joints, and (2) it returns the kinetic energy to a larger and therefore slower-moving object. Here the eccentric firing begins to occur in the larger postural muscles, slowing the horizontal rotation and forward flexion of the spine. This phase might therefore be considered *anticocking*. At the completion, the pitcher lifts his ipsilateral foot, becoming again a large object rotating over the foot and being acted upon by gravity. Gravity is now acting to decelerate the angular momentum. During the next phase the pitcher resumes the two-leg stance, using his

muscles to achieve this posture. When there remains much energy to dissipate, the pitcher may take one or two steps forward to gain additional time over which to accomplish this task.

To the physician, this means that for the transmission of energy from the ground to the thrown object and back again, it is essential that the muscles fire properly. The scapula must reposition itself constantly as a platform; the rotator cuff is always functioning to seat the humeral head within the glenoid for maximum efficient energy transfer; and, of course, the static stabilizers establish end points for these motions.[21, 23, 35, 37] When the static stabilizers begin to break down, the rotator cuff muscles and the scapular rotators function beyond their usual limits, leading to fatigue. Their endurance is insufficient to absorb these additional demands. The position of the humeral head is not maintained within the glenoid. The player attempts to overcome this handicap by changing his body mechanics. This faulty technique then accentuates and contributes to additional pathological change.[15, 16]

If the thrower places his contralateral foot in an exaggerated externally rotated position during early cocking, his pelvis and torso are forced into beginning their forward rotation earlier. The shoulder muscles must bring the arm forward in line with the rest of the throwing mechanism. This results in early fatigue of the shoulder muscles, allowing the pitcher to drop his elbow. The dropped elbow, in combination with the hyperextended shoulder, increases the valgus forces across the elbow, leading to separate clinical and pathological sequelae.

Conversely, if a thrower does not externally rotate his contralateral hip enough, he prevents forward rotation of the torso, increasing the relative horizontal adduction of the shoulder relative to the trunk and increasing the stresses and retention of kinetic energy in the posterior portion of the shoulder.

Shoulder pathology itself contributes to faulty technique. In an athlete with a subluxing shoulder, there is a tendency to protect the shoulder against an exaggerated horizontal extension and external rotation by delaying the protraction of the scapula. This, in addition to decreased use of some of the more powerful internal rotators, produces a less effective throw.[16] In addition, because of the decreased protraction and elevation of the scapula, the same throwing motion produces more relative glenohumeral elevation and horizontal adduction and internal rotation, leading to impingement.

Impingement and Instability in the Athlete

The shoulder in the young athlete must be viewed from a special perspective. Shoulder function and stability are more closely related to dynamic muscle actions than to static anatomy.[38, 48] Because stability and function are so inter-related, most sports injuries to the shoulder are related to instability. The shoulder joint is designed for mobility rather than stability and is delicately balanced between the two, making it susceptible to injury when subjected to athletic demands.[1, 25] This is particularly true of sports requiring arm elevation to 90 degrees. The four joints of the shoulder (glenohumeral, scapulothoracic, sternoclavicular, and acromioclavicular) are a complex array whose subtle inter-relationships produce an extraordinary range of motion. Pathology in any one will disrupt high-level shoulder function.

As discussed in the previous section, the glenohumeral joint is particularly vulnerable because upper extremity sports put tremendous stresses on its stabilizing mechanisms: the glenohumeral contact area enhanced by the glenoid labrum, the static stabilizers (ligamentous labral complex), and the dynamic stabilizers (rotator cuff muscles).

Given the complex controlling mechanisms and tremendous demands imposed by upper extremity sports, it is not surprising that a small deficiency has a cumulative effect on the shoulder. Sports that require overhead and throwing maneuvers stress the tissues to near their physiological limits. If this stress is applied at a rate that is greater than the rate of tissue repair, such repetitive insults can produce progressive damage to the shoulder. A shoulder exercising at or near these physiological limits without proper warmup, mechanics, and conditioning will eventually break down from overuse. Although this chronic type of attritional pathology is the more common pattern, we do see acute injuries as well in which a single episode of stress disrupts the tissue integrity.

A final review of the stabilizing mechanisms of the shoulder: The scapular rotators (i.e., the trapezius, rhomboids, and serratus anterior) place the glenoid in the optimal position for the activities being performed; the rotator cuff muscles center the humeral head in the most stable position in the glenoid while providing maximal available leverage; and the ligamentous labral capsular complex—especially the inferior glenohumeral ligament—provides restraint at the margin of the joint. Overuse with overhead activities may stretch or injure the static stabilizers. The instability, in turn, disrupts the synchronous firing of the scapular rotators and rotator cuff muscles. The latter must now attempt to contain the humeral head on their own. Injury leads to muscle asynchrony, which contributes to additional injury. When the arm is now in the abducted and externally rotated position and the humeral head subluxes anteriorly, the rotator cuff is compressed and abraded between the acromion, the coracoacromial ligament, and the humeral head. These impingement problems are therefore secondary to the instability.

Historically, rotator cuff damage and anterior instability have been thought of and treated as different entities.* Acromioplasty for rotator cuff impingement

and tears gave inconsistent results in athletes.[43] Repair of the cuff combined with acromioplasty in the young athletic population provided pain relief but did not always return the athlete to his former competitive status. Indeed, these postsurgical results worsened as the patient's skill level increased. Most of these poor results are probably a consequence of missed diagnoses in that instability was the primary cause of the patient's problem. In these patients, the labrum is not visualized well during the open cuff procedure and not visualized at all in patients without cuff tears.

Studying the shoulder in the laboratory and with the arthroscope has led to an awareness of the relationship between rotator cuff damage and glenohumeral instability. These studies suggest that anterior instability often represents the primary lesion, whereas rotator cuff impingement and tears are secondary.

RELOCATION TEST

A diagnosis in throwing and overhand athletes under the age of 35 will often be based on subtle findings. The physical examination may be confusing in that the impingement signs are generally obvious, whereas the subluxation signs are subtle. The most sensitive test we have found has been the "relocation test." As will be recalled, for an apprehension test the patient's arm is abducted and externally rotated, and a gentle, anteriorly directed force is applied to the humeral head. The relocation test is performed using the following sequence of maneuvers: with the patient supine, the arm is placed in the position of apprehension, i.e., abduction and external rotation, while gently pushing anteriorly on the humeral head (Fig. 26-2). This ma-

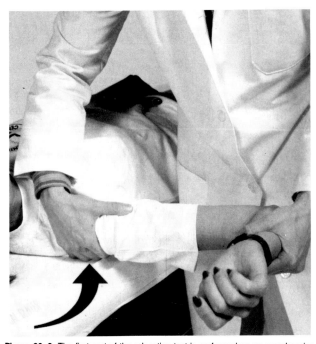

Figure 26–2. The first part of the relocation test is performed as an apprehension test: abduct and externally rotate the arm while pushing gently anteriorly on the humeral head. This usually is uncomfortable for a patient with anterior subluxation.

*See references 1, 13, 24, 25, 30, 41, 43, 44.

neuver generally produces pain (not apprehension) in a patient with subluxation. The test is then repeated with a posteriorly directed force on the humeral head, which reduces the head to its normal position (Fig. 26–3). Patients with primary impingement may have no change in their pain, whereas patients with instability and secondary impingement are now able to tolerate maximal external rotation when the humeral head is returned to its reduced position.

ETIOLOGY OF SHOULDER PAIN IN THROWING ATHLETES

Athletes who have shoulder pain and who are involved in overhead sports can be divided into four groups based on the history, physical examination, and arthroscopic findings: Group I—pure impingement; Group II—instability secondary to anterior ligament and labral injury with subsequent impingement; Group III—instability secondary to hyperelastic capsular ligaments and tissues with secondary impingement; and Group IV—pure anterior instability (Fig. 26–4).

Pain Secondary to Pure Impingement

In the first group are athletes with pure impingement and a history of overhead activity with superior shoulder pain. Generally, these patients have positive impingement signs, negative apprehension signs, and no change on the relocation test. Examination under

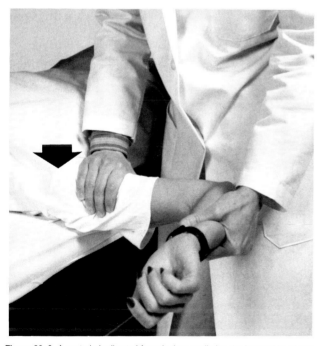

Figure 26–3. A posteriorly directed force is then applied to the humeral head with the arm remaining in the abducted and externally rotated position. Patients with impingement may have no change in pain, whereas patients with instability are now able to tolerate the external rotation with the humeral head maintained in a reduced position.

anesthesia reveals a joint that is stable upon stress testing. Arthroscopically, these patients may have an undersurface cuff tear but will have a normal labrum and glenohumeral ligaments. Because of their repetitive overhand activities, however, they have developed overgrowth of the inferior aspect of the acromion and narrowing of the subacromial space. In our experience, this group includes a very small number of patients who are usually over age 35. This group should be placed on a rotator cuff strengthening and stretching program. The conservative program lasts six months with exercises, rest, and anti-inflammatory medications. Rest does not mean placing the arm in a sling; this would simply lead to further contracture of the rotator cuff. Rest means abstaining only from the offending sport and other motions that aggravate the pain. If conservative care fails, our recommended treatment is an arthroscopic acromioplasty with resection of the coracoacromial ligament and subdeltoid bursa. Depending on the skill and judgment of the surgeon, this can be done with a standard open operative procedure. In these patients the undersurface of the rotator cuff may show signs of wear. An arthroscopic "housecleaning debridement" of this area is usually not necessary. Such debridement does not promote healing of the cuff and does not treat the pathological process of impingement. Overzealous debridement can lead to thinning and the creation of a weakened area in the cuff that could later progress to a full-thickness tear. This group of athletes is relatively small and seems to be diminishing in size as our ability to deliver kinesiologically sound conditioning programs improves.

Pain Secondary to Instability Due to Anterior Ligament and Labral Injury with Secondary Impingement

Group II patients have instability due to chronic anterior capsular ligament and labral injury with secondary impingement. Clinically, these patients have positive impingement signs and will experience pain when the apprehension test is performed. The pain is then relieved with the relocation test. Under anesthesia, they may have an unstable shoulder, but this instability is so subtle that it often goes undetected. Arthroscopic findings usually show an anterior labral tear and/or a deficient anteroinferior glenohumeral ligament. The posterior examination may show a small defect in the posterior humeral head cartilage, similar to a Hill-Sachs lesion, and posterior labral damage. The rotator cuff may show some damage or fraying. Conservative care emphasizes strengthening the rotator cuff and the scapular rotators. Most patients in this group will improve on such a program; those whose damage is considerable will not. Proper treatment for the latter group is an operative repair of their capsular labral complex. An isolated acromioplasty procedure is contraindicated because it can lead to further glenohumeral instability.

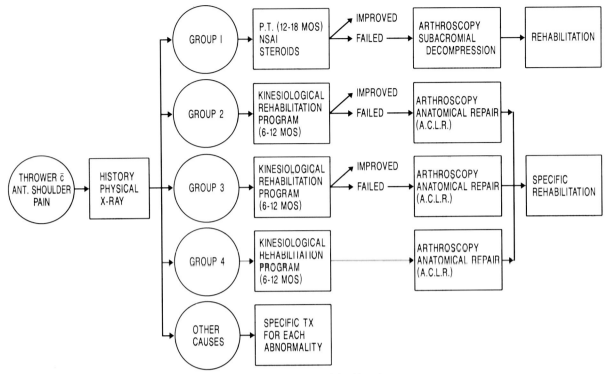

Figure 26–4. Classification of shoulder pain.

Pain Secondary to Instability Due to Hyperelastic Capsular Ligaments with Secondary Impingement

Group III patients are those with instability due to hyperelasticity with subsequent impingement. Like Group II, these patients have positive impingement signs, demonstrate pain with the apprehension test, and have pain relief with the relocation test. These athletes usually have ligamentous laxity and may demonstrate increased thumb flexion and abduction, and hyperextension of the elbows, knees, and metacarpophalangeal joints, in addition to increased shoulder range of motion. The involved shoulder can be subluxated easily, often in more than one direction. Usually, positive impingement signs are caused by irritation of the rotator cuff and biceps tendon. Examination under anesthesia commonly reveals laxity of both shoulders but usually more so on the dominant, involved extremity. At arthroscopy the anterior labrum is intact, although it may be hypoplastic with a redundant anterior capsule and lax inferior glenohumeral ligament. There may also be fraying of the rotator cuff, but this is often absent or minimal. The major arthroscopic finding is that the humeral head can easily be manipulated over and around the intact labrum. Initial treatment for this group includes a physical therapy program designed to tighten the shoulder by strengthening the rotator cuff muscles and the scapular rotators. This program is similar to the program for impingement alone. If this fails after at least six months, a capsular labral reconstruction is performed to improve function. Again, an acromioplasty procedure is contraindicated as it can lead to further glenohumeral instability.

Pain Secondary to Pure Instability Without Secondary Impingement

Group IV patients are those with pure instability without impingement. There is often a history of a single traumatic episode, e.g., sliding back to base with the arm outstretched to beat the tag. This group demonstrates negative impingement signs, pain with apprehension testing, and relief of pain with the relocation test. At the time of arthroscopy, the rotator cuff is normal but there is obvious labral damage and, possibly, posterior humeral head lesions caused by the subluxing humeral head. As in Groups II and III, proper treatment is a capsular labral reconstruction. Physical therapy for these patients has only a small chance of success.

Instability should always be considered as a source of shoulder pain in throwing and overhand athletes with a history of overuse in sports. The instability is subtle and may require an experienced examiner. The examination under anesthesia may be compared with the "normal" shoulder. Under anesthesia, the humeral head usually can be translated farther posteriorly than anteriorly. Hawkins and colleagues have reported that posterior translation of up to 50 per cent of the humeral head in the glenoid can be normal.[18] The examination under anesthesia may elicit clicks, which signify labral damage in addition to the instability. Arthroscopy is often necessary to obtain a better understanding of these athletic shoulders. At the time of arthroscopy, pathology may be found in the anterior labrum, anterior capsule, inferior glenohumeral ligament, posterohumeral head, or posterior labrum. Many of these findings are too subtle to be appreciated on computed tomography (CT) or magnetic resonance imaging (MRI) investigations, at least at our present level of radiological sophistication.

Proper diagnosis allows the problem to be approached through physical therapy and correction of inappropriate kinematics. Early in the course of the disease this approach may prove sufficient. Postoperatively, rehabilitation and conditioning are necessary to restore performance and prevent recurrence.

REHABILITATION FOR ROTATOR CUFF PROBLEMS

Most rotator cuff problems in athletes can be treated nonsurgically.[22] Rest is the initial treatment; *this does not mean immobilization*. In the athlete, this means the cessation of the overhead activity that is causing the symptoms, e.g., throwing a baseball or spiking a volleyball. Stretching and strengthening exercises that are specific to the rotator cuff need to be emphasized during this initial rehabilitation program so that the rotator cuff and the capsular complex do not become contracted. However, *stretching in general should be done judiciously and only for muscle groups with demonstrable tightness*. The potential for overzealousness needs to be recognized and avoided. *Anterior stretching should be done only if it is certain that no anterior instability, subtle or overt, exists. If doubt exists, the following three exercises should be deleted from the rehabilitation protocol*.

Stretching exercises, if necessary, are performed in the supine position on an exercise table with the athlete holding a 2- to 5-pound weight in the involved extremity. The first exercise begins with the arm in the 90/90 position—90 degrees of shoulder abduction and 90 degrees of elbow flexion (the cocking position of throwing)—and with as much external rotation as possible. The athlete's shoulder should be at or over the edge of the table to ensure that movement at the glenohumeral joint is not restricted (Fig. 26–5). This exercise is performed as a static stretch, allowing gravity to elongate the tissues gradually.

The second stretching exercise is also done in a supine position (Fig. 26–6). The shoulder is elevated 135 degrees in the frontal plane with the elbow extended and the shoulder externally rotated. Again, the shoulder must be at the table's edge, free to move into as much horizontal extension and external rotation as possible. The same 2- to 5-pound weight is used. The next progression of the stretching is to put the arm in 180 degrees of elevation, as far overhead as possible, with the palm toward the ceiling and the elbow extended (Fig. 26–7). This may require the athlete to lie diagonally across the table so that the shoulder is positioned over the edge.

The posterior portion of the shoulder capsule can be stretched with the athlete in the standing position (Fig. 26–8). The shoulder is placed in 90 degrees of elevation, and the opposite hand is used to pull the shoulder into horizontal adduction. Finally, the inferior capsule can be stretched with the arm as far overhead as possible and with the elbow flexed, by pulling the elbow behind the head as much as possible (Fig. 26–9).

After the shoulder has been mobilized, the next component of rehabilitation of the rotator cuff is strengthening. Separate exercises for each of the rotator cuff muscles have been designed. These exercises should be performed initially with a 1- to 2-pound

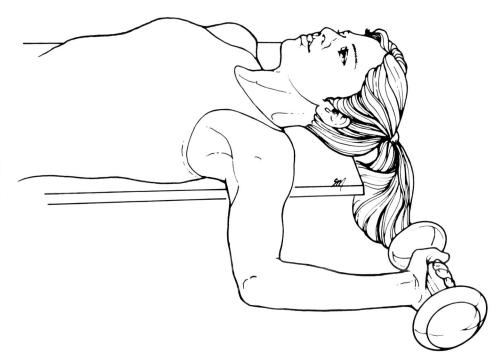

Figure 26–5. Static stretching exercise with the shoulder abducted 90 degrees and the elbow flexed 90 degrees will stretch the anterior shoulder capsule and soft tissues.

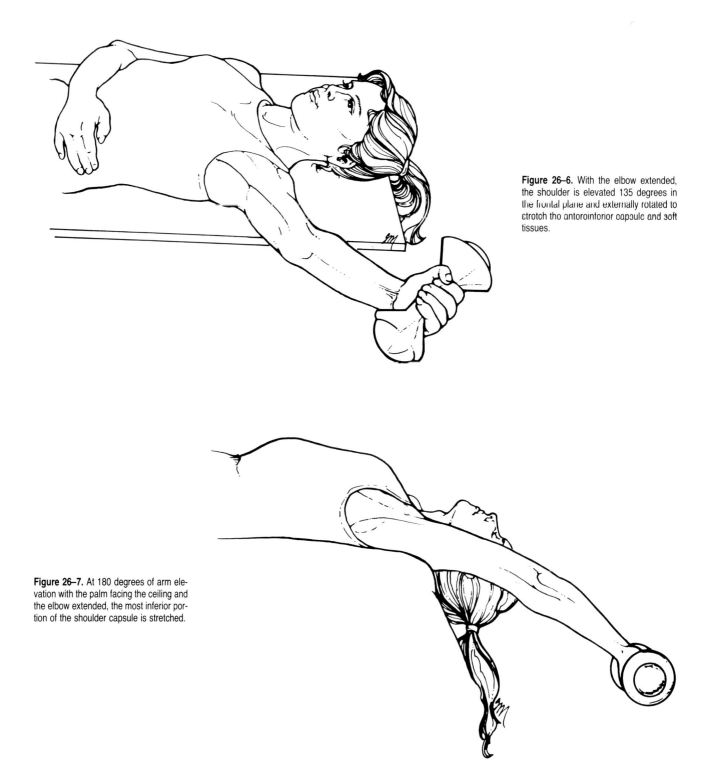

Figure 26–6. With the elbow extended, the shoulder is elevated 135 degrees in the frontal plane and externally rotated to stretch the anteroinferior capsule and soft tissues.

Figure 26–7. At 180 degrees of arm elevation with the palm facing the ceiling and the elbow extended, the most inferior portion of the shoulder capsule is stretched.

weight, progressing up to a 5-pound weight. Only the well-muscled athlete will need to progress up to 10 pounds with these exercises. Additional repetitions rather than increasing weights is the rule with rotator cuff exercises.

The supraspinatus can be exercised selectively with the athlete seated or standing and with the shoulders elevated 70 degrees, in horizontal flexion of 30 degrees and full internal rotation (Fig. 26–10). This places the shoulder movement in the plane of the scapula and strengthens the supraspinatus selectively. While in this position, the athlete raises his arms from 10 or 20 degrees of elevation to 70 or 80 degrees. It is important not to raise the arm above 90 degrees, as this can cause increased impingement symptoms. Again, the initial exercises are with light weights of 1 to 2 pounds and progress to 5 or 10 pounds. More weight is seldom necessary.

The athlete can then exercise the infraspinatus and teres minor muscles while lying on the side with the arm held next to the body and the elbow flexed 90 degrees (Fig. 26–11). The exercise is started with the forearm against the abdomen. The arm is then brought up into external rotation with the elbow remaining close to the body. As the weight is brought back to the initial position, the external rotators work eccentrically to control this motion.

The subscapularis muscle is exercised in the supine position, again with the arm held close to the side and the elbow flexed to 90 degrees (Fig. 26–12). Beginning with maximum external rotation, the arm is moved into maximum internal rotation, again returning the arm slowly to the starting position. This exercise can

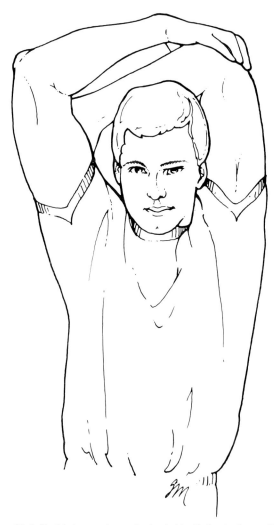

Figure 26–9. The inferior capsule can also be stretched in the standing position by elevating the arm overhead as far as possible with the elbow flexed, and pulling the arm behind the head as far as possible.

also be done while lying on the involved side with the arm slightly forward of the trunk and the elbow flexed to 90 degrees. The forearm is brought up and across the chest.

In addition to strengthening the rotator cuff muscles with weights, surgical tubing of varied resistances can be used. It is important to deal with each muscle individually and to emphasize both the stretching and the strengthening aspects of the rehabilitation program as necessary. Without proper strengthening of the entire shoulder complex, the rotator cuff will fatigue and become irritated from overuse. If the rotator cuff and capsule do not have an adequate length, microscopic tears will occur from the overhead motion necessary in competition. Due caution must be exercised before stretching is begun. Only after the rotator cuff has been strengthened properly and has adequate length, if appropriate, should the patient return to his or her regular athletic activity.

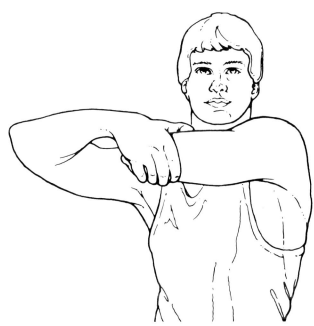

Figure 26–8. In the standing position, the posterior portion of the shoulder capsule and soft tissues can be stretched by placing the arm in 90 degrees of elevation and using the opposite hand to pull the shoulder into horizontal adduction.

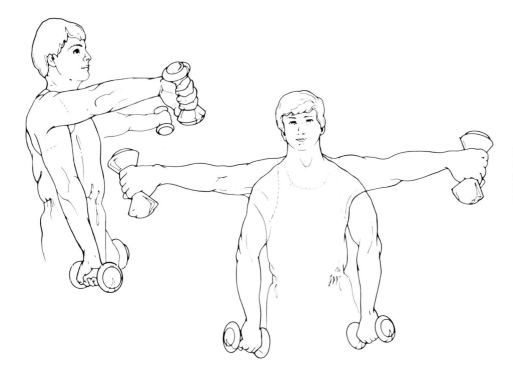

Figure 26–10. Selective strengthening of the supraspinatus muscle can be achieved by performing diagonal shoulder lifts with the arms in 30 degrees of forward flexion and full internal rotation.

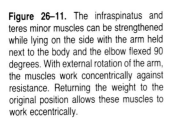

Figure 26–11. The infraspinatus and teres minor muscles can be strengthened while lying on the side with the arm held next to the body and the elbow flexed 90 degrees. With external rotation of the arm, the muscles work concentrically against resistance. Returning the weight to the original position allows these muscles to work eccentrically.

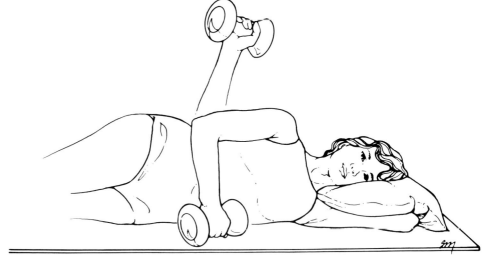

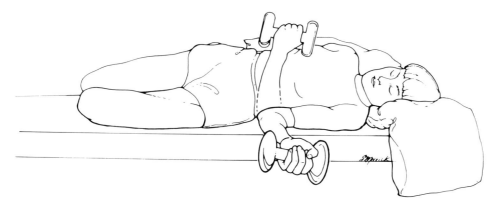

Figure 26–12. The subscapularis muscle is strengthened in a sidelying position with the involved side down and slightly forward of the trunk with the elbow flexed 90 degrees. Moving from a position of maximum external rotation into maximum internal rotation and then returning to the original starting position requires both concentric and eccentric supscapular muscle contraction.

REHABILITATION FOR ANTERIOR INSTABILITY

The rehabilitation for anterior shoulder instability will vary in length depending on (1) the degree of shoulder instability or laxity, (2) whether the condition is acute or chronic, (3) strength and range of motion status, and (4) performance/activity demands. The treatment program is outlined in three phases. In all exercises during Phases I and II, there must be no undue stress on the anterior joint capsule. An isokinetic strength and endurance test is scheduled in Phase III, along with the addition of a progressive throwing program as needed.

Phase I

1. Modalities as needed (heat, ice, electrotherapy, etc.).
2. Range-of-motion exercises as tolerated. For shoulder abduction and external rotation, avoid stress to the anterior joint capsule by positioning the shoulder in the scapular plane (approximately 20 to 30 degrees forward of the coronal plane). Shoulder hyperextension is contraindicated.
3. Shoulder stretch: the posterior cuff and capsule only and only as necessary.
4. Mobilization (posterior glides) only as necessary.
5. Active shoulder internal and external rotation exercises with surgical or rubber tubing. The arm is positioned at the side with the elbow flexed at 90 degrees. Avoid excessive stress to the anterior joint capsule by limiting external rotation to the 45-degree range (as tolerated).
6. Supraspinatus exercise in the scapular plane.
7. Active shoulder flexion exercise through available range of motion.
8. Active shoulder abduction exercise to 90 degrees. Maintain the shoulder in the scapular plane to avoid placing stress on the anterior joint capsule.
9. Shoulder extension exercise, lying prone or standing and bending at the waist. Avoid hyperextension by not allowing the arm to extend beyond the plane of the body.
10. Shoulder shrug exercise—avoid traction in the glenohumeral joint between repetitions to limit excessive inferior glide of the humeral head.
11. Active horizontal adduction exercise—perform supine with the starting position in the scapular plane.
12. Active shoulder internal/external rotation—progress to free weights. For external rotation, perform sidelying with the involved side up. For internal rotation, perform lying on the side with the involved side down and slightly forward of the trunk and the elbow flexed to 90 degrees. Avoid placing excessive stress on the anterior joint capsule by limiting movement to 45 to 50 degrees.
13. Forearm strengthening exercises (elbow, wrist).

Phase II

1. Continue posterior cuff/capsule stretch, mobilization, and range-of-motion exercises (only as necessary).
2. Continue shoulder strengthening with surgical tubing and/or free weights. Emphasize the eccentric phase of contraction.
3. Add isokinetic strengthening exercise for internal/external rotation of the shoulder. Use higher speeds, e.g., 200 degrees per second or more. Exercise with the arm at the side. Maintain the shoulder in 15 to 20 degrees of flexion and avoid painful external rotation.
4. Add an arm ergometer for endurance exercise.
5. Add pushups. Movement should be pain free and progress through levels of difficulty: wall, modified (on knees), and military (on toes). Avoid placing stress on the anterior joint capsule by maintaining proper alignment of the shoulders and elbow at the starting position. Do not lower the body beyond the elbows.
6. Add total body conditioning with the emphasis on strength and endurance. Include flexibility exercises only as needed.

Phase III

1. Continue posterior cuff/capsule stretching as needed.
2. Continue to increase isotonic and isokinetic exercises. For shoulder internal and external rotation, position the upper extremity at zero degrees at first; progress to 45 degrees, then to 80 to 90 degrees of shoulder abduction as tolerated. Some patients will be rehabilitated completely with more safety in the zero-degree position. Gradually increase the stress to the anterior joint capsule by exercising in the shoulder position specific to the sport (as tolerated).
3. Add isokinetic exercises for shoulder flexion and extension, abduction and adduction, and horizontal abduction and adduction. Take precautions to avoid excessive stress to the anterior joint capsule.
4. Add chin-ups.
5. Continue the arm ergometer for endurance.
6. Perform the isokinetic strength and endurance test as tolerated. The shoulder should be pain free and have no swelling.
7. Begin a progressive shoulder throwing program: an isokinetic test for shoulder internal and external rotation should demonstrate at least 90 per cent strength and 90 per cent endurance compared with the uninvolved side before proceeding with the throwing program. Advance through the throwing sequence as needed.
8. Begin practicing drills specific to the sport and team position.

If the rehabilitative program fails, surgery is generally indicated.

SURGICAL PROCEDURES

Bristow Operation

For many years, the Bristow operation (designed by Helfet and modified by May) has been popular as a treatment for anteriorly dislocating shoulders; we include a detailed description here because it is still the procedure of choice for a number of surgeons. Within the last 5 to 10 years, however, we have had the opportunity to study the procedure more carefully. As other procedures have been developed, indications for the Bristow operation have been narrowed considerably. Our primary indications for the Bristow procedure are for nondominant shoulders in throwers and for shoulders in athletes whose primary activity is not in overhead sports. It works best with nondominant shoulders with multiple dislocations in which there is considerable bony loss.

The loss of 6 to 10 degrees of external rotation following the Bristow procedure renders it unsatisfactory in the treatment of the dominant arm of a thrower. Even a minimal decrease in motion usually prevents the patient from returning to high-level participation.

The Bristow procedure has been criticized for several reasons, such as complications with the screw (loosening, migration, breakage), its ineffectiveness in treating the subluxating shoulder, neurovascular injuries, nonunion of the transferred coracoid, and so on. Our opinion, developed over the last few years, is that a technically competent surgeon can perform the procedure without significant complications. If the surgeon lacks the skill or the equipment to perform this procedure, then perhaps it is inappropriate. The choice between the Bristow operation and other soft tissue procedures may become purely academic as the surgeon's skill and equipment allow him or her to perform the capsulolabral reconstructions in which no muscles are removed and no changes in the anatomical relationships occur. An athlete treated with this procedure will be able to throw and perform overhead activities and will not risk the complications noted above. Indeed, we anticipate that as the range of indications narrows for the Bristow procedure and widens for the capsulolabral reconstruction, the former will probably go out of vogue.

The Magnuson-Stack and Putti-Platt procedures are not recommended for the athlete's dominant throwing arm under any circumstances. These tighten the shoulder so much that the athlete is left with limited mobility.

We have not found the Bristow procedure to be successful in subluxing shoulders or in hyperelastic patients. Better procedures have been developed for many patients who would have been candidates for this operation in the past. The evolution of these newer techniques allows us to be more exacting in our selection of patients.

The following is a detailed description of the Bristow procedure, adherence to which minimizes complications. The procedure is easily performed supine with an arm board. A folded towel should be placed under the scapula. Using a modified axillary approach (Fig. 26–13), the deltopectoral interval is identified and developed with the cephalic vein retracted laterally. The clavipectoral fascia is likewise incised. The conjoined tendon with 1/4 inch of bone is removed with a curved osteotome (Fig. 26–14) and allowed to retract distally. Care must be taken to identify and protect the musculocutaneous nerve. The remaining bleeding bone edge may be rubbed with bone wax, if necessary, to secure hemostasis. The subscapularis can be divided in line with its fibers with electrocautery between its upper two-thirds and lower one-third, beginning just medial to the bicipital groove (Fig. 26–15). Anatomical dissections performed in our laboratory have shown this interval to lie in the internervous plane between the upper and lower subscapular nerves. This is a safe interval for dissection, therefore, as the branches of the upper subscapular nerve supply innervation to the upper two-thirds of the subscapularis muscle and the lower subscapular nerve innervates the lower one-third of the muscle.[28a]

The capsule is separated from the subscapularis and incised in line with the subscapular interval. A blunt-tipped, three-pronged retractor is placed anteriorly on the scapular neck so that the following steps can be performed without cartilage damage (Fig. 26–16). The anterior glenoid rim is debrided down to bleeding bone. Using a 3.2-mm drill, a hole is created across the glenoid, parallel to the joint (Fig. 26–17). Using a depth gauge, measure the depth, add the bony block height, and subtract 5.0 mm. The block is then shaped to fit snugly against the prepared surface and secured in position with the appropriately sized malleolar screw (Fig. 26–18).

The inferior capsular flap is now pulled up and sutured to the superior capsular flap just lateral to the bony block (Fig. 26–19). Incising the inferior capsule at the glenoid rim may facilitate a tighter capsular closure if there is marked anteroinferior capsular redundancy. The shoulder is put through its range of motion. If it appears too tight, the conjoined tendon can be partially released in a controlled fashion to allow additional motion. Bleeding is controlled, and the muscles are allowed to return to their anatomical position. The wound is closed in the usual manner.

Postoperatively, the arm is placed in a sling; Codman's exercises begin the next day. Motion is encouraged out of the sling within the middle of the shoulder's range. Care is taken to avoid forced abduction and external rotation until healing progresses. Light weights are used to regain strength, again in the midportions of the range only. Strong abduction and external rotation are to be avoided lest the screw be dislodged; also avoid using the biceps against resistance. The bony block heals after three months, and more vigorous stretching and strengthening can be initiated.

The purpose of this procedure is to reinforce the middle and inferior capsule and glenohumeral ligament system. By transferring the tip of the coracoid process

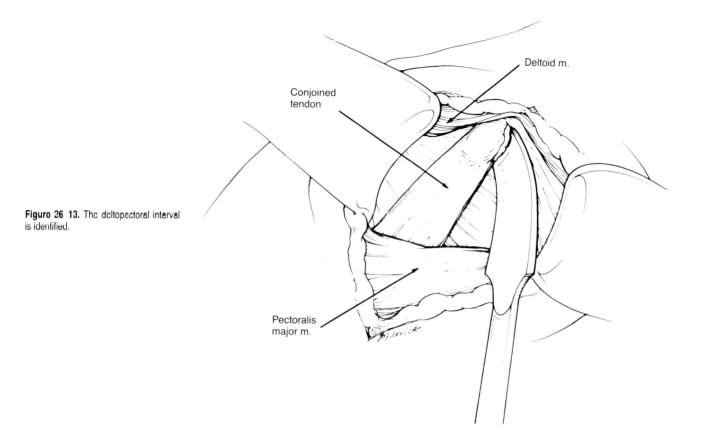

Figure 26-13. The deltopectoral interval is identified.

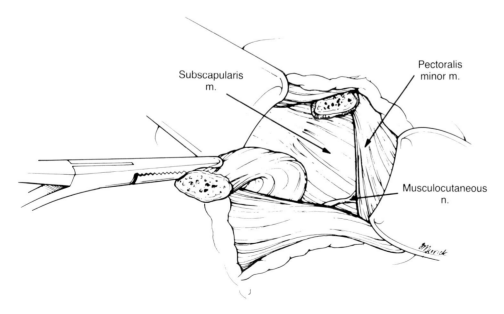

Figure 26–14. The conjoined tendon with 1/4 inch of bone is removed with a curved osteotome.

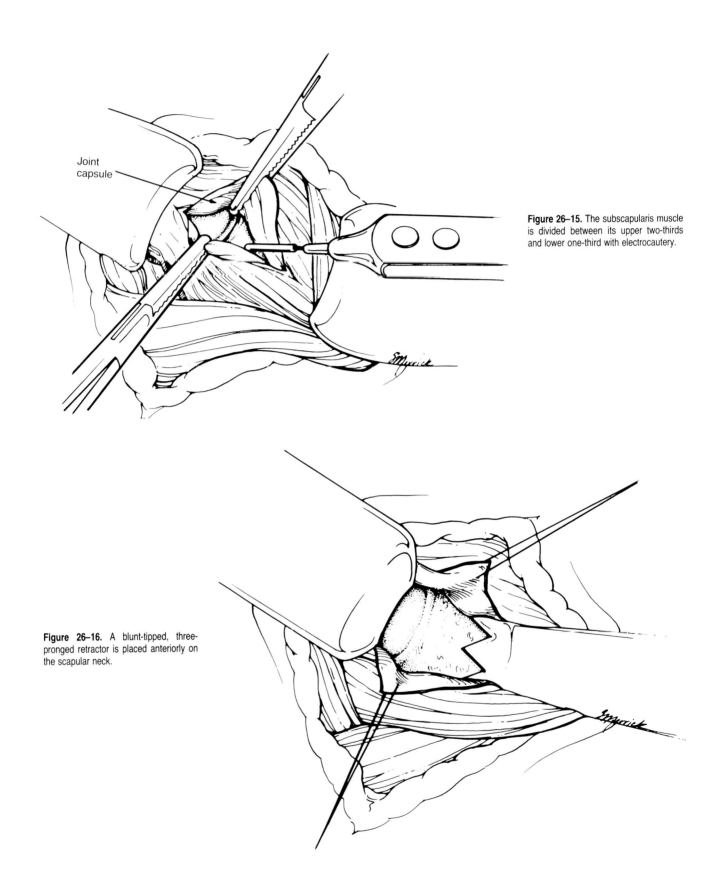

Joint
capsule

Figure 26–15. The subscapularis muscle is divided between its upper two-thirds and lower one-third with electrocautery.

Figure 26–16. A blunt-tipped, three-pronged retractor is placed anteriorly on the scapular neck.

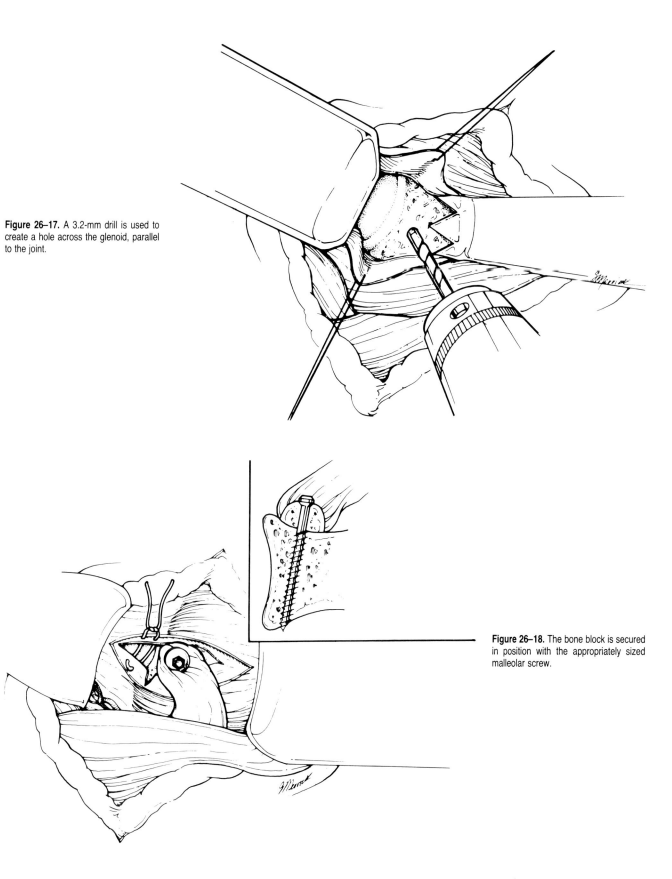

Figure 26–17. A 3.2-mm drill is used to create a hole across the glenoid, parallel to the joint.

Figure 26–18. The bone block is secured in position with the appropriately sized malleolar screw.

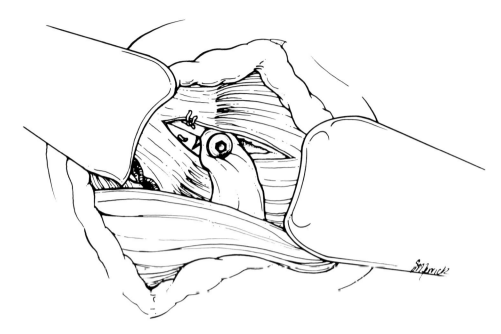

Figure 26–19. The inferior capsular flap is pulled up and sutured to the superior capsular flap just medial to the bony block.

with the attached compound tendon, the inferior portion of the subscapularis muscle is effectively tethered during abduction and external rotation of the arm. The superior excursion of this portion of the subscapularis muscle tendon unit is prevented, thus providing stability.

Arthroscopy

Any discussion of sports medicine raises the question of the proper place of arthroscopy in the management of shoulder problems. Properly used, the arthroscope is an invaluable tool that provides capabilities, especially in diagnosis, not afforded by other tools.

As with arthroscopy of other joints, shoulder arthroscopy can be divided into three main groups of procedures: (1) diagnostic, (2) those that remove unwanted materials, and (3) those that attempt to reconstruct various structures.

In our experience, the history, physical examination, and routine x-rays are diagnostic in at least 80 per cent of cases. The arthroscopic examination can be extremely valuable and can confirm the exact nature of the disease. For example, is a subluxing shoulder secondary to labral detachment or a stretched capsule? Is there any rotator cuff disease? Arthroscopy is superior to MRI and other radiographic techniques in its degree of resolution in viewing intra-articular structures. In cases of instability, arthroscopy allows positioning of the shoulder to observe subluxation. These positions cannot be achieved in the MRI gantry.

The question arises as to whether diagnostic arthroscopy can be performed under the same anesthesia with the open procedure without increasing the risk of infection. We believe that any increased risk stems from fluid extravasation into the surrounding soft tissues. We therefore limit diagnostic arthroscopy in these cases to the posterior portal only, limit the length of

the procedure to a maximum of five minutes, and then proceed with the operative procedure. If more portals are necessary, if more time is needed, or if excessive edema is noted, the open procedure is delayed.

Not only is diagnostic arthroscopy helpful in the treatment of the injured shoulder in the athlete, but arthroscopic removal of unwanted materials can often be the definitive procedure. Materials to be removed may include torn labrum, loose bodies, rheumatoid synovium, pus from pyarthrosis in the joint or in its subacromial bursa, and so on. If the material removed was formerly part of a stabilizing structure (e.g., labrum), the patient must be cautioned that although one symptomatic problem has been addressed (torn labral fragment), a second problem (an instability) may be unmasked and may require a second surgery. Parenthetically, we do no more rotator cuff debridement than is necessary for visualization of tears.

With regard to arthroscopic reconstructions, we regard them as techniques in development. The success rate of stapling, in the best of hands, is 80 per cent compared with 93 to 95 per cent for the Bankart and Bristow procedures performed openly. The apparent advantage of reduced early postoperative morbidity is less striking when one considers that these open procedures are among the least painful in shoulder surgery. Moreover, the length of time of postoperative immobilization is no different whether open or arthroscopic stabilization procedures are performed. Therefore, arthroscopic procedures do not shorten the recovery time for these individuals.

The ideal procedure for all athletes will repair and reinforce the anterior capsule and build up the anterior rim while simultaneously adjusting the laxity of the capsule. We now believe that a capsulolabral reconstruction often offers the most satisfactory answer to the problem of the pathological high-performance shoulder.[20]

Capsulolabral Reconstruction

The anterior capsulolabral reconstruction was devised for overhead throwing athletes with dominant arm involvement, who have documented anterior instability and in whom conservative treatment has failed.

Technique

The patient is placed supine on the operating table with the arm positioned on a Parker table or on two arm boards. To create stability and prominence of the humeral head, two or three folded surgical towels are placed along the vertebral border adjacent to the scapula. This will elevate the scapula and provide room to sublux the humeral head posteriorly for access to the anterior glenoid. Below the level of the coracoid, a 6- to 8-cm skin incision is made in line with a midaxillary skin fold in the relaxed skin tension lines. The skin is undermined in all directions, exposing the deltopectoral fascia and interval. Meticulous hemostasis is required for proper visualization. The anterior deltoid, cephalic vein, pectoralis major, and deltopectoral groove are identified. The deltopectoral fascia is split in line with the cephalic vein and freed along its pectoral border. Using Goulet retractors, the deltopectoral groove is opened while retracting the cephalic vein laterally with the deltoid and the pectoralis major medially. The lateral border of the conjoined tendon is identified and freed from surrounding tissues. The conjoined tendon is retracted medially with a long, narrow Richardson retractor. The superior border of the subscapularis is identified by the recess; the inferior border is identified by the anterior humeral circumflex vessels. Internal and external rotation of the humeral head helps to delineate the superior and inferior margins.

With the arm in external rotation (protecting the long head of the biceps) and using coagulating electrocautery, the subscapularis tendon is split in line with its fibers in its lower third (Fig. 26–20). Kocher clamps are then placed on the superior and inferior margins of the subscapularis to provide tension while the dissection progresses. Using a No. 15 surgical blade, the interval between the capsule and subscapularis is sharply defined. This is most easily accomplished at the myotendinous junction where the tendon and capsule are not so adherent. Meticulous dissection to define this interval is paramount. By lifting the superior and inferior edges, the interval may be more readily identified near the muscle border. Further separation superiorly, inferiorly, and medially is obtained by using a soft-tissue elevator. Improved exposure to the capsule is obtained by placing a blunted, three-pronged pitchfork retractor onto the scapular neck, preceded by a modified self-retaining, long-tonged Gelpi retractor placed beneath the superior and inferior margins of the cut subscapularis muscle and tendon. Better exposure to the joint capsule and the underlying glenohumeral joint can now be appreciated.

Near the center of the humeral head, a transverse capsulotomy is made parallel to the split in the subscapularis at approximately midjoint level and extended medially toward the bony glenoid rim, creating a superior and inferior flap. The capsulotomy is extended into a T by incising the capsule superiorly along the glenoid margin and inferiorly, taking care to protect the axillary nerve (Fig. 26–21). The "T-ing" of the capsule may need to be extended in either direction, depending on the redundancy of the capsule and the shift necessary to tighten it. With the completion of

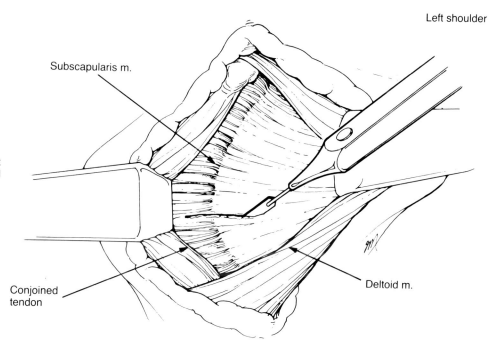

Figure 26–20. The subscapularis is split at the junction of the upper two-thirds and the lower one-third.

Subscapularis m.

Left shoulder

Conjoined tendon

Deltoid m.

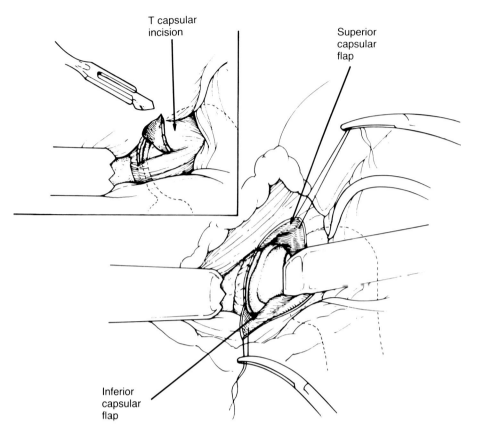

Figure 26–21. The capsulotomy is extended into a T.

the T capsulotomy, a narrow humeral-head retractor can be positioned in the joint. The point of the retractor should be situated on the posterior rim, taking care not to injure the articular cartilage of the glenoid fossa; in the proper position, the retractor can be used to lever the head posteriorly with minimal force. With both the subscapularis pitchfork and humeral-head retractors in proper position, the retraction can be balanced between the instruments. This provides good exposure to the anterior glenoid and scapular neck.

The operation is now tailored to the patient's degree of laxity. Based on the amount of observed laxity, a decision can usually be made during the operating procedure as to how the capsular flaps will be sutured onto the anterior glenoid rim. Leaving a small (1-mm) rim of capsule attached to the anterior glenoid, the soft tissue medial to the glenoid is incised sharply. It is then elevated sufficiently to allow for preparation of three anchoring bone holes along the anterior glenoid. The preparation of the glenoid neck allows proper visualization and placement of the holes and enables the repaired capsule to heal to bone. Using a right-angle drill or modified Bankart instruments, the bone holes are made in the anterior glenoid (Fig. 26–22). The drill is angled toward the anterior glenoid, aiming for an exit just inside the lip of the bony rim. The center hole is made first, followed by an inferior and then a superior hole. After drilling through the glenoid, the drill should be withdrawn by rotating the running drill toward the glenoid neck. This will facilitate insertion of the suture by approximating the U-shaped curve

of the needle. Tension is then placed on the stay suture in the inferior capsular flap to approximate its final position. Starting with the inferior hole, a No. 1 nonabsorbable Ethibond suture on a cutting needle is passed from outside to just inside the glenoid bony rim and through the capsule from outside to inside. The suture is then brought out through the capsule and through the middle hole in the glenoid rim, creating a horizontal mattress suture configuration. Another No. 1 nonabsorbable suture is inserted through the middle hole from outside to inside the glenoid rim and from outside to inside the capsular flap. This suture is passed back through the capsule and out through the superior hole (Fig. 26–23). The sutures are then tied to the neck of the glenoid. The inferior flap should lie down inside the anterior glenoid in an inverted fashion; this acts to recreate a reinforced labrum. The shift is reinforced by pulling the superior flap down over the inferior flap, using a pants-over-vest technique. The previously placed sutures can now be passed with a free needle through the superior flaps and tied on the outside (Fig. 26–24). This maneuver reinforces the anterior capsule at the site of the prior anterior instability (Fig. 26–25). The residual capsulotomy is then closed using simple vertical stitches (Fig. 26–26). The arm, in 20 degrees of forward flexion, should be abducted and externally rotated to determine the range of motion possible without disrupting the repair. Ideally, this safe zone allows 90 degrees of abduction and 45 degrees of external rotation. With the Gelpi self-retaining retractor removed, the subscapularis muscle

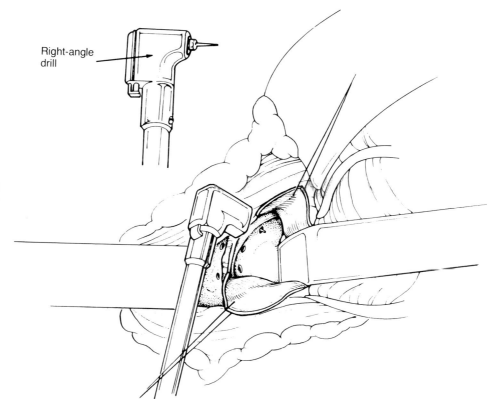

Right-angle drill

Figure 26–22. A right-angle drill is used to make three separate holes in the anterior glenoid rim.

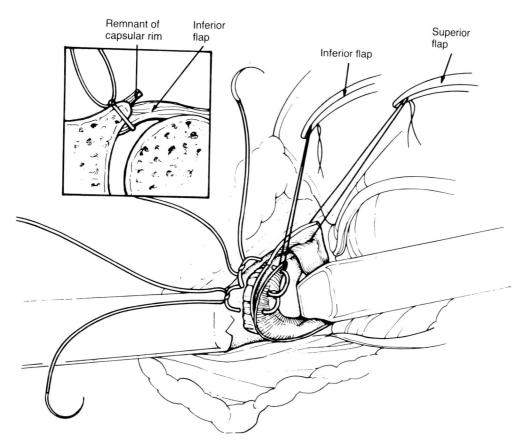

Remnant of capsular rim

Inferior flap

Inferior flap

Superior flap

Figure 26–23. The inferior capsular flap is shifted superiorly within the joint.

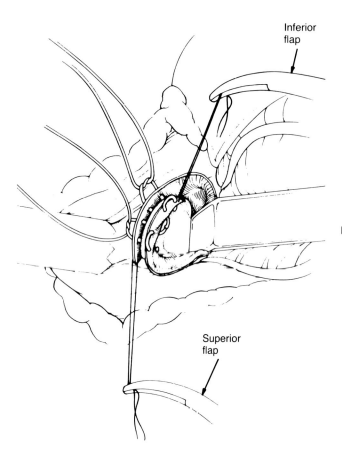

Figure 26–24. The superior capsular flap is shifted distally outside the joint.

Figure 26–25. The anterior capsule is now reinforced at the site of the prior anterior instability.

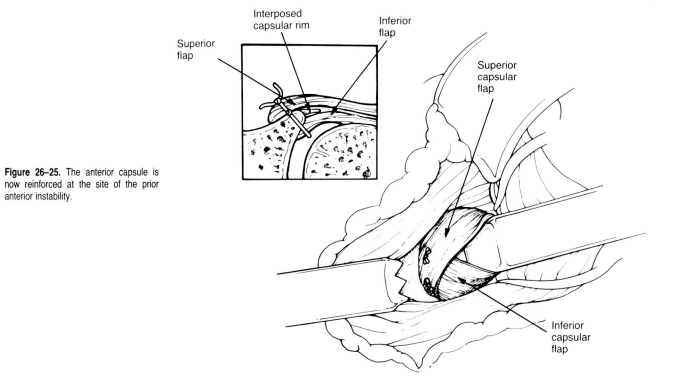

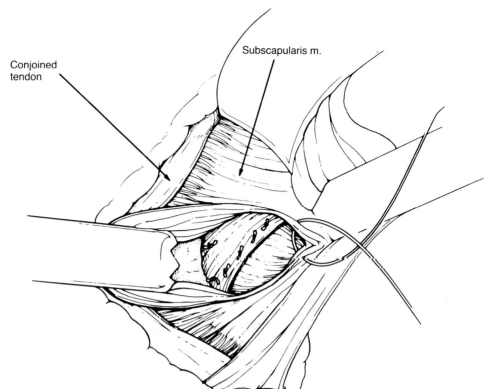

Conjoined
tendon

Subscapularis m.

Figure 26–26. The residual capsulotomy is closed with simple vertical stitches.

falls into place. The edges are reapproximated with simple inverted stitches. The subcutaneous tissue is approximated, and the skin is closed with a subcuticular running suture and Steri-Strips. A compression dressing is applied. The arm is placed in an abduction splint that should support the arm near 90 degrees of abduction and slight external rotation to allow healing in a more optimal position for postoperative motion.

Postoperative Rehabilitation Program

The patient is immobilized in an abduction brace (Fig. 26–27) for two weeks. The postoperative position is important: to regain full range of motion afterwards, the shoulder should be in 90 degrees of abduction, 30 degrees of forward flexion, and 45 degrees of external rotation. This is the optimal position for the throwing athlete; it places the shoulder in external rotation and prevents tightening of the anterior and inferior capsule. The abduction brace may be removed for gentle passive abduction, flexion, and external rotation twice daily and to allow the shoulder to adduct. Abduction–external rotation is performed in the plane of the scapula (20 to 30 degrees forward flexion). External rotation is not forced. The patient begins isometric adduction–forward flexion exercises and also active elbow flexion-extension strengthening exercises. Two weeks after surgery, the abduction splint is discontinued. Gentle range-of-motion exercises are continued with active internal rotation with the arm at the side to the neutral position, using surgical tubing as toler-

ated. Work on external rotation as tolerated, without placing so much stress on the capsule that the sutures are jeopardized. Shoulder shrugs are used to strengthen the trapezius.

Four to five weeks after surgery, sidelying external rotation exercises are begun, as well as supraspinatus-strengthening exercises. Shoulder abduction should be at 90 degrees by this time. Six to eight weeks after surgery, the continuing strengthening exercises are performed with emphasis on the rotator cuff muscles. At two to four months the weights are increased. By two months the patient should have full range of motion. Isokinetic strengthening and endurance shoulder flexion and abduction exercises are begun, using the faster speeds (240 degrees per second). At two and one-half months wall pushups begin, progressing to modified pushups on the knees and then military pushups. The arms are positioned at 70 to 80 degrees of abduction and the body is not lowered to the floor; this would place the shoulder in extension, stressing the anterior capsule. At four months the isokinetic strengthening exercises are performed at different speeds, again with emphasis on the higher speeds. An isokinetic test is usually performed at this point. The test is done over a three-day period so that the shoulder will not fatigue. If the isokinetic test indicates adequate strength and endurance (90 per cent or more of the other shoulder), the athlete may begin the throwing program. Five months after surgery, chin-ups are allowed and the throwing program progresses. At six months the strengthening and endurance exercises are

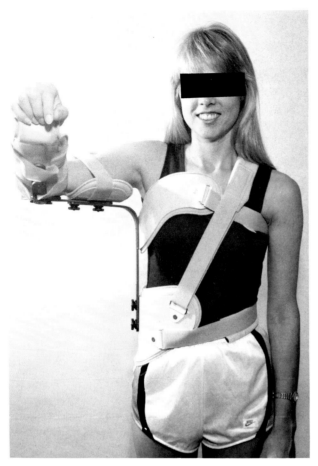

Figure 26–27. Postoperative splinting in 90-degree abduction, 30-degree forward flexion, and 45-degree external rotation.

continued with emphasis on the muscles needed specifically for the sport of interest, without neglecting total body conditioning.

Progressive Throwing Program

The program delineated here covers two and one-half to three months. For less serious shoulder injuries, it can be accelerated. At each step, the following three processes must be performed.

1. Warmup: Use heat as a warmup prior to stretching and throwing (hot pack, whirlpool, hot shower, etc.). The heat promotes soft tissue flexibility, increases circulation, and activates some of the natural lubricants of the body.

2. Stretching: Perform shoulder stretches after heat and then proceed with the throwing program.

3. Cool down: Apply ice after throwing to decrease cellular damage and lessen the inflammatory response to microtrauma.

Step 1. Toss the ball (no wind-up) 30 to 40 feet. Work out three to five times, 10 to 15 minutes per session, for a one-week period.

Step 2. Lob the ball (playing catch with little or no wind-up) no more than 30 feet. Continue three to five times, 10 to 15 minutes per session, for one week.

Step 3. Increase the distance to 40 to 50 feet while still lobbing the ball (easy wind-up). Schedule alternate days for the throwing and strengthening program. Increase the throwing time to 15 to 20 minutes per session, two to three times for one week.

Step 4. Increase the distance to 60 feet while still lobbing the ball, with an occasional straight throw at not more than half speed. Increase the throwing time to 20 to 25 minutes per session, two to three times per week.

Step 5. Perform long, easy throws from the midoutfield (150 to 200 feet), getting the ball barely back to home plate on five to six bounces. This is to be performed for 20 to 25 minutes per session on two consecutive days. Then rest the arm for one day. Repeat three times over a nine-day period, then progress to the next step if able to complete this sequence without pain or discomfort: throw two days, rest one day, throw two days, rest one day, etc.

Step 6. Perform long, easy throws from the deepest portion of the outfield, with the ball barely getting back to home plate on numerous bounces. This is to be performed for 25 to 30 minutes per session on two consecutive days. Rest for one day. Repeat the same routine over a nine-day period and progress to the next step if there is no pain or discomfort.

Step 7. Perform stronger throws from the midoutfield, getting the ball back to home plate on three to four bounces. Do this for 30 to 35 minutes per session on two consecutive days. Rest for one day. Repeat the same routine over a nine-day period. If there is no pain or discomfort, progress to the next step.

Step 8. Perform short, crisp throws with a relatively straight trajectory from the short outfield back to home plate on one bounce. These throws are to be performed for no more than 30 minutes on two consecutive days. Rest one day. Repeat over a nine-day period.

Step 9. Continue with the body conditioning program, i.e., strength, flexibility, and endurance. For days in which both strengthening and throwing are performed, schedule throwing in the morning and strengthening in the afternoon. If able to throw without pain or discomfort, proceed to the next step.

Step 10. Return to throwing from the normal position (i.e., the mound). The throw should be at 1/2 to 3/4 speed, with emphasis on technique and accuracy. Throw for two consecutive days, then rest for one day. A throwing session should not last longer than 25 minutes. Repeat this sequence three times over the next nine days, then advance to the next step if there is no pain or discomfort.

Step 11. Throw from the normal position at 3/4 to full speed. Throw for two consecutive days and rest for one day; continue this sequence for nine days. Sessions should not last longer than 30 minutes.

Step 12. Simulate a game-day situation for six innings. Warmup with an appropriate number of pitches and throw for an average number of innings, taking the usual rest breaks between innings. Repeat this simulation a couple of times with a three- to four-day rest between simulations.

Posterior Shoulder Problems in the Athlete

INSTABILITY

Athletes very rarely suffer a posterior shoulder dislocation. Commonly, they present with repeated episodes of posterior shoulder subluxation. This occurs in one of two ways: (1) from overuse, which stretches out the posterior capsule, or (2) from one traumatic episode that results in subluxation with stretching of the posterior capsule, which then recurs with repeated use of the shoulder. For example, a pitcher will stress his posterior capsule repeatedly in the follow-through phase of throwing. If he overthrows or does not warm up properly or limits his follow-through by poor lower-body mechanics, he can injure the posterior capsule, which will lead to repeated subluxation. Another example is a quarterback who falls on his outstretched hand while being tackled and feels something pull in the posterior aspect of his shoulder. He may or may not feel that his shoulder came out of the joint. When he recovers from this acute injury, he notices that he has posterior pain with throwing and cannot throw with the same velocity. On examination he may have pain over the posterior shoulder joint, but he may also present with pain over the biceps and rotator cuff, as in a typical impingement syndrome. It may take a number of examinations on different occasions to ascertain that the problem is instability rather than impingement. Usually, the position of pain is in forward flexion at 90 degrees and internal rotation. It may also be possible to sublux the shoulder in this position. If this is not possible, the patient should be positioned supine with the affected shoulder over the edge of the examination table; an attempt is made, while grasping the humeral head, to sublux the humeral head posteriorly. This is usually done by forward flexion and the application of a posterior longitudinal thrust to the arm in an attempt to sublux the shoulder. It must be remembered that the athlete in this group may be able to voluntarily sublux his shoulder posteriorly. He can often demonstrate the instability on a clinical examination. These athletes are usually not psychologically disturbed and do not use their shoulder instability for secondary gain. They can be treated exactly the same as the athlete who cannot voluntarily dislocate his shoulder.

Occasionally, in the well-muscled athlete the instability cannot be defined in the clinical examination. Examination under anesthesia, as well as arthroscopy, usually will be necessary to determine the correct diagnosis.

Pathological findings are different from those found with anterior instability. The true reverse Bankart lesion is usually not seen. The labrum may be shallow and poorly developed, but it is almost always intact and not torn away from the posterior glenoid. The capsule is usually redundant. The initial management of these athletes is conservative, with an extensive physical therapy program. The physical therapist is instructed to strengthen the external rotators—namely, the infraspinatus and teres minor—as well as the posterior deltoid. Biofeedback may have a place in this form of instability, as described by Beall and associates.[6] The exercise program lasts for at least six months. Coaches work on follow-through technique to allow the leg muscles to accept much of the stress that the athlete had been placing on the posterior shoulder.

Usually, with a conservative program approximately two-thirds of the athletes note subjective improvement. The instability is often not eliminated, but the functional disability is improved so that the athlete can perform without problem.[19]

Management of athletes with recurrent posterior shoulder subluxation who do not respond to conservative care is controversial. The results of surgical reconstruction for posterior instability have been disappointing.[18, 41]

Posterior Capsulorrhaphy

Our recommended procedure is a posterior capsulorrhaphy. Initially the capsulorrhaphy was performed by stapling, but in the last five years a suture technique has been used. The patient is placed on the operating table in the lateral decubitus position with the involved shoulder superior and draped free. He is held in position with a Vacupack, supporting posts, and kidney rests. The operating table is placed in slight reverse Trendelenburg position. The peroneal nerve should be protected where it crosses the neck of the fibula on the inferior leg. A saber incision is made on the superior aspect of the shoulder, beginning just posterior to the acromioclavicular joint and continuing posteriorly toward the posterior axillary fold (Fig. 26–28). This incision is usually about 10 cm in length. The subcutaneous tissues are undermined to expose the deltoid. The deltoid is split (Fig. 26–29) from an area on the spine 2 to 3 cm medial to the posterolateral corner of the acromion, distally approximately 5 to 6 cm. The deltoid should not be split below the level of the teres minor because the axillary nerve, which enters the deltoid at the inferior border of the teres minor, might be damaged. It is usually not necessary to reflect the deltoid from the spine or acromion, except occasionally in a well-muscled individual. The teres minor and infraspinatus are encountered below the fascia, deep to the deltoid. The interval between these muscles is not always apparent (Fig. 26–30). An important landmark is the raphe between the two heads of the infraspinatus, which is a bipennate muscle. This raphe should not be confused with the interval between the teres minor and the infraspinatus, which is usually below the equator of the humeral head. The interval between these two muscles is developed by blunt dissection, and retractors are placed to expose the posterior shoulder capsule (Fig. 26–31).

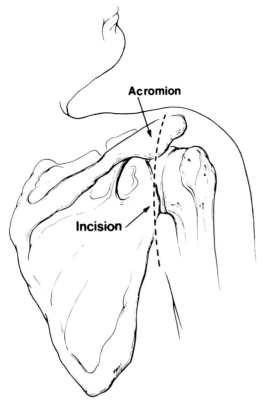

Figure 26–28. The incision is made superiorly, beginning posterior to the acromio clavicular joint and directed toward the posterior axillary fold.

The capsule needs to be freed from the muscles; this must be done by sharp dissection laterally since the capsule is adherent to the tendons of the teres minor and infraspinatus. Medially, this can be done with a periosteal elevator. Once the capsule is sufficiently freed from the overlying muscles, a transverse arthrotomy is made into the posterior capsule from lateral to medial, down to but not into the labrum. The joint is

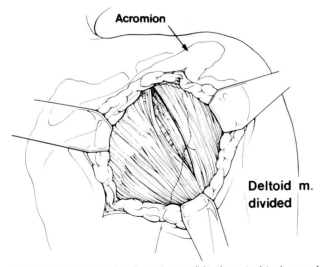

Figure 26–29. The deltoid is split 2 to 3 cm medial to the posterolateral corner of the acromion.

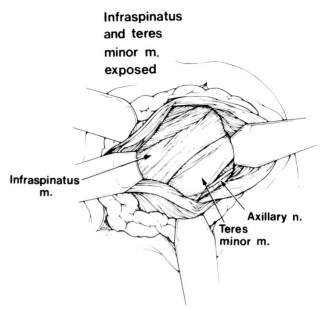

Figure 26–30. The teres minor and infraspinatus muscles are exposed; the axillary nerve enters the deltoid below the teres minor.

inspected. Two capsular flaps are developed by T-ing the capsule parallel to the glenoid and just adjacent to the labrum. These are tagged with suture to control the flaps. The inferior capsular flap must be carefully developed because of the close proximity of the axillary nerve. If the labrum is intact, as is usually the case, the sutures can be placed directly into the labrum. If the labrum is torn, it needs to be reflected so that bone holes can be made and sutures passed directly through the bone, as is done in a Bankart repair anteriorly. The inferior capsule flap is then advanced superiorly and medially and attached to the glenoid labrum with No. 1 Ethibond sutures (Fig. 26–32). This usually eliminates the posterior as well as any inferior instability. The superior capsular flap is then sutured over the inferior flap by advancing it inferiorly and medially (Fig. 26–33). There may still be a transverse gap in the capsule laterally; this is closed with interrupted mattress sutures. The teres minor and infraspinatus fall together and usually do not need any sutures. The deltoid fascia, which has been split, is then repaired (Fig. 26–34).

Postoperatively, the patient's arm and shoulder are immobilized in a position of 30 degrees of abduction and neutral rotation for three weeks.

Postoperative Rehabilitation Program

Isometric exercises are begun in the immediate postoperative period for the deltoid and the rotator cuff muscles. After three weeks of isometric exercise, active and active-assisted range of motion is begun. The emphasis is on elevation in the scapular plane of the body and on regaining rotation. From four to six weeks postoperatively, no motion is performed in the sagittal plane—i.e., forward flexion—to avoid placing in-

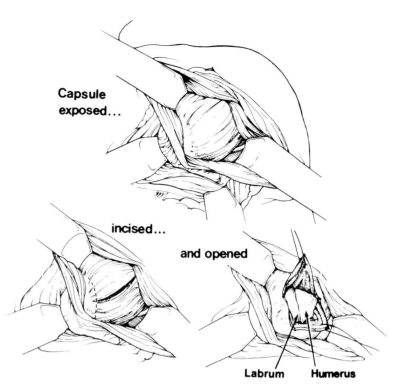

Figure 26–31. The capsule is exposed; a transverse arthrotomy is made in the posterior capsule from lateral to medial. Two capsular flaps are developed by "T-ing" the capsule parallel to the glenoid and adjacent to the labrum.

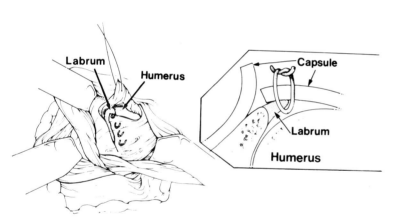

Figure 26–32. The inferior capsular flap is advanced superiorly and medially and attached to the labrum.

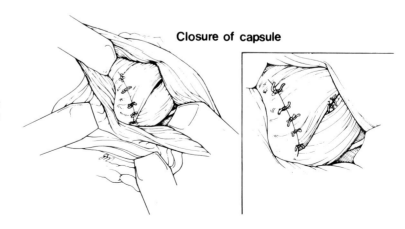

Figure 26–33. The superior flap is sutured over the inferior flap by advancing it inferiorly and medially. The lateral split in the capsule is closed with interrupted mattress sutures.

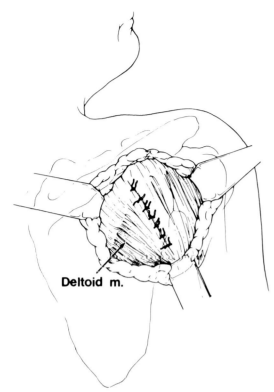

Figure 26–34. The deltoid fascia, which has been split, is repaired.

creased stress on the newly repaired posterior capsule and soft tissues. At six weeks, forward flexion is allowed. At 12 weeks, resistance beyond 90 degrees of elevation can be added to increase strength and endurance. Attention should be focused on regaining synchrony of the scapular rotators, rotator cuff, and deltoid. When this is firmly re-established, the athlete may return to his sport. It will usually take another six months to develop the endurance necessary to return to competitive throwing.

Posterior shoulder repair can allow an athlete to return to his former throwing ability. Many athletes with posterior instability have little functional disability other than in their sport. The difficulty of returning to competitive throwing should not be underestimated; however, with careful surgical selection and meticulous rehabilitation, return is possible.

POSTERIOR LESIONS

Throwing athletes commonly have posterior glenoid spurs visible on x-rays. These may or may not be symptomatic. Bennett described calcification in the posterior aspect of the shoulder.[7] The symptom complex included pain referred to the posterior deltoid; it should be noted that not every pitcher had the lesion. The size of this lesion was not related to the symptoms. Occasionally, such lesions are noted in asymptomatic shoulders. Symptoms may develop gradually with increasing severity or, alternatively, may have a sudden

onset. Bennett described an x-ray view to demonstrate the spur—an anteroposterior view of the glenohumeral joint with the machine tilted 5 degrees cephalad and the arm positioned in abduction and external rotation, as in the cocking position of throwing. The scapula is then rotated to a position that shows the exostosis on the inferior glenoid. A conventional axillary lateral view often shows the bone spur in this area as well.

In our experience the lesion itself is often asymptomatic. However, when there is a fracture in the spur or a fibrous union at its base, the resultant symptoms will interfere with pitching. Rest in these cases results in pain-free motion during normal activities and exercise. A return to pitching, however, causes severe pain by the third inning. We believe that the motion imparted to the spur during the act of pitching at full velocity causes the irritation that produces pain.

These athletes usually respond to conservative care, which includes not only rest but also anti-inflammatory medication and steroid injections. Athletes whose pain prevents them from throwing effectively have responded to an operative approach with resection of the spur either arthroscopically or through the same deltoid-splitting approach described earlier. By exposing the capsule between the infraspinatus and teres minor, the capsule is opened and the spur identified and removed. The athlete usually can return to competitive throwing about six months after surgery. The etiological process is probably a traction phenomenon on the posterior glenoid. Lombardo and colleagues reported four cases with successful return to competition after spur removal.[31]

Acromioclavicular Joint Problems

Acromioclavicular joint disease occurs in athletes who participate in sports requiring weightlifting or repetitive overhead activity, or in athletes sustaining direct trauma to this area. This is a chronic condition, and arthritic changes can develop. Most athletes who have failed a course of anti-inflammatory medication and injection respond well to the removal of the distal 1/4 inch of the clavicle, as described by Mumford.[33a] Baseball pitchers, hockey players, and weightlifters have been treated successfully without loss of function, strength, or motion following the procedure.[10]

Acute injury to the acromioclavicular joint is common in collision sports such as football or hockey. Typically, a player falls on the point of the shoulder, either by being tackled or by making a tackle; hockey players are checked into the boards. The treatment is controversial, but it is our opinion that athletes do better with a nonoperative approach. This is true whether the injury is Grade I, II, or III. No attempt is made to reduce the shoulder with an apparatus or splint. The shoulder is immobilized in a sling for comfort for a few days to a week, and then a rehabilitation program is begun. The athlete in football or hockey can usually return to play in about three to four weeks, even after a Grade III dislocation. We have operated only on those Grade III injuries in which the deformity would interfere with activity.

Residual weakness after closed treatment had been studied.[14, 34, 50] A recent study conducted in our office evaluated 20 athletes with Grade III acromioclavicular dislocations treated conservatively.[45] No strength deficits were noted at the lower isokinetic speeds of 60 degrees and 120 degrees per second. The only deficit noted was a slight decrease in shoulder extension at 120 degrees per second. These athletes had minor subjective complaints about their shoulders but denied functional difficulties.

Occasionally, an athlete will have late problems with pain over the acromioclavicular area from a previous injury. These athletes usually have developed degenerative changes after a Grade I or II dislocation. A Mumford procedure is the treatment of choice. Athletes requiring such a procedure should be advised that there is a risk of loss of maximum bench press strength and possible weakness of shoulder flexion and extension. Pain relief is excellent, however, as is the rate of return to competitive sports, including pitching.[10]

A transverse cut is made over the acromioclavicular joint, the clavicle is identified, and the periosteum is elevated with a small elevator. A power saw is used to remove 1/4 inch of the distal clavicle. The shoulder is tested through its arc of motion to ensure that the clavicle is no longer impinging against the acromion. There is a tendency among surgeons to remove too much bone. The edges are smoothed and a piece of Gelfoam is sutured into the wound, closing the interval. A pursestring suture is then placed in the soft tissues of the enlarged joint space, and the tissues are drawn down into this space. The subcutaneous tissue and skin are closed in the usual fashion, and the arm is placed in a sling for comfort.

Motion is encouraged immediately in the postoperative period. Most patients can return to their athletic activities within four months; baseball pitchers usually require six months.

Neurological Problems

QUADRILATERAL SPACE SYNDROME

Cahill and Palmer described the quadrilateral space syndrome in 1983.[9] The axillary nerve is compressed by fibrous bands in the quadrilateral space. Compression occurs when the athlete abducts and externally rotates the arm, as in the cocking motion in throwing. The athlete presents with posterior shoulder pain, usually in the area of the teres minor. The pain is exacerbated in the abducted and externally rotated position. The neurological examination is usually normal. Electromyographic studies are not helpful. The diagnosis is confirmed by an arteriogram of the subclavian artery, which visualizes the posterohumeral circumflex artery as it passes through the quadrilateral space. The posterohumeral circumflex artery is patent when the arm is at the side and occludes when the arm is brought into the abducted and externally rotated position. It is helpful to perform comparative studies on both arms to look for anatomical variation. In the athlete with this condition, rest and cortisone injections in this area may help to relieve the pressure on the axillary nerve. If the symptoms persist, an operative decompression of the quadrilateral space is indicated. This can be performed through a posterior approach, going inferior to the deltoid and releasing the teres minor tendon to decompress the axillary nerve.[8] The results have been favorable in the athlete.

SUPRASCAPULAR NERVE ENTRAPMENT

Suprascapular nerve entrapment occurs most often at the suprascapular notch area in the general population. In the athlete, however, the nerve is often entrapped distally as it passes around the base of the acromion to innervate the infraspinatus. The supraspinatus muscle is spared. Athletes present with varied pain symptoms, often misdiagnosed as tendinitis. On close examination there is obvious atrophy of the infraspinatus muscle. It should be noted that the supraspinatus is minimally involved, if at all. This condition is seen in high-level, hard-throwing pitchers. It has been our experience that if the nerve lesion is at the scapular spine, the condition does not respond well to surgical management.

The infraspinatus is not completely denervated. We have had good results with maximizing the residual infraspinatus muscle function with a daily exercise program to allow the high-level athlete to return to major league pitching. This is consistent with findings that, in throwing, the infraspinatus is seldom called upon for more than 30 to 40 per cent of its maximum strength.[17] Therefore, if the infraspinatus can be maximized to perform near this reduced level, pitching at the previous level of competition is possible.

Vascular Problems

AXILLARY ARTERY

Wright described occlusion of the axillary artery when the arm was brought overhead.[51] He believed that the second portion of the axillary artery was occluded by pressure of the overlying pectoralis minor muscle. This occlusion can be observed in a normal individual and can be demonstrated by angiography. Tullos and associates described occlusion of the axillary artery during pitching;[46] they thought that transient occlusion of the axillary artery was due to the stretching of the pectoralis minor that occurred with each pitch. In rare instances, sufficient local trauma occurred over time to produce intimal damage and subsequent thrombosis. The axillary vein may also be involved.

The clinical presentation includes a variety of signs and symptoms, which are often nonspecific. The diagnosis is difficult. The athlete may complain of fatigue and muscle ache, lack of endurance, or intermittent paresthesia. He may report increased fatigue and loss of control. If there are no objective findings, the symptoms may be dismissed as minor or psychosomatic. Alternatively, presentation can include loss of pulses, cyanosis, and decreased skin temperature with claudication—symptoms that make the diagnosis evident. When the diagnosis is suspected, an arteriogram is usually necessary for confirmation. Vascular surgery relieves the blockage, by either excision with reanastomosis or a bypass graft. In one well-known case involving a professional baseball pitcher, progression of the thrombus resulted in a cerebrovascular accident with subsequent partial paralysis.

AXILLARY VEIN THROMBOSIS

Thrombosis of the axillary vein was originally described by Paget in 1875 and by van Schrocther in 1884.[2] This condition has been called "effort thrombosis" because of its association with a forceful event that produces injury to the vein. It usually occurs in active, athletic individuals and is usually preceded by strenuous effort or repetitive action. The athlete presents with pain and swelling in the arm. Objectively, there may be venous distention involving the upper extremity with secondary cyanosis. A venogram will confirm the diagnosis. The treatment is usually conservative, with rest and elevation. Anticoagulation is used in the initial phases to avoid progression of the thrombus. Following the initial episode, the athlete may continue to complain of exertional claudication.

Vogel and Jensen reported a college swimmer suffering effort thrombosis of the subclavian vein.[49] They believed that this was an unusual presentation of a thoracic outlet syndrome, although various provocative maneuvers did not cause any alteration in the radial pulse. A venogram revealed complete occlusion of the subclavian vein in the area of the first rib. Treatment consisted of intravenous streptokinase, heparin, and Coumadin. After four months, the first rib was removed and the patient became asymptomatic. Vogel and Jensen thought that the most common site of compression of the subclavian vein was between the first rib and the clavicle in the costoclavicular area, but that the tendons of the pectoralis minor as well as the head of the humerus can also compress the axillary vein on its anterior aspect with shoulder adduction. In establishing the diagnosis, it is important that the physical findings during the examination be exacerbated by exercising the arm.

The Shoulder in Swimming

Kennedy and Hawkins reported that approximately 3 to 4 per cent of Canadian swimmers complained of shoulder pain, agreeing with Macnab and Rathbun who found an avascular area at the supraspinatus insertion on the humerus in the area of the biceps as it passes over the humeral head.[26, 27, 32] Swimmers in training may swim 10,000 meters a day, six days a week, twelve months a year, which exposes this vulnerable area in the shoulder to an overuse syndrome.

The shoulder mechanics in the different strokes are slightly different, as described by Richardson and coworkers.[39] The upper-extremity propulsion power in all strokes derives from adduction and internal rotation of the shoulder using the pectoralis major, subscapularis, teres major, and latissimus dorsi muscles. Coaches teach their swimmers not to drop their elbows during the pull-through or recovery phases because this places the internal rotators at a mechanical disadvantage by increasing the posture of relative external rotation.

Hand paddle training usually exacerbates shoulder pain. The purpose of the hand paddle is to increase hand resistance in the water by increasing the load and the time spent in the pull-through phase.

Prevention of injury must include decreasing distance and exercising the posterior structures of the shoulder, emphasizing the external rotators (to balance the hypertrophied internal rotators) and the scapular rotators. If a scapular lag develops from fatigue, the swimming motion is altered in such a way as to impinge the anterior structures.

The swimming athlete usually presents with anterolateral pain that is diffuse in nature, reporting that the pain usually occurs during the recovery and pull-through phases of the stroke. The most common treatment for competitive swimmers is conservative: ice, decreased distance, heat, rest, ultrasound, oral medication, and, rarely, steroid injection. At present it does not appear that surgery to remove the coracoacromial ligament or an acromioplasty is compatible with continued high-level participation.

Swimmers also commonly present with "bicipital tendinitis." This is only a small part of the problem; if treatment is directed only to the biceps tendon, symptoms will persist because there is almost always involvement of the rotator cuff.[39]

Although the strokes are different, remarkable similarities exist in the shoulder motions of free-style swimming, the butterfly, and the backstroke. All three use adduction with internal rotation and abduction with external rotation. Forward flexion and extension while the arm is in abduction is minimal, and decreased body roll with increased abducted flexion and extension of the shoulder may be a factor in producing symptoms. A breast stroker who complains of shoulder pain is probably using one of the other three strokes during the majority of the practice session, and it is this practice stroke that is causing the symptoms.

Stroke modification can sometimes help to relieve the impingement syndrome. In free-style swimming, the middle fingers should enter the water first. If the thumb enters the water first, there is too much internal rotation of the shoulder, which may cause an impingement syndrome. Conversely, by increasing elbow height in the recovery phase and increasing body roll, an impingement syndrome can sometimes be relieved.

Swimmers tend to have increased motion in their shoulders, and many can also sublux their shoulders. Often an asymptomatic posterior subluxation is present. These swimmers tend to overdevelop their internal rotators and neglect the external rotators. If the athlete has symptoms of subluxation, a conservative program that strengthens the external rotators is warranted. Surgery is seldom indicated.

Kennedy and colleagues reported on swimmers with positive apprehension signs, most frequently in the backstroke.[26, 27] They wrote that the swimmer may be subluxing the shoulder anteriorly when he enters his flip turn. At this stage, the shoulder is in full abduction and external rotation and the hand is used to push off the wall. Shoulder cineradiography found that the humeral head was subluxing anteriorly onto the rim of the glenoid. On examination, the athlete commonly has an apprehension sign and the shoulder can be subluxed anteriorly. The swimmer has three alternatives: (1) tolerate the apprehension and the minor discomfort that occurs in the active phase of the backstroke turn, (2) change the format of the turn, or (3) consider surgical intervention. Although Kennedy and associates recommended a Putti-Platt procedure, we believe that this is unlikely to help a competitive swimmer. Surgery should only be considered as a last resort, and the procedure of choice is an anterior capsulolabral reconstruction.

McMasters also reported anterior glenolabral damage in swimmers.[33] He described a patient population with labral injuries producing functional instability without anatomical instability. This group can occasionally be helped by arthroscopically resecting the damaged part of the labrum. However, the patient should be warned that the labral debridement may actually increase the instability. We also believe that a capsulolabral reconstruction may be warranted. McMasters thought that the best surgical candidate was one with minimal or no apprehension in abduction and external rotation. He believed that the pain was due to the labrum's catching during the swimming motion with its internal rotation and adduction. He reported dramatic relief of symptoms from debridement of the damaged labrum and that converting such a patient into a subluxer was infrequent. It must be remembered that the group of patients who can be helped by arthroscopic surgery is very select. By and large, instability in a swimmer usually results from overuse and should be treated conservatively.

Conclusion

Sports medicine has evolved rapidly. Goals have changed and techniques have improved. We have come to focus on the overhead throwing athlete as the template for specific shoulder pathology. The intricacies of shoulder kinematics and musculoskeletal interaction require additional study before we can achieve a satisfactory level of understanding. The concept of return to function involves much more stringent criteria in this population; we are only beginning to approach this goal.

Acknowledgments • The authors acknowledge with gratitude the important contribution of C. E. Brewster, R.P.T., who provided the detailed descriptions of the rehabilitation programs so essential to successful care. D. Moynes Schwab provided invaluable assistance in the writing of this chapter.

References

1. Aamoth GM, and O'Phelan EH: Recurrent anterior dislocation of the shoulder: a review of forty athletes treated by subscapularis transfer. Am J Sports Med 5:188, 1977.
2. Adams JT, and Deweese JA: "Effort" thrombosis of the axillary and subclavian veins. J Trauma 11:923, 1970.
3. Atwater AE: Biomechanics of overarm throwing movements and of throwing injuries. Exerc Sport Sci Rev 7:43–85, 1979.
4. Atwater AE: Cinematographic analysis of overarm and sidearm throwing patterns. Am Assoc Health Phys Ed Rec. Abstracts 1968, p 81.
5. Barnes DA, and Tullos HS: An analysis of 100 symptomatic baseball players. Am J Sports Med 6:62–67, 1978.
6. Beall SM, Dufenbach G, and Allen A: Electromyographic biofeedback in the treatment of voluntary posterior instability of the shoulder. Am J Sports Med 15:175–178, 1987.
7. Bennett GE: Elbow and shoulder lesions of baseball players. Am J Surg 98:484–488, 1959.
8. Brodsky JW, Tullos HS, and Gartsman GM: Simplified posterior approach to the shoulder joint. J Bone Joint Surg 69A:773–774, 1987.
9. Cahill BR, and Palmer RE: Quadrilateral space syndrome. J Hand Surg 8:65–69, 1983.
10. Cook FF, and Tibone JE: The Mumford procedure in athletes—an objective analysis of function. Am J Sports Med. 16(2):97–100, 1988.
11. Dominquez RH: Coracoacromial ligament resection for severe swimmer's shoulder. In Erikson B (ed): Swimming Medicine IV. Baltimore: University Park Press, 1978, pp 110–114.
12. Gainor BJ, Piotrowski G, Puhl J, et al: The throw: biomechanics and acute injury. Am J Sports Med 8:114–118, 1980.
13. Garth WP, Allman FL, and Armstrong WS: Occult anterior subluxation of the shoulder. Am J Sports Med 15(6):579–585, 1987.
14. Glick JM, Milburn LJ, Haggerty JF, and Nishimoto D: Dislocated acromioclavicular joint: follow-up study of 35 unreduced acromioclavicular dislocations. Am J Sports Med 5(6):264–270, 1977.

15. Glousman RE, Jobe FW, Tibone JE, et al: Dynamic EMG analysis of the throwing shoulder with glenohumeral instability. J Bone Joint Surg 70A:220–226, 1988.

16. Glousman RE: The relationship of instability to rotator cuff damage—conservative and surgical repair. AAOS Course in Athletic Injuries to the Shoulder, September 1987, Beverly Hills, California.

17. Gowan ID, Jobe FW, Tibone JE, et al: A comparative EMG analysis of the shoulder during pitching. Am J Sports Med 15(6):586–590, 1988.

18. Hawkins RJ, Koppert G, and Johnston G: Recurrent posterior instability (subluxation) of the shoulder. J Bone Joint Surg 66A:169–174, 1984.

19. Hurley JA, Anderson TE, Dear W, et al: Posterior shoulder instability: surgical vs non-surgical results. Orthop Trans 11:458, 1987.

20. Jobe FW, Giangarra CE, Glousman RE, et al: Relationship of instability and impingement in throwing athletes: review of the anterior capsulolabral reconstruction. Paper presented at ASES, Las Vegas, Nevada, February, 1989.

21. Jobe FW, Moynes DR, Tibone JE, et al: An EMG analysis of the shoulder in throwing and pitching: a second report. Am J Sports Med 12:218–220, 1984.

22. Jobe FW, and Moynes DR: Delineation of diagnostic criteria and a rehabilitation program for rotator cuff injuries. Am J Sports Med 10(6):336–339, 1982.

23. Jobe FW, Tibone JE, Perry J, et al: An EMG analysis of the shoulder in throwing and pitching: a preliminary report. Am J Sports Med 11(1):3–5, 1983.

24. Jobe FW, and Jobe CM: Painful athletic injuries of the shoulder. Clin Orthop 173:117–124, 1983.

25. Jobe FW: Rotator cuff problems in the athlete. Paper presented at AAOS Specialty Day AOSSM, Atlanta, Georgia, February 1988.

26. Kennedy JC, and Hawkins RJ: Swimmer's shoulder. Phys Sports Med 2:34–38, 1974.

27. Kennedy JC, Hawkins RJ, and Krusoff WB: Orthopedic manifestations of swimming. Am J Sports Med 6:309–322, 1978.

28. King JE, Brelsford H, and Tullos HS: Analysis of the pitching arm of the professional baseball pitcher. Clin Orthop 67:116–123, 1969.

28a. King W, and Perry J: Personal communication, 1989.

29. Lindner E: The phenomenon of the freedom of lateral deviation in throwing. In Biomechanics II. Baltimore: University Park Press, 1971, pp 240–245.

30. Lombardo SJ, Kerlan RK, Jobe FW, et al: The Modified Bristow procedure for recurrent dislocation of the shoulder. J Bone Joint Surg 58A:256–261, 1976.

31. Lombardo SJ, Jobe FW, Kerlan RK, et al: Posterior shoulder lesions in throwing athletes. Am J Sports Med 5:106–110, 1977.

32. Macnab I, and Rathbun JB: The microvascular pattern of the rotator cuff. J Bone Joint Surg 52B:544–553, 1973.

33. McMasters WC: Anterior glenoid labrum damage: a painful lesion in swimmers. Am J Sports Med 14:383–387, 1986.

33a. Mumford EB: Acromioclavicular dislocations. J Bone Joint Surg 23:799–802, 1941.

34. Nelson G, Wojtys E, and Goldstein S: Operative vs nonoperative treatment of acromioclavicular separations. Paper presented at AAOS Specialty Day AOSSM, Atlanta, Georgia, 1988.

35. Nuber GW, Gowan ID, Moynes DR, and Antonelli D: EMG analysis of classical shoulder motion. Trans Orthop 11, 1986.

36. Nuber GW, Jobe FW, Perry J, et al: Fine wire electromyography analysis of muscles of the shoulder during swimming. Am J Sports Med 14:7–11, 1986.

37. Perry J: Anatomy and biomechanics of the shoulder in throwing, swimming, gymnastics and tennis. Symposium on injuries to the shoulder in the athlete. Clin Sports Med 2:247–270, 1983.

38. Poppen NK, and Walker PS: Normal and abnormal motion of the shoulder. J Bone Joint Surg 58A:195, 1976.

39. Richardson AR, Jobe FW, and Collins HR: The shoulder in competitive swimming. Am J Sports Med 8:159, 1980.

40. Rockwood CA: Editorial: shoulder arthroscopy. J Bone Joint Surg 70A:639–640, 1988.

41. Rowe C, and Zarins B: Recurrent transient subluxation of the shoulder. J Bone Joint Surg 63A:863–871, 1981.

42. Samuelson RE, and Miller E: Posterior dislocations of the shoulder. Clin Orthop 32:69–86, 1964.

43. Tibone JE, Elrod B, Jobe FW, et al: Surgical treatment of tears of the rotator cuff in athletes. J Bone Joint Surg 68A:887–891, 1986.

44. Tibone JE, Jobe FW, Kerlan RF, et al: Shoulder impingement syndrome in athletes treated by anterior acromioplasty. Clin Orthop 188:134–140, 1985.

45. Tibone JE, Sellers R, and Tonino P: Strength testing of third degree AC separations. Submitted for publication.

46. Tullos HS, Erwin WD, Woods WG, et al: Unusual lesions of the pitching arm. Clin Orthop 88:169, 1972.

47. Tullos JS, and King JE: Throwing mechanism in sports. Orthop Clin North Am 4:709–720, 1973.

48. Turkel SJ, Panio MW, Marshall JL, and Girgis FG: Stabilizing mechanisms preventing anterior dislocation of the glenohumeral joint. J Bone Joint Surg 63A:1208–1217, 1981.

49. Vogel CM, and Jensen JE: 'Effort' thrombosis of the subclavian vein in a competitive swimmer. Am J Sports Med 13:269–272, 1985.

50. Walsh W, Peterson DA, Shelton G, and Neumann RD: Shoulder strength following acromioclavicular injury. Am J Sports Med 13:152, 1985.

51. Wright IS: The neurovascular syndrome produced by hyperabduction of the arm. Am Heart J 29:1, 1945.

Fractures and Dislocations of the Shoulder in Children

Ralph J. Curtis, Jr., M.D.
Charles A. Rockwood, Jr., M.D.

Fractures of the Proximal Humerus

DEVELOPMENTAL ANATOMY

Embryonic development of the shoulder has been described in detail in earlier chapters of this text. The proximal humerus begins to form a cartilaginous anlage at approximately five weeks' gestation. At six or seven weeks, the glenohumeral joint is formed when a cavity develops between the humerus and scapula. By the beginning of the fetal period, the components of the shoulder region are adult in configuration. They progressively enlarge and mature throughout this phase. By birth, the primary epiphyseal center for the proximal humerus has appeared. On rare occasions, the epiphysis has begun to ossify by this time. Ossification of the proximal humeral epiphysis usually occurs by the sixth postnatal month. Two additional centers develop. The greater tuberosity appears between seven months and three years of age, while the lesser tuberosity appears approximately two years later. These centers coalesce to become a single ossification center by age five to seven years.[14, 17, 19, 20, 39, 56]

The proximal humeral physis is quite important, contributing 80 per cent of the longitudinal growth of the humerus.[4, 14, 15, 51] Its shape is unique, having an inferior concavity, the apex of which is somewhat posteromedial. It is important that there be a strong posteromedial periosteum adjacent to this apex. This contour remains essentially the same throughout growth, so injury does not cause significant deformity.[4, 9, 56] This is unlike the proximal femur, in which the relative size and shape of the bone change as skeletal maturation takes place. The proximal humeral physis usually closes between ages 19 and 22.[19, 39, 56] This has recently been challenged, and newer data cite closure of the physis in girls as occurring between ages 14 and 17, while in boys this occurs between ages 16 and 18.[14, 44]

SURGICAL ANATOMY

Fractures involving the proximal humeral physis tend to occur through the zone of hypertrophy adjacent to the zone of provisional calcification.[13, 46] Fractures in this region rarely bother or disturb physeal growth as this region is distal to the actively proliferating cells of the growth plate. There is tremendous potential for remodeling of these fractures owing to the large contribution to growth of the humerus from this physis.[4, 14, 15, 37]

The proximal humeral physis is asymmetrical, and the apex of the physis is somewhat posteromedial with a strong posteromedial periosteum. Most fractures in this region show anterior and lateral displacement of the shaft fragment that protrudes through the weaker periosteum at this point. The strong posteromedial periosteum remains attached distally, often with a metaphyseal bony fragment.* On occasion the periosteum of this region, along with the biceps tendon, can become interposed between the displaced metaphyseal fragment and the remaining epiphyseal fragment, leading to difficulty in reduction.[30, 55, 58]

---

*See references 1, 2, 5, 9, 13, 14, 35, 37.

Fractures at the level of the proximal humerus allow the head fragment to be rotated into flexion, abduction, and external rotation by the intact rotator cuff. The distal fragment, often displaced anterolaterally through the weaker periosteum, is additionally displaced proximally and adducted by the pectoralis major.[13, 16, 24, 26] These anatomical factors should be remembered when attempting reduction of a completely displaced fracture.

INCIDENCE

Fractures of the proximal humerus in children are somewhat unusual. They actually represent less than 1 per cent of all fractures in children, and only 3 to 6 per cent of all epiphyseal fractures.[*] This is the fourth most common epiphyseal fracture reported in a large series from the Mayo Clinic.[44]

When the frequency of these fractures is observed by age, we note that the adolescent is most commonly affected.[†] This probably reflects the greater frequency of participation in sports and activities that make this age group prone to high-energy trauma. Fractures of the proximal humeral physis in the newborn are the second most common age distribution.[‡] Only clavicular fractures occur more frequently in the neonate.

Fractures in the neonate and early childhood period are commonly the Salter-Harris Type I injuries. By contrast, children from ages 5 to 11 years sustain metaphyseal fractures more commonly than those involving the physeal plate. This is most likely due to the rapid growth phase that occurs in the metaphyseal area in this age group, which leads to relative weakness and, therefore, to a higher incidence of fracture in this region. Salter-Harris Type II fractures do occur, but infrequently. In the adolescent, 75 per cent of these fractures are Salter-Harris Type II; Type I fracture occurs in approximately 25 per cent.[§]

Proximal humeral fractures can also occur through the unicameral bone cyst found most often in the proximal metaphysis. This fracture is best treated by a short period of immobilization. Occasionally, resolution of the cyst occurs in conjunction with fracture healing.

MECHANISM OF INJURY

In the newborn, fractures of the proximal humerus are attributable to trauma during delivery. If the arm becomes hyperextended or excessively rotated as the baby passes through the birth canal, fracture can occur.[¶] The most common mechanism of injury reported in the older child is a fall on the outstretched hand. This indirect force is transmitted proximally through the arm across the metaphysis, driving it anteriorly and laterally.[*] Neer and Horowitz were of the opinion that a direct blow to the posterolateral aspect of the shoulder was the most common mechanism.[37] Williams has described six potential mechanisms of injury to describe proximal humeral fractures in children.[60]

CLASSIFICATION

Fractures of the proximal humerus can be classified by *location*, by degree of *displacement*, and by degree of *stability*. From the standpoint of treatment, both the degree of initial displacement as well as the degree of stability are important. The classification described by Neer and Horowitz is commonly used.[37] They have classified fractures according to the degree of displacement. Their classification is as follows:

Grade I   less than five mm
Grade II   to one-third the width of the shaft
Grade III to two-thirds the width of the shaft
Grade IV   greater than two-thirds the width of the shaft, including total displacement

Fractures can be classified as either stable or unstable. This determination, combined with the grade of displacement and the age of the patient, is used in determining the mode of treatment.

In classifying these fractures by location, we can also note that these fractures of the proximal humerus are either metaphyseal or those involving the physis. In subclassifying physeal involvement, fractures in this area are well described by the Salter-Harris classification.[46] Salter-Harris I fractures are the most common in neonates and represent, in addition, 25 per cent of fractures that occur in adolescents. Salter-Harris Type II fractures make up the remaining 75 per cent in adolescents. The metaphyseal fragment is most frequently posteromedial in the region of the thick periosteal sleeve. There is only a single reported case of a Salter-Harris Type III fracture. This occurred in association with a dislocation in a 10-year-old child.[10] Salter-Harris Type IV injury is hypothesized by Dameron and Rockwood to occur with an open injury.[14] Salter-Harris Type V injuries of the proximal humerus are extremely rare.

Stress fractures involving the proximal humeral physis and metaphysis have been described (Fig 27–1). This usually occurs as the result of repetitive stress such as throwing. It has been described in adolescent baseball pitchers and is treated with rest and cessation of the offensive activity.[7, 54]

---

*See references 3, 5, 14, 22, 23, 34, 37, 38, 41, 43, 49, 52.
†See references 3, 5, 14, 22, 37, 38, 41, 49, 52.
‡See references 5, 8, 12, 21, 23, 25, 29, 34, 43, 47, 50, 53.
§See references 5, 14, 22, 27, 37, 38, 43, 45, 52.
¶See references 12, 13, 21, 29, 34, 47, 50, 53.

*See references 4, 5, 13, 14, 22, 43, 51, 58.

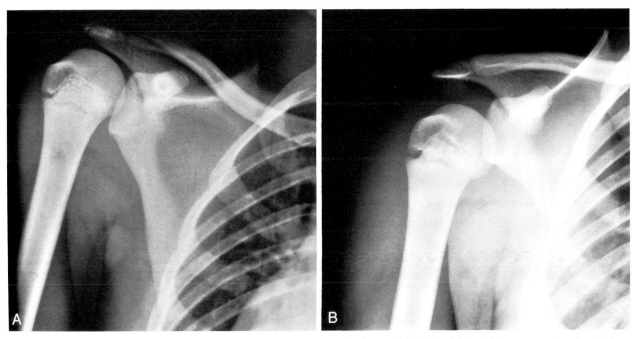

Figure 27–1. This 13-year-old Little League baseball pitcher complained of right shoulder pain of two weeks' duration. *A*, This original anteroposterior radiograph shows a suggestion of widening at the lateral physis. *B*, The patient was allowed to continue pitching and demonstrates displacement of this proximal humeral stress fracture.

SIGNS AND SYMPTOMS

Clinically, in the neonate, the diagnosis of a fracture of the proximal humerus is sometimes difficult. The child will often present with a pseudoparalysis of the arm. The arm is held motionless at the side in the extended position. The newborn may even be febrile. The differential diagnosis in a child with this presentation would include clavicle fracture, brachial plexus injury, and infection, as well as proximal humeral fracture.[14, 20, 43]

As with most fractures in the older child, the patient complains of pain and dysfunction. There is often substantial swelling and ecchymosis in the area with a typical deformity. The arm is shortened with the shaft fragment prominent anteriorly. The arm is usually supported at the elbow and held tightly applied to the thorax. Any attempt at range of motion is limited by pain. A careful evaluation of the neurological and vascular status is required.[14, 37, 43, 45]

RADIOGRAPHIC FINDINGS

In the neonate, diagnosis by x-ray of proximal humerus fractures is somewhat difficult. Often, ossification in the proximal humeral physis is not present at the time of birth.[34, 61] X-ray in this particular situation would be nonrevealing. Subtle changes in the relationship of the humeral shaft to the scapula with comparison side to side can be helpful. Clinical correlation is perhaps the most important factor. The use of arthrog-

raphy has been described and can successfully outline the displaced epiphyseal fragment.*

As with all other areas of the shoulder, radiographic evaluation in two planes at 90 degrees to each other is essential. An anteroposterior view, as well as a lateral view, either in the axillary or the transscapular lateral position, is necessary. Comparison with the opposite side can be helpful when fractures with minimal displacement are suspected. The asymmetrical proximal humeral physis can be very confusing when distinguishing fracture from normal physis.[14, 37, 61]

TREATMENT

With regard to treatment of proximal humeral fractures in children, three main factors must be considered: age of the patient, degree of displacement, and degree of stability.

At no other physis in the body is there a larger contribution to longitudinal growth than at the proximal humeral physis. Approximately 80 per cent of the longitudinal growth for the humerus occurs in this area.[4, 15, 20, 39] Therefore, there is tremendous potential for remodeling of fractures in this region (Fig. 27–2). This potential is inversely proportional to the age of the patient. Varus malalignment and shortening are not uncommon as a result of treatment of proximal humeral fractures. Because of the wide range of motion of the glenohumeral joint, significant residual varus

---

*See references 2, 8, 11, 14, 19, 37, 56.

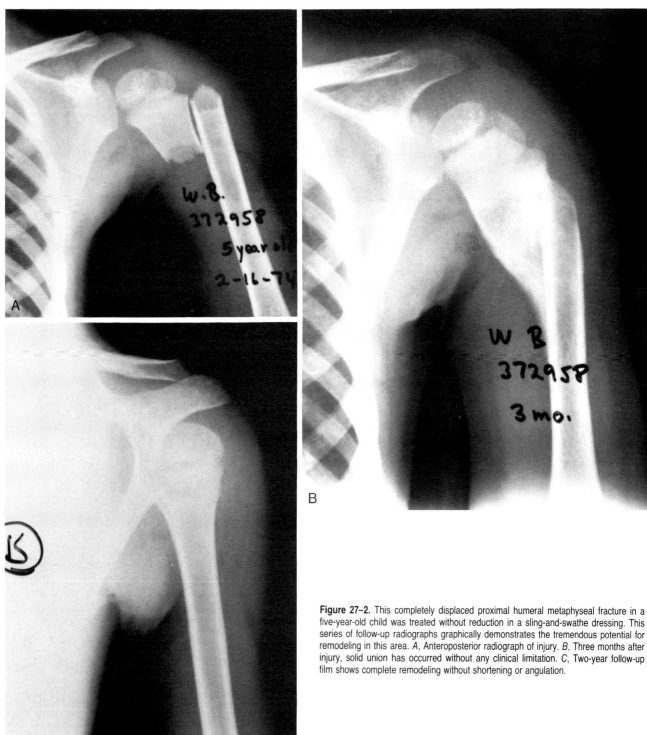

Figure 27–2. This completely displaced proximal humeral metaphyseal fracture in a five-year-old child was treated without reduction in a sling-and-swathe dressing. This series of follow-up radiographs graphically demonstrates the tremendous potential for remodeling in this area. *A,* Anteroposterior radiograph of injury. *B,* Three months after injury, solid union has occurred without any clinical limitation. *C,* Two-year follow-up film shows complete remodeling without shortening or angulation.

deformity causes no functional limitation. Shortening in these fractures is well accommodated by the upper extremity because of its independent functioning and non–weight-bearing status. Therefore, significant malalignment or shortening in this fracture can be consistent with a good result.[4, 14]

Fractures that occur in newborns and infants up to age one are almost all Salter-Harris Type I injuries. As was previously discussed, it is very difficult to assess the degree of displacement radiographically in these fractures when the proximal humeral epiphysis has not ossified (Fig. 27–3). Clinical assessment becomes extremely important. The use of arthrography can be helpful. During the clinical exam, longitudinal traction with gentle manipulation while the arm is flexed 90 degrees and abducted 90 degrees can reduce this fracture. Most will be stable. The arm can then be immobilized to the trunk with a soft sling-and-swathe dressing. The arm should be protected after reduction for approximately two weeks or until clinical symptoms indicate adequate healing.[14]

For children less than age 12, a slightly more aggressive approach to treatment is often indicated. Pa-

tients less than five most commonly have fractures involving the physis, whereas the older child often has metaphyseal involvement. This is explained by the relative weakness of the metaphysis owing to rapid growth at the proximal humerus between ages 5 and 12. Most fractures in this age group are Grades I and II, and uniformly the literature agrees they can be treated by a short period of immobilization followed by progressive, gradual mobilization (Fig. 27–4).*

Grades III and IV displacements warrant further attention. Most authors would agree that attempts at gentle reduction for these displaced fractures would be necessary. Dameron and Rockwood have given us guidelines for an acceptable reduction based upon age.[14] They feel fractures of the proximal humerus between the ages of one and five should have some degree of apposition and less than 70 degrees of angulation. Ages 5 through 12 require 50 per cent apposition and less than 40 to 45 degrees angulation (Fig. 27–5).

---

*See references 3, 11, 14, 30, 35, 43, 49, 52, 59.

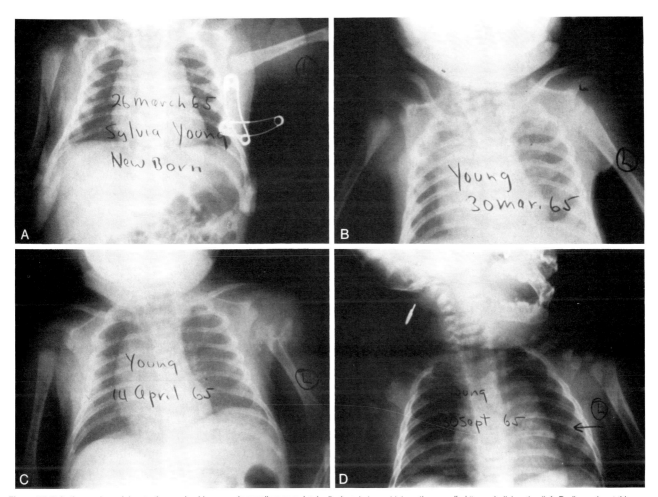

Figure 27–3. In the newborn, injury to the proximal humerus is usually a completely displaced physeal injury, the so-called "pseudodislocation." *A,* Radiographs at this age are sometimes misleading owing to lack of ossification in the proximal epiphysis. *B,* Closed manipulation can be performed by applying longitudinal traction and gentle posterior pressure over the proximal humerus. *C,* At two and a half weeks, abundant callus is present and the patient is clinically asymptomatic. *D,* Six-month follow-up radiograph shows no asymmetry compared with the opposite side.

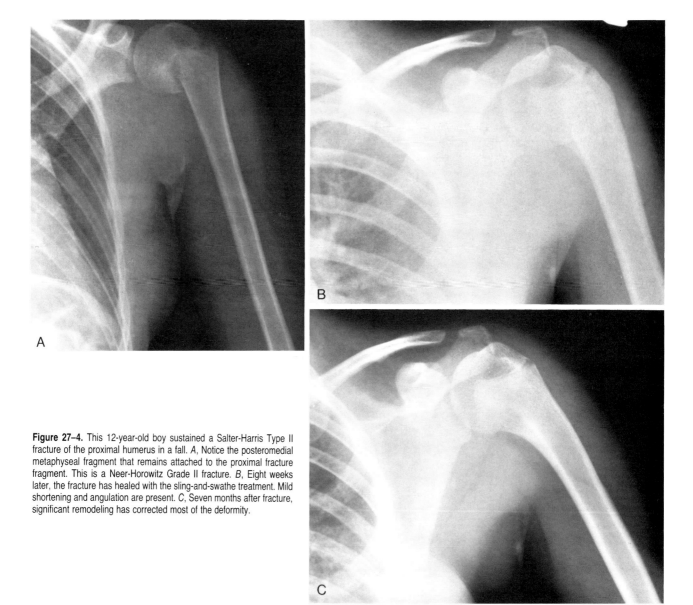

Figure 27–4. This 12-year-old boy sustained a Salter-Harris Type II fracture of the proximal humerus in a fall. *A*, Notice the posteromedial metaphyseal fragment that remains attached to the proximal fracture fragment. This is a Neer-Horowitz Grade II fracture. *B*, Eight weeks later, the fracture has healed with the sling-and-swathe treatment. Mild shortening and angulation are present. *C*, Seven months after fracture, significant remodeling has corrected most of the deformity.

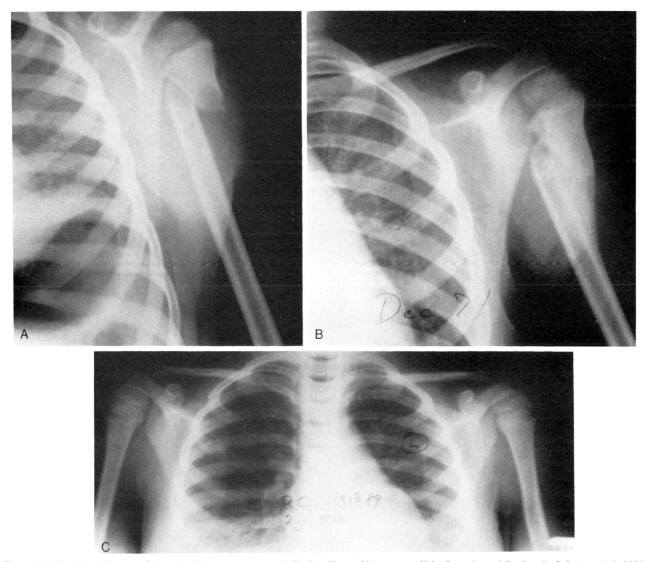

Figure 27–5. Metaphyseal fractures of the proximal humerus are common in the 6- to 10-year-old age group, with healing and remodeling the rule. *A,* Anteroposterior initial injury radiograph demonstrates a completely displaced metaphyseal fracture of the proximal humerus in an eight-year-old. *B,* Rapid healing has taken place with treatment in a sling and swathe. This is an eight-week follow-up x-ray. *C,* Complete remodeling is seen in this anteroposterior film taken at two-year follow-up.

Closed reduction can be accomplished in most cases with a combination of local anesthesia and intravenous sedation. General anesthesia is also acceptable, but in cases that require casting because of instability, this is more difficult to apply while the patient is asleep. Manipulative reduction is accomplished with longitudinal traction in which the distal fragment is flexed 90 degrees and abducted 90 degrees.

If the reduction is found to be stable, a simple sling-and-swathe or collar-and-cuff dressing is applied (Fig. 27–6).[18] If the fracture is found to be unstable, several methods of immobilization have been used. A shoulder spica-type cast with the arm maintained in the "salute" position is popular (Fig. 27–7). Commercial abduction splints can be used as well. The hanging arm cast has been described by some authors, but its use presents difficulty in maintaining a reduction achieved by manipulation. Skeletal traction with an olecranon pin can also be used. This requires diligent daily observation

of position of the traction to carefully maintain reduction. Retrograde percutaneous pinning with smooth Kirschner wires can be accomplished with the use of image intensification control.[28] Pins can be removed after fracture stability is obtained in three to four weeks. Temporary immobilization by any of these methods is maintained for two to four weeks, during which time partial stability at the fracture site has been obtained (Fig. 27–8). Fractures in this age group usually require six to eight weeks to gain solid stability in healing, and remodeling occurs over the next year.

In the adolescent, fractures more commonly involve the proximal humeral physis. In this age group, there is less potential for remodeling, so a more accurate reduction is required. The exact definition of an acceptable reduction is poorly documented. Closed manipulation may become necessary for the displaced Grade III or IV fractures. Fractures in this age group are also more likely to have some element of instability

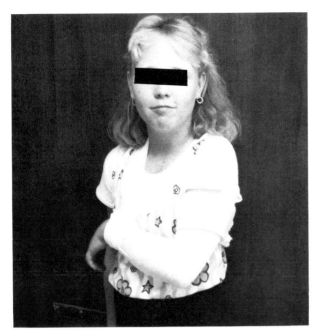

Figure 27-6. Clinical photograph of a nine-year-old girl wearing a homemade sling and swathe used in the treatment of proximal humerus fractures. A stockinette is padded at pressure points with cast padding and held in position with safety pins.

following reduction. In addition, interposition of the biceps tendon-periosteum complex can lead to difficulty with closed reduction. For fractures that are deemed to be in acceptable position and for those that are stable once reduction has been accomplished, a collar-and-cuff or sling-and-swathe–type dressing is ac-

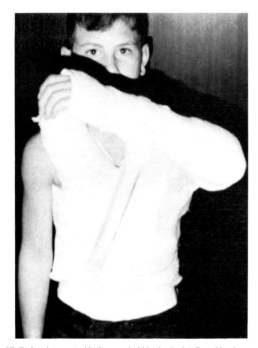

Figure 27-7. A spica cast with the arm held in the "salute" position is sometimes used for the unstable proximal humerus fracture in adolescents. (Reproduced with permission from Rockwood CA, and Green DP (eds): Fractures (3 vols), 2nd ed. Philadelphia: JB Lippincott, 1984.)

ceptable. For fractures that show some degree of instability after reduction, the arm can be maintained in the abducted "salute" position with spica cast or abduction splints as previously described. Other acceptable alternatives are skeletal traction or percutaneous pin fixation. Immobilization time usually requires six to eight weeks.

INDICATIONS FOR OPERATIVE TREATMENT

As in most children's fractures, operative treatment is only rarely required. There are numerous reports that provide evidence that nonoperative treatment is effective for all but a few exceptions in proximal humeral fractures.*

Surgical debridement is required in the case of open fractures. These fractures may be stable following debridement, and internal fixation is usually not indicated. In the rare case of fracture with neurovascular compromise, open reduction and internal fixation of an unstable fracture is indicated.

For the displaced fracture that demonstrates considerable instability after reduction, retrograde percutaneous pinning can be an acceptable alternative. This is accomplished under image intensification control, using smooth Kirschner wires or Steinmann pins. These implants are removed in three to four weeks as fracture stability is obtained.

Unique to fractures of the proximal humerus is the possibility for biceps tendon and periosteum interposition that prevents adequate reduction.[55] Even with this soft tissue block, an acceptable alignment can often be obtained following manipulation. If not, open reduction can be required for removal of the interposed soft tissues (Fig. 27–9). The rare Salter-Harris Types III and IV fractures, because of their intra-articular nature, would require accurate open reduction and internal fixation to restore joint congruity.[10] Percutaneous pinning with smooth Steinmann pins is the fixation of choice. These pins are usually removed at three to four weeks.

AUTHORS' PREFERRED METHOD OF TREATMENT

In neonates and children less than one year old, the diagnosis is made clinically. X-rays are rarely useful. If the fracture is determined to be significantly displaced, a gentle closed manipulation can be performed by applying longitudinal traction with the shoulder flexed and abducted 90 degrees. A sling-and-swathe dressing is used to immobilize the arm until comfortable.

In children from approximately 12 months to 5 years, an acceptable position would be any apposition and angulation up to 70 degrees. For the older child, ages 5 to 12 years, 50 per cent apposition and 50 degrees

*See references 3, 4, 8, 11, 14, 16, 22, 26, 30, 37, 49.

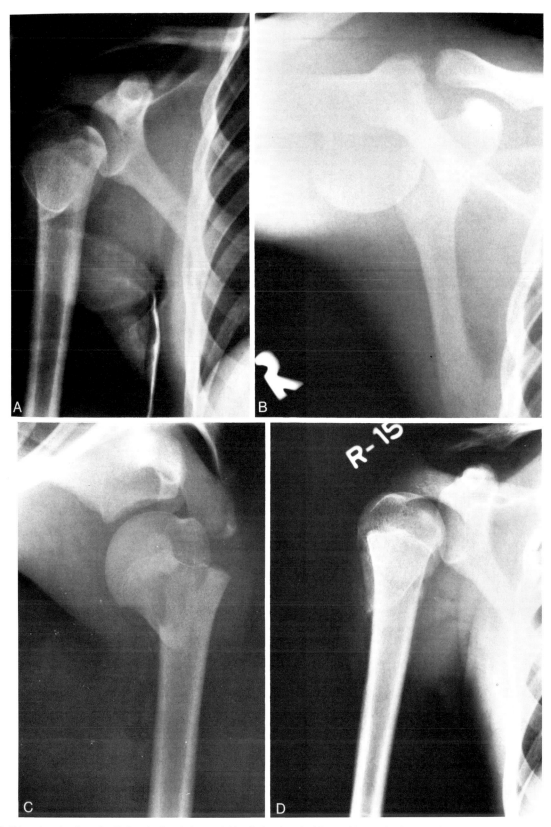

Figure 27-8. This series of radiographs displays treatment of an unstable, displaced proximal humeral fracture in olecranon pin traction. *A,* Anteroposterior radiograph demonstrates severe shortening with rotation of the proximal fragment. *B,* Axillary lateral view shows shortening and complete displacement. *C,* This view shows reduction with olecranon pin traction. *D,* X-ray three weeks after injury shows that reduction has been maintained as traction is slowly lowered to position the arm at the patient's side.

Illustration continued on following page

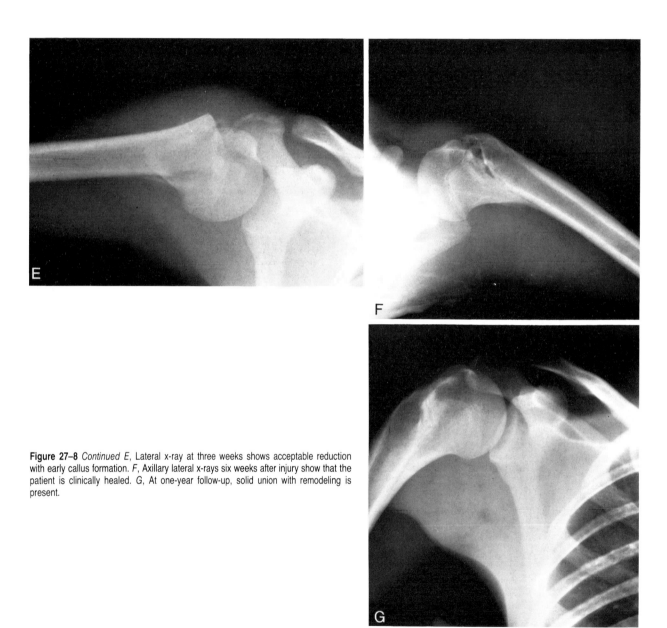

Figure 27–8 *Continued E*, Lateral x-ray at three weeks shows acceptable reduction with early callus formation. *F*, Axillary lateral x-rays six weeks after injury show that the patient is clinically healed. *G*, At one-year follow-up, solid union with remodeling is present.

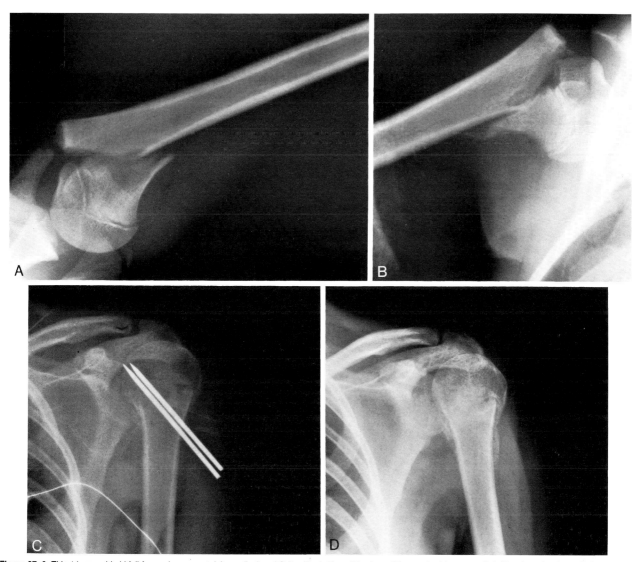

Figure 27–9. This 14-year-old girl fell from a horse, sustaining a displaced Salter-Harris Type II fracture of the proximal humerus. *A,* Axillary lateral radiograph demonstrates original displacement. *B,* She returned three weeks after closed reduction and treatment with a sling-and-swathe immobilization with recurrent displacement. *C,* Open reduction with removal of interposed soft tissue and retrograde pinning with two threaded Steinmann pins was then performed. *D,* Anteroposterior radiograph after pin removal six weeks after injury.

angulation is acceptable. A sling-and-swathe or modified Velpeau immobilization is usually all that is necessary. Only for the most unstable fractures would a short period of abduction treatment be required. We prefer the modified shoulder spica described by Rockwood.* This uses a long-arm cast attached by a broom stick to a plaster of Paris waist and belly band. For those patients who are not ambulatory, olecranon pin traction can be used.

In the adolescent, certainly a more accurate reduction is required. A position consistent with a Neer Grade II fracture would be acceptable. If instability is present, a modified shoulder spica cast or percutaneous pinning is preferred.

COMPLICATIONS

The proximal humeral fracture in children is rarely associated with complications of a significant nature. However, as with proximal humeral fractures in the adult, neurovascular injury can occur. This should be recognized early so that appropriate reduction and potential vascular surgery can be accomplished. Neurological dysfunction of a permanent nature is rare.

Although nonunion has not been identified as a problem, malunion does occur (Fig. 27–10). Several authors have described humeral shortening, varus angulation, and restricted shoulder movement as complications.[3, 4, 24, 33, 37] Humeral shortening can occur with all grades of fracture, but up to three to four cm shortening is well tolerated in the upper extremity. Malunion with varus angulation is also well tolerated because of the wide range of glenohumeral motion normally present.

*Personal communication.

Glenohumeral Subluxation and Dislocation

DEVELOPMENTAL ANATOMY

The reader is referred to the section in this chapter entitled "Fractures of the Proximal Humerus" and to earlier chapters on shoulder anatomy.

SURGICAL ANATOMY

As has previously been discussed, the proximal humerus and glenoid articulate to form the shoulder joint itself. This joint is biomechanically designed to accommodate the wide range of motion necessary to perform upper extremity function. To accomplish this range of motion, the capsule of the glenohumeral joint is redundant inferiorly. The articular surface of the humerus is approximately three times the size of the relatively flat glenoid. Therefore, there is very little bony constraint inherent in this joint. The primary constraint for the joint is the capsular-ligamentous complex. The anterior glenohumeral ligaments reinforce the anterior capsule. Interestingly enough, this complex capsular-ligamentous structure has to provide stability and yet allow for the demands of such a wide range of motion. The largest of these ligaments, the anteroinferior glenohumeral ligament is placed within the inferior redundant area and is designed to tighten as the arm is abducted and externally rotated. This becomes the primary site of pathology in shoulder instability.[70, 89, 100] In many cases the anteroinferior glenohumeral attachment to glenoid and labrum is stripped from the anterior neck of the glenoid, the so-called Bankart or Perthes lesion (Fig. 27–11).[100]

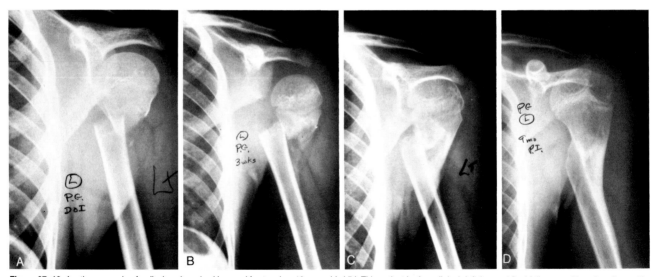

Figure 27–10. Another example of a displaced proximal humeral fracture in a 10-year-old child. This patient had no clinical deficiency at final follow-up, although radiographic shortening and angulation were still present. *A,* Anteroposterior radiograph of injury shows a displaced fracture. *B,* Early callus formation is present at three weeks. Treatment is with a sling-and-swathe dressing. *C,* Fracture has healed solidly by eight weeks with significant angulation and shortening. *D,* By nine months some remodeling has occurred.

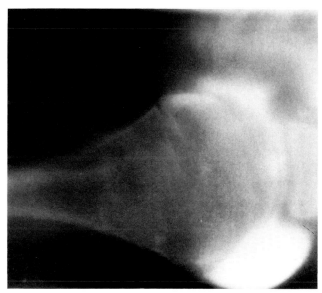

Figure 27–11. Arthrotomogram of the glenohumeral joint in the axillary lateral plane demonstrates leakage of dye along the anterior glenoid neck. This is the so-called Bankart or Perthes lesion.

The humeral attachment of the capsule is approximately along a line consistent with the region of the anatomical neck. This places it proximal to the physeal line, except for a small area on the medial side that extends distally along the shaft of the humerus. As in other joints, the strong capsular attachment to the epiphysis makes the physis the weak link, which explains why fractures of the proximal humerus are so much more common than dislocations of the shoulder joint in children.[67, 70, 88, 92, 97, 98]

The rotator cuff tendons, including subscapularis in the front, as well as supraspinatus, infraspinatus, and teres minor posteriorly, are closely applied to the capsule of the joint. They perform a very important function as secondary stabilizers of the joint. This comes into play especially when addressing rehabilitation and prevention of recurrent glenohumeral dislocation.[70]

INCIDENCE

The treatment of shoulder instability has been a major topic in the recent literature, yet shoulder dislocations in children under 12 years old has been rarely reported.* Most of the major authors on fractures and dislocations in children barely touch on the subject.[63, 94, 95, 98, 103, 106] There are several case reports of true glenohumeral dislocations in children under 12; however, a large series has not been reported.† Rowe's 1956 article reviewing 500 dislocated shoulders revealed that only 8 patients were under age 10.[98] In the same group, 99 were between ages 10 and 20.[98] Rock

wood has reported a large series of patients, predominantly in the adolescent age group, with recurrent dislocation.[70] Certainly as the child reaches the adolescent period, instability becomes a much more common problem. Most major series on the natural history and treatment of shoulder instability include cases of adolescent patients.* This has been dealt with extensively in the chapter on adult dislocations in this text.

CLASSIFICATION

Two basic classification schemes can be used to classify dislocations of the shoulder in children. The most common classification used is that based on the direction or location of the dislocation. More useful, however, is a classification describing the etiology of the dislocation. This classification system is similar to that used for adults but takes into account congenital and developmental problems unique to children.[70]

Site of Dislocation

1. Anterior
2. Posterior
3. Inferior (luxatio erecta)

As with dislocations of the shoulder in adults, the anterior dislocation in children is also the most common. Posterior dislocations as well as luxatio erecta are uniquely uncommon. McNeil and Freundlich, as well as Laskin and Sedlin, have reported rare cases of luxatio erecta in children.[72, 82, 86] Several isolated reports of posterior dislocation have been documented as well.[71, 76, 85, 89, 104]

Etiology

1. Traumatic
2. Atraumatic
   A. Voluntary
   B. Involuntary
      (1) Congenital abnormality or deficiencies of bone or soft tissues
      (2) Hereditary joint laxity problems, such as Ehler-Danlos syndrome
      (3) Developmental joint laxity problems
      (4) Emotional and psychiatric disturbances

MECHANISM OF INJURY

Anterior dislocations predominate in the traumatic type of dislocations. There should be evidence of significant trauma in these cases. The mechanism is similar to that observed in the adult. A fall on the outstretched hand forces the arm into abduction and external rotation, levering the humeral head out an-

---

*See references 63, 67, 77, 80, 89, 90, 101, 103, 106.
†See references 64, 71–74, 77, 84, 90, 105.

*See references 62, 66, 70, 80, 87, 89, 97, 102, 105.

teriorly. This can occur in motor vehicle accidents, falls from a height, fights, or contact sports.[63, 70, 95, 101]

Traumatic posterior dislocations occur much less frequently. In many cases, there is a history of violent trauma with the arm in a position of flexion, internal rotation, and adduction. The other common mechanisms that can produce posterior dislocations are convulsions and electroshock. In these cases, the shoulder is dislocated posteriorly by the violent contraction of the shoulder internal rotators.[70, 104, 240]

In the neonatal period, pseudodislocation with traumatic epiphyseal separation is common.[64, 75] True traumatic dislocation of the shoulder is extremely rare, and most cases have underlying congenital and neuromuscular defects or infection.*

Atraumatic shoulder instability is probably more common in both children and adolescents than is readily recognized.[70, 88, 89, 99] Cases of dislocation or subluxation without a clear, significant traumatic history should arouse suspicion. Inherent joint laxity is the underlying element that allows the shoulder to be dislocated either voluntarily or involuntarily as the result of a minimally traumatic event. In the voluntary dislocator, conscious selective firing of muscles while antagonists are inhibited, combined with arm positioning, allows the shoulder to dislocate. Patients with voluntary subluxation or dislocation have very little pain associated with the dislocation and can always experience spontaneous reduction (Fig. 27–12).[70, 83, 88, 89, 99]

SIGNS AND SYMPTOMS

In traumatic anterior dislocation, the patient presents with a painful swollen shoulder with the arm held in an abducted, externally rotated position. There is obvious deformity. The shoulder is somewhat hollow beneath the prominent squared-off acromion laterally. The humeral head can be palpated in an anterior and inferior position. Careful examination of the neurological and vascular status is necessary. Specific attention to the axillary nerve function is indicated. The axillary nerve sensory distribution is along the lateral upper arm, while the motor innervation is to the deltoid and teres minor muscles.

Traumatic posterior dislocation is much less common and causes pain in the shoulder region with a flat anterior appearance and posterior fullness. The arm is held internally rotated across the chest. A hallmark of the posterior dislocation is the lack of shoulder external rotation and inability to supinate the forearm. Once again, the neurovascular status should be checked closely. History of convulsion or electric shock would be consistent with a posterior dislocation.

In the neonatal period, traumatic separation of the

_____
*See references 64, 67–69, 73, 74, 81, 92, 94, 103, 107.

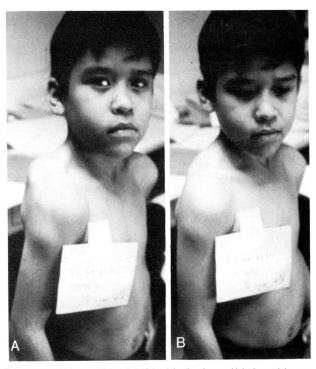

Figure 27–12. Voluntary dislocation of the right glenohumeral joint in an eight-year-old boy. *A*, Dislocated. *B*, Reduced. (Reproduced with permission from Rockwood CA, and Green DP (eds): Fractures (3 vols), 2nd ed. Philadelphia: JB Lippincott, 1984.)

upper humeral physis, the so-called pseudodislocation of the shoulder, can mimic exactly an anterior dislocation.[75] In our review of the literature, we have not documented a case of a true traumatic dislocation of the shoulder occurring with childbirth.[64, 74]

The most notable initial finding in patients with atraumatic shoulder instability is the relative lack of pain associated with subluxation or dislocation. Even in cases of involuntary atraumatic dislocation, the minor pain associated with actual dislocation subsides within a few hours. Many of these episodes of subluxation and dislocation can occur on multiple occasions and usually spontaneously reduce. Clinical evidence of multiple joint laxity and multidirectional instability of the opposite shoulder should be established on clinical exam.[70, 88, 99] The characteristics noted in patients with multidirectional instability of the shoulder include laxity in the normal shoulder and signs of generalized ligamentous laxity including hyperextension at the elbows, knees, and metacarpophalangeal joints. Multidirectional instability at the shoulder is characterized by a positive sulcus sign and translation of a significant degree on the anterior and posterior drawer test.[70]

The sulcus sign is a dimpling of the skin below the acromion as manual longitudinal traction applied to the arm produces inferior subluxation of the humeral head. The drawer test, schematically diagrammed in Figure 27–13, manually tests excessive translation of the humeral head in the anterior to posterior plane.

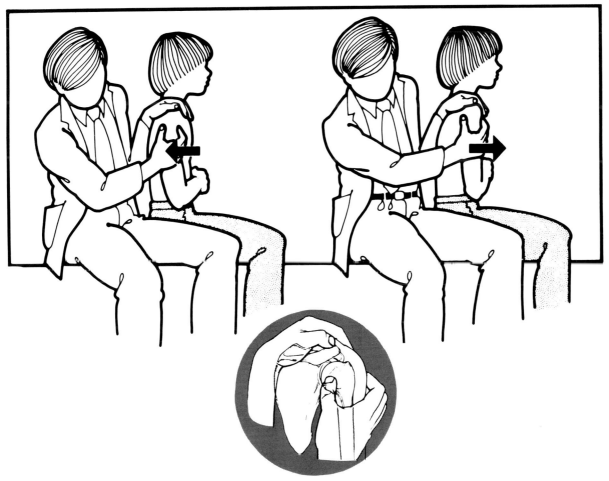

Figure 27-13. Drawer test. The examiner, seated next to the patient, uses one hand to grip the humeral head to translate it anteriorly and posteriorly while stabilizing the scapula with the opposite forearm and hand.

RADIOGRAPHIC FINDINGS

Traumatic lesions on plain radiography are similar to those found in the adult (Fig. 27–14).[70, 97] The Hill-Sach's compression lesion on the posterolateral aspect of the humeral head is the most common (Fig. 27–15). Bony injury to the anterior glenoid rim can be inferred by a double density at the anterior-inferior glenoid margin on the anteroposterior film (Fig. 27–16). However, the axillary lateral and West Point lateral views will demonstrate this lesion much more clearly. Normal radiographs are usually found in cases of atraumatic dislocation. The inferior component of multidirectional instability can be demonstrated by applying weight to the arm during the radiograph (Fig. 27–17).

TREATMENT

An acute dislocation of the shoulder should undergo closed reduction by one of the standard accepted techniques. For anterior dislocation, many reduction techniques have been previously described.[63, 70, 95] A

prereduction neurological exam is essential for comparison with postreduction status. Light sedation can be used and is followed by a traction-countertraction maneuver. The Stimson maneuver and the Steel maneuver are equally effective.[205] Postreduction x-rays are required, as well as a detailed examination of the neurological status. Immobilization following closed reduction is suggested in a sling and swathe for four to six weeks. Similarly, for the posterior dislocation, a closed reduction can be performed with traction in line with the deformity followed by gentle external rotation. Immobilization should be with the arm in a neutral or slightly externally rotated position. This may require use of a spica cast.[70, 85, 104]

The true incidence of recurrence after traumatic shoulder dislocation in a child is difficult to assess because of the rarity of the injury.* Rowe has reported a 100 per cent recurrence rate in children ages 1 to 10 and a 94 per cent recurrence rate for adolescents.[98] Rockwood has reported only a 50 per cent recurrence

---

*See references 63, 70, 77, 80, 89–91, 103, 106.

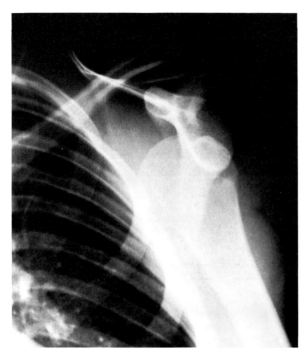

Figure 27–14. Common radiographic appearance of an anterior dislocation of the shoulder.

rate in 8 cases between 13.8 and 15.8 years of age.[70] Wagner and Lyne have reported an 80 per cent recurrence rate in 10 cases with clearly open epiphyses.[105] Many series on the natural history of shoulder dislo-

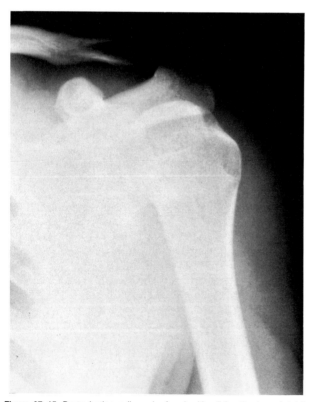

Figure 27–15. Postreduction radiograph of a shoulder dislocation in a skeletally immature adolescent. Note the large posterolateral compression fracture of the humeral head, or Hill-Sachs lesion.

cations in adolescents and young adults reveal recurrence rates in the 80 to 90 per cent range.[79, 85, 87, 97, 102]

The actual indications, therefore, for surgical intervention in children have not been established. For cases of recurrent dislocation, standard soft tissue procedures, such as the Putti-Platt, Bankart, and Magnuson-Stack, have been used.[70, 76, 87, 97] Barry and associates[66] have described the effective use of the coracoid transfer for recurrent anterior instability in adolescents.

Treatment of the atraumatic dislocator would appear to be a more difficult task. Most authors emphasize the necessity of careful diagnosis in these cases. Rockwood, Neer, and Rowe, among others, have described a vigorous rehabilitation program as the initial treatment of choice.[62, 70, 88, 89, 99] Strengthening of the rotator cuff and deltoid is stressed and was successful in a large percentage of cases. Most would agree that surgical intervention would be entertained only after failing a strict 6- to 12-month rehabilitation program. Neer and Foster have described an operative procedure specifically designed to eliminate capsular redundancy and multidirectional instability.[89]

AUTHORS' PREFERRED METHOD OF TREATMENT

The most important problem that faces the physician in dealing with shoulder dislocations in children is to establish whether the dislocation is truly traumatic or atraumatic in nature. This should be done by careful history of the event that caused the dislocation, as well as a good past history, combined with physical examination to elicit any evidence of multidirectional instability or a congenital or developmental problem. Care should be taken to identify the voluntary dislocator, who should be treated nonoperatively in essentially 100 per cent of cases.

When the child presents with a dislocated shoulder, either anterior or posterior, adequate radiographic diagnosis should be made. Care should be taken to perform a neurovascular examination followed by closed reduction. We prefer either the traction-countertraction method under light sedation or gentle manipulative reduction as described by Steel.[70] Immobilization after reduction for anterior dislocation should include a sling for a period of four weeks. For the posterior dislocation, the arm should be placed in a neutral or slightly externally rotated position for a similar time period. This may require a modified shoulder spica cast to complete this task.

When considering operative intervention for recurrent *traumatic* dislocation in a child, one should consider that the recurrence rate reported in the literature is at least 50 per cent or higher.[79, 88, 98] The parents should be counseled early on that the rate of recurrence is quite high. We personally would hesitate to intervene after a first dislocation; however, with established recurrence, surgical intervention is indicated. Capsular shift reconstruction as described by Rockwood is used with repair of a Bankart lesion if necessary.[70] The use

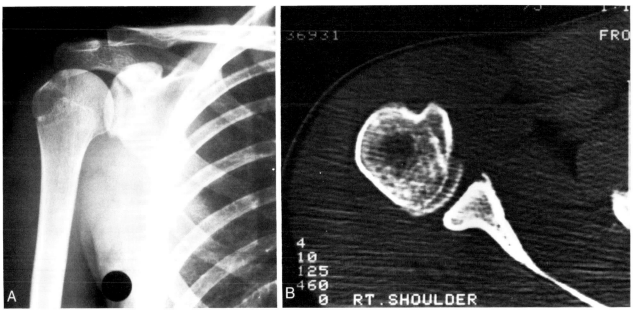

Figure 27–16. *A*, Anteroposterior radiograph of a 14-year-old boy with recurrent anterior subluxation. Notice the presence of a Hill-Sachs compression fracture on the humeral head and a subtle double density at the anteroinferior glenoid rim. *B*, CT scan shows this to be an avulsion-type bony injury of the anterior glenoid.

of metal about the shoulder should be avoided because of reported complications.[65, 109]

For the *atraumatic* dislocator, reduction can be accomplished for an acute dislocation in a similar fashion to that described above. If multidirectional laxity or congenital dysplasia is identified, the diagnosis of atraumatic dislocation is confirmed. These patients should be treated with a vigorous rehabilitation pro-

gram. Rotator cuff strengthening done below the horizontal is used.[70] The exercise is best performed using light Theraband and progressing to the pulley and weight apparatus (Fig. 27–18). Only for definite recurrence in the face of a 6- to 12-month supervised rehabilitation program would we consider surgical intervention for the child with atraumatic recurrent dislocation. Again, the voluntary dislocator should not be considered a surgical candidate, and psychiatric evaluation may be more appropriate. A capsular procedure described by Neer or the capsular shift technique described by Rockwood can be used to surgically eliminate the laxity of the joint capsule in a circumferential manner.[70, 89] This technique in the atraumatic dislocator requires special attention to detail.

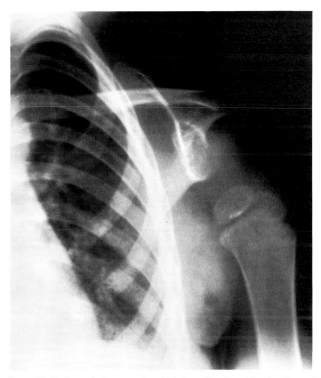

Figure 27–17. Dramatic demonstration of inferior subluxation of the glenohumeral joint in a patient with multidirectional instability. The clinical correlate is the "sulcus sign."

Fractures of the Clavicle and Injuries to the Sternoclavicular and Acromioclavicular Joints

GENERAL

Developmental Anatomy

The clavicle is the first bone to appear in the human embryo at about postovulatory day 35. The crown-rump measurement is 12 to 15 mm when precursor mesenchymal cells separate from the scapular arch. The central portion of the clavicle forms by intramembranous ossification, and, therefore, the clavicular shaft is considered to be membranous bone.[112, 113, 119, 124–126]

The clavicle is also the first bone to ossify *in utero*. Ossification begins at two areas. First, it begins at the junction of the central and lateral one-third and, sec-

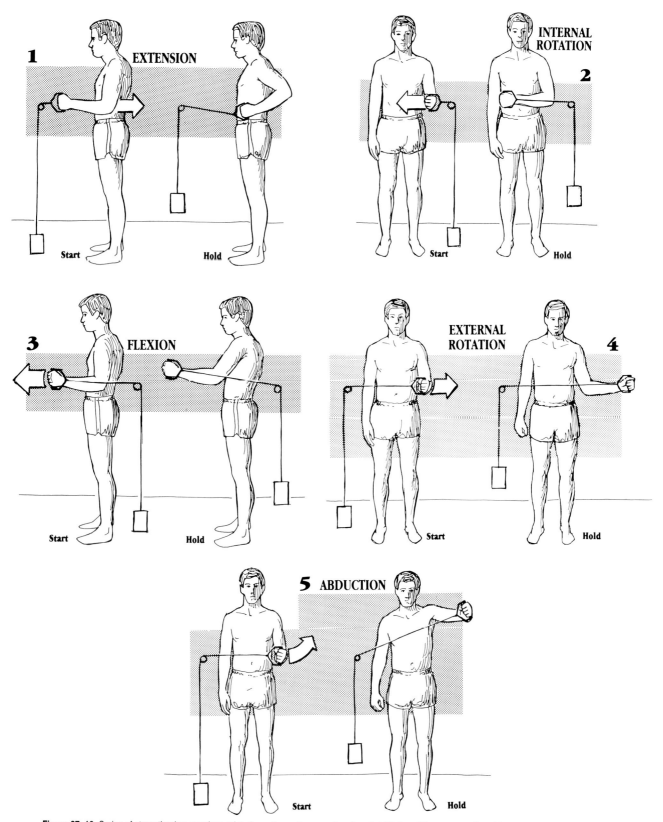

Figure 27–18. Series of strengthening exercises using the pulley and rope system for rehabilitation of the rotator cuff and three components of the deltoid.

ond, at the junction between the central and medial one-third. By 45 days *in utero*, these two ossification centers fuse to form one mass of clavicular shaft that predominates in growth to age five years. Cartilaginous growth plates develop medially and laterally with the medial physis providing most of the longitudinal growth for the bone. Up to 80 per cent of the length of the clavicle is contributed by the sternal physis.[119, 124, 126] Ossification in the medial epiphysis occurs from 12 to 19 years of age, and fusion occurs from 22 to 25 years. The lateral or acromial epiphysis is usually very inapparent radiographically and has very little longitudinal growth. It rarely develops a secondary ossification center and fuses to the clavicle by age 19.*

SURGICAL ANATOMY

The clavicle, when viewed from above, has a double curve, convex anteriorly in the medial two-thirds and convex posteriorly in the lateral one-third. When viewed from the front, it is flat and almost completely straight. The clavicle is weak at the junction of the two curves. On cross-sectional anatomy, the distal two-thirds of the bone is flat, and in the medial one-third, it is triangular and bulbous.[110, 124, 137, 144] The clavicle is the bony link between the upper extremity and the axial skeleton. It serves to anchor the scapula and provides a rigid base for muscular attachments that stabilize the shoulder for arm function. The trapezius, deltoid, sternocleidomastoid, and pectoralis major muscles all attach to the clavicle. Without clavicular stability, the weight of the arm tends to protract the scapula bringing it forward, medial, and downward. In addition, the clavicle forms the roof of the thoracic outlet. It therefore provides protection for the subclavian and axillary vessels, the brachial plexus, and the superior lung.[110, 137, 144]

Sternoclavicular Joint

The sternoclavicular joint is a diarthrodial joint made up of the large medial end of the clavicle, the sternum, and the first rib. It is extremely incongruous and has very little bony stability in and of itself. A fibrocartilaginous disc or meniscus covers most of the articular surface to provide a cushion within this incongruous joint. A strong series of ligaments bind the joint together. The intra-articular disc ligament is a dense fibrous structure that arises from the first rib and hemisects the joint, either completely or incompletely, attaching anteriorly and posteriorly to the strong capsular ligaments. The anterior portion of the capsular ligament is heavier and stronger than the posterior portion. This anterior capsular ligament provides the primary support against upward and anterior displacement of the medial clavicle. The capsular ligaments attach predominantly to the epiphysis of the medial

clavicle. The physis lies outside the joint capsule itself, and, therefore, in Salter-Harris type injuries, the weak link is through the physis.[112, 120, 154] The joint is further protected by interclavicular and costoclavicular ligaments that contribute to the maintenance of "poise of the shoulder" (Fig. 27–19).[172]

The epiphysis at the medial end of the clavicle is the last of the long bones to appear, as well as the last to close. The medial clavicular epiphysis ossifies between the 18th and 20th years. Fusion to the shaft occurs between the 23rd and 25th years.[124, 133, 147, 164] Certainly then, with this fact in mind, it can be recognized that many of the so-called sternoclavicular dislocations are injuries through the medial physeal plate.[112, 120, 162]

The sternoclavicular joint is positioned immediately anterior to many structures exiting the mediastinum. The innominate artery and vein, the vagus and phrenic nerves, as well as the trachea and esophagus, all pass immediately posterior to the region of the sternoclavicular joint. Displaced fractures of the medial clavicle that are posterior can impinge upon these structures, causing immediate and life-threatening emergency.[110, 131, 151, 165]

It should be remembered that the sternoclavicular joint is freely moveable with capabilities of 30 to 35 degrees of upward clavicular elevation, 35 degrees of motion in the anterior to posterior plane, and 45 to 50 degrees of rotation about the long axis of the clavicle. This articulation is extremely important, providing the only true articulation between the upper extremity and the axial skeleton.[110]

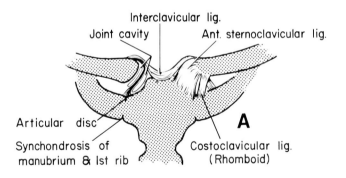

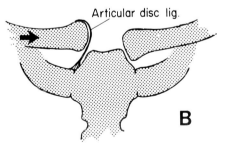

Figure 27–19. *A,* Schematic drawing of the anatomy of the sternoclavicular joint. Note the heavy ligamentous structure and articular disc. *B,* The articular disc ligament provides a checkrein for medial displacement of the clavicle. (Reproduced with permission from Rockwood CA, and Green DP (eds): Fractures (3 vols), 2nd ed. Philadelphia: JB Lippincott, 1984.)

---

*See references 119, 120, 124, 126, 133, 147, 164.

Acromioclavicular Joint

The lateral one-third of the clavicle is surrounded by an extremely thick periosteal tube that remains intact circumferentially all the way to the acromioclavicular joint. It is important that the very strong coracoclavicular ligaments attach firmly to the inferior portion of this periosteal sleeve. At the distal extent of the clavicle, a secondary ossification center is present, although this usually remains as an unossified epiphysis. When it does become ossified, the fusion process to the shaft occurs over a very short time sequence and is rarely seen on x-ray.[147, 213] The acromioclavicular joint is a diarthrodial joint.[208] In the adult, an intra-articular disc forms to cover the distal clavicle. The joint is surrounded by a relatively weak capsule supported superiorly and inferiorly by acromioclavicular ligaments that, in a child, blend with the thick periosteum of the distal clavicle. The primary stabilizing ligaments are the strong conoid and trapezoid portions of the coracoclavicular ligaments. They arise from the coracoid and attach to the undersurface of the distal clavicle and periosteum. As one might imagine from this anatomical configuration, fracture in this region would be more common than dislocation. In the younger patient this thick periosteal tube usually remains intact inferiorly and distally along with the supporting ligamentous structures. Therefore, even displaced fractures have a tremendous potential for remodeling (Fig. 27–20).[115, 205]

CLAVICULAR SHAFT

Incidence

The clavicle is the most frequently fractured bone in children. Over 80 per cent of clavicle fractures that occur in children are within the shaft of the bone. Fortunately, clavicle fractures in children commonly progress to rapid union with few complications. Little rehabilitation is required to predict an excellent prognosis for full functional return.*

Because of the thick periosteum surrounding the clavicle in children, clavicular fractures are most commonly nondisplaced or angulated greenstick-type fractures. The thick periosteal tube tends to protect against displacement. Displaced fractures are rare but do occur more commonly in high-energy, direct blows.[160] Plastic deformation has been reported to occur and may be difficult to detect.[116]

Mechanism of Injury

Fractures of the clavicular shaft in children are most frequently caused by indirect force. Often the child falls on an outstretched hand, transmitting the force through the arm to the clavicle. The strong ligamentous attachments both medially and laterally protect these

_____

*See references 112, 115, 120, 134, 153, 154, 162, 167.

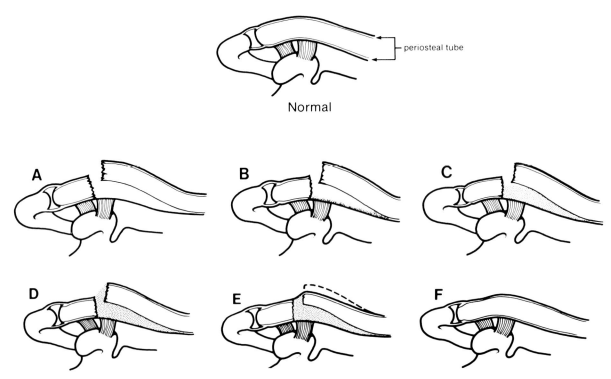

Figure 27–20. Phases of healing in fractures of the distal clavicle in children. *A,* The clavicular shaft herniates through the periosteal tube with fracture. *B,* The coracoclavicular ligaments remain in continuity with the inferior portion of the periosteal tube. *C, D,* Periosteal callus is formed within the tube to stabilize the fracture. *E,* Remodeling occurs with resorption of the superior prominence of the shaft fragment. *F,* Final remodeling with good stability is achieved. (Reproduced with permission from Rockwood CA, and Green DP (eds): Fractures (3 vols), 2nd ed. Philadelphia: JB Lippincott, 1984.)

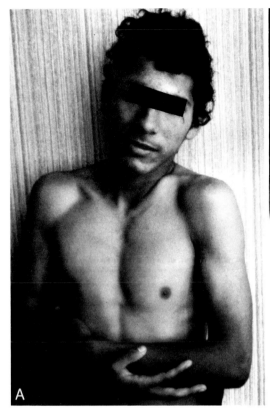

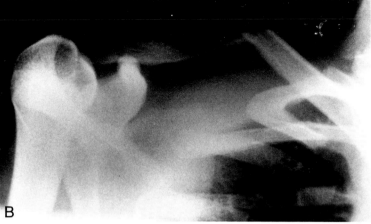

Figure 27–21. *A*, Clinical photograph of a young patient with a clavicle fracture. Note that the arm is supported by the good hand at the elbow and the head is tilted to the side of the fracture. *B*, Corresponding radiograph shows the clavicle fracture.

areas, thus exposing the relatively unprotected shaft to fracture.[120, 153, 154] Fractures can also occur by direct blows to the subcutaneous bony shaft. Recent articles propose that this may be the most common mechanism of injury.[160] Fractures caused by direct blows are more often complete and displaced owing to greater energy necessary to cause fracture. They can be associated with injuries to the underlying neurovascular and pulmonary structures.[131, 142, 143, 150, 165, 170]

Birth fractures can occur in the clavicular shaft at the time of delivery. When the infant is forced through a relatively narrow pelvic inlet, greenstick fractures of the clavicular shaft occur. These fractures are of little consequence but are the most frequent neonatal fracture.[117, 123, 153, 155]

Signs and Symptoms

In the neonate, clavicular fractures are often first noticed as a swelling, which represents healing callus several days after the fracture. Most of the children have little discomfort and require essentially no treatment. Some neonates, however, demonstrate pseudoparalysis or lack of voluntary movement of the entire arm.[117, 120, 139, 157] The differential diagnosis would include true birth injury to the brachial plexus, acute osteomyelitis of the shoulder region, and fracture of the proximal humeral physis, in addition to clavicular fracture. Physical examination will reveal crepitus, swelling, and tenderness. The diagnosis is confirmed radiographically. It must be remembered that clavicle

fractures in the neonate can coexist with brachial plexus injuries.[131, 155, 157]

In the older child, symptoms vary with the degree of displacement. The complaint of pain and clinical findings of local swelling, tenderness, and deformity are most common. The child supports the affected side with the opposite hand under the elbow (Fig. 27–21). The shoulder is often drooping forward, and the head is turned to the affected side because of spasm in the sternocleidomastoid muscle. If the fracture is complete, the proximal fragment will be displaced posteriorly and superiorly by the pull of the sternocleidomastoid and trapezius muscles. In the acute fracture, examination to exclude injury to the underlying vascular structures and brachial plexus should be performed initially. Venous distention, absent pulses, or an expanding hematoma at the fracture site should be of concern.[120]

In many children, there will be a delay of complaints or symptoms after clavicle fracture. In this late presentation visible or palpable callus is commonly present. Appropriate history, clinical tenderness, and radiographs are essential to distinguish fracture from congenital pseudarthrosis or cleidocranial dysostosis. Congenital pseudarthrosis of the clavicle is a developmental defect most often affecting the middle third of the right clavicle (Fig. 27–22). This probably occurs *in utero* as a result of pressure from the subclavian artery. The bony ends are smooth and hypertrophic. This entity is not painful.*

---

*See references 111, 128, 138, 141, 148, 152, 166.

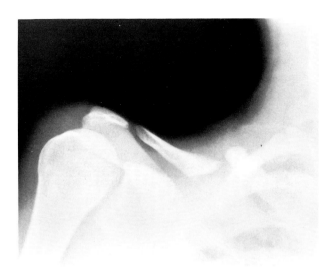

Figure 27–22. Congenital pseudarthrosis of the clavicle. This patient is asymptomatic but has noted clinical deformity.

Cleidocranial dysostosis is an hereditary abnormality that affects membranous bone formation, most commonly the clavicle. There is often absence of the distal one-third. Uncommonly, the central one-third is involved with characteristic tapering and attenuation of the ends near the defect.[121, 122] Other bony defects, including those involving the cranium, pubis, mandible, and vertebrae, occur.

Radiographic Findings

The standard x-ray technique for clavicular fractures in children includes a routine anteroposterior view with appropriate soft tissue penetration.[120] This will reveal the vast majority of fractures without further study. Difficult fractures for making a radiographic diagnosis include fractures of the medial end of the clavicle and nondisplaced fractures. Bony overlap with the sternum, spine, and ribs can obscure the medial fractures. Nondisplaced fractures can be overlooked by overlap with the second rib or even slight motion by the child during exposure.

Normally, there is a soft tissue shadow that parallels the superior border of the clavicle. If this shadow is elevated or asymmetrical, a fracture should be suspected (Fig. 27–23).[159] A cephalic tilt view or lordotic view with the x-ray tube angled upward some 30 to 40 degrees can be helpful. If clinical suspicion warrants further evaluation in the face of negative plain films, tomograms or CT scan should be used. However, these specialized techniques are rarely required. Often routine shoulder x-rays are overexposed for adequate visualization of distal clavicle fractures or injuries of the acromioclavicular joint. A soft tissue technique is often necessary to demonstrate injuries in this region.

Treatment

A large variety of splints, bandages, and dressings have been used to treat fractures of the clavicular shaft

in children. A few of these are illustrated in Figure 27–24.[114, 120] The key point to be made, however, is that virtually all clavicle shaft fractures in children can be treated by nonoperative means.

In the neonate, complete fractures are distinctly uncommon. This is probably because of the increased flexibility of the bone and thick periosteal cover that are characteristic at this age. This thick periosteal tube helps explain the predictably rapid remodeling that occurs. Neonates require no treatment other than a soft bandage to bind the arm to the thorax for a few days.[115, 120, 134, 136, 151, 153]

In patients up to 12 years of age, reduction, even in displaced fractures, is not required. A soft figure-of-eight immobilization either made from stockinette or the commercial variety can be used (Fig. 27–25). Immobilization for three to six weeks is usually necessary for clinical union. Parents should be warned that a "bump" will appear as healing callus forms, but remodeling over 6 to 12 months is the rule (Fig. 27–26).[120]

In the older child, 12 years of age to maturity, a well-padded figure-of-eight harness is usually the immobilization of choice. Even in this older age group, nonunion is extremely rare, and most fractures that heal, even with moderate displacement or angulation, do not cause symptoms or impair function. The tendency for remodeling over a period of 9 to 12 months is still great in this age group. Gross displacement and severe angulation can be treated by gentle manual closed manipulation under intravenous sedation or hematoma block. The patient is placed supine on a table with a bolster in between the shoulders. Gentle, upward, backward, and lateral pressure is applied to the distal fragment to accomplish reduction. In this

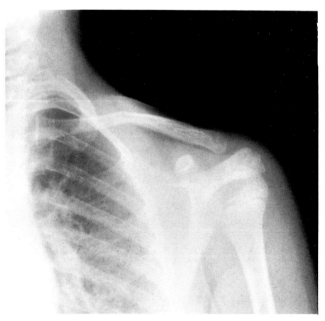

Figure 27–23. Greenstick fracture of the clavicle in an eight-year-old girl who had fallen on her outstretched arm. Note the soft tissue swelling superiorly at the fracture site. This is often a key to the diagnosis of the minimally displaced fracture.

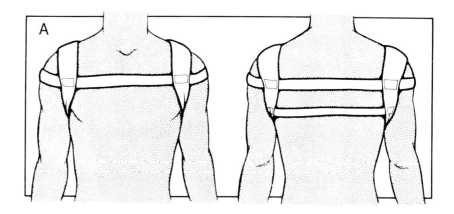

Figure 27–24. *A–F,* Various methods that historically have been used to immobilize fractures of the clavicle. (Reproduced with permission from Rockwood CA, and Green DP (eds): Fractures (3 vols), 2nd ed. Philadelphia: JB Lippincott, 1984.)

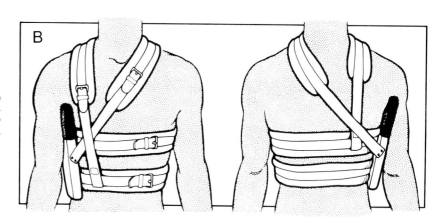

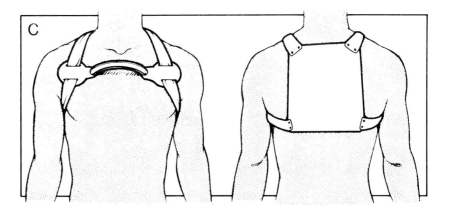

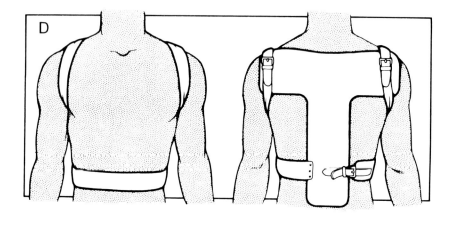

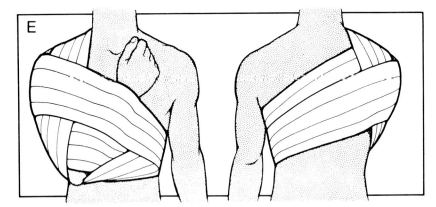

Figure 27–24 *Continued*

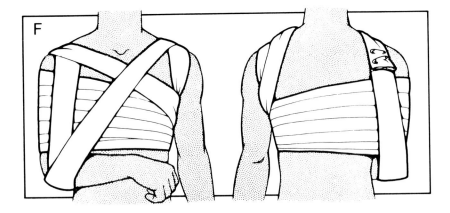

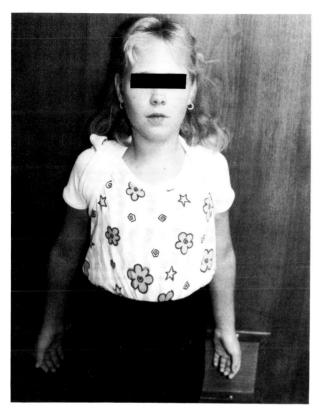

Figure 27–25. A commercial figure-of-eight sling is used to hold the shoulders up and back for both comfort and reduction.

age group, immobilization time averages six to eight weeks.

Indications for Operative Treatment

There are truly only two reasons for operative treatment of acute clavicular fractures in children: first, for debridement of open fractures and second, for stabilization of fractures associated with neurovascular complications.[131, 150, 171] A third possible indication would be for open reduction of a grossly displaced fracture that was irreducible by closed means in an older child. This type of fracture has been noted to occur because of buttonholing of the proximal fragment through trapezius muscle.[132]

Authors' Preferred Method of Treatment

During infancy, symptomatic treatment is used. If movement of the extremity elicits pain, the arm is bound to the thorax with a soft dressing for five to seven days. Children under age six are treated in a simple "homemade" figure-of-eight dressing. The figure-of-eight dressing is made by filling a stockinette with cast padding and attaching it to itself with safety pins. The dressing is tightened as needed for comfort only. Reduction is not required because of the tremendous potential for remodeling in this age group. Length of immobilization is usually three weeks.

In the 6-year to 12-year age group, a similar attitude of benign neglect can be taken toward reduction. We recommend the use of a commercial figure-of-eight dressing. It is tightened daily, as comfort allows, obtaining some element of reduction. Clinical union may require three to six weeks.

For the adolescent age 12 to 16 years, more attention to reduction may be required when dealing with a markedly displaced fracture. Reduction can be accomplished under mild sedation or hematoma block. The patient is placed supine upon a table with a bolster between the scapulae, allowing the shoulders to fall backward by gravity. Gentle manipulation at the fracture site can then be accomplished. A commercial figure-of-eight splint is then used to hold reduction. Clinical union requires six to eight weeks.

A return to contact sports activities is delayed in this older age group until the patient gains clinical union with full motion and strength. Solid radiographic evidence for healing is also required. This may take 8 to 12 weeks.

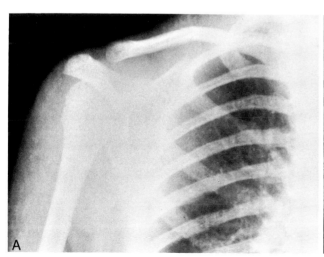
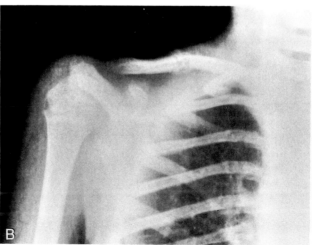

Figure 27–26. *A,* This greenstick fracture of the clavicle was misinterpreted on the original radiograph. *B,* The child presented one week later with continued pain and an enlarging mass at the fracture site. The follow-up radiograph demonstrates the healing "mass" of callus.

Open fractures are treated by irrigation and debridement followed by delayed closure and then immobilization by the methods previously described. The rare fracture associated with neurovascular injuries is treated by intramedullary pinning with threaded Hagie or Steinmann pins.

Complications

Neurovascular complications in children's clavicular fractures are rare but have been reported.[131, 142, 143, 165, 170] Prompt recognition and appropriate surgical or medical management are the keys to optimizing outcome. Vascular occlusion secondary to abundant callus formation does not appear to be a problem.

Because of the tremendous remodeling potential in children, malunion does not present a problem. Parents should be warned ahead of time of the prominent callus formation that will occur. They should realize that remodeling often takes 9 to 12 months.

Clavicular nonunion is distinctly rare in children.* The reported incidence of nonunion in all ages is 1 to 3 per cent. Those cases reported in children are in the adolescent age group, with the youngest being age 12 years.[146]

MEDIAL END OF CLAVICLE AND STERNOCLAVICULAR JOINT

Incidence

Fractures of the medial end of the clavicle are extremely rare in children. Rockwood reports that they constitute less than 1 per cent of all fractures of the clavicle in children.[120] Rowe has stated that they account for only 6 per cent of clavicle fractures.[154] Fractures of the shaft in this medial region are much less common than injuries to the medial physeal plate. Sternoclavicular dislocations have been reported, although most commonly Salter-Harris Type I and II injuries through the medial physis mimic such an injury in a child.[174, 176, 183, 189, 192, 198] As we recall from the anatomy in this region, the medial physis does not close until age 22 to 25 years (Fig. 27–27).

Mechanism of Injury

An indirect force with a relatively short lever arm applied to the anterior point of the shoulder can cause fracture in the region of the medial clavicle. This is the most common mechanism of injury for fracture as well as sternoclavicular dislocation. The point of application of force laterally will describe the direction of displacement at the medial end. If the shoulder is compressed and rolled forward, a posterior displacement occurs. If the shoulder is compressed and forced posteriorly, anterior displacement occurs.[120] This can

---

*See references 127, 129, 140, 145, 146, 163, 170.

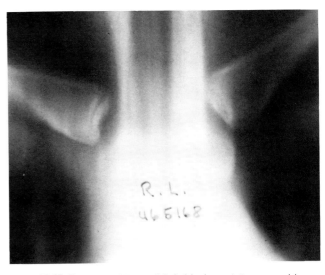

Figure 27–27. Tomogram of the medial clavicle demonstrates open epiphyses. These epiphyses do not fuse to the clavicular shaft until age 22 to 25. (Reproduced with permission from Rockwood CA, and Green DP (eds): Fractures (3 vols), 2nd ed. Philadelphia: JB Lippincott, 1984.)

happen in contact sports, such as football, when a player at the bottom of the pile has one shoulder on the ground while the opposite shoulder is compressed.

Injuries to the medial clavicle can occur by direct blows as well. These directly applied forces often produce nondisplaced or posteriorly displaced fractures.

Classification

Basically, three categories of injury occur at the medial clavicle. Certainly, the most common is the Salter-Harris type injury, either Type I or Type II (Fig. 27–28). Fractures of the medial shaft of the clavicle occur as well but are much less common. Sternoclavicular dislocations have been reported, but many were probably unrecognized Salter-Harris type fractures.[120, 174, 176, 183, 189, 198]

Further classification of the Salter-Harris type physeal injuries is based upon the direction of displacement

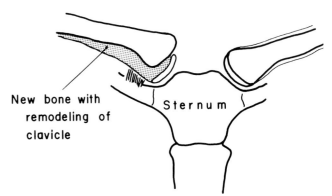

Figure 27–28. Diagram depicting a Salter-Harris Type I injury to the medial clavicular physis. Healing is by periosteal new bone with significant potential for remodeling.

of the shaft fragment. The epiphysis usually stays with the sternum with or without a small metaphyseal fragment. The shaft is then displaced either anteriorly or posteriorly. Certainly, anterior displacement is the most common.

Signs and Symptoms

Common clinical signs of fracture or dislocation are apparent. There is pain and swelling in the region. The head is often tilted toward the side of injury. The injured arm is supported across the chest. Deformity is somewhat difficult to characterize because of the swelling. Many of these injuries that are nondisplaced will show up late, with already visible or palpable callus.

Anteriorly displaced fractures and dislocations are the most common and are apparent on exam (Fig. 27–29). The posterior Salter-Harris type injury is sometimes difficult to diagnose clinically.[178–182, 188, 191, 192, 194] Often, marked swelling disguises the posterior deformity. Careful palpation along the superior sternum may allow one to ascertain the relative position of the medial clavicle (Fig. 27–30). Venous congestion or diminished pulses in the ipsilateral arm, as well as breathing difficulties, choking sensations, and difficulty swallowing, should be taken extremely seriously. They may represent impingement upon structures of the mediastinum by a posteriorly displaced fragment.

Radiographic Findings

The sternoclavicular joint and medial clavicle region are difficult to visualize by plain radiography. The midline position in the body allows overlapping radiographic shadows with the sternum, ribs, spine, and structures of the mediastinum. In addition, this is a difficult area to visualize by two radiographic views at 90 degrees to each other.

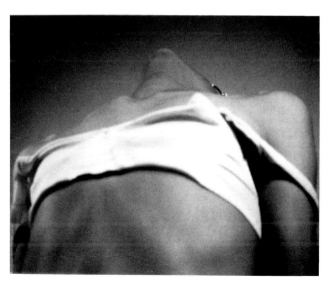

Figure 27–29. Clinical photograph demonstrating anterior displacement of a medial clavicular injury on the right.

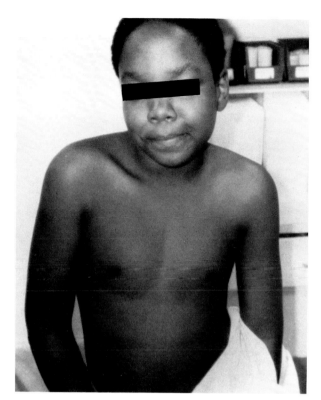

Figure 27–30. Posterior displacement of a medial clavicular injury. Notice the loss of contour of the left clavicle compared with the normal right side.

Many special radiographic views have been described. A simple, effective technique using tangential x-ray is the so-called serendipity view described by Rockwood.[120] It is a 40-degree cephalic tilt view (Fig. 27–31). The sternoclavicular joint and medial clavicle are projected away from the other structures that cause bony overlap. Comparison can be made from the involved side to the uninvolved side on the same film. This is helpful in diagnosis of the nondisplaced medial shaft fracture, as well as in demonstrating the direction of displacement of the shaft component of a Salter-Harris fracture or dislocation. With the fairly ready availability of sophisticated radiographic techniques such as CT scan and tomography, the diagnosis of fractures and dislocations in this area has been simplified. Tomography is excellent in demonstrating fractures of the medial clavicle.[177, 185] Tomograms can also help define the direction of displacement. CT scanning is a very accurate and excellent technique for defining pathology in this difficult region.[177, 184, 185] Differentiation of fractures from dislocation, as well as direction and degree of displacement, is readily accomplished with the CT scan. In addition, location of displaced fragments as they relate to structures of the mediastinum can be assessed (Fig. 27–32).

Treatment

As with other children's fractures about the shoulder, medial clavicular fractures either of the shaft or growth plate have a tremendous potential for healing

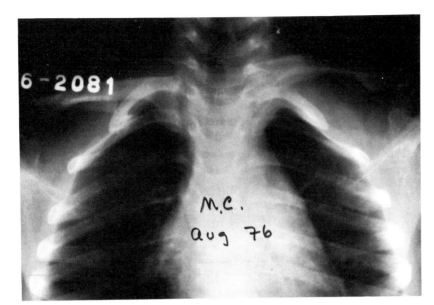

Figure 27–31. Serendipity view of the medial clavicles. This 40-degree tangential radiograph demonstrates an anterior dislocation of the left sternoclavicular joint. (Reproduced with permission from Rockwood CA, and Green DP (eds): Fractures (3 vols), 2nd ed. Philadelphia: JB Lippincott, 1984.)

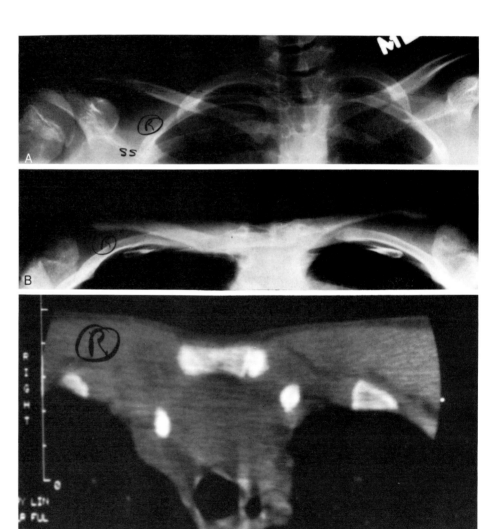

Figure 27–32. Posterior sternoclavicular dislocation of the right medial clavicle. *A*, Plain anteroposterior radiograph shows asymmetry but is difficult to interpret. *B*, Tangential view demonstrates posterior displacement. *C*, CT scan clearly demonstrates the injury as well as the relationship of the displaced medial clavicle to the mediastinal structures.

and remodeling. Many of these fractures if nondisplaced are discovered late when callus formation is already present. Little more than symptomatic treatment is indicated in these cases.

For the anteriorly displaced fracture or Salter-Harris type injury that mimics sternoclavicular dislocation, closed reduction can be performed. With appropriate local or general anesthesia, the patient is placed supine on a table with a bolster in between the shoulders. Longitudinal traction on the arm is then applied with the arm abducted 90 degrees. Gentle posterior pressure at the point of the shoulder as well as at the displaced fracture site will usually accomplish reduction. Immobilization is then accomplished by holding the shoulders back with a well-padded figure-of-eight dressing. Some authors prefer plaster figure-of-eight casting. A sling is used for comfort if necessary. Length of immobilization is from two to four weeks. Many of these fractures or dislocations will be unstable after reduction. Despite this instability, open reduction for the purpose of internal fixation is hazardous and unnecessary.[120, 175] Even when left with fairly substantial residual displacement, the tremendous remodeling potential discussed earlier does not warrant operative treatment. Case reports of pin migration, including deaths from broken pins that migrate into the innominate artery, lung, and heart, are present in the literature.[175] Chronic instability or nonunion of a fracture in this area is not reported.

Fractures with posterior displacement can require emergency reduction.[120, 178–182, 188, 191, 194] Most important, a careful examination to reveal impingement of mediastinal structures is in order. If reduction is necessary, the patient is placed on his back with a bolster in the midback region between the shoulders. After appropriate anesthesia, lateral traction is applied to the arm. The area overlying the medial clavicle is prepared, and a towel clip can then be used percutaneously to grab the posteriorly displaced medial clavicle, pulling laterally and anteriorly to accomplish reduction. An audible snap or pop often occurs. Reduction is uniformly stable. Rapid healing and remodeling is definitely the rule. A figure-of-eight dressing is used for immobilization for three to four weeks.

Authors' Preferred Method of Treatment

Nonoperative treatment is used in anteriorly displaced injuries of the medial clavicle and sternoclavicular joint (see Fig. 27–31). The tremendous remodeling potential is taken into consideration. Closed reduction under hematoma block is rarely performed in the adolescent with a markedly displaced anterior physeal fracture. A figure-of-eight splint is used until adequate comfort is obtained. This requires two to four weeks in most cases.

The only indication for more vigorous intervention would be in the case of posterior displacement of a medial clavicular injury with obvious compromise of mediastinal structures. If no evidence of impingement on mediastinal structures is evident, careful observation is undertaken. Repeat radiographs will often demonstrate periosteal new bone along the posterior and inferior medial clavicle, and further healing and remodeling is the rule. If mediastinal compression is present, attempted closed reduction under appropriate anesthesia is warranted. Only if this closed reduction failed would open reduction be considered. We do not use internal fixation at the medial end of the clavicle because of the well-documented high incidence of complications associated with this technique.

LATERAL END OF THE CLAVICLE AND ACROMIOCLAVICULAR JOINT

Incidence

Injuries to the lateral end of the clavicle and acromioclavicular joint occur in the general population more frequently than injuries to the medial end.[120, 205, 215] Rowe described 52 cases of acromioclavicular joint injury out of 1603 shoulder girdle injuries reviewed.[154] Distal clavicular fractures represent 10 to 12 per cent of all fractures of the clavicle.[154, 199] Incidence data for these injuries in children are not given. Because of the unique anatomy of this area in children, there is likely a higher percentage of fracture and pseudodislocation rather than true acromioclavicular dislocation.[206, 207, 218]

Mechanism of Injury

Sports injuries and falls predominate as causes for injury.[199, 205, 206] Both fractures and dislocations in the region of the lateral clavicle are caused by a blow to the point of the shoulder. As the shoulder strikes the ground, the acromion and scapula are driven inferiorly while the clavicle remains extended by the action of the sternoclavicular joint. Failure occurs either through the bone of the distal clavicle or through the periosteal tube around the distal clavicle. This same mechanism applies in those rare cases of true acromioclavicular dislocation.

Classification

The most common injury at the lateral end of the clavicle is a fracture that represents either a metaphyseal fracture or a Salter-Harris Type I or II fracture. The Salter-Harris fracture is often difficult to confirm radiographically since the distal clavicular epiphysis is only rarely ossified.[213] In either case, the distal clavicle is stripped from its distal periosteal tube, allowing the proximal fragment to protrude. The periosteal tube remains intact on its inferior surface in connection with the coracoclavicular ligaments. With or without surgical replacement of the clavicle into the periosteal tube, the potential for healing and remodeling is tremendous. Therefore, unlike the unstable adult fracture medial to the coracoclavicular ligaments, these fractures regain stability through the intact periosteum-ligament complex with healing (see Fig. 27–20).[205]

Classification of injuries to the acromioclavicular joint is similar to the adult classification.[205] Certainly, children older than approximately 15 years of age can have a truly adult-type injury. However, in most children, injuries to the acromioclavicular joint are not true dislocations, but rather fractures involving the distal clavicle. The common denominator is that there is a disruption of the periosteal tube allowing the distal clavicle to be displaced. The remaining tube is usually in continuity with the intact coracoclavicular ligaments. The classification in children, therefore, is based upon the position of the distal clavicle and accompanying injury to the periosteal tube, rather than injury to ligaments. Acromioclavicular joint injuries in children older than 15 should be considered to be adult in character.

Rockwood has classified injuries to the distal clavicle and acromioclavicular joint as follows (Fig. 27–33).[205]

Type I: Mild ligamentous sprain of the acromioclavicular ligaments without disruption of the periosteal tube. X-rays in this case are normal and the distal clavicle is stable by exam.

Type II: Partial disruption of the dorsal periosteal tube with some instability at the distal clavicle. Radiographically, there is slight widening of the acromioclavicular joint but no change in the coracoclavicular interval.

Type III: Large dorsal longitudinal split in the periosteal tube with gross instability of the distal clavicle. Although similar to adult acromioclavicular dislocations, these oftentimes are pseudodislocations in that they represent Salter-Harris Type I injury to the distal clavicular epiphysis. X-rays reveal superior displacement of the clavicle in relation to the coracoid of at least 25 per cent, and up to 100 per cent, the normal coracoclavicular distance (Fig. 27–34).

Type IV: Similar to the Type III injury, but the distal clavicle is buttonholed through the trapezius muscle fibers with the distal end completely buried in muscle. On the anteroposterior projection x-ray, there is widening of the acromioclavicular joint but little superior migration similar to a Type II dislocation. Actually, if an axillary radiograph is obtained, posterior displacement of the distal clavicle can be visualized.[210]

Type V: Complete dorsal periosteal split with subcutaneous dislocation of the distal end of the clavicle.

Type VI: Inferior dislocation of the clavicle beneath the coracoid.[209]

Other injuries can mimic injuries to the distal clavicle and acromioclavicular joint. Separation of the common physis for the base of the coracoid and the upper glenoid fossa or avulsion of the accessory ossification center on the dorsal surface of the coracoid with intact coracoclavicular ligaments can present as distal clavicular injuries (Fig. 27–35).[212, 214] Care should be taken to rule out these possibilities with appropriate radiographs. Dislocation of the acromioclavicular joint has been described in conjunction with dislocation medially and, thus, represents a complete dislocation of the clavicle.[201, 204]

Signs and Symptoms

Type I and II injuries demonstrate mild local swelling, local tenderness, and occasional ecchymosis. Some restricted motion is present secondary to pain. In the displaced injuries, there is obvious deformity present. In Type III and V injuries, the distal end of the clavicle is quite prominent superiorly. This is not because the clavicle is elevated, but rather because the remainder of the upper extremity sags with its own weight. Swelling and ecchymosis are present. The patient supports the elbow with the opposite hand. Motion is avoided owing to pain. In Type IV injuries, the distal end of the clavicle is prominent posteriorly as it is impaled in the belly of the trapezius muscle.[200, 210] In the rare Type VI injury, the top of the shoulder is flattened and ecchymotic. The acromion is quite prominent, and the distal end of the clavicle cannot be palpated. A thorough neurological exam should be performed to exclude injury to the brachial plexus in all cases.

Radiographic Findings

X-ray techniques for the distal clavicle vary from standard shoulder views based upon the decreased mass in this region. Unlike x-rays to visualize the glenohumeral joint, x-rays for the region of the distal clavicle require a soft tissue technique to adequately demonstrate fractures and displacement. An anteroposterior view may be all that is necessary to visualize fractures, but the axillary lateral view and the 20-degree cephalic tilt view will help demonstrate the type of injury present in most cases.

Stress x-rays are performed as described for adult injuries to the acromioclavicular joint.[205] By measuring the coracoclavicular distance on the anteroposterior x-ray, the particular classification of injury can be ascertained. In the Type I injury, there is no difference by comparison with the normal shoulder. In Type II distal clavicle injuries there is less than 25 per cent increase in the coracoclavicular distance with slight widening of the acromioclavicular joint. For the Type III injury, the displacement is 25 to 100 per cent. Type V injuries are represented by greater than 100 per cent increase in the coracoclavicular distance.[205] If an x-ray reveals an inferiorly displaced scapula relative to the clavicle without an increase in the coracoclavicular interval, a fracture of the base of the coracoid should be suspected. This fracture can best be demonstrated by using a Stryker notch view (Fig. 27–36).

Treatment

There is general agreement now that fractures of the distal clavicle and acromioclavicular joint injuries in

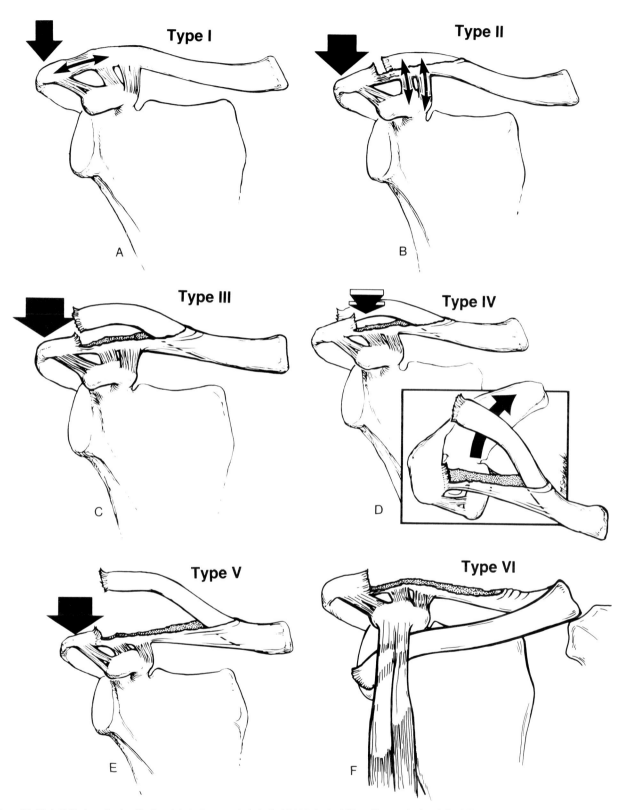

Figure 27–33. *A–F*, Rockwood's classification of clavicular–acromioclavicular joint injuries in children. (See text for description.) (Reproduced with permission from Rockwood CA, and Green DP (eds): Fractures (3 vols), 2nd ed. Philadelphia: JB Lippincott, 1984.)

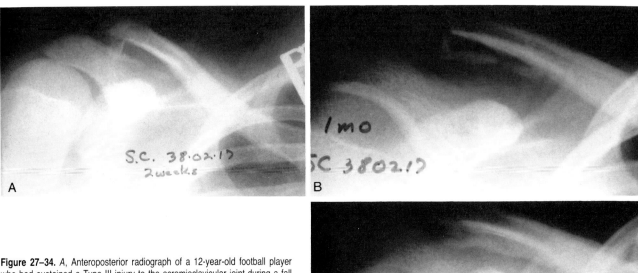

Figure 27–34. *A*, Anteroposterior radiograph of a 12-year-old football player who had sustained a Type III injury to the acromioclavicular joint during a fall on the point of his shoulder two weeks earlier. Notice the early appearance of new bone in the remaining periosteal tube. *B*, At one month clinical symptoms have subsided and additional callus has formed. *C*, Six months after injury, the entire periosteal tube is filled with new bone and significant remodeling is under way.

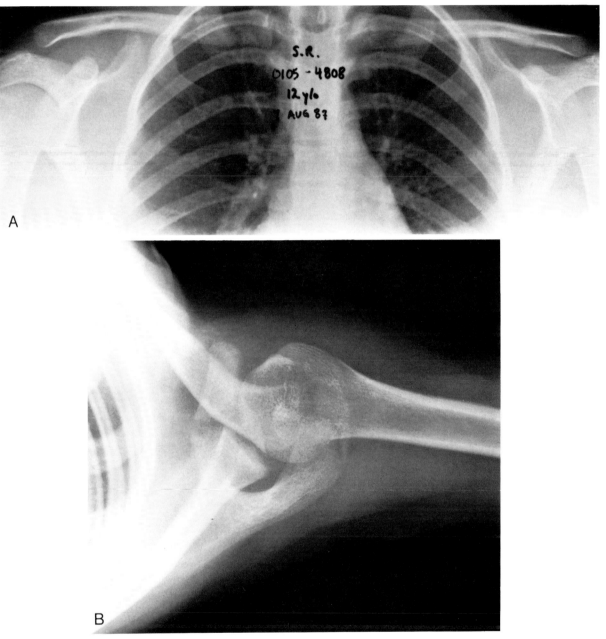

Figure 27–35. From clinical examination, this 12-year-old boy was thought to have a distal clavicular–acromioclavicular joint injury after falling on his right shoulder. *A,* Comparison anteroposterior views of both shoulders reveal a slight depression of the right scapula but no difference in comparative coracoclavicular distances. *B,* Axillary lateral view demonstrates the condition to be a fracture of the base of the coracoid.

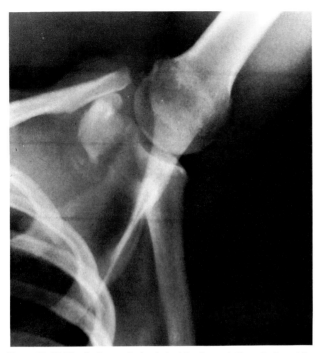

Figure 27-36. The Stryker notch view is best for demonstrating a fracture at the base of the coracoid.

children represent, in most cases, herniation of the clavicle from its periosteal tube. With the tremendous potential for periosteal new bone formation and remodeling, Dameron and Rockwood suggest that reduction either by closed or open means is unnecessary.[205] Healing will usually take place in less than six to eight weeks, and remodeling occurs during the first year. They would reserve surgical reduction for the Types IV, V, and VI acromioclavicular injuries. Others, such as Falstie-Jensen and Mikkelsen, have reported that superior results are obtained by replacing the displaced distal clavicle within the periosteal tube followed by internal fixation.[207] Ogden also suggests a greater attempt at reduction with fixation if necessary for distal clavicular physeal injuries.[216]

Eidman and associates concluded from a series of 25 cases in children under age 16 that true adult-type acromioclavicular dislocation is rare under age 13.[206] Although all patients in this group were treated surgically, they recommended that nonoperative treatment be used for children under age 13.

Certainly there is great controversy in the adult literature on how best to approach a Grade III acromioclavicular dislocation. Reports in the recent literature indicate that even in adults, nonoperative results for Grade III injuries are acceptable in terms of motion, strength, and function.[202, 221] This would certainly seem to provide further evidence to support a conservative approach to these injuries in children.

Authors' Preferred Method of Treatment

We prefer to treat fractures of the distal clavicle and Type I and Type II injuries to the acromioclavicular joint in children nonoperatively. One can expect healing of the fracture by periosteal new bone formation with remodeling of the fracture deformity (Fig. 27-37). Patients are treated symptomatically with contrast soaks and early range of motion. A sling is used for comfort. Mild analgesic medications are used as needed for pain. Healing time depends on the age of the patient.

Type III injuries to the acromioclavicular joint in children up to the age of 15 can be treated in a similar fashion. A three- to four-week period of symptomatic treatment with progressive mobilization is indicated. Return to activities is allowed when full motion and strength are regained. Closed reduction is not attempted, and the Kenny Howard–type sling is not

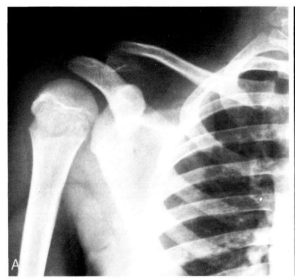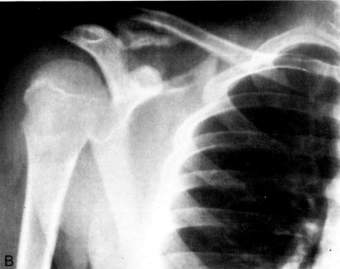

Figure 27-37. *A,* Anteroposterior radiograph demonstrates a distal clavicle fracture in a six-year-old boy. *B,* At one month, abundant periosteal new bone has formed in the remaining periosteal tube.

used. Because the acromioclavicular ligaments and distal periosteal tube remain intact, we prefer to treat fracture of the base of the coracoid nonoperatively.

Type IV, V, and VI injuries may be treated with a closed reduction, but if this is unsuccessful, then a surgical repair is undertaken. If the distal clavicle can be replaced into the periosteal tube and is stable with imbrication, no internal fixation is used. If unstable, a temporary coracoclavicular lag screw is used in the older child and transacromial wires are used in the young child. The fixation device is removed at three to six weeks, followed by appropriate protection and mobilization.

Scapula

DEVELOPMENTAL ANATOMY

Development of the scapula is by multiple ossification centers (Fig. 27–38). Their appearance is highly variable in terms of chronological appearance. At birth, only the body of the scapula is usually ossified. At approximately one year, an ossification center develops for the coracoid process. By age 10, an ossification center that combines for the base of the coracoid, as well as the upper one-fourth of the glenoid, develops.[231] This center fuses with the remainder of the scapula by age 16. There are often multiple centers of ossification present for the coracoid. At puberty, two to five ossification centers develop in the acromion and fuse by approximately age 22. Failure of fusion of one of these centers leads to the familiar variant called "os acromiale" (Fig. 27–39).[232] At puberty as well, the center for the vertebral border and inferior angle of the scapula, as well as a horseshoe shaped epiphysis for the lower three-fourths of the glenoid, appears. All of these fuse by age 22.[224, 225, 230, 233, 240, 242]

SURGICAL ANATOMY

From a practical standpoint, the various growth centers that form within the scapula are of little clinical consequence except to confuse the unwary surgeon on radiographic exam.[230] Many physes are present and can mimic fracture, especially in the region of the coracoid and acromion. Anomalies of the scapula are also not uncommon to further add to the confusion on radiographic exam.[232, 233, 237, 238, 240, 241] Clinical exam and x-ray comparison of the uninvolved side is useful.[224]

From its position on the posterolateral thorax, the scapula gives rise to 17 muscular attachments. It is highly mobile and provides approximately 60 degrees of rotation through its articulation with the thorax. Scapular contributions to the glenohumeral and acromioclavicular joints provide a firm foundation for shoulder function.[237, 242] Most scapular fractures actually represent avulsion by ligaments that support these joint structures.[226, 228]

CLASSIFICATION

Scapular fractures in children are uncommon.[223–225, 234] They will be classified by the area of location within the scapula. Fractures of the body, glenoid, acromion, and coracoid will be discussed.

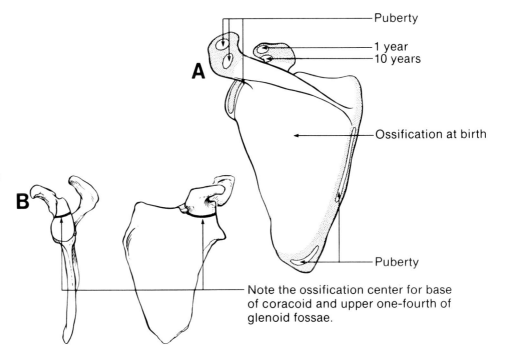

Figure 27–38. *A, B,* Multiple ossification centers of the scapula.

Puberty
1 year
10 years
Ossification at birth
Puberty
Note the ossification center for base of coracoid and upper one-fourth of glenoid fossae.

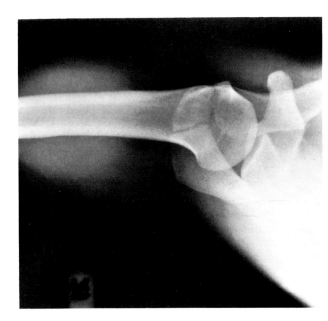

Figure 27-39. Unfused os acromiale seen on the axillary lateral view. This can be mistaken for an acute fracture of the acromion, which is a very rare injury in a child.

Figure 27-40. Fractures of the body of the scapula are usually associated with high-energy injuries. *A*, Anteroposterior radiograph shows a displaced body fracture. *B*, True scapular lateral view.

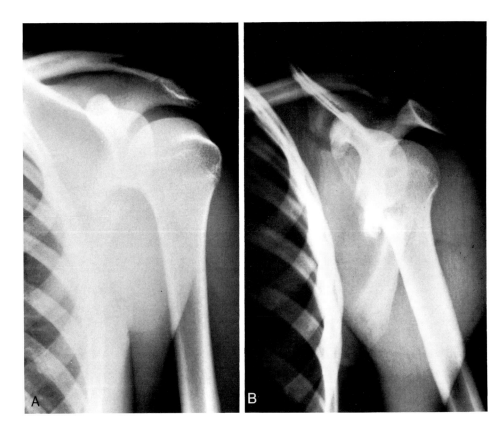

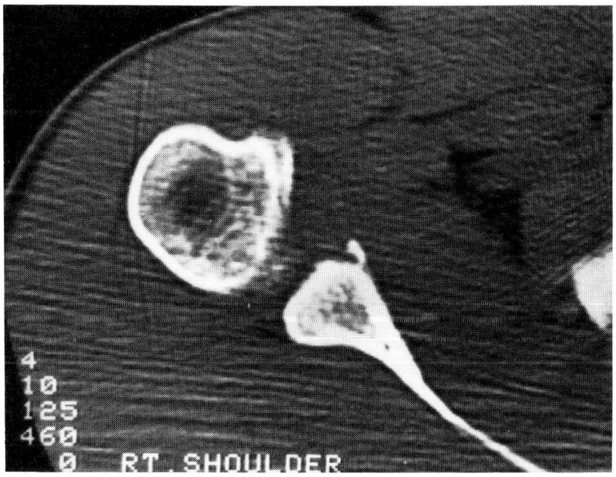

Figure 27-41. Displaced fractures of the anterior glenoid are associated with dislocations of the glenohumeral joint. A CT scan is very good at assessing this lesion.

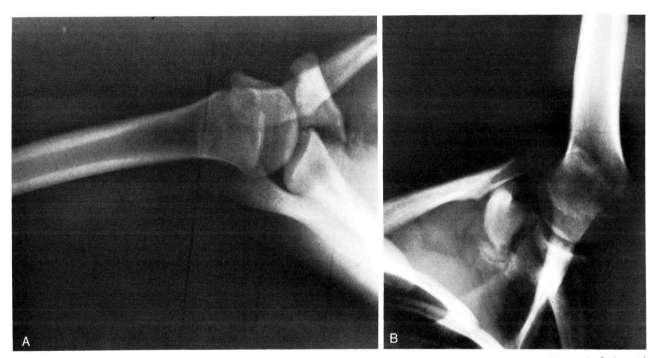

Figure 27-42. Fractures of the base of the coracoid are best seen on the Stryker notch view. A, Axillary lateral view of injury. B, Healing callus shown on the Stryker notch view.

MECHANISM OF INJURY, SIGNS AND SYMPTOMS, TREATMENT

Fractures of the Body of the Scapula

These fractures are relatively uncommon in children. The body of the scapula is fractured as the result of a severe direct blow as occurs in motor-vehicle accidents or falls from great heights (Fig. 27–40). They are often associated with rib, cervical spine, and clavicular fractures. In addition, injuries to the brachial plexus, internal organs, and lungs must be ruled out carefully. Treatment is nonoperative and includes rest and immobilization followed by progressive mobilization similar to treatment for the adult injury. Most important is the recognition of associated injuries. Four to six weeks is often required for healing. Remodeling will occur as in other children's fractures.[*] As in the adult, injury to the suprascapular nerve can occur with scapular fractures involving the suprascapular notch region.[236]

Dislocation of the scapula has been reported more frequently in the adult literature. Only a single case in a child has been reported by Nettrour and associates.[235] It is reasonable to assume that this injury would be associated with severe trauma and has the potential for neurovascular catastrophe.

Fractures of the Glenoid

The importance of these fractures is that they are often associated with severe traumatic dislocation of the shoulder.[224, 225, 226] Certainly fractures of the anterior glenoid rim are the most common, and yet, they are very uncommon in children (Fig. 27–41). Fractures involving the superior one-fourth of the glenoid can be associated with avulsion fractures of the coracoid through their common epiphysis. Large anterior glenoid fragments may require open reduction and internal fixation if associated with an unstable dislocation of the glenohumeral joint.[224, 226, 227, 243, 244] Other intra-articular fractures, even when associated with substantial displacement, seem to be well tolerated when treated nonoperatively with remodeling the rule.[224, 234]

Fractures of the Acromion

These fractures can result from a direct, severe force to the point of the shoulder.[224, 234, 239] They are extremely rare. They are treated by rest for five to seven days, followed by progressive range of motion. One should remember that failure of fusion of one of the multiple acromial epiphyses can lead to os acromiale.[232] This should not be mistaken for fracture. It can lead to problems with impingement in the older adolescent athlete who uses the arm for overhead sports such as pitching, swimming, and serving in tennis.

---

*See references 223, 224, 229, 234, 239, 243, 244.

Fractures of the Coracoid

These fractures have been discussed in conjunction with fractures of the distal clavicle. A hard fall on the point of the shoulder can result in minor injury to the acromioclavicular ligaments with fracture at the base of the coracoid (Fig. 27–42). This usually occurs through the common physis of the coracoid base and superior one-quarter of the glenoid.[224, 228, 231, 245] Occasionally, the fracture involves only a superior sliver of bone from the coracoid. As the acromioclavicular ligaments are stretched, the coracoclavicular ligaments remain intact, and the result is an avulsion fracture. The fracture is easily missed on routine shoulder views and is best seen on the Stryker notch view.[224] Treatment is usually nonoperative with supportive measures.

References

Fractures of the Proximal Humerus

1. Aitken AP: Fractures of the proximal humeral epiphysis. Surg Clin North Am 43:1573–1580, 1963.
2. Aufranc OE, Jones WN, and Bierbaum BE: Epiphyseal fracture of the proximal humerus. JAMA 207:727–729, 1969.
3. Aufranc OE, Jones WN, and Butler JE: Epiphyseal fracture of the proximal humerus. JAMA 213:1476–1479, 1970.
4. Baxter MP, and Wiley J: Fractures of the proximal humeral epiphysis: their influence on humeral growth. J Bone Joint Surg 68B(4):570–573, 1986.
5. Blount WP: Fractures in Children. Baltimore: Williams & Wilkins, 1954, pp 21–25.
6. Bourdillon JG: Fracture-separation of the proximal epiphysis of the humerus. J Bone Joint Surg 32B:35–37, 1950.
7. Cahill BR, Tullos HS, and Fain RH: Little League shoulder. J Sports Med 2:150–153, 1974.
8. Campbell J, and Almond HGA: Fracture-separation of the proximal humeral epiphysis. J Bone Joint Surg 59A:262–263, 1977.
9. Chapchal G (ed): Fractures in Children. New York: Thieme-Stratton, 1979.
10. Cohen BT, and Froimson AI: Salter III fracture dislocation of the glenohumeral joint in a 10-year-old. Orthop Rev 15(6):403–404, 1986.
11. Conwell EH: Fractures of the surgical neck and epiphyseal separations of the upper end of the humerus. J Bone Joint Surg 8:508, 1926.
12. Cumming WA: Neonatal skeletal fractures. Birth trauma and child abuse? J Can Assoc Radiol 30:30, 1979.
13. Dameron TB, and Reibel DB: Fractures involving the proximal humeral epiphyseal plate. J Bone Joint Surg 51A:289–297, 1969.
14. Dameron TB, and Rockwood CA: Fractures and dislocations of the shoulder. In Rockwood CA et al (eds): Fractures in Children. Philadelphia: JB Lippincott, 1984, pp 589–607.
15. Digby KH: The measurement of diaphyseal growth in proximal and distal directions. J Anat Physiol 50:187–188, 1916.
16. Fraser RL, Haliburton RA, and Barber JR: Displaced epiphyseal fractures of the proximal humerus. Can J Surg 10:427–430, 1967.
17. Gardner E: The prenatal development of the human shoulder joint. Surg Clin North Am 43:1465–1470, 1963.
18. Gilchrist DK: A stockinette-Velpeau for immobilization of the shoulder girdle. J Bone Joint Surg 49A:750–751, 1967.
19. Grant JCB: An Atlas of Anatomy, 6th ed. Baltimore: Williams & Wilkins, 1972.
20. Gray DJ, and Gardner E: The prenatal development of the human humerus. Am J Anat 124:431, 1969.
21. Haliburton RA, Barber JR, and Fraser JL: Pseudo-dislocation: an unusual birth injury. Can J Surg 10:455, 1967.

22. Hohl JD: Fractures of the humerus in children. Orthop Clin North Am 7:557–571, 1976

23. Horak J, and Nilsson BE: Epidemiology of fracture of the upper end of the humerus. Clin Orthop Rel Res 112:251, 1975.

24. Howard NJ, and Eloesser L: Treatment of fractures of the upper end of the humerus: an experimental and clinical study. J Bone Joint Surg 16:1–29, 1934.

25. Jeffrey CD: Fracture separation of the upper humeral epiphysis. Surg Gynecol Obstet 96:205–209, 1953.

26. Kohler R, and Trillaud JM: Fracture and fracture separation of the proximal humerus in children: report of 136 cases. J Pediatr Orthop 3:326, 1983.

27. Landin LA: Fracture patterns in children. Acta Orthop Scand [Suppl] 202:1, 1983.

28. Lee HG: Operative reduction of an unusual fracture of the upper epiphyseal plate of the humerus. J Bone Joint Surg 26:401–404, 1944.

29. Lemperg R, and Lilliequist B: Dislocations of the proximal epiphysis of the humerus in newborns. Acta Paediatr Scand 59:377–380, 1970.

30. Lentz W, and Jeuser P: The treatment of fractures of the proximal humerus. Arch Orthop Traum Surg 96:282–285, 1980.

31. Levin GD: A valgus angulation fracture of the proximal humeral epiphysis. Clin Orthop 116:155–157, 1976.

32. Lorenzo FT: Osteosynthesis with Blount's staples in fractures of the proximal end of the humerus. J Bone Joint Surg 37A:45–48, 1955.

33. Lucas LS, and Gill JH: Humerus varus following birth injury to proximal humeral epiphysis. J Bone Joint Surg 29:367–369, 1947.

34. Madsen ET: Fractures of the extremities in the newborn. Acta Obstet Gynaecol Scand 34:41, 1955.

35. McBride EO, and Sisler J: Fractures of the proximal humeral epiphysis and juxta-epiphyseal humeral shaft. Clin Orthop Rel Res 38:143–153, 1965.

36. Merten DF, Kirks DR, and Ruderman RJ: Occult humeral epiphyseal fracture in battered infants. Pediatr Radiol 10:151, 1981.

37. Neer CS, and Horowitz BS: Fractures of the proximal humeral epiphyseal plate. Clin Orthop Rel Res 41:24–31, 1965.

38. Nilsson S, and Svartholm F: Fracture of the upper end of the humerus in children. Acta Chir Scand 130:433–439, 1965.

39. Ogden JA, Conologue GJ, and Jensen P: Radiology of postnatal skeletal development: the proximal humerus. Skeletal Radiol 2:153–160, 1978.

40. O'Neill JA Jr, Meacham WF, Griffin PP, and Sawyers JL: Patterns of injury in the battered child syndrome. J Trauma 13:332, 1973.

41. Peterson CA, and Peterson HA: Analysis of the incidence of injuries to the epiphyseal growth plate. J Trauma 12:275–281, 1972.

42. Poland J: Traumatic Separation of the Epiphyses in General. London: Smith, Elder, 1898.

43. Rang M: Children's Fractures, 2nd ed. Philadelphia: JB Lippincott, 1983, pp 143–151.

43a. Rockwood CA Jr, Wilkins KE, and King RE (eds): Fractures in Children. Philadelphia: JB Lippincott, 1984, pp 577–607.

44. Rose SH, Melton LJ, Morrey BF, et al: Epidemiologic features of humeral fractures. Clin Orthop 168:24, 1982.

45. Salter RB: Textbook of Disorders and Injuries of the Musculoskeletal System. Baltimore: Williams & Wilkins, 1970, pp 439–440.

46. Salter RB, and Harris WR: Injuries involving the epiphyseal plate. J Bone Joint Surg 45A:587–622, 1963.

47. Scaglietti O: The obstetrical shoulder trauma. Surg Gynecol Obstet 66:868–877, 1938.

48. Sharrard WJW: Paediatric Orthopaedics and Fractures, Vol. II. Edinburgh: Blackwell Scientific Publications, 1979, pp 940–943, 1500–1508.

49. Sherk H, and Probst C: Fractures of the proximal humeral epiphysis. Orthop Clin North Am 6:401–413, 1975.

50. Shulman BH, and Terhune CB: Epiphyseal injuries in breech delivery. Pediatrics 8:693, 1951.

51. Smith FM: Fracture separation of the proximal humeral epiphysis. Am J Surg 91:627–635, 1956.

52. Tachdjian MO: Paediatric Orthopaedics. Philadelphia: WB Saunders, 1972, pp 1555–1560.

53. Truesdale ED: Birth Fractures and Epiphyseal Dislocations. New York: Paul B. Hoeber, 1917.

54. Tullos HS, and Fain JW: Little Leaguer's shoulder: rotational stress fracture of the proximal epiphysis. J Sports Med 2(3):152–153, 1974.

55. Visser JO, and Rietberg M: Interposition of the tendon of the long head of biceps in fracture separation of the proximal humeral epiphysis. Netherlands J Surg 32:12–15, 1980.

56. Warwick R, and Williams P: Gray's Anatomy, 35th British ed. Philadelphia: WB Saunders, 1973.

57. Watson-Jones R: Fractures of the neck of the humerus. In Fractures and Joint Injuries. Baltimore: Williams & Wilkins, 1955, pp 471–474.

58. Weber BG, Brunner C, and Freuler F: Treatment of Fractures in Children and Adolescents. New York: Springer-Verlag, 1980, pp 87–129.

59. Whitman R: A treatment of epiphyseal displacements and fractures of the upper extremity of the humerus designed to assure definite adjustment and fixation of the fragments. Ann Surg 47:706–708, 1908.

60. Williams DJ: The mechanisms producing fracture separation of the proximal humeral epiphysis. J Bone Joint Surg 63B:102–107, 1981.

61. Zimmer EA: Kohler's Borderland of the Normal and Early Pathologic in Skeletal Roentgenology, 10th ed. (Translated by JT Case.) New York: Grune & Stratton, 1961.

Subluxations and Dislocations of the Glenohumeral Joint

62. Aronen JG, and Regan K: Decreasing the incidence of recurrence of first time anterior shoulder dislocation with rehabilitation. Am J Sports Med 12(4):283–291, 1984.

63. Asher MA: Dislocations of the upper extremity in children. Orthop Clin North Am 7:583–591, 1976.

64. Babbitt DP, and Cassidy RH: Obstetrical paralysis and dislocation of the shoulder in infancy. J Bone Joint Surg 50A(7):1447–1452, 1968.

65. Bach FR, O'Brien SJ, Warren RF, and Leighton M: An unusual neurological complication of the Bristow procedure: a case report. J Bone Joint Surg 70A(3):458–460, 1988.

66. Barry TP, Lombardo SJ, Kerlan RK, et al: The coracoid transfer for recurrent anterior instability of the shoulder in adolescents. J Bone Joint Surg 67A(3):383–386, 1985.

67. Blount WP: Fractures in Children. Baltimore: Williams & Wilkins, 1955.

68. Chung MK, and Nissenbaum MM: Congenital and development defects of the shoulder. Orthop Clin North Am 6:381, 1975.

69. Cozen L: Congenital dislocation of the shoulder and other anomalies. Arch Surg 35:956–966, 1937.

70. Dameron TB, and Rockwood CA: Fractures and dislocations of the shoulder. In Rockwood CA et al (eds): Fractures in Children. Philadelphia: JB Lippincott, 1984, pp 659–676.

71. Foster WS, Ford TB, and Drez D: Isolated posterior shoulder dislocation in a child. Am J Sports Med 13(3):198–200, 1985.

72. Freundlich BD: Luxatio erecta. J Trauma 23(5):434–436, 1983.

73. Green NE, and Wheelhouse WW: Anterior subglenoid dislocation of the shoulder in an infant following pneumococcal meningitis. Clin Orthop 135:125–127, 1978.

74. Grieg DM: True congenital dislocation of the shoulder. Edinburgh Med J 30:157–175, 1923.

75. Haliburton RA, Barber JR, and Fraser RL: Pseudodislocation: an unusual birth injury. Can J Surg 10:455–462, 1967.

76. Hawkins RJ, Koppert G, and Johnston G: Recurrent posterior instability (subluxation) of the shoulder. J Bone Joint Surg 66A(2):169–174, 1984.

77. Heck CC, Jr: Anterior dislocation of the glenohumeral joint in a child. J Trauma 21:174–175, 1981.

78. Hernandez A, and Drez D: Operative treatment of posterior shoulder dislocations by posterior glenoidplasty, capsulorrha-

phy and infraspinatus advancement. Am J Sports Med *14*(3):187–191, 1986.

79. Hovelius L: Anterior dislocation of the shoulder in teenagers and young adults. J Bone Joint Surg *69A*(3):393–399, 1987.

80. Hovelius L, Erikson GK, Fredin FH, et al: Recurrences after initial dislocation of the shoulder. J Bone Joint Surg *65*(3):343–349, 1983.

81. Kuhn D, and Rosman M: Traumatic, nonparalytic dislocation of the shoulder in a newborn infant. J Pediatr Orthop *4*:121, 1984.

82. Laskin RS, and Sedlin ED: Luxatio erecta in infancy. Clin Orthop *80*:126–129, 1971.

83. Lawhon SM, Peoples AB, and MacEwen GD: Voluntary dislocation of the shoulder. J Pediatr Orthop *2*:590, 1982.

84. Lichtblau PO: Shoulder dislocation in the infant. Case report and discussion. J Fla Med Assoc *64*:313, 1977.

85. May VR, Jr: Posterior dislocation of the shoulder: habitual, traumatic and obstetrical. Orthop Clin North Am *11*:271, 1980.

86. McNeil EL: Luxatio erecta: letter to the editor. Ann Emerg Med *13*(6):490, 1986.

87. Miller LS, Donahue JR, Good RP, and Staerk AJ: The Magnuson-Stack procedure for treatment of recurrent glenohumeral dislocation. Am J Sports Med *12*(2):133–137, 1984.

88. Neer CS II: Involuntary inferior and multidirectional instability of the shoulder: etiology, recognition, and treatment. AAOS Instr Course Lect *34*:232–238, 1985.

89. Neer CS II, and Foster DR: Inferior capsular shift for involuntary inferior and multidirectional instability of the shoulder. J Bone Joint Surg *62A*:897–908, 1980.

90. Nicastro JF, and Adair DM: Fracture-dislocation of the shoulder in a 32-month-old child. J Pediatr Orthop *2*:427, 1982.

91. Norwood L, and Terry GC: Shoulder posterior subluxation. Am J Sports Med *12*(1):25–30, 1984.

92. Ogden JA: Skeletal Injury in the Child. Philadelphia: Lea & Febiger, 1982, pp 227–228.

93. Pettersson H: Bilateral dysplasia of the neck of the scapula and associated anomalies. Acta Radiol Diagnosis *22*:81–84, 1981.

94. Pollen AG: Fractures and Dislocations in Children. Baltimore: Williams & Wilkins, 1973.

95. Rang M: Children's Fractures, 2nd ed. Philadelphia: JB Lippincott, 1983.

96. Richards RR, Hudson AR, Bertoia JT, et al: Injury to the brachial plexus during Putti-Platt and Bristow procedures: a report of eight cases. Am J Sports Med *15*(4):374–380, 1987.

96a. Rockwood CA Jr, Wilkins KE, and King RE (eds): Fractures in Children. Philadelphia: JB Lippincott, 1984, pp 659–676.

97. Rowe CR: Anterior dislocation of the shoulder: prognosis and treatment. Surg Clin North Am *43*:1609–1614, 1963.

98. Rowe CR: Prognosis in dislocation of the shoulder. J Bone Joint Surg *38A*:957–977, 1956.

99. Rowe CR, Pierce DS, and Clark JG: Voluntary dislocation of the shoulder. J Bone Joint Surg *55A*:445–459, 1973.

100. Rowe CR, Zarins B, and Ciullo JV: Recurrent anterior dislocation of the shoulder after surgical repair. J Bone Joint Surg *66A*(2):159–168, 1984.

101. Sharrard WJW: Paediatric Orthopaedics and Fractures. Oxford: Blackwell Scientific Publications, 1971.

102. Simonet WT, and Cofield RH: Prognosis in anterior shoulder dislocation. Am J Sports Med *12*(1):19–24, 1984.

103. Tachdjian MO: Paediatric Orthopaedics. Philadelphia: WB Saunders, 1972.

104. Vastamaki M, and Solonen KA: Posterior dislocation and fracture dislocation of the shoulder. Acta Orthop Scand *51*:479–484, 1980.

105. Wagner KT, and Lyne ED: Adolescent traumatic dislocations of the shoulder with open epiphyses. J Pediatr Orthop *3*:61–62, 1983.

106. Weber BG, Brunner C, and Freuler F: Treatment of Fractures in Children and Adolescents. Berlin: Springer-Verlag, 1980, pp 94–95.

107. Wickstrom J: Birth injuries of the brachial plexus. Treatment defects in the shoulder. Clin Orthop *23*:187–196, 1962.

108. Wickstrom J, Haslam ET, and Hutchinson RH: The surgical management of residual deformities of the shoulder following birth injuries of the brachial plexus. J Bone Joint Surg *37A*:27–36, 1955.

109. Zuckerman JD, and Matsen FA: Complications about the glenohumeral joint related to the use of screws and staples. J Bone Joint Surg *66A*(2):175–180, 1984.

Fractures of the Clavicle and Injuries to the Sternoclavicular and Acromioclavicular Joints

110. Abbott LD, and Lucas DG: The function of the clavicle. Ann Surg *140*:583–599, 1954.

111. Alldred AJ: Congenital pseudarthrosis of the clavicle. J Bone Joint Surg *42B*:312–319, 1963.

112. Allman FL: Fractures and ligamentous injuries of the clavicle and its articulation. J Bone Joint Surg *49A*:774, 1967.

113. Andersen H: Histochemistry and development of the human shoulder and acromioclavicular joints with particular reference to the early development of the clavicle. Acta Anat *55*:124–165, 1963.

114. Billington RW: A new (plaster yoke) dressing for fracture of the clavicle. Southern Med J *24*:667–670, 1931.

115. Blount WP: Fractures in Children. Baltimore: Williams & Wilkins, 1955.

116. Bowen AD: Plastic bowing of the clavicle in children. J Bone Joint Surg *65A*:403, 1983.

117. Cohen AW, and Otto SR: Obstetric clavicular fractures. J Reprod Med *25*:119–122, 1980.

118. Copeland SM: Total resection of the clavicle. Am J Surg *72*:280–281, 1946.

119. Corrigan GE: The neonatal clavicle. Biol Neonat *2*:79–92, 1959.

120. Dameron TB, and Rockwood CA: Fractures and dislocations of the shoulder. *In* Rockwood CA et al (eds): Fractures in Children. Philadelphia: JB Lippincott, 1984, pp 624–653.

121. Fairbanks HAT: Atlas of General Affections of the Skeleton. Edinburgh: E & S Livingstone, 1951.

122. Fairbanks HAT: Cranio-cleido dysostosis. J Bone Joint Surg *31B*:608–617, 1949.

123. Farkas R, and Levine S: X-ray incidence of fractured clavicle in vertex presentation. Am J Obstet Gynecol *59*:204–206, 1950.

124. Fawcett J: The development and ossification of the human clavicle. J Anat *47*:225–234, 1913.

125. Gardner E: The embryology of the clavicle. Clin Orthop *58*:9–16, 1968.

126. Gardner E, and Gray DJ: Prenatal development of the human shoulder and acromioclavicular joints. Am J Anat *92*:219–276, 1953.

127. Ghormley RK, Black JR, and Cherry JH: Ununited fractures of the clavicle. Am J Surg *51*:343–349, 1941.

128. Gibson DA, and Carroll N: Congenital pseudarthrosis of the clavicle. J Bone Joint Surg *52B*:629–643, 1970.

129. Gumley GJ, and Jupiter JJ: Clavicle non-union — a review of management and presentation of a stable bone graft. Orthop Trans *9*:29, 1985.

130. Hamilton FH: Fractures of the clavicle. *In* A Practical Treatise of Fractures and Dislocations. Philadelphia: Henry C. Lea, 1866, pp 177–199.

131. Howard FM, and Shafer SJ: Injuries to the clavicle with neurovascular complications: a study of fourteen cases. J Bone Joint Surg *47A*:1335–1346, 1965.

132. Jablon M, Sutker A, and Post M: Irreducible fractures of the middle-third of the clavicle. J Bone Joint Surg *61A*:296–298, 1979.

133. Jit I, and Kulkarni M: Times of appearance and fusion of epiphysis at the medial end of the clavicle. Indian J Med Res *64*(5):773–792, 1976.

134. Key JA, and Conwell HE: Fractures of the clavicle. *In* The Management of Fractures, Dislocations and Sprains. St. Louis: CV Mosby, 1946, pp 495–512.

135. Lester CW: The treatment of fractures of the clavicle. Ann Surg *89*:600–606, 1929.

136. Liechtl R: Fracture of the clavicle and scapula. *In* Weber BG,

Brunner C, and Freuler F (eds): Treatment of Fractures in Children and Adolescents. New York: Springer-Verlag, 1980, pp 88–95.

137. Ljunggren AE: Clavicular function. Acta Orthop Scand 50:261–268, 1979.

138. Lloyd-Roberts GC, Apley AG, and Owen R: Reflections upon the aetiology of congenital pseudarthrosis of the clavicle. J Bone Joint Surg 57B:24–29, 1975.

139. Madsen ET: Fractures of the extremities in the newborn. Acta Obstet Gynecol Scand 34:41–74, 1955.

140. Manske DJ, and Szabo RM: The operative treatment of midshaft clavicular non-unions. J Bone Joint Surg 67A:1367, 1985.

141. Marsh HO, and Hazarian E: Pseudarthrosis of the clavicle. J Bone Joint Surg 52B:793, 1970.

142. Miller DS, and Boswick JA: Lesions of the brachial plexus associated with fractures of the clavicle. Clin Orthop 64:144, 1969.

143. Mital MA, and Aufranc OE: Venous occlusion following greenstick fracture of the clavicle. JAMA 206:1301–1302, 1968.

144. Moseley HG: The clavicle: its anatomy and function. Clin Orthop 58:17–27, 1968.

145. Neer CS II: Nonunion of the clavicle. JAMA 172:1006–1011, 1960.

146. Nogi J, Heckman JD, Hakala M, and Sweet DE: Non-union of the clavicle in a child. A case report. Clin Orthop 110:19, 1975.

147. Ogden JA, Conologue GJ, and Bronson ML: Radiology of postnatal skeletal development, III. The clavicle. Skeletal Radiol 4:196–203, 1979.

148. Owen R: Congenital pseudarthrosis of the clavicle. J Bone Joint Surg 52B:644–652, 1970.

149. Oxnard CE: The architecture of the shoulder in some mammals. J Morph 126:249–290, 1968.

150. Penn I: The vascular complications of fractures of the clavicle. J Trauma 4:819–831, 1964.

151. Pollen AG: Fractures and Dislocations in Children. Baltimore: Williams & Wilkins, 1973.

152. Quinlan WR, Brady PG, and Regan BF: Congenital pseudarthrosis of the clavicle. Acta Orthop Scand 5:489–492, 1980.

153. Rang M: Clavicle. In Children's Fractures, 2nd. ed. Philadelphia: JB Lippincott, 1983.

153a. Rockwood CA Jr, Wilkins KE, and King RE (eds): Fractures in Children. Philadelphia: JB Lippincott, 1984, pp 608–652.

154. Rowe CR: An atlas of anatomy and treatment of midclavicular fractures. Clin Orthop 58:29–42, 1968.

155. Rubin A: Birth injuries: incidence, mechanism and end result. Obstet Gynecol 23:218–221, 1964.

156. Salter RB: Textbook of Disorders and Injuries of the Musculoskeletal System. Baltimore: Williams & Wilkins, 1970, pp 439–440.

157. Sanford HN: The Moro reflex as a diagnostic aid in fracture of the clavicle in the newborn infant. Am J Dis Children 41:1304–1306, 1931.

158. Sayre L: A simple dressing for fracture of the clavicle. Am Pract 4:1, 1871.

159. Snyder L: Loss of accompanying soft tissue shadow of clavicle with occult fracture. Southern Med J 72:243, 1979.

160. Stanley D, Trowbridge EA, and Norris SH: The mechanism of clavicular fractures: a clinical and biomechanical analysis. J Bone Joint Surg 70B(3):461–464, 1988.

161. Stimson LA: A Practical Treatise on Fractures and Dislocations, 8th ed. Philadelphia: Lea & Febiger, 1917.

162. Tachdjian MO: Paediatric Orthopaedics. Philadelphia: WB Saunders, 1972.

163. Taylor AR: Non-union of fractures of the clavicle: a review of thirty-one cases. J Bone Joint Surg 51B:568, 1969.

164. Todd TW, and DiErrico J Jr: The clavicular epiphyses. Am J Anat 41:25–50, 1928.

165. Tse DHW, Slabaugh PB, and Carlson PA: Injury to the axillary artery by a closed fracture of the clavicle. J Bone Joint Surg 62A:1372, 1980.

166. Wall JJ: Congenital pseudarthrosis of the clavicle. J Bone Joint Surg 52A:1003–1009, 1970.

167. Watson-Jones R: Fractures of the clavicle. In Fractures and Joint Injuries. Baltimore: Williams & Wilkins, 1955, pp 460–462.

168. Wilkins R, and Johnston RM: Ununited fractures of the clavicle. J Bone Joint Surg 65A:773, 1983.

169. Wilson JC: Fractures and dislocations in children. Pediatr Clin North Am 14:659–662, 1967.

170. Yates DW: Complications of fractures of the clavicle. Injury 7:189–193, 1976.

171. Zenni EJ, Krieg JK, and Rosen MJ: Open reduction and internal fixation of clavicular fractures. J Bone Joint Surg 63A:147–151, 1981.

Medial End of Clavicle

172. Bearn JG: Direct observations on the function of the capsule of the sternoclavicular support. J Anat 101:159, 1967.

173. Booth CM, and Roper BA: Chronic dislocation of the sternoclavicular joint. Clin Orthop 140:17, 1979.

174. Brooks AL, and Henning GD: Injury to the proximal clavicular epiphysis. J Bone Joint Surg 54A:1347, 1972.

175. Clark RL, Milgram JW, and Yawn DH: Fatal aortic perforation and cardiac tamponade due to a Kirschner wire migrating from the right sternoclavicular joint. South Med J 67:316, 1974.

176. Denham RH, and Dingley AF: Epiphyseal separation of the medial clavicle. J Bone Joint Surg 49A:1179, 1967.

177. DePalma JM, Gilula LA, Murphy WA, and Sagel SS: Computed tomography of the sternoclavicular joint and sternum. Radiology 138:123, 1981.

178. Elting JJ: Retrosternal dislocations of the clavicle. Arch Surg 104:35, 1972.

179. Greenlee DP: Posterior dislocation of the sternal end of the clavicle. JAMA 125:426, 1944.

180. Heinig CF: Retrosternal dislocation of the clavicle: early recognition, x-ray diagnosis and management. J Bone Joint Surg 50A:830, 1968.

181. Kennedy JC: Retrosternal dislocation of the clavicle. J Bone Joint Surg 31B:74, 1949.

182. Lee FA, and Gwinn JL: Retrosternal dislocation of the clavicle. Radiology 110:631, 1974.

183. Lemire L, and Rosman M: Sternoclavicular epiphyseal separation with adjacent clavicular fracture. J Pediatr Orthop 4:118, 1984.

184. Levisohn EM, Bunnell WP, and Yuan HA: Computed tomography in the diagnosis of dislocations of the sternoclavicular joint. Clin Orthop 140:12, 1979.

185. Lourie AA: Tomography in the diagnosis of posterior dislocation of the sterno-clavicular joint. Acta Orthop Scand 51:579, 1980.

186. Lowman CL: Operative correction of old sternoclavicular dislocation. J Bone Joint Surg 10:740, 1928.

187. Lunseth PA, Chapman KW, and Frankel VH: Surgical treatment of chronic dislocation of the sterno-clavicular joint. J Bone Joint Surg 57B:193, 1975.

188. McKenzie JMM: Retrosternal dislocations of the clavicle. A report of two cases. J Bone Joint Surg 45B:138, 1961.

189. Nettles JL, and Linscheid RL: Sternoclavicular dislocations. J Trauma 8:158, 1968.

190. Omer GE: Osteotomy of the clavicle in surgical reduction of anterior sternoclavicular dislocation. J Trauma 7:584, 1967.

191. Paterson DC: Retrosternal dislocation of the clavicle. J Bone Joint Surg 43B:90, 1961.

192. Rockwood CA: Dislocations of the sternoclavicular joint. AAOS Instr Course Lect 24:144, 1975.

192a. Rockwood CA Jr, Wilkins KE, and King RE (eds): Fractures in Children. Philadelphia: JB Lippincott, 1984; pp 624–628.

193. Salvatore JE: Sternoclavicular joint dislocation. Clin Orthop 58:51, 1968.

194. Selesnick FH, Jablon M, Frank C, and Post M: Retrosternal dislocation of the clavicle. J Bone Joint Surg 66A:297, 1984.

195. Simurda MA: Retrosternal dislocation of the clavicle: a report of four cases and a method of repair. Can J Surg 11:487, 1968.

196. Stein AH: Retrosternal dislocation of the clavicle. J Bone Joint Surg 39A:656, 1957.

197. Tyler HDD, Sturrock WDS, and Callow FMC: Retrosternal dislocation of the clavicle. J Bone Joint Surg 45B:132, 1963.
198. Wheeler ME, Laaveg SJ, and Sprague BL: S-C joint disruption in an infant. Clin Orthop 139:68, 1979.

Lateral End of Clavicle

199. Allman FL: Fractures and ligamentous injuries of the clavicle. J Bone Joint Surg 42B:312–319, 1963.
200. Barber FA: Complete posterior acromioclavicular dislocation. Orthopaedics 10(3):493–496, 1987.
201. Beckman T: A case of simultaneous luxation of both ends of the clavicle. Acta Chir Scand 56:156–163, 1923.
202. Bjerneld H, Hovelius L, and Thorling J: Acromioclavicular separations treated conservatively. Acta Orthop Scand 54:743–745, 1983.
203. Browne JE, Stanley RF, and Tullos HS: Acromioclavicular joint dislocations: comparative results following operative treatment with and without primary distal clavisectomy. Am J Sports Med 5:258, 1977.
204. Buckfield CT, and Castle ME: Acute traumatic dislocation of the clavicle. J Bone Joint Surg 66A:379, 1984.
205. Dameron TB, and Rockwood CA: Fractures and dislocations of the shoulder. In Rockwood CA et al (eds): Fractures in Children. Philadelphia: JB Lippincott, 1984, pp 624–653.
206. Eidman DK, Siff SJ, and Tullos HS: Acromioclavicular lesions in children. Am J Sports Med 9(3):150–154, 1981.
207. Falstie-Jensen S, and Mikkelsen P: Pseudodislocation of the acromioclavicular joint. J Bone Joint Surg 64B:368–369, 1982.
208. Gardner E, and Gray DJ: Prenatal development of the human shoulder and acromioclavicular joints. Am J Anat 92:219–276, 1953.
209. Gerber C, and Rockwood CA: Subcoracoid dislocation of the lateral end of the clavicle. J Bone Joint Surg 69A(6):924–927, 1987.
210. Gunther WA: Posterior dislocation of the clavicle. J Bone Joint Surg 31A:878, 1949.
211. Gurd FB: The treatment of complete dislocation of the outer end of the clavicle: a hitherto undescribed operation. Ann Surg 113:1094–1097, 1941.
212. Hall RH, Isaac F, and Booth CR: Dislocation of the shoulder with special references to accompanying small fractures. J Bone Joint Surg 41A:489–494, 1959.
213. Kohler A, and Zimmer EA: Borderlands of Normal and Early Pathologic in Skeletal Roentgenology, 3rd Am ed. (Translated by SP Wilke.) New York: Grune & Stratton, 1968, pp 156–159.
214. Montgomery SP, and Lloyd RD: Avulsion fracture of the coracoid epiphysis with acromioclavicular separation: report of two cases in adolescents and review of literature. J Bone Joint Surg 59A:963–965, 1977.
215. Neer CS II: Fractures of the distal third of the clavicle. Clin Orthop 58:43–50, 1968.
216. Ogden JA: Distal clavicular physeal injury. Clin Orthop 188:68–73, 1984.
217. Rauschning W, Nordesjo LO, Nirdgren B, et al: Resection arthroplasty for repair of complete acromioclavicular separations. Arch Orthop Trauma Surg 97:161, 1980.
218. Rockwood CA: Fractures of outer clavicle in children and adults. J Bone Joint Surg 64B:642, 1982.
218a. Rockwood CA Jr, Wilkins KE, and King RE (eds): Fractures in Children. Philadelphia: JB Lippincott, 1984, pp 627–631.
219. Roper BA, and Levack B: The surgical treatment of acromioclavicular dislocations. J Bone Joint Surg 64B:597, 1982.
220. Taft TN, Wilson FC, and Oglesby JW: Dislocation of the acromioclavicular joint. J Bone Joint Surg 69A(7):1045–1051, 1987.

221. Walsh WM, Peterson DA, Shelton G, and Neumann RD: Shoulder strength following acromioclavicular injury. Am J Sports Med 13(3):153–161, 1985.
222. Weber BG, Brunner C, and Freuler R: Treatment of Fractures in Children and Adolescents. New York: Springer-Verlag, 1980, p 89.

Fractures of the Scapula

223. Asher MA: Dislocations of the upper extremity in children. Orthop Clin North Am 7(3):583–591, 1976.
224. Dameron TB, and Rockwood CA: Fractures and dislocations of the shoulder. In Rockwood CA et al (eds): Fractures in Children. JB Lippincott, Philadelphia, 1984, pp 653–659.
225. DePalma AF: Surgery of the Shoulder, 2nd ed. Philadelphia: JB Lippincott, 1973, p 28.
226. Hall RH, Isaac F, and Booth CR: Dislocation of the shoulder with special reference to accompanying small fractures. J Bone Joint Surg 41A:489–494, 1959.
227. Hardegger FH, Simpson LA, and Weber BG: The operative treatment of scapular fractures. J Bone Joint Surg 66B:725, 1984.
228. Heyse-Moore GH, and Stoker DJ: Avulsion fractures of the scapula. Skel Radiol 9:27, 1982.
229. Imatani RJ: Fractures of the scapula: a review of 53 fractures. J Trauma 15:473–478, 1975.
230. Kohler A, and Zimmer EA: Borderlands of Normal and Early Pathologic in Skeletal Roentgenology, 3rd Am ed. (Translated by SP Wilke.) New York: Grune & Stratton, 1968, pp 156–159.
231. Kuhns LR, Sherman MP, Poznanski AK, and Holt JF: Humeral head and coracoid ossification in the newborn. Radiology 107:145–149, 1973.
232. Liberson R: Os acromiale: a contested anomaly. J Bone Joint Surg 19:683–689, 1937.
233. McClure JG, and Raney B: Anomalies of the scapula and related research. Clin Orthop 110:22–31, 1975.
234. McGahan JP, Rab GT, and Dublin A: Fractures of the scapula. J Trauma 20:880, 1980.
235. Nettrour LF, Krufky EL, Mueller RE, and Raycroft JF: Locked scapula: intrathoracic dislocation of the inferior angle. J Bone Joint Surg 54A:413–416, 1972.
236. Nunley MA, and Bedini SJ: Paralysis of the shoulder subsequent to comminuted fracture of the scapula. Phys Ther Rev 40:442–447, 1960.
237. Owen R: Bilateral glenoid hypoplasia: report of five cases. J Bone Joint Surg 35B:262–267, 1953.
238. Pettersson H: Bilateral dysplasia of the neck of the scapula and associated anomalies. Acta Radiol Diagnosis 22:81–84, 1981.
238a. Rockwood CA Jr, Wilkins KE, and King RE (eds): Fractures in Children. Philadelphia: JB Lippincott, 1984, pp 653–659.
239. Rowe CR: Fractures of the scapula. Surg Clin North Am 43:1565, 1963.
240. Samilson RL: Congenital and developmental anomalies of the shoulder girdle. Orthop Clin North Am 11:219–231, 1980.
241. Sutro CJ: Dentated articular surface of the glenoid: an anomaly. Bull Hosp J Dis 28:104–108, 1967.
242. Warwick R, and Williams PL: Gray's Anatomy, 35th Br ed. Philadelphia: WB Saunders, 1973, p 322.
243. Weber BG, Brunner CH, and Freuler F: Treatment of Fractures in Children and Adolescents. Berlin: Springer-Verlag, 1980, pp 94–95.
244. Wilber MC, and Evans EB: Fractures of the scapula. J Bone Joint Surg 59A:358–362, 1977.
245. Zilberman Z, and Rejouitsky R: Fracture of the coracoid process of the clavicle. Injury 13:203, 1981.

CHAPTER

28

Special Problems with the Child's Shoulder

Kaye E. Wilkins, M.D.

Brachial Plexus Injuries

During a five-year period at the University of Pennsylvania Hospital in Philadelphia, Rubin observed 116 injuries occurring at birth.[57] This amounted to a rate of one injury per 143 deliveries. Of the five most common birth injuries, injuries to the brachial plexus was third (Table 28–1). In the pediatric age group, almost all of the injuries to the brachial plexus occur at the time of parturition. In the older child, they usually are the result of very severe trauma, such as a motor vehicle accident or being thrown from a motorized cycle. Occasionally they result from severe child abuse. This discussion will be limited to those occurring at the time of delivery.

Over the years birth injuries to the brachial plexus have been described in various terms. Prior to the 1900s they were named after those who were actually credited with their early description, i.e., Erb-Duchenne paralysis[59] and Klumpke paralysis.[18] Initially Duchenne used the term "laceration brachial birth palsy."[18] In 1905 Clark and associates published their extensive work in which they titled the condition "brachial birth palsy."[18] Sever in 1916 coined the term "obstetric paralysis."[59] Scaglietti later classified the various causes of "birth palsy."[58] He believed that birth palsy was a clinical symptom of the child's inability to move the upper extremity owing to shoulder trauma

Table 28–1. INCIDENCE OF BIRTH INJURIES

Clavical fracture	43
Facial nerve injury	21
Brachial plexus injury	**18**
Intracranial hemorrhage	13
Fracture of the humerus	7
TOTAL	116

Adapted and reprinted with permission from Rubin A: Birth injuries: incidence, mechanism and end results. Obstet Gynecol 23:218–221, 1964.

at birth. This could be the result of a central neurological lesion or a fracture of the clavicle or proximal humerus. Obstetrical paralysis was thought to be only one of the many causes of birth palsy. In his extensive monograph on the subject published in 1966, Gjorup used the term "obstetrical lesion of the brachial plexus."[24] Leffert has utilized the term "congenital brachial palsy" for those injuries occurring after a difficult delivery.[40]

In this discussion we will use the term *brachial plexus injury of the newborn* (BPIN).

HISTORICAL REVIEW

The extensive works of Clark and coworkers,[18] Gjorup,[24] and Sever[59] provide very complete reviews of the early description of this entity prior to 1900. Much of the following historical description has been excerpted from their works. The original references, most of which are not in English, can be found in their articles. Smellie is credited with first describing the condition in 1768 in his "A collection of preternatural cases and observations in midwifery." The cause was attributed to a prolonged intrauterine compression of the upper extremity against the pelvis. Actually, however, Danyau in 1851 was the first to describe the actual pathology in a child who had paralysis of the upper extremity after delivery and who died at the age of eight days. A *post mortem* examination of the infant revealed extensive hemorrhage around the brachial plexus.

Duchenne in 1872 in his monograph *l' Ectrilisation Locallisse* recorded the case of Danyau and four others and recognized the effect of traction on the upper extremities in the creation of the paralysis. He described in detail the classical clinical picture of the condition. Two years later Erb demonstrated with electrical studies that pressure of the junction of the fifth and sixth cervical nerve roots, i.e., "Erb's point," produced the characteristic group of paralyzed muscles. He believed that the paralysis was due to the Prague method of gripping the infant in which the delivery fingers were hooked over the back of the child's neck, placing both compression and traction forces on the brachial plexus (Fig. 28–1).

In 1884 Augusta Déjérine-Klumpke described a lesion in adults involving mainly the lower portion of the brachial plexus with the characteristic claw hand, meiosis, and enophthalmos. Although this specific paralytic pattern had been originally described by Flaubert in 1827, Klumpke's contemporaries named this pattern in the infant after her. The term "Klumpke's paralysis" has persisted into the present literature.

Following these original descriptions of BPIN, much of the work during the ensuing years involved defining the etiology and ascribing various modalities of therapy. These studies are discussed in more detail in the following sections on the pathogenesis and treatment of BPIN.

PATHOGENESIS

Etiology

In his original case in 1851, the pathological findings of a profound and extensive hemorrhagic infiltration

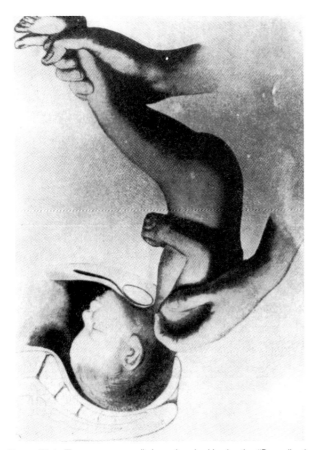

Figure 28–1. The pressures applied on the shoulder by the "Prague" grip. (Reproduced with permission from Sever JW: Obstetric paralysis. Am J Dis Child 12:541–578, 1916.)

were thought by Danyau to be due to some type of compressive force against the brachial plexus, possibly by the forceps used during delivery. Duchenne, however, believed that traction was probably a major factor in the cases he had described, since forceps had not been used in the delivery. Erb still subscribed to the compressive theory and believed that the clavicle, by applying direct pressure against the plexus during a forceful delivery, was the offending agent. Thus, prior to 1900 the common factors said to produce the injuries were (1) backward pressure on the nerves by the clavicle on the transverse processes of the vertebrae and first rib; (2) hyperextension of the arms in breech presentation; (3) direct pressure on the nerves by the forceps; and (4) tension on the nerve roots.[18]

Taylor, in his extensive report with Clark and Prout in 1905, produced experimental evidence showing that traction was the only force producing the lesion in the nerves.[18] Anatomically they demonstrated that the clavicle could never be shown to produce direct pressure against the nerves; even if it did, it would have compressed distally rather than proximally. By the same token, hyperextension alone did not place significant pressure or stretch on the brachial plexus. These authors also demonstrated that the forceps could not extend sufficiently caudad to apply direct pressure on the plexus.

In their experimental work on newborn infant cadavers, Taylor and coworkers were able to reproduce the lesion previously described with traction alone on the plexus.[18] Any form of traction that tended to separate the head from the shoulder seemed to apply a constant tensile force on the upper plexus. Soon after this original report, Taylor actually felt the upper roots of the plexus give way under his fingers as he was performing a difficult breech delivery. The infant subsequently expired; an autopsy revealed stretching and thinning at the junction of the fifth and sixth cervical nerve roots.[66]

Eleven years later, Sever reproduced these same findings in infant cadavers. The clavicle actually appeared to provide some protection to the plexus. With the head and shoulder forcibly separated, the two upper cords were said to stand out like violin strings (Fig. 28–2). The suprascapular nerve, having less freedom of movement, appeared to fail first. With the clavicle intact it was difficult to completely tear the two nerves at Erb's point. The primary lesion appeared to be rupture of the sheath only. If the force was increased, avulsion of the fifth and sixth nerve roots from the cord appeared to occur next. The lower roots were very difficult to put on stretch without abducting or hyperextending the arm. Fracture of the clavicle allowed the shoulder to drag more on the plexus, predisposing it to greater traction forces. Rotation or abduction of the head did not appear to have much effect on the tension applied to the plexus.[59]

The only other theory espoused during this time was that originally proposed by Lange in 1912.[69] He postulated that the primary lesion was a laceration of the shoulder capsule with release of hemorrhagic fluid

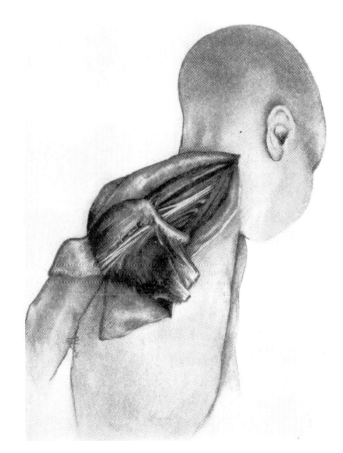

Figure 28–2. When the head and neck are separated, considerable tension is applied to the junction of the fifth and sixth cervical roots. (Reproduced with permission from Sever JW: Obstetric paralysis. Am J Dis Child *12*:541–578, 1916.)

anteriorly, which secondarily involved the brachial plexus. In the United States this theory was supported by both Thomas[69] and Ashurst.[4] They believed that anterior dislocation or subluxation of the shoulder was the primary precipitating factor and that all treatment should be directed toward repair of this shoulder pathology. This theory was still partially supported almost 20 years later by Scaglietti, who thought that the posterior subluxation and retroversion seen in these patients later was a result of injury to the cartilaginous epiphysis at birth.[58] In his experimental work on infant cadavers, Sever was unable with forceful manipulation to rupture the joint capsule, dislocate the humeral head, or separate the proximal humeral physis.[59]

Thus there seems to be ample evidence that the nerves are ruptured following the stretching of the plexus. Wickstrom, in his experimental studies on infant cadavers, found that the lower roots, when placed on stretch, were able to be ruptured with half the force necessary to rupture the upper root.[71, 72] Recent investigators doing primary nerve repairs have confirmed the presence of these torn nerves, with the lesion being usually confined to the upper plexus.[12, 22, 37]

PATHOLOGY

Anatomical Location

The structure of the brachial plexus along with the muscles innervated by the specific roots is depicted in

Figure 28–3. In the series of cases explored surgically, the anatomical location consistently involved at least the roots of the fifth and sixth cervical nerves.[12, 18, 22, 37, 40, 68] There was a rupture of the roots or a neuroma in continuity. In almost all cases the suprascapular nerve was involved. There did not appear to be any isolated lower nerve root lesions. Avulsion of the upper roots was rare, whereas the lower roots were almost always avulsed. In those lesions that were complete, a combination of both ruptures and avulsions of the roots was usually present.[40] The frequency of the lesions and their location in those undergoing surgery is shown in Figure 28–4.

Microscopic Pathology

In those patients explored during recent years, there is some selectivity regarding spontaneous versus no recovery, and only those patients with complete lesions are now explored surgically. A truer picture of the microscopic lesions can be gleaned from the earlier work of Taylor and associates in which almost all lesions were explored with very little selectivity.[18, 66, 68] They recognized that many lesions were incomplete, with the nerve bundles being pulled apart at different levels. In the milder incomplete lesions the supporting sheaths first gave way, producing a hematoma that infiltrated the epineurium, perineurium, and nerve bundles (Fig. 28–5). Over time this hemorrhage was thought to organize into fibrous tissue, producing a constricting band across the torn nerve bundle (Fig.

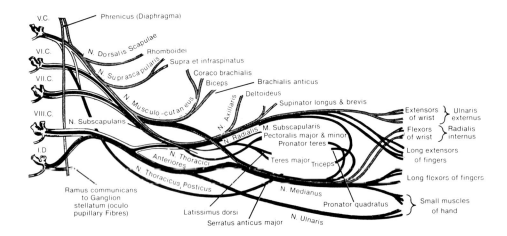

Figure 28–3. Semidiagrammatic scheme of the brachial plexus demonstrating the nerve supply to the muscles of the upper extremities. (Reproduced with permission from Taylor AS: Conclusions derived from further experience in the surgical treatment of brachial birth palsy. Am J Med Sci *146*:836–856, 1913.)

Figure 28–4. Patterns of placement of the sural nerve grafts in 20 patients. Absence of the nerve roots indicates those that were avulsed. (Reproduced with permission from Boome RS, and Kaye JC: Obstetrical traction injuries of the brachial plexus. J Bone Joint Surg *70B*:571–576, 1988.)

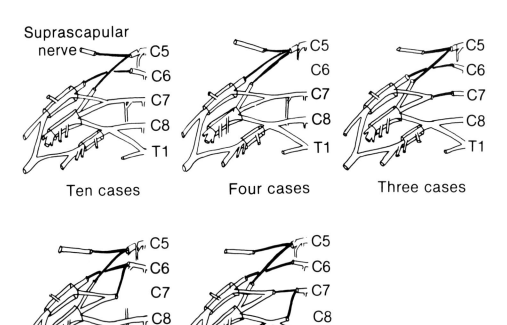

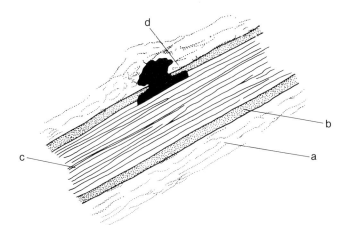

Figure 28–5. A schematic representation of the pathology in the incomplete lesions. Initial rupture of the perineural sheath produces a hematoma (d) involving the epineurium (a), perineurium (b) and nerve bundles (c). (Reproduced with permission from Clark LP, Taylor AS, and Prout TP: A study of brachial birth palsy. Am J Med Sci *130*:670–707, 1905.)

28–6). Repair of the nerve sheath was believed to take place before regeneration of the nerve fibers. If the nerve sheath had buckled inward into the nerve fibers, as the sheath healed it would produce a strangulation effect, preventing regeneration of those fibers. In addition to the scarring within the nerve bundles themselves, considerable thickening of the surrounding cervical fascia was also found.[18]

The various types of lesions are summarized in the classification proposed by Aitken (Table 28–2).[3] The range of lesions begins with the mild Type I stretching of the brachial plexus with good or complete recovery. In Type II lesions, some of the fibers are ruptured with hemorrhage, producing mild to moderate residual weakness and contracture. In the severe Type III lesions, many fibers are ruptured and nerve roots avulsed, producing severe residua. More recent surgical reports have shown that there can be a mixture of these types of lesions throughout the brachial plexus, involving the individual roots and trunks.[12, 22, 40]

Associated Conditions

In most instances the injury to the brachial plexus occurs as a single isolated condition. However, other conditions associated with birth trauma can occur simultaneously with sufficient frequency to deserve mention.

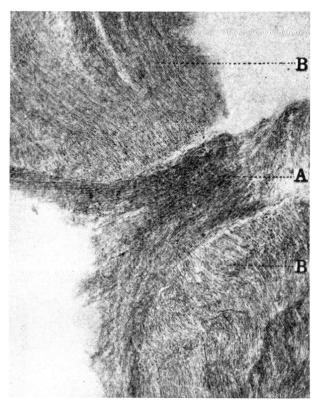

Figure 28–6. Photomicrograph demonstrating the constricting fibrous tissue *(A)* across the torn nerve fibers *(B)*. (Reproduced with permission from Clark LP, Taylor AS, and Prout TP: A study of brachial birth palsy. Am J Med Sci *130*:670–707, 1905.)

Facial Nerve Injury

Probably the most common associated condition is a paralysis of the facial nerve, which is associated with forceps delivery. This is usually indicative of a difficult delivery. In a recent series Greenwald and coworkers found that this occurred in 10 per cent of his cases.[28]

Torticollis

In some cases, idiopathic infantile muscular torticollis is also thought to have some association with birth trauma. Zancolli found only a 2.7 per cent incidence of torticollis in his series.[76] Suzuki and coworkers, however, found when they examined their patients with brachial plexus injuries closely that there was some evidence of torticollis in 51 per cent of the cases.[64]

Table 28–2. CLASSIFICATION OF NERVE LESIONS

Pathology	Recovery	Muscles
Type I: Mild stretching of plexus, with or without absorption of hemorrhage	Complete	No residual signs or symptoms Slight weakness
Type II: Moderate rupture of a few fibers with hemorrhage	Fair to poor	Definite weakness Mild degree of contracture
Type III: Severe rupture of many fibers with hemorrhage	Poor to minimal	Affected limb shorter than the normal by more than 3 cm Muscular wasting, trophic and sensory changes

Modified with permission from Aitken J: Deformity of the elbow joint as a sequel to Erb's obstetrical paralysis. J Bone Joint Surg *34B*:352–365, 1952.

In the breech-presentation infants the incidence was 80 per cent. The more severe the paralysis, the higher was the incidence of torticollis. The torticollis was seen on the same side as the brachial plexus lesion in 95 per cent of their cases.[64] However, these findings have not been confirmed by other investigators. The only other series in which there was a high incidence was Middleton's, with an incidence of about 20 per cent.[49]

Spasticity

Aston found that three of his cases developed spasticity in the lower extremities.[5] This has been noted by others as well.[13, 28] Autopsy studies have demonstrated neuronal damage with focal hemorrhage for a considerable distance in the cervical and thoracic cord.[1] It appears that this occurs in those individuals who are more severely involved with root avulsions.

Other Fractures

The most common fracture was that of the clavicle, which occurred in 13 per cent of the cases of Greenwald and associates.[28] Fractures of the proximal humerus and humeral shaft are also seen.

Other Nerve Injuries

In severe lower root injuries, involvement of the first thoracic root can interfere with sympathetic nerve function, producing a Horner's syndrome with the characteristic meiosis and enophthalmos. Involvement of the fourth cervical root can produce a phrenic nerve paralysis with associated paralysis of the hemidiaphragm.

Secondary Effects

Muscle Weakness and Paralysis

In the upper lesions, the muscles supplied by the fifth and sixth cervical roots are either weakened or paralyzed completely (see Fig. 28–3). A graphic representation of the involved muscles supplied by these nerve roots is shown in Figure 28–7. This results clinically in an inability to raise or abduct the arm due to paralysis of the deltoid and supraspinatus. External rotation is limited owing to paralysis of the infraspinatus and teres minor. The shoulder is held in internal rotation by the teres major, subscapularis, and latissimus dorsi, which are functional but contracted due to lack of opposition.

The elbow lacks flexion owing to weakness of the biceps, brachialis, and supinator. This also accounts for the forearm being contracted in pronation.[59] In the wrist there is weakness of the dorsiflexors of both the carpus and fingers (Fig. 28–8).

The next most common pattern of BPIN involves all of the nerve roots. In addition to the lesions of the upper roots, the wrist and finger flexors are involved,

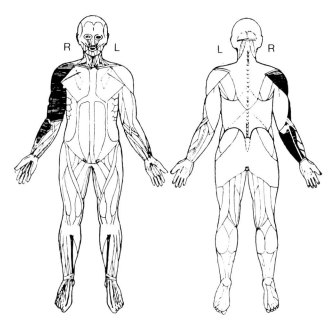

Figure 28–7. The pattern of muscles involved *(dark shading)* in the typical upper root level of BPIN. (Reproduced with permission from Sever JW: Obstetric paralysis. Am J Dis Child *12*:541–578, 1916.)

making the hand useless. The wrist is usually in ulnar deviation as well.

In rare cases only the seventh and eighth cervical and first thoracic nerve roots are involved, with relative sparing of the upper roots. This pattern of nerve loss

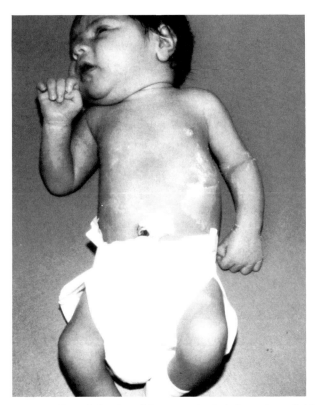

Figure 28–8. The typical posture of the upper extremity in the newborn with an upper root injury.

produces the typical Klumpke's paralysis, with the forearm supinated, the wrist dangling in dorsiflexion, and the characteristic "hooked" finger contractures (Fig. 28–9). For all practical purposes, isolated lesions of only the eighth cervical and first thoracic roots are not seen.[40]

Shoulder Contractures

In the typical upper root lesion the shoulder is held in adduction and internal rotation and slight forward flexion. The scapula is rotated on the coronal plane by the weight of the arm and the pull of the biceps.[5] This posture is produced by weakness of the abductors (deltoid and supraspinatus) and the external rotators (infraspinatus and teres major), allowing the active internal rotators (teres major, subscapularis, and latissimus dorsi) to become contracted and shortened owing to lack of opposing forces.[59] Moore thought that the anterior portion of the deltoid was strong, while the posterior portion was paralyzed.[50] With persistence of these unbalanced muscle forces, secondary contractures and osseous deformities develop (Fig. 28–10). The posterior deltoid is atrophied. The subscapularis and pectoralis major become contracted; the infraspinatus becomes lengthened and atrophied as well. As a result of this constant tension there is persistent internal rotation of the humeral head, producing a posterior subluxation. In addition, the anterior capsule becomes contracted and the posterior capsule is stretched. Weakness of the infraspinatus contributes to the posterior capsular insufficiency.

The shoulder is actually abducted when the scapular humeral relationships are examined. When the arm is forcibly adducted to the chest and the humerus is externally rotated, there is a forward elevation of the superior corner of the scapula that makes it more prominent, producing the so-called "scapular sign of Putti"[58] (Figs. 28–11 and 28–12). Aston has termed this rotation of the scapula "contractural winging" to distinguish it from the paralytic type seen with serratus anterior paralysis.[5]

Over time the humeral head becomes retroverted, which Zancolli describes as a posterior epiphyseolysis of the proximal humerus.[76] This persistent internal rotation causes the medial aspect of the humeral head to become flattened. On the scapular side the glenoid fossa becomes hypoplastic and sclerotic and may even form a "saddle" type of joint with the depressed humeral head.[76]

In addition to the aforementioned characteristic deformities, other deformities can rarely occur. Probably the best classification of shoulder deformities is that of Zancolli, in which he places them in four subgroups.[76] The first group has only the typical adduction, internal rotation, and flexion soft tissue contractures with a congruous joint. In the second group there is the development of the typical bony deformities of the humeral head and glenoid. Both of these common deformities have been discussed previously. These two groups are the result of the muscle imbalance forces produced by the upper root paralysis. The remaining two subgroups contain deformities that result from iatrogenic factors. In the third group, the shoulder is

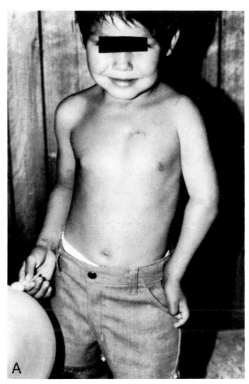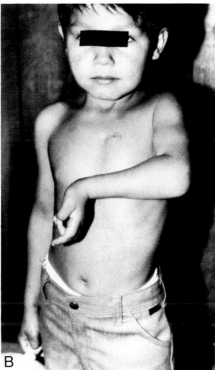

Figure 28–9. The usual posture of the arm with a lower root lesion with the elbow extended (A) and flexed (B).

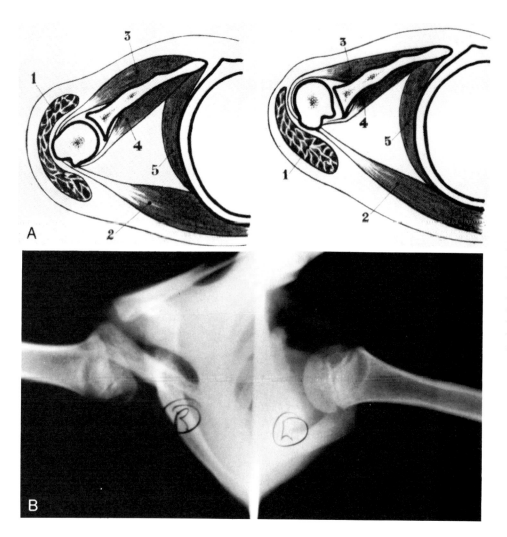

Figure 28–10. Shoulder deformities. *A,* Horizontal section comparing the normal shoulder (left) with the shoulder affected with an upper root lesion (right). 1, deltoid; 2, pectoralis major; 3, infraspinatus; 4, subscapularis; 5, serratus anterior. *B,* Radiographs of both shoulders, showing the retroversion of the humeral head on the right. (Reproduced with permission from Scaglietti O: The obstetrical shoulder trauma. Surg Gynecol Obstet *66*:868–877, 1938.)

Figure 28–11. The humerus is truly abducted when it is compared with the scapula *(A).* Adduction of the arm and external rotation of the scapula elevates the superior margin *(B).* (Reproduced with permission from Zancolli EA: Classification and management of the shoulder in birth palsy. Orthop Clin *12*:433–457, 1981.)

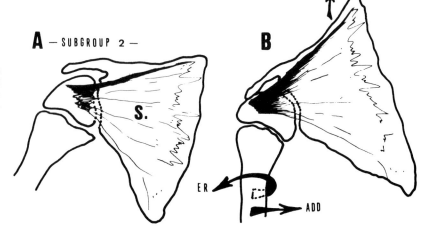

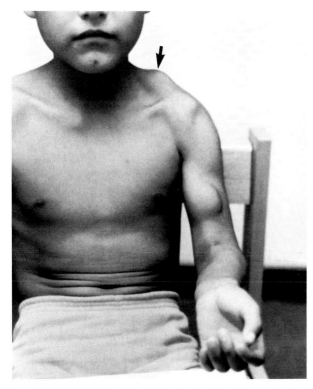

Figure 28–12. Clinical picture demonstrating the elevation of the superior border of the scapula *(arrow)* with external rotation of the humerus and adduction of the arm—the "scapular sign of Putti."

held in external rotation and abduction. There may be a subcoracoid or anteroinferior dislocation of the shoulder. This is usually the result of being placed in a "Statue of Liberty" splint or of vigorous anterior surgical release procedures.[6, 41, 76] In this type of deformity, the scapular sign of Putti is produced by internal rotation with adduction rather than with the usual external rotation. Radiographically the humeral epiphysis overlaps the inferior border of the glenoid because it is inferiorly subluxed.[76] In the fourth group, an isolated contracture of the supraspinatus muscle produces a pure abduction contracture.

In addition to the bony changes seen in the glenohumeral joint, secondary bony changes occur in the coracoid and acromion as well. The acromion bends forward and downward to hook over the front of the posteriorly subluxed humeral head. This hooking increases with age and varies directly with the degree of posterior subluxation. The clavicle is shorter and curves more acutely than on the opposite side.[59] The coracoid is markedly elongated owing to the pull of the contracted coracobrachialis muscle.[60]

Elbow Deformities

The major deformities are seen in soft tissue and are due to muscle imbalance. Since the triceps receives more innervation from the seventh cervical root, there may be only partial weakness compared with a more profound weakness of the brachialis, biceps, and su-

pinators. Thus the elbow is held in slight flexion and pronation. Over time the elbow flexors and anterior capsule become contracted. The partial weakness of the triceps appears to prevent it from completely stretching out these anterior capsular contractures.[15, 34, 62] Such soft tissue contractures are usually seen to some degree, even in cases with considerable recovery (Fig. 28–13).

The bony changes are less consistent. Sever in 1916 mentioned that dislocation of the radial head may occur only occasionally.[59] After many more years of experience, in a review article in 1940 he mentioned that "roentgenograms of the elbow practically never show bony changes of importance." He disputed that there was a bony change in the olecranon fossa limiting flexion.[62] Other authors have noted significant bony changes ranging from subluxation to complete dislocation of the radial head.[2, 3] The most extensive review of the development of radial head changes was that by Aitken.[3] He described changes occurring as early as seven weeks, including a clubbing of the proximal radial metaphysis and early bowing of the ulna in the sagittal plane. Over time the radial head developed an anterior notch, subsequently becoming dislocated and flattened anteriorly (Figs. 28–14 and 28–15). Aitken also noticed isolated anterior radial head dislocations that resembled the so-called congenital dislocation of the radial head seen without paralysis (Fig. 28–16).[3] In his series the incidence of posterior dislocation of the radial head was 25.4 per cent versus only 5.6 per cent for the anterior dislocation.[3] A third type of bony elbow deformity in which there was a relentless medial dislocation of both the radius and ulna was described by Adler and Patterson.[2]

These bony changes appeared to have been the result of the overaggressive use of the original Fairbank

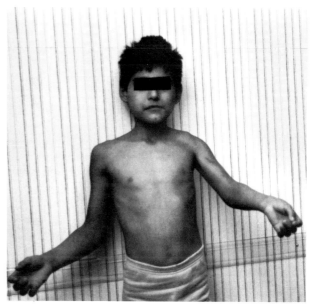

Figure 28–13. Persistent elbow flexion contracture in a 13-year-old patient who sustained a BPIN on the left arm. There is still a fixed supination contracture of the forearm.

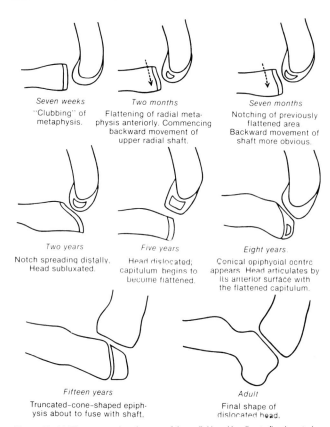

Seven weeks
"Clubbing" of metaphysis.

Two months
Flattening of radial metaphysis anteriorly. Commencing backward movement of upper radial shaft.

Seven months
Notching of previously flattened area Backward movement of shaft more obvious.

Two years
Notch spreading distally, Head subluxated.

Five years
Head dislocated; capitulum begins to become flattened.

Eight years
Conical epiphyoial ocntre appears. Head articulates by its anterior surface with the flattened capitulum.

Fifteen years
Truncated-cone-shaped epiphysis about to fuse with shaft,

Adult
Final shape of dislocated head.

Figure 28–14. The progressive changes of the radial head leading to fixed posterior subluxation in patients who were treated with braces for BPIN. (Reproduced with permission from Aitken J: Deformity of the elbow joint as a sequel to Erb's obstetrical paralysis. J Bone Joint Surg *34B*:352–365, 1952.)

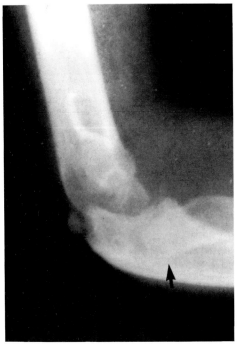

Figure 28–15. Radiograph of a young patient who was treated with a brace in early infancy, showing the posterior dislocation and deformity of the radial head *(arrow).*

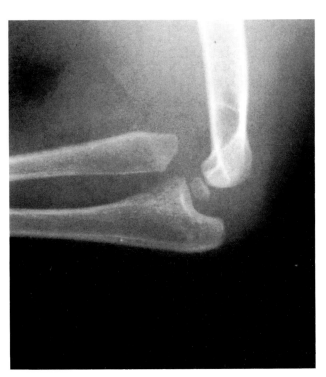

Figure 28–16. Radiograph of a patient with BPIN who had the rarer type of anterior dislocation of the radial head.

splint, which held the elbow in 90 degrees of flexion with the forearm fully supinated.[20] Aitken postulated that placing the elbow at 90 degrees against a partially active triceps caused the primary bowing of the ulna, which led to the secondary posterior subluxation of the radial head (Fig. 28–17).[3] All cases with this posterior subluxation were treated with the old Fairbank brace. In none of the untreated cases was this deformity found.[3] Dislocation of the radial head after use of the Fairbank brace was also noted by Adler and Patterson[2] and in one of the cases treated by this author (see Fig. 28–15).

The cause of the rarer anterior dislocation remains unexplained.

Radiographic Changes

In the previous sections on shoulder and elbow deformities, mention is made of some of the bony changes that are seen radiographically. Kattan and Spitz[36] have summarized these changes in their article. In the newborn the proximal humerus lies more distant to the glenoid. The development of the proximal epiphyseal ossification center is retarded. As it ossifies, the epiphyseal center is lateral to that of the greater tuberosity because of the internal rotation of the humerus. The diaphragm may be elevated if there is phrenic nerve paralysis. The acromion is elongated, hooked, and flared on its end. The clavicle and glenoid are underdeveloped. There is posterior subluxation of the humeral head, and the coracoid process becomes elongated.[36]

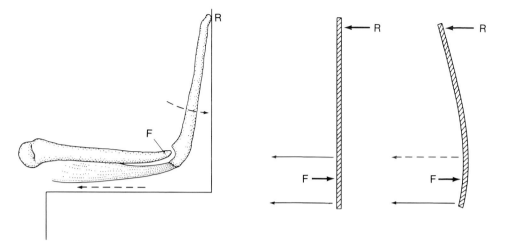

Figure 28–17. Forcing the forearm against a partially active triceps produces a bowing of the proximal ulna. (Reproduced with permission from Aitken J: Deformity of the elbow as a sequel to Erb's obstetrical paralysis. J Bone Joint Surg 34B:352–365, 1952.)

INCIDENCE

Overall Incidence

The overall incidence of BPIN ranges from a low of 0.25 to 2.60 per 1000 live births (Table 28–3). This can be misleading, however, because there may be many factors that affect the overall incidence, such as body habitus varying among ethnic groups and the quality of care both prenatally and at the time of delivery. The important consideration in the overall incidence is: Has it changed? When Adler and Patterson compared their overall incidence in 1938 versus 1962, there was an almost fivefold decrease (see Table 28–3).[2] Greenwald and coworkers, on the other hand, found that their overall incidence remained about two per 1000.[28] It was their impression, however, that the number of severe cases had decreased. Thus the overall morbidity may be decreasing. This also reflects my experience in 15 years in San Antonio. During the first seven or eight years, I saw many patients who required surgical correction for their deformities. In the past five years these cases have been rare. This may also reflect more aggressive nonoperative treatment in early infancy. The overall decrease in morbidity has also been recognized by both Hardy and Specht in their recent series.[30, 63]

There has been some variance in the incidence of males versus females and right versus left among the many series reported. In an effort to obtain a more accurate overall incidence, 11 series were combined for a total of 2095 cases (Table 28–4). The incidence in males is only 3 per cent greater than in females. The right side is more involved in only 15 per cent of cases; 5 per cent present with bilateral involvement.

Contributing Factors

Breech Deliveries

The incidence of BPIN in infants who are breech presentations is markedly increased. Rubin found a 17-fold increase in the incidence of BPIN with breech presentations.[57] In Vassalos and colleagues' series BPIN was 10 times more frequent with breech delivery.[70] The incidence of bilateral cases is also higher in breech deliveries.[2, 58]

Other Birth Risk Factors

Levine and associates developed a risk assessment profile for those individuals more likely to sustain a brachial plexus injury during delivery.[44] These factors included shoulder dystocia, infant weight greater than 4000 gm, mid or low forceps deliveries, and first pregnancies. The cut-off figure for birth weight seems to be 4000 gm. In the 200,000 births examined from Washington state, McFarland and coworkers found the risk to be 2.5 times greater in those infants weighing 4000 to 4500 gm. Infants heavier than 4500 gm had an additional threefold increase in incidence. In fact, these

Table 28–3. OVERALL INCIDENCE OF BRACHIAL PLEXUS INJURIES

Author(s)	Year	Incidence per 1,000 Births
Adler and Patterson[2]	1938	1.56
	1962	0.38
Gordon et al[26]	1973	1.89
Greenwald et al[28]	1984	2.00
Hardy[30]	1981	0.87
Levine et al[44]	1984	2.60
Specht[63]	1975	0.57
Vassalos et al[70]	1968	0.25

Table 28–4. STATISTICS OF BRACHIAL PLEXUS INJURIES

Total cases	2095	100%
Males	1079	51.5%
Females	1016	48.5%
Right	1183	55%
Left	860	40%
Both sides	108	5%
Breech presentation	389	19%

Data combined from references 5, 7, 12, 13, 24, 28, 30, 31, 60, 65, 70, and 73.

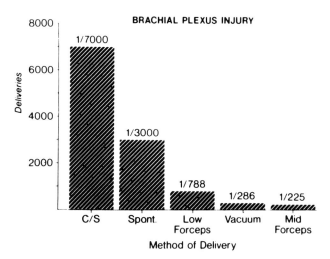

Figure 28–18. The incidence of Erb's palsy by method of delivery. (Reproduced with permission from The American College of Obstetricians and Gynecologists. McFarland LV, Raskin M, Daling JR, and Benedetti TJ: Erb/Duchenne's palsy: a consequence of fetal macrosomia and method of delivery. Obstet Gynecol 68:784–788, 1986.)

authors felt that the incidence was high enough to justify cesarean section for all infants estimated to weigh more than 4500 gm.[48]

Among the methods of delivery, the incidence was least in cesarean section and highest in mid forceps (Fig. 28–18). One would expect that cesarean section would totally protect the infant from BPIN. McFarland and associates found four cases associated with BPIN that were delivered by cesarean section. They theorized that in some cases a forceful vaginal delivery had been attempted or that the injury occurred when the infant was extracted at surgery.[48]

Levine and colleagues found that the infants with BPIN had lower Apgar scores and were more often delivered using spinal or epidural anesthesia after a prolonged second stage of labor.[44] Having had a previous infant with BPIN may also be a risk factor. Gordon and associates found that 14 per cent of the mothers in their series had had previous infants with BPIN.[26]

DIAGNOSIS

Clinical Presentation

Usually the diagnosis is very obvious. The infant fails to move the extremity. Initially it is limp, with only some active finger and wrist flexion. The extremity is held internally rotated next to the trunk, with the hand held in the characteristic "policeman's tip" position.[59] Often there is tenderness just proximal to the clavicle. Taylor believed that severe induration in this area was indicative of avulsed roots.[67] The differential diagnosis includes fractures about the shoulder, spastic hemiplegia, or an infectious process in the shoulder area.

With fractures of the clavicle there is usually local tenderness and swelling at the midpoint of the clavicle. Ultrasonography may be useful in localizing the frac-

ture itself. Fracture of the proximal humeral physis is extremely rare but can occur as a result of extreme force applied to the arm during delivery. With this concomitant injury localized swelling and crepitus in the shoulder area usually is found. Fracture of the shaft of the humerus may also produce this picture of "pseudoparalysis." With this injury there may be a transient radial nerve paralysis, which serves only to confuse the issue. Again, the swelling and tenderness are localized over the humeral shaft. Radiographs may be helpful with fractures of the shaft of the the humerus but may not help with fracture of the proximal physis owing to the lack of ossification in the epiphysis. In all of these fracture patterns there is voluntary elbow flexion, which can usually be elicited with a strong stimulus distally.

In spastic hemiplegia, the ipsilateral lower extremity usually is involved as well. Infectious processes, i.e., septic arthritis or proximal humeral osteomyelitis, may be difficult to differentiate. Usually these conditions are not symptomatic at birth but develop in the first few days or weeks of life.

Electrodiagnostic Studies

Very few investigators have found the electromyograph (EMG) useful as a diagnostic tool. It is very difficult to use in small infants. Usually it is more useful in determining the extent of the injury and the presence or absence of recovery. Eng, who specializes in physical medicine, found it very useful in her evaluation of patients, using it as a baseline to determine the extent and severity of the injury.[19] She found that the extent of involvement did not always correlate with the rapidity or delay in recovery; the EMG return appeared to precede the clinical return by at least a month. It may be that part of her success was her wide clinical experience with the EMG in her practice. Chung and Nissenbaum found the EMG to be of only limited value in questionable cases. They used it primarily in the posterior cervical muscles in cooperative children.[17] Recent workers, using the EMG to try to identify recovery as a basis for surgical exploration and repair, have found it less reliable than simple clinical observation.[12, 22] Kawabata and coworkers found that intraoperative electrophysiological examination of root sensory evoked potential, nerve action potential, and evoked muscle response were useful to understand the extent of the lesion and were helpful in decision making regarding nerve reconstruction.[37]

Myelographic Studies

The use of the myelogram has been proposed in attempting to determine the presence or absence of root avulsion. Recently, however, in their cases involving surgical exploration, Boome and Kaye found that the myelographic findings correlated so poorly with operative findings that they have abandoned it as a diagnostic tool.[12] Kawabata and coworkers increased

POSTGANGLIONIC   PREGANGLIONIC

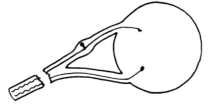
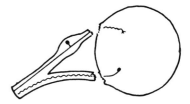

Figure 28–19. Types of brachial plexus traction lesions. Motor axon degeneration is found in the postganglionic type and motor axon preservation in the preganglionic type. (Reproduced with permission from Bonney G: The value of axon responses in determining the site of lesions in traction injuries of the brachial plexus. Brain 77:588–609, 1954.)

—— NORMAL AXONS

~~~ DEGENERATE AXONS

their accuracy by combining routine preoperative metrizamide myelography with computed tomographic (CT) myelography.[37] They found that a pseudomeningocele and root sleeve defects, although reliable in diagnosing root damage, did not necessarily indicate complete avulsion.

Histamine Response

Bonney in 1954 reported on the use of the peripheral axon responses in differentiating between pre- and postganglionic injuries.[11] In the complete peripheral nerve lesions (postganglionic), the axon responses to histamine and cold vasodilation are absent. In those that are avulsions, i.e., preganglionic lesions, the peripheral nerves and their attachment with the ganglions are intact, allowing the axon response to remain positive (Fig. 28–19).[11] Kawabata and associates found that these responses were 80 per cent reliable in their preoperative evaluation for nerve repair.[37] These axon responses appear to be more useful in evaluating traumatic brachial plexus injuries in adults.

RECOVERY AND PROGNOSIS

A tremendous variation exists in the literature regarding the rate of full recovery (Table 28–5). Some of the more optimistic recent articles reflect a trend toward less severe lesions. Brown has emphasized that many of the more recent studies are prospective and that milder forms are included that probably were not included in the older follow-up studies.[16] In his series,

Table 28–5. PERCENTAGE OF PATIENTS ACHIEVING FULL RECOVERY

Author(s)	Year	Percentage
Aitken[3]	1952	16.0
Wickstrom[72]	1962	13.4
Adler and Patterson[2]	1967	7.0
Bennett and Harrold[7]	1976	75.0
Hardy[30]	1981	80.0
Greenwald et al[28]	1984	95.7

Hardy reported full recovery in 80 per cent at 13 months.[30] In a more recent series by Greenwald, the rate of full recovery was an almost unbelievable 95.7 per cent.[30] In the earlier series by Aitken in which he classified the severity of the lesion into three types, only 17 of 106 patients recovered completely. The same was true for Wickstrom's series, in which only 13.4 per cent achieved full recovery.[72]

The review by Tada and coworkers gives a more accurate picture of the recovery rate in untreated individuals.[65] They reported a detailed serial evaluation of patients over a five-year period. In the overall group there was rapid recovery of useful motor function in upper root lesions and of the upper roots in cases of total arm involvement. There was very poor recovery of the lower roots in total arm involvement. Of their cases with myelographic evidence of root avulsion, 70.4 per cent had useful sensory recovery and one-third had useful motor recovery. These authors concluded that even without treatment useful function can be expected, even with severe lesions.[65]

The quality of life appears to be quite good even in those patients who had persistent functional disability. In their series Adler and Patterson found that although only 7 per cent of their patients achieved full recovery, almost all were gainfully employed and had successful married lives.[2] One was employed as a professional baseball player; another patient with bilateral whole-arm involvement was a supervisor of a milk-distributing company. None of their patients was on welfare.[2] Because many infants had low Apgar scores at delivery, Gordon and coworkers performed psychological studies at eight months and four years and found that they were normal.[26]

Eng had raised the concern that early neuronal deprivation might affect future extremity function.[19] In their most recent study, however, Greenwald and associates demonstrated that the tendency toward normal right-handedness persisted even if the right extremity had been involved initially.[28]

Investigators have always felt the desire to predict which patients will achieve good recovery. As early as 1925, Sever noted that the presence of unequal pupils and persistence of a wrist drop for longer than six weeks indicated a poor prognosis.[60] Gjorup reviewed the European literature, which agreed that the prognosis was always poor in those who had Klumpke's pattern of involvement.[24] More recently, Bennett and Harrold in 1976 concluded that there was no way to predict early those who would recover.[7] In their series they noticed that those patients in whom the suprascapular nerve was involved did not achieve full recovery. They postulated that the suprascapular nerve, because of its course and flexion distally in the suprascapular notch, is more vulnerable to neurotmesis.[7]

TREATMENT

The cornerstone of the initial treatment in all cases is nonoperative management.[33] This is designed to maintain the flexibility of the active muscles until recovery of the affected muscles occurs. Operative measures are designed for two purposes: (1) to correct both the soft tissue and bony deformities that develop from contractures, and (2) more recently, there has been an emphasis on the early repair of the nerves in order to ensure recovery.

Nonoperative Management

Massage and Range of Motion

Initially the infant is simply supported passively, and no range-of-motion exercises are initiated until the early traumatic neuritis subsides. Placing the arm in a sling or swathe with a collar and a cuff helps to support the shoulder and decreases the tension on an irritated plexus. After 10 to 14 days, each joint in the extremity is then carried through a passive range of motion to maintain flexibility. The active muscles are gently stretched, including the wrist and finger flexors, elbow extensors, pronators of the forearm, internal rotators, and adductors of the shoulder. To stretch the shoulder muscles, the mother must be taught to stabilize the scapula so that the motion is produced at the glenohumeral rather than the scapulothoracic joint. Patterson, who was a strong believer in physical therapy, believed that many of the cases requiring surgical release were the result of inadequate physical management.[53] In his program only one in ten patients required surgery for relief of deformities. He emphasized that lack of success often was due to the parents' failure to appreciate the importance of frequent treatments at home. In addition, a program of close supervision and follow-up is necessary to ensure that the parents understand the therapy being performed.[53] In some instances, ignorance, inexperience, or lack of financial resources inhibits the success of this early nonoperative program.

Active Exercises

Once the child is old enough to obey commands and interact with adults, active exercises in the form of play activities are initiated. Sever advocated a very innovative program in which nursery rhymes were sung with each exercise.[62] For example, to stimulate elbow flexion the parent and child sing:

Up, down, up, down,
This is the way we go to town.
What to buy? To buy a fat pig.
Home again, home again rig a gig gig.

To stimulate circumduction one sings:

Grind the coffee,
Grind the coffee,
Grind, grind, grind.

This program was combined with many other games designed to stretch contracted muscles and strengthen weakened muscles.

Forceful Manipulation

Ashurst in 1918 believed this lesion was not completely due to primary neurological injury but was the result of extensive soft tissue injury around the shoulder. He recommended forceful manipulation of the shoulder under anesthesia at about six months to reduce the dislocation, followed by plaster immobilization.[4] Fortunately, this method of treatment never achieved any measure of popularity.

Electrical Stimulation

Duchenne was one of the first to advocate electrical stimulation of the paralyzed muscles. This was later abandoned because the stimulus often frightened the children. Electrical stimulation was most extensively used by Chung and Nissenbaum[17] and Eng.[19] Eng advocated a galvanic current strong enough to produce a forceful contracture; her program even included the use of home stimulation by the parents. It might be noted that even with this aggressive program, only 30 per cent of patients achieved full recovery. These appear to be the only articles in the literature advocating the use of electrostimulation.

Braces and Splints

Credit is given to Fairbank for the use of the so-called "Statue of Liberty" splint.[20] It was originally designed to immobilize the shoulder in the corrected position after his extensive anterior soft tissue release of the shoulder. In those patients treated early, Sever recommended the use of a plaster slab or cast to hold the shoulder abducted 90 degrees and externally rotated 90 degrees, with the elbow flexed 90 degrees and the forearm supinated (Fig. 28–20).[63] His rationale was the removal of gravity tension forces from the paralyzed muscles, which was believed to hasten their recovery; it was also believed to prevent shoulder subluxation and acromial overgrowth.[59] The use of a Sever brace in very early infancy was also popularized by Boorstein who reported on its use in over 200 cases

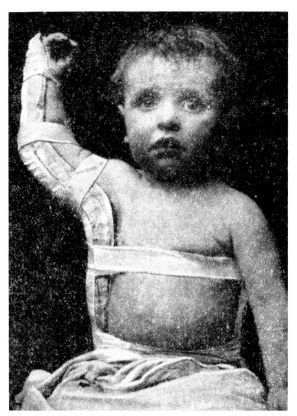

Figure 28–20. Plaster cast devised by Sever for treatment of infants with BPIN. (Reproduced with permission from Sever JW: Obstetrical paralysis. Pub Health Nursing *32*:187–199, 1940.)

(Figs. 28–21 and 28–22). He provided some evidence that patients treated with the brace had better results than those treated without it.[13, 14]

It soon became evident that many problems were associated with too-aggressive use of the brace. The major problem was stiffness after the brace was used as the only treatment. In Adler and Patterson's series, when brace treatment was supplemented with physical therapy no iatrogenic contractures occurred.[2] They pointed out that the parents often cannot be depended on to supplement the use of the brace with a passive range-of-motion program.[2] As mentioned earlier, aggressive bracing produced an abduction, external rotation contracture of the shoulder, and in some cases inferior subcoracoid dislocations.[6, 41, 76] In addition, the brace affected the elbow, creating subluxation and dislocation of the radial head (see the section Elbow Deformities). In an effort to prevent these elbow deformities, Aitken modified the brace so that the elbow was only flexed 45 degrees and the forearm was in midpronation instead of full supination.[3] In none of the recent reports on treatment of BPIN has the use of the brace been recommended. The only current use of splints for BPIN is that advocated by Perry and coworkers;[54] this involves the use of dynamic splints to supplement absent or weakened muscles in patients with severe residua, i.e., total arm involvement. These braces are usually permanent.[54]

Operative Management

Patterson has grouped the operative procedures into three categories:[53]

1. Primary repair of the nerve lesion. Originally all the nerve lesions were explored; currently, only those that appear to have no chance to recover spontaneously are considered.

2. Correction of the secondary deformities that have developed as a result of muscle imbalances. These involve both soft tissue and bony deformities.

3. Reinforcement of weak or paralyzed muscles with tendon transplants. In many cases the deformities must be corrected first.

The discussion of these procedures is organized on a regional basis, i.e., procedures involving the shoulder followed by those on the elbow and the forearm. The principles involving primary nerve repair will be discussed last.

Shoulder Deformities

Soft Tissue Releases. The primary soft tissue deformity is contracture of the internal rotators and the anterior capsule. Historically, this was the first area approached surgically. In England, Fairbank in 1913 popularized an extensive release of the subscapularis and anterior capsule; the pectoralis major was only

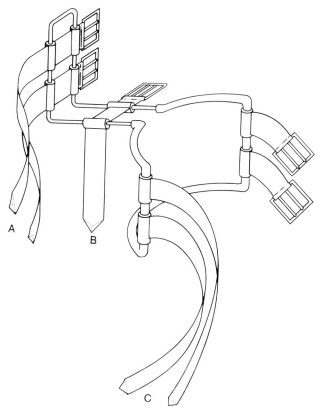

Figure 28–21. Schematic drawing of the Fairbank splint: *(A)* forearm strap, *(B)* arm strap, *(C)* chest strap. (Reproduced with permission from Gilmour J: Notes on the surgical treatment of brachial birth palsy. Lancet *209*:696–699, 1925.)

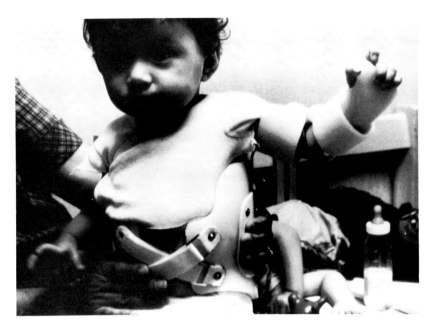

Figure 28–22. An infant with a Fairbank-type splint.

partially lengthened.[20] At Boston Children's Hospital, Sever further popularized this approach but did not open the capsule out of fear of creating postoperative adhesions and stiffness.[59] He cut the entire tendon of the pectoralis major and subscapularis unless there was anterior subluxation, in which case it was not divided. This was followed by cast and then splint immobilization. If it blocked anterior reduction of the humeral head, the acromion was osteotomized. In some cases partial release of the origins of the short head of the biceps and coracobrachialis was performed. Sever reported on his first 500 cases of BPIN in 1916.[59] Nine years later his series had increased to 1100 cases with 70 operative procedures.[60] He modified the procedure slightly, releasing the tip of the coracoid process to allow distal retraction of the coracobrachialis and short head of the biceps. He did note that postoperatively it was difficult for the patient to internally rotate the shoulder. This procedure was accepted as the standard by other authors.[13, 14, 23] Follow-up studies, however, demonstrated a high incidence of recurrence due to the absence of active external rotation of the shoulder.

Tendon Transfer. Many investigators have tried to substitute functioning muscles for those muscles paralyzed or weakened by nerve injuries. Unfortunately, the success of these procedures has been limited somewhat by the fact that often the transplanted muscles may not be fully functional or by the presence of secondary deformities. The two major muscle functions that are lost with upper root lesions are external rotation and abduction of the shoulder. Since these motions are not totally separate or pure, a single isolated muscle transfer may not fully correct the deficiency.

External Rotation Transfer. The first attempt at improving external rotation was the capsular reattachment procedure reported in 1932 by Kleinberg.[39] He released the subscapularis and then tightened the lateral capsule and external rotator cuff attachments anteriorly on the humerus; this was intended to both strengthen these muscles and act as a checkrein on internal rotation. Since he was transferring an already weakened muscle, the procedure's effects were limited and it was never accepted by his colleagues as a workable transfer. Moore noticed that the anterior deltoid often was strong in these patients. He devised a procedure in which this portion was transplanted posteriorly to the spine of the scapula to convert it to more of an external rotator.[50, 51]

At about the same time L'Episcopo reported that he had achieved good results with the Sever anterior release but had noticed a return of internal rotation.[43] He believed that something was needed to restore active external rotation. The subscapularis was the greatest offender in producing internal rotation, he thought, but would be technically difficult to transfer because of its anatomical location and short tendon. In his original report in 1934 he transferred only the teres major tendon to the posterior aspect of the proximal humerus to change it from an internal to an external rotator of the shoulder.[42] He also emphasized that this must be performed with the Sever operation. In a later report in 1939 L'Episcopo modified the procedure slightly by transferring both the teres major and latissimus dorsi tendons (Figs. 28–23 and 28–24).[43] In cases in which there was retroversion of the humeral head, he performed a rotational osteotomy of the humerus above the insertion of the deltoid. This procedure has enjoyed wide acceptance by the orthopedic community.[5, 40, 71, 72, 74, 76] Leffert, in 20 years of experience with the procedure, has noted considerable parent and patient satisfaction.[40] Although it did not produce a strong shoulder, there was marked improvement in active external rotation. In many cases in which substitution patterns had been established preoperatively, a vigorous program of physical therapy was necessary to eliminate these motions.[40]

As with any successful procedure, each new worker

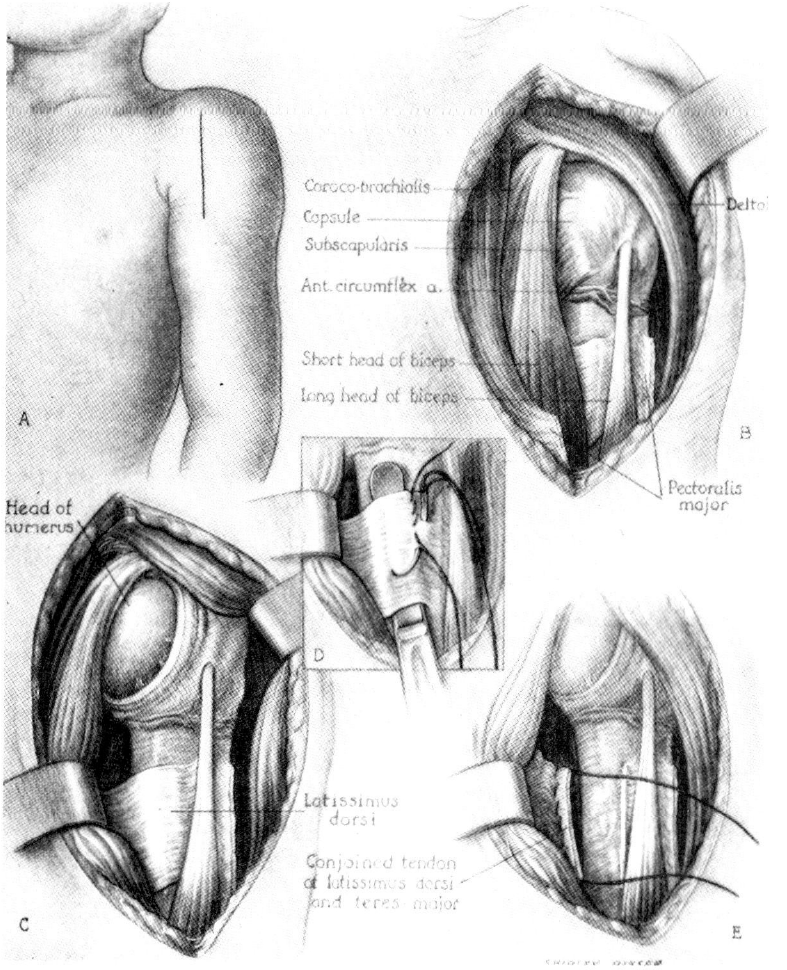

Figure 28–23. The anterior approach for the L'Episcopo procedure. *A*, The incision. *B*, The deep anterior structures after the pectoralis major has been cut. *C*, In the original description both the anterior capsule and subscapularis were cut, exposing the head of the humerus. *D*, Presuturing the conjoined tendon of the latissimus dorsi and teres major. *E*, Release of the conjoined tendon. (Reprinted by permission from the *New York State Journal of Medicine*, copyright by the Medical Society of the State of New York. From L'Episcopo JB: Restoration of muscle balance in the treatment of obstetrical paralysis. NY State J Med *39*:357–363, 1939.)

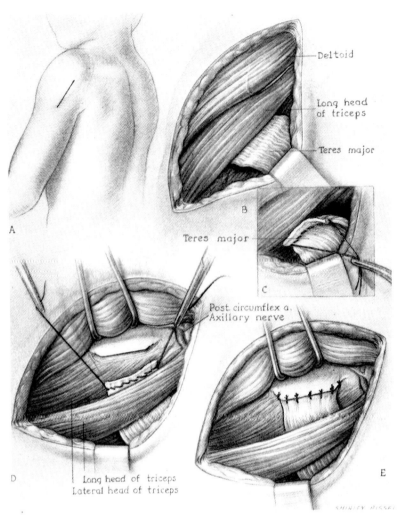

Figure 28–24. The posterior approach for the L'Episcopo procedure. *A,* Posterior incision parallel to the posterior deltoid. *B,* Exposure of the relaxed teres major posterior to the long head of the triceps. *C,* The conjoined tendons of the teres major and latissimus dorsi are pulled out of the posterior incision by their sutures. *D,* The conjoined tendons are passed under the long head of the triceps. *E,* The tendons are sutured to an anterior periosteal flap. (Reprinted by permission from the *New York State Journal of Medicine,* copyright by the Medical Society of the State of New York. From L'Episcopo JB: Restoration of muscle balance in the treatment of obstetrical paralysis. NY State J Med 39:357–363, 1939.)

adds his or her own modifications; thus, there have been many variations of the original L'Episcopo procedure. Zachary used a single incision entering the back of the humerus through the standard posterior approach of Henry.[74] The tendon of the latissimus was transferred to a slot in the origin of the lateral head of the triceps to give it a more effective mechanical advantage. In some patients a weakness of internal rotation was noticed because the pectoralis major and subscapularis had been tenotomized. To allow some preservation of this function, Green and Tachdjian[27] and Chung and Nissenbaum[17] lengthened the pectoralis major by Z-plasty rather than sectioning it. In addition, the elongated coracoid was removed and the acromion osteotomized. Zancolli uses a single axillary approach.[76] He lengthens the tendon of the latissimus dorsi and leaves its attachment on the humerus; this portion is then circled posteriorly around the proximal humerus and sutured back to its proximal end. The pectoralis major, which is released initially, is transferred up to the distal end of the subscapularis (Fig. 28–25). He emphasized that for this procedure to be successful the joint must be congruous. If the head is retroverted, he believed that the L'Episcopo procedure

was contraindicated because it would produce a late anteroinferior subluxation of the head that was more disabling than the original posterior subluxation.[76] Aston, in evaluating the Texas Scottish Rite experience, found that those patients in whom the anterior release procedures were supplemented with the latissimus and teres major tendon transfers functioned better than those who had only the release procedures.[5]

Abduction Transfer. Some workers have attempted to improve abduction of the shoulder as well. In 1927 Mayer described removing the trapezius off the distal clavicle, acromion, and distal scapular spine and attaching it to a fascial tube, which was then passed over the deltoid and attached to the humerus at the distal insertion of the deltoid.[46] This procedure was modified over the years by broadening the fascial attachment to simulate the shape of the deltoid.[47] The procedure could not be used if any subluxation of the shoulder was present; in addition, it required an abduction splint for six months. Ober transferred the origins of the long head of the triceps and the short head of the biceps up to the acromion in an attempt to improve abduction strength.[52] This procedure had limited effectiveness because these muscles often were not fully functional.

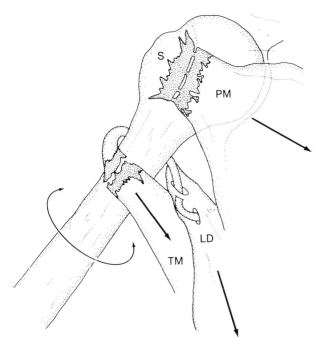

Figure 28–25. Zancolli's modification of the L'Episcopo procedure. The teres major (TM) is left intact. The distal portion of the Z-plasty of the latissimus dorsi (LD) has been passed posteriorly around the shaft of the humerus and sutured to the proximal portion. The pectoralis major (PM) is sutured to the insertion of the subscapularis (S). (Reproduced with permission from Zancolli EA: Classification and management of the shoulder in birth palsy. Orthop Clin North Am 12:433–457, 1981.)

Hoffer and coworkers transferred the conjoined tendon of the latissimus dorsi and teres major into the rotator cuff in an attempt to obtain both external rotation and abduction. Rather than performing an anterior release, they stretched the contracted anterior capsule with a series of preliminary shoulder spica casts. In their 11 patients they had an average gain of 64 per cent of active abduction and 45 per cent of external rotation.[32]

Proximal Humeral Osteotomy. One of the major problems seen in older children is secondary internal rotation of the humeral head (retroversion). Scaglietti believed that this was due to any injury to the proximal physis at birth.[58] In an effort to improve the function of the internally rotated upper extremity, numerous authors have advocated a simple external rotational humeral osteotomy. Early in this century there were two schools of thought regarding treatment of the secondary effects of BPIN. In England and the United States the anterior release procedures were popularized by the work of Fairbank and Sever.[20, 59–62] On the European Continent Vulpis and Lange espoused the humeral osteotomy; this procedure was introduced in the United States in a report by Rogers in 1916.[56] It seems to have been the Italian authors who popularized it in America. L'Episcopo mentioned its use briefly with his tendon transfer if the shoulder joint was incongruous.[43] Scaglietti and Putti combined it with the Sever release in an attempt to relocate the humeral head.[58] Zancolli, however, believed that it was a mistake to try to reconstruct the already deformed shoulder joint.[76] He noted that if the head was directed

posteriorly and was reduced with an anterior release or if external rotation transfers were performed, over time they would often progress to the more disabling anteroinferior subluxation or external rotation abduction contracture.[76] His criteria for doing the derotation osteotomy included an internal rotation abduction contracture in the shoulder, a positive Putti scapular sign with external rotation, and posterior subluxation of the humeral head on radiographs. Almost 70 per cent of the patients in his surgical group underwent this procedure.

In a more recent review, Goddard and Fixsen reported 10 cases in which only one child was independent in daily activities preoperatively.[25] Postoperatively nine achieved independence. They also noted improvement in forearm function since external rotation of the upper humerus brought the flexed, pronated distal portion into a better position, allowing it to be used for more activities. The most important improvement was the ability to move the hand to the mouth.

Almost all authors have recommended that the osteotomy be done proximally to the insertion of the deltoid.[25, 58, 71, 76] This allows the deltoid to be externally rotated, placing the stronger anterior deltoid in a more advantageous mechanical position. Postoperatively, Blount, Rogers, and Scaglietti simply maintained the extremity in a spica cast with no internal fixation.[8, 9, 56, 58] In fact, Blount actually added some anterior angulation of the distal fragment, which he thought increased the patient's ability to raise the upper extremity anteriorly (Fig. 28–26).[9] He performed the procedure by percutaneous osteolysis. Goddard and Fixsen used

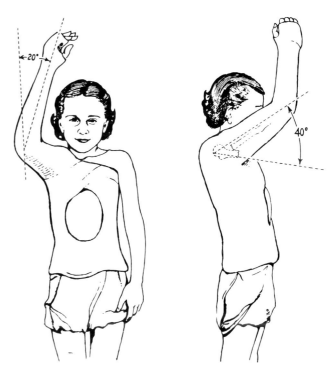

Figure 28–26. The position of the patient postoperatively after Blount's drill osteoclasis. The 40 degrees of anterior angulation is not apparent cosmetically and improves forward flexion. (Reproduced with permission from Blount WP: Osteoclasis of the upper extremity in children. Acta Orthop Scand 32:374–382, 1962.)

an intramedullary rod supplemented with spica cast fixation.[25] The most popular method of fixation appears to be a small plate with compression.[71, 72, 76] The accepted position of correction is when external rotation is complete with the shoulder abducted 90 degrees and the hand can approach the anterior abdomen without producing a scapular sign of Putti.[76] It is important that the external rotation not be overcorrected.

Internal Rotation Procedures. In those patients who have undergone either too-vigorous treatment with the Statue of Liberty splint or anterior release and external rotation muscle transfers, the result can be an external rotation abduction contracture with or without anteroinferior dislocation of the humeral head. Zancolli has managed these individuals with a posterior release and reduction of the shoulder if the joint is not deformed (Fig. 28–27).[76] In those patients with a deformity of the humeral head, a simple internal derotational humeral osteotomy is performed.[76]

Arthrodesis. Fusion of the glenohumeral joint is considered as a salvage type of procedure. Kleinberg reported its use in a case in 1924.[38] It appeared, however, that the major benefit came from simply placing the extremity in external rotation and abduc-

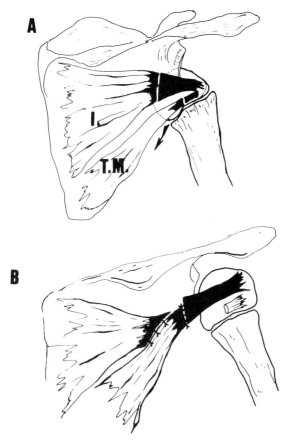

Figure 28–27. Zancolli's posterior release. *A,* The infraspinatus (I) and teres minor (TM) muscles are cut at different levels. *B,* The teres minor is sutured to the distal infraspinatus tendon. The humeral head is usually reduced with simple internal rotation. The capsule is left intact. (Reproduced with permission from Zancolli EA: Classification and management of the shoulder in birth palsy. Orthop Clin North Am *12*:433–457, 1981.)

tion. Wickstrom also found that although the function of the extremity was improved after the arthrodesis, there was sufficient weakness of the extrascapular muscles to limit the excursion of the pectoral girdle.[72] Unfortunately, patients who are candidates for arthrodesis have such extensive involvement that all their shoulder muscles are weakened, which compromises the end result.[16]

Elbow and Forearm Deformities

Elbow Flexion. Lack of full elbow extension usually does not constitute a significant disability. The major disability appears to be this deficiency coupled with a supination deformity in more extensively involved individuals. Blount, using his percutaneous osteoclasis technique, performed a transverse osteotomy of the distal humeral metaphysis to obtain greater elbow extension.[9] Sever corrected the disability with soft tissue, subperiosteal lengthening of the anterior muscles coupled with lengthening of the biceps tendon.[62]

Forearm Supination. Patients with extensive involvement of either entire nerve roots or the lower roots often have their forearm fixed in supination, which results in very limited function in the hand. The deformity of the forearm places the palm of the hand in a position useless for anything more than (perhaps) carrying objects. A weakened hand is much more useful if the forearm is partially pronated because the functional part of the hand faces the working surface of tables and desks. The simplest way to correct this supination deformity is an osteotomy of the forearm. Blount has found his percutaneous osteoclasis to be useful in the midshaft of the radius and ulna.[8, 10] In some of the higher lesions, the forearm has remained in a pronated condition. Correcting the internal rotation of the shoulder often will improve the function sufficiently to render the lack of supination less of a problem. Sever in his cases often performed a simple release of the pronator teres to allow the supinators to become effective.[61] L'Episcopo[43] and Adler and Patterson[2] have advocated more extensive forearm tendon transfers to try to improve active pronation.

Hand and Wrist Procedures. Procedures to improve hand and wrist function are often individualized according to the functional muscles available or the contracture present, or both. It is beyond the scope of this text to discuss these procedures in detail; they are extensively covered in the standard textbooks on hand surgery.

Primary Nerve Repair

Early Work. It has always seemed that the most logical way to treat BPIN was primarily to repair the nerves. This was the major thrust of many of the early workers. In 1905, Clark and associates reported extensively on the results of early exploration and primary repair in seven cases.[18] They had a 30 per cent mortality rate in these first cases. By 1913, Taylor had increased his experience to 43 cases.[67] It was his opinion that the earlier the repair was done, the better. Three months was the optimum time—before the scar formation either had constricted the partially intact bundles or had consolidated, making the primary repair more difficult. The repair consisted of a simple end-to-end suture that was covered with a Cargile membrane to inhibit the late invasion of scar. The most difficult part, as far as the patient was concerned, was that postoperative immobilization called for the head and neck to be held close to the shoulder to protect the nerve repair; this required the use of a special dressing and brace (Fig. 28–28).

For some reason nerve repair did not seem to achieve a widespread popularity at this time, probably because a critical review of these repairs demonstrated, as Sever stated, "no brilliant results."[60] In the light of current knowledge, Taylor probably operated on many patients who would have improved without surgery. His enthusiasm and supposedly good results passed, and there was an almost 40-year interval in which very few authors advocated primary nerve repair. In fact, in his extensive review of the literature up to 1966 Gjorup stated, "It would appear reasonable to conclude, therefore, that obstetrical brachial plexus lesion cannot be remedied by neurosurgical procedures."[24]

Microsurgical Repair. The development of microsurgical repair with nerve grafts renewed interest in the primary repair of the plexus. Nerve grafting was attempted in adults with traumatic lesions by Seddon in 1947, but his results were considered mediocre; they were so poor, in fact, that in his Watson-Jones address to the Royal College of Surgeons in 1963 he recom-

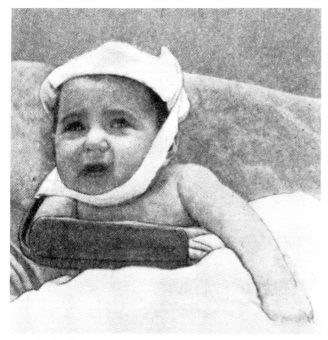

Figure 28–28. Taylor's postoperative brace used to approximate the shoulder to the neck to protect the postoperative nerve repair. (Reproduced with permission from Taylor AS: Conclusions derived from further experience in the surgical treatment of brachial birth palsy. Am J Med Sci *146*:836–856, 1913.)

mended that the procedure be abandoned.[31] Gilbert and coworkers have gained extensive experience in recent years in the primary repair of lesions of the brachial plexus in infants.[21, 22] In their review of previous series without nerve repair, it became apparent that if there is no deltoid or biceps recovery by the third month, the result is almost always very poor. Since the deltoid is difficult to test in small infants, they relied almost exclusively on biceps recovery. They found that their clinical examination for recovery was much more useful than the electromyograph. Their indications for exploration were (1) a completely flail arm with a Horner's syndrome after one month, because of the uniformly poor outcome in these cases, and (2) absence of biceps function after three months. (They cautioned that if there was slight return in four to five months, surgery should be performed because the outcome was still very poor.)

Their technique involves a supraclavicular approach with several nerve grafts. The grafts are secured by a fibrin glue rather than fine sutures. It was emphasized that the inferior roots need to be explored aggressively even if the incidence of avulsion in this area is high. The rare lower root rupture, if found, can be repaired with a better outcome than the almost nonexistent spontaneous recovery that is the rule. Their results are quite impressive. In the C5–C6 lesion they had nearly 80 per cent near-normal results versus an expected recovery of almost zero. Boome and Kaye in South Africa and Kawabata and coworkers in Japan have also found that the three-month period of no recovery is a useful indication for surgical intervention.[12, 37] Although their series were not as long term as those of Gilbert and colleagues, their early results were comparable.

Postoperative immobilization in these more recent cases is less drastic than with the earlier work of Taylor (see Fig. 28–28).[66] The patient is in a body jacket for only three weeks.

Author's Preferred Method of Treatment

Early Treatment

Usually I simply place the arm in a Jacksonville sling when asked to see the patient after delivery. I avoid any manipulation at that time because of the irritability of the plexus. At about two weeks I sit down with the parents and go over a program of passive stretching, starting at the fingers and progressing to the glenohumeral joint. The flexors of the fingers and wrist are fully stretched. The forearm is supinated and the elbow is both flexed and extended. The shoulder is the most difficult joint to manipulate because the parents must stabilize the scapula. The primary aim is to stretch the internal rotators. The parent must stabilize the scapula with one hand and externally rotate the humerus with the elbow flexed at 90 degrees. Ideally this is done with each diaper change. The major goal is to maintain the passive range of motion of all the joints. At about six months of age, when the child can begin to interact with the parents, active exercises are initiated that encourage the use of the weakened muscles. Each exercise needs to be individualized for the specific muscle groups to be strengthened; usually these must take the form of games rather than specific repetitive exercises.

Patients who fail to demonstrate any significant recovery in their biceps by three months of age are referred to a colleague for consideration for surgical repair of the plexus. My experience is that in most cases of BPIN, the child's ability to recover useful function of the extremity is quite good if the parents faithfully carry out an aggressive stretching and exercise program. Useful function is defined as having enough external rotation and shoulder abduction to raise the hand to the mouth and the top of the head (Fig. 28–29). Standard operative procedures cannot accomplish much more than this.

Treatment of Late Effects

The real disability usually is seen in infants who do not receive early treatment and who end up with internal rotation contractures. These children usually recover at least 70 to 80 per cent of shoulder abduction. If there is an internal rotation contracture of at least 30 degrees, it is practically impossible for the child to move the hand to the face or the top of the head without leaning the head forward in an awkward motion (Fig. 28–30). Usually these patients have such significant bony changes that glenohumeral incongruity is already present. I have found that a single derotational osteotomy of the humerus changes the position of the hand so that it can be placed on the head postoperatively (Fig. 28–31).

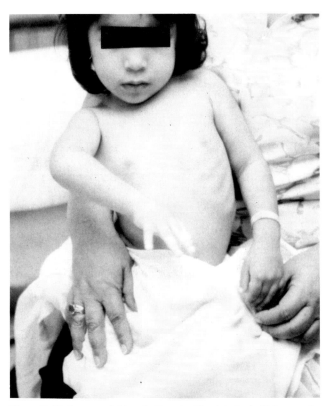

Figure 28–30. Even though this patient has shoulder abduction to 75 degrees, she is unable to put her hand to her mouth because of a 45-degree internal rotation contracture.

The osteotomy is secured with a four-hole compression plate. I usually make the osteotomy as far proximal as possible. I have not noticed any problem postoperatively if the osteotomy is performed proximal to the deltoid insertion. The arm is externally rotated enough to provide at least 30 to 45 degrees of

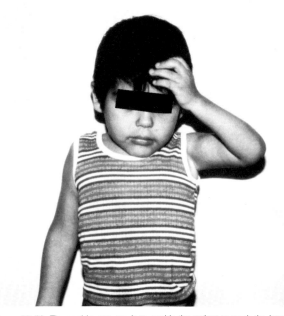

Figure 28–29. The goal in recovery is to enable the patient to reach the hand to the head or mouth.

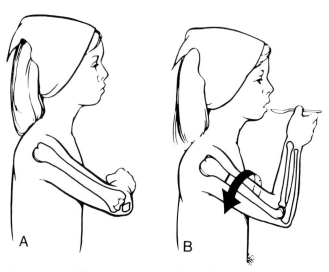

Figure 28–31. *A,* With limited abduction and forward flexion, the internal rotation contracture prevents the forearm and hand from reaching the face. *B,* Derotating the humerus approximately 90 degrees enables the hand to be brought to the head and face. (Modified from Ling CM: The influence of age on the results of open sternomastoid tenotomy in muscular torticollis. Clin Orthop Rel Res *116*:144, 1976.)

external rotation; at least the same amount of internal rotation must remain. Postoperatively the patient is immobilized for one month in a shoulder spica cast in the Statue of Liberty position to decrease the rotational stresses on the small plate (Fig. 28–32). Follow-up for as long as 10 years has shown that these patients continue to maintain sufficient external rotation to raise their arms above their heads (Fig. 28–33).

Torticollis

Torticollis is a deformity characterized by the approximation of the mastoid process to the sternoclavicular joint. The deformity almost always is unilateral; in the rare cases where it is bilateral, it produces a resultant forward inclination of the cervical spine and head.

Torticollis is derived from the two Latin terms *tortus*, which means twisted, and *collum*, which refers to the neck. In the literature it is synonymous with many other terms. German authors referred to it as *caput obstipum* or *collum obstipum*, indicating some obstetric etiology.[98, 118, 126] The terms *fibromastosis colli* or *collum distortum* have also been used to describe the condition.[117]

As with many other medical conditions, Hippocrates is said to have been one of the first authors to describe

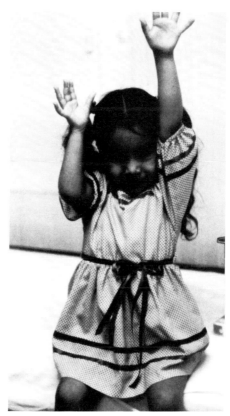

Figure 28–33. View of the patient in Figure 28–30, two years postoperative, demonstrating the continuing ability to reach the arm above the head.

the pathogenesis of this condition. In the statue that immortalizes Alexander the Great in the British Museum, one sees the classic torticollis except for the facial distortion.[126] The first description of the surgical management of torticollis, an open section of the sternomastoid muscle, was supplied by Isaac Minnius in Germany in 1641.[138] In the United States cases were reported in Boston as early as 1841 and 1842 by John Warren and John Brown, respectively.

CLASSIFICATION

Torticollis can be classified into many types. Probably the most complete classification is that of Chandler and Altenberg (Table 28–6).[88] It includes all types for all ages and is based primarily upon the etiology. Because of its completeness it has stood the test of time. For purposes of simplification I will classify torticollis according to the age of onset of the pathology. *Infantile* or *idiopathic* types become manifest during the first year of life. *Late onset–acquired* types are those that develop later as either a temporary or permanent condition. This discussion will be limited to the classic infantile form. Other types that develop in the first year of life will be discussed in the section on differential diagnosis. Space does not permit more than a brief discussion of the late onset–acquired type.

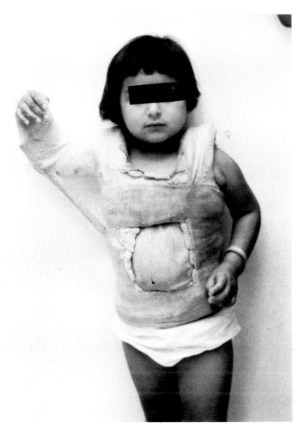

Figure 28–32. The position of the upper extremity in the "Statue of Liberty" cast used to decrease the rotational stresses upon the humeral plate postoperatively.

Table 28–6. CLASSIFICATION OF TORTICOLLIS

1. **Structural**
   a. Osseous
      Hemivertebrae
      Congenital fusion of cervical vertebrae deformity
      Malformation of skull and vertebral processes
      Cervical rib
      Pterygium colli
      Compensatory to structural defects of dorsal and lumbar spine
      Klippel-Feil syndrome
      Spina bifida
      Postrachitic
      Sprengel's
   b. Myogenic
      Congenital absence of cervical muscles
      Congenital hypertrophy
2. **Paralytic**
   Anterior poliomyelitis
   Spastic paralysis
   Postinfections (neuritis)
   Post-traumatic
   Other nerve lesions
   Erb's
   Spasmodic
3. **Vascular**
   Congenital
   Anterior scalenus syndrome
4. **Infections**
   Cervical adenitis
   Retropharyngeal abscess
   Mastoiditis
   Infections of cervical vertebrae
   Arthritis and synovitis
   Cutaneous infection
   Infections of congenital cysts and diverticula
   Spontaneous dislocation of cervical vertebra

   Fasciitis
   Retrotonsilar abscess
   Otitis media
   Myositis
   Spondylitis
   Meningitis
5. **Traumatic**
   Fractures and dislocations of cervical spine
   Fracture of cranial base
   Trauma of cervical fascia, muscles, nerves, etc.
   Fracture of clavicle and scapula
6. **Functional**
   Hysterical
   Spasmodic torticollis?
7. **Ocular**
   Visual defects, corneal scars, etc.
   Muscular
8. **Aural**
   Deafness
   Vestibular
9. **Scar Formation**
   Burns
   Trauma
   Lupus, etc.
10. **Neoplastic (Local or Central)**
    Osseous
    Myogenic
    Lymphatic
    Vascular
    Nerve
11. **Congenital**
    Posture in utero
    Trauma at birth
    Ischemia? of muscle

Reproduced with permission from Chandler FA, and Altenberg A: Congenital muscular torticollis. JAMA 125:476–483, 1944.

The major infantile type represents the classic picture of the conversion of the distal sternocleidomastoid muscle into fibrous tissue. It may present in early infancy as a large local mass (sternomastoid tumor) with or without a true fixed torticollis. In other instances the presence of a mass may or may not be appreciated in infancy, and there is the slow development of a fixed torticollis due to a fibrous contracture of the sternocleidomastoid. This form usually is referred to as congenital muscular torticollis; however, Sarnet and Morrissy believed that it should be termed idiopathic because of its still undetermined etiology.[129]

Other types of torticollis in which there is no contracture of the sternocleidomastoid develop during infancy (Table 28–7). These will be discussed later under the differential diagnosis.

Table 28–7. CLASSIFICATION OF INFANTILE TORTICOLLIS

Congenital or idiopathic muscular
Ocular
Osseous deformities
Sandifer syndrome
Paroxysmal torticollis in infancy
Posterior fossa tumors
Fibrodysplasia ossificans progressiva
Congenital myogenic deformities

Anatomy of the Sternocleidomastoid Muscle

In the classic infantile type of torticollis, the primary pathological process involves only the sternocleidomastoid muscle. Thus it is important to have a clear knowledge of the anatomy of this unique muscle in attempting to understand the pathophysiology of this disorder and its surgical treatment. The article by Chandler and Altenberg[88] and the textbook by Jones[106] constitute the best sources on the anatomy of the sternocleidomastoid muscle.

Muscle

The sternocleidomastoid is composed of two major divisions, each of which has its own subdivisions. Each division has its own separate head of origin, but they insert as a composite head.

The *sternal head* arises as a rounded tendon from the sternum and is composed of three subdivisions: the superficial sterno-occipital, the superficial sternomastoid, and the deep sternomastoid (Fig. 28–34). The *clavicular head* arises as a mixture of tendinous and muscular fibers from the superior aspect of the inner third of the clavicle. It is composed of two subdivisions, the cleido-occipital and the deep cleidomastoid. These two heads combine proximally to insert as a continuous band of fibers from the tip of the mastoid process

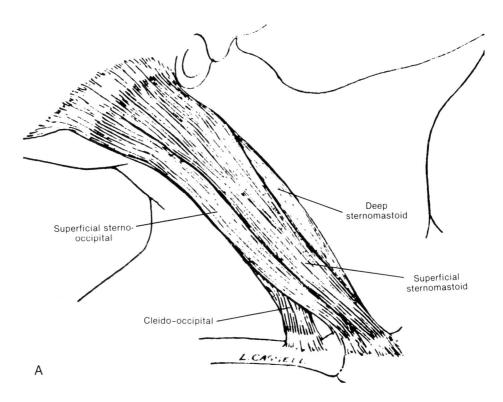

A

Figure 28–34. *A,* External view of the right sternocleidomastoid muscle. *B,* Deep view shows its relationship to the spinal accessory nerve. (Reproduced with permission from Chandler FA, and Altenberg A: Congenital muscular torticollis. *JAMA 125:*476–483, 1944. Copyright 1944, American Medical Association.)

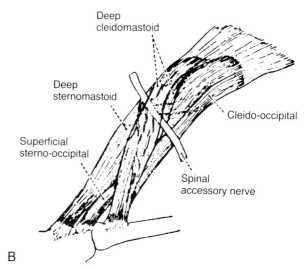

B

anteriorly to the insertion of the trapezius posteriorly on the superior nuchal line.

Nerve Supply

The main motor supply is from the spinal accessory nerve, which is composed of accessory nerves from the vagus and segments of the upper five cervical nerves. This nerve leaves the skull via the jugular foramen, where it courses with the carotid artery and the internal jugular vein. It passes through the deep surface of the sternocleidomastoid muscle between the cleidomastoid and sterno-occipital portions. The small intramuscular rami of the nerve must pass through the sternal head before they reach the clavicular head (Fig. 28–35).

Arteries

The arterial supply to the sternocleidomastoid is quite extensive, arising from five or more arterial sources (Fig. 28–36).

Veins

The venous drainage of the sternocleidomastoid is far more extensive than its arterial supply (Fig. 28–37). The muscle drains into all the major veins of the neck. In addition to the surface connection, there is also a maze of connections within the muscle itself.

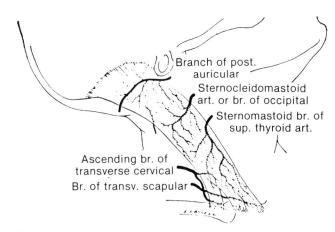

Figure 28–36. The multiple arteries supplying the sternocleidomastoid muscle. (Reproduced with permission from Chandler FA, and Altenberg A: Congenital muscular torticollis. JAMA 125:476–483, 1944. Copyright 1944, American Medical Association.)

Actions and Motions

Contraction of one side of the sternocleidomastoid turns the face to the opposite side and depresses the ear on the same side toward the shoulder. This rotation of the neck is opposed by the contralateral trapezius. If the trapezius and sternocleidomastoid contract together on the same side, the face and head rotate at the sagittal axis. Contraction of both muscles extends the neck. Secondarily the sternocleidomastoid aids respiration by fixing or elevating the thoracic cage.

INCIDENCE

The overall incidence of infantile torticollis ranges from 0.3 per cent to 0.5 per cent.[90, 92, 100, 137] There is a wide variation in the various series, however, as to the incidence of right versus left lesions, males versus females, and breech presentations. In order to obtain

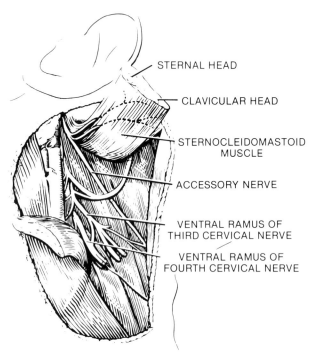

Figure 28–35. The motor rami of the spinal accessory nerve to the sternocleidomastoid first enter the sternal head and pass through its bellies before reaching the clavicular head. (Reproduced with permission from Sarnat HB, and Morrissy RT: Idiopathic torticollis: sternocleidomastoid myopathy and accessory neuropathy. Muscle Nerve 4:374–380, 1981.)

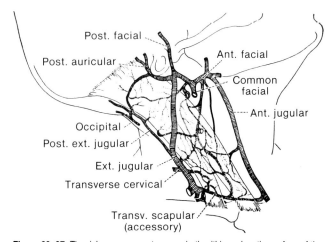

Figure 28–37. The rich venous anastomoses both within and on the surface of the sternocleidomastoid muscle. (Reproduced with permission from Chandler FA, and Altenberg A: Congenital muscular torticollis. JAMA 125:476–483, 1944. Copyright 1944, American Medical Association.)

a clearer picture of the overall incidence of these factors, I have combined the data from 1528 cases in 12 major series.* In this combined series the incidence in the sexes was nearly equal, i.e., 52 per cent females and 48 per cent males.

The right and left sides were almost equal, with 54 per cent of the cases involving the right side. In their series Coventry and Harris noticed some correlation between laterality and the fetal presentation.[90] Infants who presented in the vertex position showed a two-to-one left-to-right side ratio; in those with breech presentation the ratio was reversed, i.e., two to one right to left. This significant increase in right-sided lesions in breech presentation was also noted by Ling and Low[113] and Macdonald.[118] Eight of the 232 cases in Morrison and MacEwen's series occurred in infants delivered by cesarean section;[123] six of these eight were breech presentations. In the overall series of 1528 cases, only three were bilateral. In most of the individual series at least 50 per cent of the infants were from primiparous mothers.

Associated Conditions

Congenital Dislocation of the Hip

There is still some disagreement on the association of torticollis with congenital dislocation of the hip. This may be due to the fact that some authors differentiated between radiographic dysplasia and frank dislocation. In 49 patients Weiner found four cases (8.2 per cent) of torticollis with frank dislocation;[139] three of these four were breech. In an early study from the Alfred I. Du Pont Institute, Hummer and MacEwen looked at both frank dislocation and dysplasia.[103] In a total of 70 patients with torticollis, four (5 per cent) had frank dislocations and 10 (15 per cent) had subluxation or dysplasia, for a total of 20 per cent with some type of congenital hip disorder. In a later review of 232 patients with torticollis from the same institution, the overall incidence for both dysplasia and dislocation was 14 per cent.[123] Hummer and MacEwen found no significant statistical relationship between the side of the torticollis and the side of the hip pathology.[103] Other authors reported that frank dislocation was either absent or very low in their series.[104, 137]

Since there is a higher than expected incidence of congenital dislocation of the hip with torticollis, a very careful clinical examination must be performed on the hips in all these infants. *In those who are breech presentation, imaging procedures such as plain radiographs or ultrasonography should be performed regardless of the results of the clinical examination.*

Brachial Plexus Injuries

Again, the reported association with brachial plexus injuries of infancy is quite variable. Suzuki and co-

workers examined all their cases of brachial plexus injuries very closely for evidence of torticollis.[136] They found that there was evidence of some degree of torticollis in as many as 51 per cent of these cases; in those patients who were breech presentations the incidence was 80 per cent. They also found that in 95 per cent of cases the torticollis was on the same side as the brachial plexus injury. This is in sharp distinction from the findings of others. Chandler, who had over 200 cases of torticollis, reported only three with brachial palsy lesions.[87] Of their 271 cases, Armstrong and colleagues had only one with a brachial plexus injury.[78] Thus, although there is some relationship between these two conditions and birth trauma and while there is a higher incidence of breech presentation with these two conditions, apart from the report of Suzuki and associates there does not appear to be a consistent relationship between torticollis and brachial plexus injuries.

Oligohydramnios

In a prospective study, Dunn found that maternal oligohydramnios was a frequent condition in infants with torticollis. It was also noted to occur in association with bilateral renal anomalies that produced fetal anuria.[92]

ETIOLOGY

Most of the controversy concerns this aspect of torticollis. Despite the numerous specimens obtained at surgery for this condition and the various experimental studies, a clear consensus regarding the etiology of this condition still has not been reached. Numerous theories have been proposed to identify the cause of the condition. These theories will be discussed in detail from the least to the most plausible.

Fetal Development. Reye believed that the presence of fibrosis throughout the entire muscle that was continuous with the tendinous origins and insertions was evidence of absence of fetal development. He theorized that this may have been due to a primary defect in development of the muscle anlage.[127]

Infection. Practically no support exists for this theory. Most of the authors who proposed it—Whitman, Mikulicz, Kader, and Ulbee—wrote around the turn of the century. The theory holds that the sternocleidomastoid was traumatized and subsequently seeded by an infection that produced a myositis. Another infectious theory proposed that torticollis was a form of congenital syphilis.[100]

Heredity. Numerous isolated reports exist of family members of affected infants also being afflicted. These percentages are quite small, however; the highest was 10.4 per cent, reported by Ippolito and colleagues in Italy.[104] The details of their cases were not outlined. In other major series the number of cases was less than 3 per cent.[80, 88, 123, 138] Some ethnic or racial groups (namely, blacks and Malaysians) have been found to

---

*See references 78, 86, 88, 90, 93, 100, 104, 110, 118, 123, 131, 136.

have a lower incidence in some series.[108, 112] Suzuki and associates believed that since the breech presentation was such a factor in the etiology of the disorder in their cases, the hereditary aspect was the predisposition toward breech deliveries.[136]

In one case described in twins by Campbell and Peora, the opposite sides were involved.[85] Only one other report of torticollis in twins has appeared in the English-language literature.[133] Jones has pointed out that the absence in the literature of a detailed report of torticollis in a father and his offspring, and the equal incidence in males and females, make it unlikely to be an autosomal dominant trait.[106] Thus there is little evidence that hereditary factors play much of a part in the etiology of this disorder.

Myopathy. The advent of histochemical examination has provided many answers to the diseases of muscles. As a result, some workers have used this method of analysis to see if it provides any answers to the etiology of torticollis. Sarnat and Morrissy examined a number of surgical specimens and noted both myopathic and neuropathic changes.[129] The myopathic changes were greater in the sternal head. It was their theory that the myopathy in the sternal head produced fibrosis that constricted the nerves coursing through it, producing a neuropathic picture in the clavicular head (see Fig. 28–35).[129] In a more recent thesis study, Braga also noticed a myopathic picture and proposed that torticollis was a localized form of congenital muscular dystrophy.[83] It seems unlikely, given the absence of other manifestations of myopathy in these patients, that the myopathy could be primary and still remain localized.

Neurogenic Causes. Again, the evidence for this theory is scant and based upon isolated reports. In one adult with the residua of infantile idiopathic torticollis, an autopsy revealed atrophy of anterior horn cells in the cervical cord; this could have been due, however, to chronic disuse.[121] Other authors have proposed a neurogenic theory because of the absence of nerve fibers in the specimens collected.[120]

Arterial Obstruction. The early acceptance of arterial obstruction as a cause of torticollis was based upon the work of Nove-Josserand and Viannay, who noticed in stillborn infants that certain arteries that supply the sternocleidomastoid did not fill with the head held in certain positions. It was their belief that various parts of the sternocleidomastoid had an isolated blood supply.[88] Subsequent work by Chandler and Altenberg demonstrated a rich anastomotic blood supply to the sternocleidomastoid (see Fig. 28–36).[88] They also pointed out that the microscopic pathology after arterial ischemia is much different from that usually seen with torticollis.

Muscle Hematoma. One of the original theories, which occasionally persists to the present, is that proposed by Stromeyer in 1838.[106] He thought that torticollis represented a rupture of the sternocleidomastoid at birth, with the development of a hematoma that progressed to fibrosis and contracture, producing the classical clinical picture. This theory enjoyed wide popularity until the early part of this century. There are many arguments against it. First, many patients are delivered by cesarean section with or without trauma.[90] Second, the mass does not develop immediately after delivery. It is never characterized by a soft, fluctuant mass such as is seen with a hematoma but by a firm, fibrous structure. Pathological specimens have failed to demonstrate much residual hemosiderin.[121] If it is a hematoma from muscle rupture, why are other adjacent muscles not affected? Brown and McDowell aspirated a number of these lesions soon after their appearance but were never able to obtain any blood.[84] One case has been documented in the literature in which there was rupture of the sternocleidomastoid with intramuscular hemorrhage and necrosis in a two-day-old infant.[128] Since this was a very early specimen, the characteristic changes of fibrosis and tumor formation were not seen.

Although the hematoma theory is logical, there appears to be no evidence to support it.

Venous Occlusion. Middleton in the late 1920s provided considerable evidence that torticollis was due to venous obstruction.[121] He was able to produce similar changes in dogs by selectively ligating the venous drainage of the sartorius muscle. The changes developed slowly, much as is seen in torticollis. The muscle, initially firm and hard, eventually changed into rigid, well-organized fibrosis. He attributed this extensive fibrosis to the edema that develops. He also pointed out that lower portions of the muscle were more vulnerable because their thin-walled vessels were more liable to be compressed with extremes of intrauterine positions. This theory of venous occlusion was accepted by some of his contemporaries; Hough, on the basis of the microscopic pathology found in his cases, stated that "this theory is the most logical and best supported explanation."[100]

Intrauterine Factors. Later in their vascular studies, Chandler and Altenberg demonstrated a very rich venous plexus around the sternocleidomastoid (see Fig. 28–37).[88] Pointing out that Middleton had based his concept of venous obstruction on there being an isolated arterial and venous supply to various parts of the sternocleidomastoid, they demonstrated that numerous vascular anastomoses existed both within and around the muscles. They also questioned how the venous obstruction could be so localized and not affect the adjoining structures. They believed that even with venous obstruction, the mass should develop soon after delivery. The absence of venous thrombosis further weakened the theory. Therefore, Chandler and Altenberg looked for other causes in their cases. They could not find one common factor but thought that a number of factors were often involved. In many of their cases they were able to demonstrate an *ante partum* torticollis on radiographs of the fetus. This finding has been confirmed by Suzuki and coworkers in their studies as well.[136] Chandler and Altenberg believed that this prolonged pathological immobilization prenatally rendered the sternocleidomastoid atrophic, shortened, and partially ischemic, making it more susceptible during delivery to trauma that would not damage a normal muscle. Such trauma resulted in a sterile, nonspecific necrosis and inflammation that subsequently developed into the hard, fibrous mass. This theory that intrauterine positions predispose the muscle to trauma at delivery has been accepted by later authors.[92, 108]

In summary, the various theories proposed in the past that have tried to identify a single etiological factor have not withstood the test of time. The multifactorial theory of the combination of abnormal intrauterine positions producing a pre-existing muscle pathology that is more susceptible to trauma at delivery appears to provide the most logical explanation.

PATHOLOGY

Although much controversy exists regarding the etiology of torticollis, there appears to be unanimity regarding the pathological findings.[78, 106, 111, 127, 138] Simply stated, there is a replacement of the muscle with fibrous tissue (Fig. 28–38). Probably the best description is that given by Chandler in 1948:[87]

These tumors consist of fusiform masses, involving part or all of the muscle belly of the sternocleidomastoid, usually in

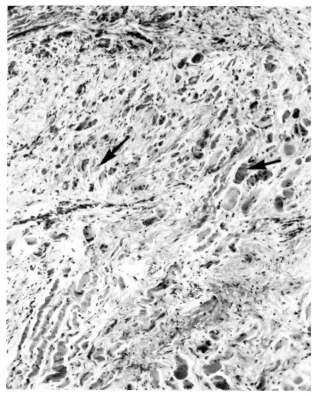

Figure 28–38. Photomicrograph of a section of the involved sternocleidomastoid muscle showing degenerating muscle fiber *(arrows)* widely separated by a diffuse infiltration of fibrous tissue. (Reproduced with permission from Armstrong D, Pickrell K, Fetter B, and Pitts W: Torticollis: an analysis of 271 cases. Plast Reconstr Surg 35:14–25, 1965.)

the middle third. The tumor is limited by the perimysium and may extend proximally and distally to involve the entire muscle substance. It is firm in consistency and separates readily from adjacent structures. Cross section reveals a white fibrocartilaginous, glistening surface which at times is slightly lobulated. In none of the specimens was there anything to suggest blood clot formation of residual blood pigment. Microscopic sections show muscle fibers in all stages of degeneration as reflected by their wide variations in staining qualities. Fibrous tissue is abundant, replacing muscle fibers to varying degrees. Occasionally normal muscle fibers survive. These are usually at the periphery of the fibrous mass.

The only deviation from this classic description was reported by Kiesewetter and coworkers, who found hemosiderin in 25 per cent of their cases. It was present in small amounts and only in a few foci about the vessels and occasionally in the macrophages. They believed, however, that extravasation of blood was a very minor feature.[108] The changes appear to be more severe in the distal portions, with the proximal end often being relatively unaffected.[84] The clavicular head also appears to be more involved.[105, 118] Although the fibrotic changes are limited to the sternocleidomastoid, the adjacent muscles may also demonstrate some secondary shortening.[100]

Other investigators have attempted to add to the classical description by performing special studies on the masses removed. Mickelson and coworkers studied the ultrastructure of the mass with the electron microscope.[120] They found that the fibrous tissue resembled mature connective tissue, similar to tendon or ligament. The fibroblasts were thought to be actively producing collagen, as evidenced by their abundant endoplasmic reticulum. The muscle changes were not believed to be unique and were characteristic of immobilization degeneration; this was theorized as being caused by the severe fibrosis. Histochemical studies by Sarnat and Morrissy[129] and Braga[83] have demonstrated myopathic changes. The etiology of these changes is still unexplained.

In some instances an exostosis or osteophyte develops at the insertion of the clavicular portion into the clavicle (Fig. 28–39). Middleton believed that this was because the fibrous scar tissue actually developed a direct relationship with the bone. This same process does not occur with the sternal attachment because the fibrosed fibers are separated from the bone by a normal tendon of insertion.[121]

TUMOR VERSUS TORTICOLLIS

There appear to be two different clinical presentations. One involves the presence of a mass or so-called sternomastoid tumor; the other is the development of wryneck or torticollis without any antecedent tumor. Some studies have demonstrated that the sternomastoid tumor may resolve completely and not progress to a fixed torticollis.[90, 102] However, careful examination of many of these individuals revealed minor degrees

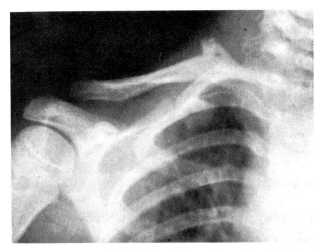

Figure 28–39. An exostosis that developed at the attachment of the clavicular head in a patient with torticollis. (Reproduced with permission from Middleton DS: The pathology of congenital torticollis. Br J Surg 18:188–204, 1930. By permission of the publishers, Butterworth & Co.)

of fibrosis or restriction of motion of the sternocleidomastoid. Other studies have followed patients with tumors carefully and found that at least 21 per cent developed a true fixed torticollis.[106, 113, 118] By the same token, when older patients with a fixed torticollis were examined and a careful developmental history was obtained, approximately 20 per cent of them had had a history of a sternomastoid tumor in early infancy.[118] When the birth histories of both groups were studied, the incidence of breech and primiparous deliveries is strikingly similar. Macdonald has grouped the muscle changes that develop into three patterns: (1) the lesion may resolve completely; (2) it may manifest as a sternomastoid tumor, which may resolve with only a minimal fibrosis; and (3) it may be clinically inapparent during early infancy but with subsequent cicatrization produce a fixed torticollis.[118]

DIAGNOSIS

Clinical Appearance

In the classical picture, a hard, smooth, firm, well-defined mass develops soon after birth in the distal aspect of the sternocleidomastoid (Fig. 28–40). In many of the large series the diagnosis is made at birth in 30 to 40 per cent of cases.[100, 123] There appears to be earlier recognition of the mass in more recent series. In Hough's cases reported in 1934, only 50 per cent were recognized in the first year of life.[100] He stated that this figure was about the same as in other contemporary series. A 1982 series from the Du Pont Institute reported that at least 82 per cent of their cases were recognized by the first three months of age. If a true fixed deformity persists, secondary deformities develop in the face and neck. A hemihypoplasia often develops on the side of the face with the affected muscle; in addition, a plagiocephaly also develops. Both of these

can develop during early infancy. The exact cause of the hemihypoplasia of the face is not clear. There is, however, a definite cause-and-effect relationship, as is demonstrated by the development of asymmetry during the torticollis and a return toward symmetry after the sternocleidomastoid contracture is released.[106]

In an effort to compensate for the fixed lateral tilt, the patient often holds the shoulder on the affected side elevated to bring the head into a more vertical position (Fig. 28–41).

Differential Diagnosis

The diagnosis of infantile or idiopathic muscular torticollis is often confirmed by the clinical examination, in which either a definite sternomastoid tumor or a fixed fibrosis of the muscle itself is found. Often, however, the infant is referred to the orthopedic surgeon with the initial diagnosis made on the basis of a head tilt alone. If the examination reveals the absence of any fixed deformity of the sternocleidomastoid, other conditions producing the classic head tilt in this age group need to be considered.

Acute Conditions

Acutely calcification of the intervertebral disc for which the etiology is unknown can cause acute neck pain and spasm, often with torticollar postures. These symptoms may persist for one to two months.[96] Acute rotary subluxation of the atlantoaxial joint will also produce a fixed head tilt. Here the radiographic appearance of the relationship of the dens to the lateral

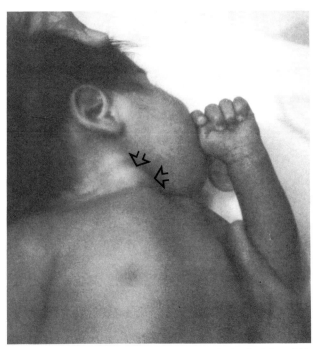

Figure 28–40. The location of the sternomastoid tumor in the distal sternocleidomastoid muscle (arrows).

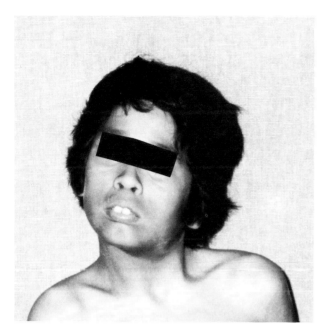

Figure 28–41. A 12-year-old male demonstrating a tight fibrotic right sternocleidomastoid muscle. There is secondary atrophy of the left side of the face. In an effort to decrease some of the effects of the fixed lateral tilt, the patient holds his left shoulder elevated. Note also that the face turns away from the tilted side.

masses is characteristic. This condition can follow either an acute rotational injury or an upper respiratory infection. These acute conditions are very rare in the infant, being seen more commonly in the older child.

Chronic Conditions

Often there is a more gradual onset of the torticollis. These conditions are often seen in infants.

Ocular Torticollis. In my experience, one of the most common causes of nonmuscular torticollis is rotary strabismus. This usually is the result of imbalance of either the superior or inferior oblique muscles or a dysfunction of the fourth cranial nerve. The torticollis usually does not become manifest until about four to six months of age when the infant starts to focus on objects. There is a full range of motion of the neck. In addition, the torticollis is often episodic. It may be especially apparent when the child is focusing on a person or an object. In the structural infantile torticollis, the face is turned away from the side of the head tilt and upwards (see Fig. 28–41). In the ocular type the face is turned slightly *toward the side of the head tilt* (Fig. 28–42). In addition, the conjugate ocular movements may be abnormal. When the infant looks toward the side of the head tilt, the contralateral eye "shoots up."[116] I have also noted that if the body is tilted in the same direction of the head tilt, i.e., the axes of the head and the trunk are in line with each other, the torticollis disappears.

Osseous Lesions. In some cases the torticollis may be fixed owing to congenital deformities of the cervical spine. Unbalanced hemivertebrae in the cervical spine

can produce a head tilt. Often there is no rotary component, just a pure lateral tilting. Radiographs usually confirm the presence of the vertebral anomalies (Fig. 28–43).

Dubousset has described a number of cases of the rare occurrence of a hemiatlas in which the development of the torticollis is progressive.[91] In early infancy the torticollis may be present but is flexible. The rotation is easily correctable, but the tilt and lateral translocation may not correct fully. The amount of correction decreases with age. In most patients there is a regional aplasia of the muscles in the nuchal concavity on the side of the tilt. Dubousset described three groups of deformities: (1) an isolated hemiatlas, (2) a hemiatlas occurring with other anomalies of the cervical spine, and (3) fusion of the atlas with the occiput with absence of one lateral mass. Although radiographs may demonstrate the deformity in the infant, good definition often is not possible until the patient is 12 to 18 months of age. Dubousset recommends early correction and surgical fusion if the deformity appears to be progressive.

Sandifer's Syndrome. Although this condition has been named after Dr. Paul Sandifer, it was originally described by Kinsbourne in 1964.[109, 135] The syndrome involves abnormal tilting or posturing of the head and neck owing to an esophagitis caused by gastroesophageal reflux with or without a hiatal hernia. The abnormal posturing is thought to be due to the discomfort the infant feels with the gastroesophageal reflux. It was emphasized by Murphy and Gellis that this condition may not always be accompanied by vomiting.[125] Diagnosis may require, in addition to an upper gastrointestinal series, more sophisticated studies such as tech-

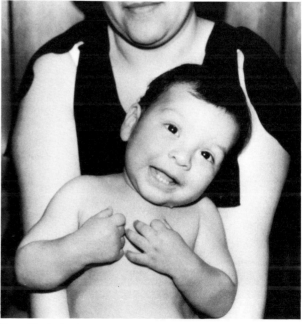

Figure 28–42. An eight-month-old with ocular torticollis. The face turns slightly *toward* the side of the head tilt.

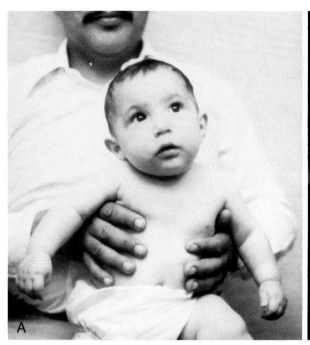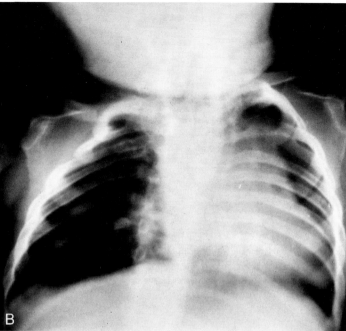

Figure 28–43. *A*, Clinical photograph of an infant with congenital hemivertebrae involving the upper thoracic and lower cervical vertebrae. *B*, Radiograph demonstrating the vertebral anomalies.

netium scintiscans, intraluminal pH monitoring, and/ or esophagoscopy. Treatment is usually medical.

Paroxysmal Torticollis of Infancy. This condition is usually seen in infants from two to eight months of age and is manifested by recurrent attacks of head tilt lasting from a few hours to a few days. It is thought to be a manifestation of the neurological disorder benign paroxysmal vertigo. These infants often develop migraine headaches and hearing loss in later life.

Posterior Fossa Tumors. These may be gradual in onset and can produce varying degrees of torticollis, which may become structural (Fig. 28–44). Often they may not become manifest until the child grows. Usually other peripheral neurological signs are present.[82]

Fibrodysplasia Ossificans Progressiva. This condition may result in enlargement of the sternocleidomastoid or other neck muscles. It is easily differentiated from the usual sternomastoid tumor by CT. In this condition there are areas of soft tissue calcification in the various cervical muscles. In infantile torticollis only the sternocleidomastoid is involved, and there is no calcification.[134]

Congenital Myogenic Lesion. Isolated cases of congenital absence of the sternocleidomastoid have been reported. This creates a head tilt away from the side of the absent muscle with some rotation toward the same side. The etiological basis for isolated absence of the sternocleidomastoid is unknown.[119]

CLINICAL COURSE

Sternomastoid Tumors

The best statistics regarding the clinical course of the sternomastoid tumor come from the longitudinal studies of Coventry and Harris, Jones, and Macdonald.[90, 106, 118] Usually the masses are initially discovered by about 2 to 4 weeks (see Fig. 28–40). The mass reaches its maximum size at about 8 to 10 weeks and usually is gone by 14 weeks (Fig. 28–45). There is often some transient facial asymmetry that begins by about 10 weeks and disappears by 24 weeks. The number of these tumors that progress to a true fixed torticollis is small. In all three studies the progression

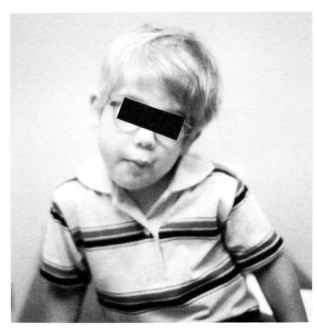

Figure 28–44. A four-year-old who had torticollis and ataxia since early infancy. Notice the presence of hemiatrophy of the face. Subsequent studies revealed the presence of a benign posterior fossa tumor.

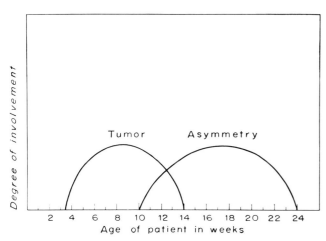

Figure 28-45. The progression and regression of the sternomastoid tumor and facial asymmetry in early infancy. (Reproduced with permission from Coventry MB, and Harris LE: Congenital muscular torticollis in infancy. J Bone Joint Surg 41A:815–822, 1959.)

of sternomastoid tumors to torticollis was nearly equal—about 13 to 15 per cent.[90, 106, 118] In Ling's and Hulbert's series the progression rate was 20 to 21 per cent.[102, 112, 113] As was mentioned earlier, many of these patients when examined clinically have some subtle loss of neck motion and minimal asymptomatic fibrosis of the sternocleidomastoid. Thus it appears that in over 80 per cent of the cases of sternomastoid tumor there is a natural regression of the lesion. This certainly has a bearing on the rationale for early surgical treatment. It could also explain the high success rate of early nonoperative management.

True Torticollis

Very little data exist on the clinical course of untreated fixed torticollis because most reports deal with the results of surgical management of this condition. In their long-term follow-up study, Canale and coworkers were able to identify four untreated cases of fixed torticollis.[86] Two were teenagers who were relatively asymptomatic despite significant facial asymmetry. Two older patients (45 and 60 years of age) also had severe facial asymmetry and troublesome discomfort localized to the contracted muscle when the head was rotated to either side; both had a compensatory thoracic scoliosis. There were no instances of cervical arthritis in any of the cases. The high incidence of facial asymmetry in other series reporting on surgical treatment in older children indicates that this is a persistent condition in untreated true torticollis.[86, 104, 112, 131]

TREATMENT

Nonoperative Management

The mainstay of nonoperative treatment is passive stretching of the affected sternocleidomastoid. In the three series reporting stretching in early infancy, the

overall success rate was about the same—70 to 80 per cent.[90, 102, 112] In Coventry and Harris' group, in which there was an aggressive and well-controlled program of physical therapy, all 24 patients had an excellent result.[90] It was noted, however, that six additional patients who received no therapy also had an excellent result. Canale and associates, in a retrospective review, compared those treated nonoperatively before six months with those treated initially from six months to a year.[86] There did not appear to be any significant difference in outcomes. They found that patients with more than 30 degrees of restriction of neck motion and facial asymmetry tended to have poor results, regardless of how or when they were treated. Children with less than 30 degrees of loss of motion or no facial asymmetry, when treated before one year of age, tended to do well with an exercise program. In addition, it was noticed that torticollis that persisted after one year failed to resolve spontaneously.[86] The poor response to stretching after one year of age was also noted by Hulbert. Twenty of 33 patients in whom nonoperative management began after one year of age required surgical intervention.[102] It has been my experience that, from a practical standpoint, it is physically very difficult to perform adequate stretching on an infant beyond six months of age. After this age the infant resists the treatment so much that it is questionable whether an effective stretching force can be applied to the sternocleidomastoid. Other methods of nonoperative treatment besides stretching have been attempted. Hough cited a treatment advocated by Rosenbaum in which the tumor was injected with a 1 per cent solution of pepsinum purissimum in Pregl's iodine solution.[100] An immediate improvement was reported in all nine of these patients. Another unique method of treatment was designed by Clarren and coworkers.[89] This involved the use of a special helmet, which was supposed to directly treat the plagiocephaly and indirectly the torticollis (Fig. 28–46); the helmet required a continuous application for two to three months. Despite a problem with parent compliance, there was a definite improvement in both the plagiocephaly and the torticollis in patients who completed the treatment.

Operative Management

Von Lackum credits Isaac Minnius with performing the first open section of the sternocleidomastoid in Germany in 1641.[138] Surgical treatment of this disorder did not achieve wide popularity until around the turn of the century. In 1891 Lorenz had advocated myorrhexis—a tearing of the muscle by very forceful manipulation.[115] This procedure caused such serious complications that it was soon abandoned.[100, 106, 132] In the early part of this century, the operative techniques became refined and surgical management became an accepted part of the treatment of this disorder. Two different approaches developed, however, which by and large were based on the surgical specialties treating the condition. General and plastic surgeons preferred

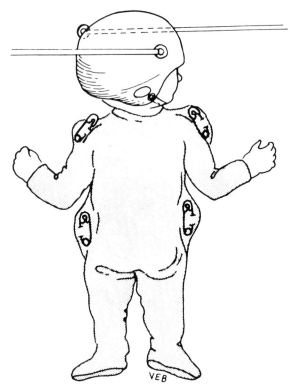

Figure 28–46. The helmet worn by infants in the treatment of torticollis and plagiocephaly. (Reproduced with permission from Clarren SK, Smith DW, and Hanson JW: Helmet treatment for plagiocephaly and congenital muscular torticollis. J Pediatr 94:43–46, 1979.)

to widely excise either the mass or the entire muscle. The orthopedic approach was to do a simple myotomy, followed by immobilization in the overcorrected position.

Resection

In 1895 Mikulicz recommended excision of the tumor and a greater portion of the muscle because of reported inadequacies of the simple myotomies performed during this era.[84, 106, 122] Subsequently some workers believed that removal of only the tumorous mass was sufficient.[88, 98, 108, 138] This was usually achieved with a distal supraclavicular incision. Others thought that since the entire muscle was pathological, the resection should be from the origin on the mastoid process to the insertion on the clavicle and sternum.[78, 84, 99, 124] This total removal was accomplished through a transverse midcollar incision at the center of the sternocleidomastoid (Fig. 28–47). Dissection can begin either proximally or distally. With this approach special care must be taken to preserve the spinal accessory nerve, which penetrates the midportion of the muscle, and the underlying vagus nerve and carotid arteries.

Most of these authors also recommended early surgical removal. In Chandler and Altenberg's series, 15 of their 26 patients were under three months, the youngest being three weeks of age.[88] As they stated,

Operative treatment of torticollis in early infancy seems to us to be fully justified, as it is a means of preventing the usual deformity instead of waiting until such deformity has developed and then attempting to correct it. The results of surgical correction in young infants have been so uniformly successful that we now feel operation is the treatment of choice in the more severe cases.

Kiesewetter and coworkers justified removal of the mass because "it is a sound pediatric surgical concept that all tumefactions in children should be considered malignant until proven otherwise histologically."[108] Brown and McDowell believed that the entire muscle needed to be removed because in their experience it was almost entirely composed of dense fibrous tissue, which later would almost certainly contract and produce facial asymmetry (Fig. 28–48).[84] Pineyro and coworkers did not believe that all the masses needed to be removed. They found that in a large number of their cases the mass resolved spontaneously. They reserved total resection for those older children in whom the entire muscle was fibrotic and in whom simple tenotomy alone would not be sufficient.[126] A major advantage of total excision was that there was little need for postoperative immobilization in the overcorrected position. Some authors even recommend no postoperative immobilization.[78, 84, 99, 108] One disadvantage, however, was that total resection produced

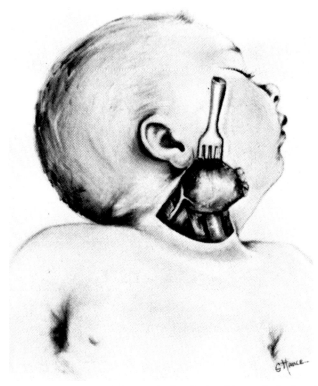

Figure 28–47. The midcervical approach allows freeing of the muscle distally and resecting it to its proximal origin. Care must be taken to preserve the underlying neurovascular structures. (Reproduced with permission from Brown JB, and McDowell F: Wry neck facial distortion prevented by resection of fibrosed sternomastoid muscle in infancy and childhood. Ann Surg 131:721–733, 1950.)

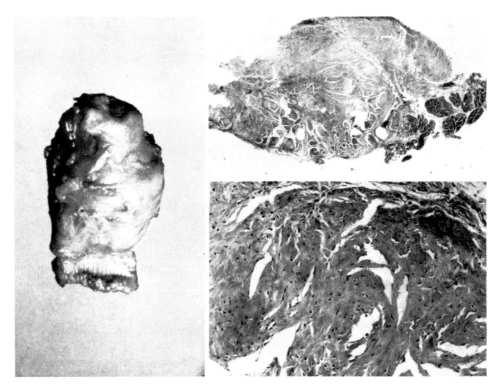

Figure 28–48. When removed early, the entire muscle grossly appears to be involved *(left)*. Low-power *(upper right)* and high-power *(lower right)* photomicrographs demonstrate almost complete replacement of the muscle bundles by fibrous tissue. (Reproduced with permission from Brown JB, and McDowell F: Wry neck facial distortion prevented by resection of fibrosed sternomastoid muscle in infancy and childhood. Ann Surg *131;*721–733, 1950.)

an absence of one side of the usual V appearance of the sternocleidomastoid columns at the base of the neck, which could have some mild cosmetic effects. None of the authors reported any weakness in cervical motion.

Myotomy

Simple myotomy followed by immobilization in the overcorrected position is the procedure preferred by the orthopedic community. This procedure is usually recommended for children over one year of age; it can produce acceptable results when performed as late as 12 years of age.[86, 104, 110, 112] The controversies regarding myotomy involve the advantages of proximal, distal, or bipolar release.

Proximal. Balkany and Mischke were the only workers who used this as their only release.[79] They found that the proximal release avoided all of the problems associated with a distal release. Postoperatively they used only halter traction for a few days, followed by a stiff cervical collar for one mouth; however, no mention was made of their results. Hellstadius and Soeur combined a proximal open release with a percutaneous distal myotomy.[97, 130] They followed this with extensive postoperative immobilization in the overcorrected position with a Minerva-type cast.

Distal. Howell in 1929 reported on the use of subcutaneous distal myotomy alone, with good results in 20 of 21 cases.[101] Soeur also had good results with the subcutaneous approach when combined with a proximal open approach.[130] He mentioned that considerable subcutaneous bleeding at the base of the neck was

sometimes a problem. Hough believed that subcutaneous myotomy was insufficient to achieve a satisfactory correction.[100] The distal myotomy is the most popular approach used.* It is usually performed open with an incision placed proximal to the clavicle.

Bipolar. Originally the bipolar approach was advocated in 1927 by Hellstadius, who performed an open mastoid release and a distal percutaneous release.[97] Twenty-three years later Soeur reported his cases using a similar approach.[130] In a more recent review, Ferkel and coworkers found that they had better results when the bipolar release was compared with a distal release alone.[93] In their long-term review of surgically treated patients, however, Canale and associates could not determine any difference between the outcomes of unipolar and bipolar releases.[86]

Postoperative Care. It is generally accepted that after myotomy some postoperative immobilization is necessary. There appears to be no consistent agreement regarding the type or length of immobilization used. Early investigators recommended aggressive immobilization with Minerva-type casts.[100, 104, 105, 130] Ippolito and colleagues believed that their good results were achieved by keeping patients in casts for at least four months.[104] More recently, the standard postoperative immobilization appears to be some type of cervical collar lined with a soft substance such as plastizote and worn for six to eight weeks.[79, 93, 110, 112, 113, 123] Another type of unusual immobilization is a tractor cap devised by Pineyro and coworkers (Fig. 28–49).[126] The most

---

*See references 77, 100, 104, 105, 110, 112, 113, 118, 123, 126.

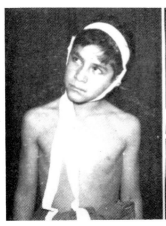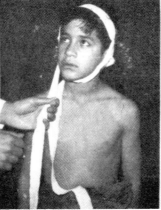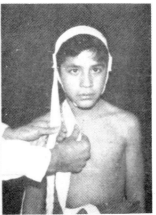

Figure 28–49. The tractor cap technique used to hold the head in the corrected position, as popularized by Pineyro. (Reproduced with permission from Pineyro JR, Yoel J, and Rocco M: Congenital torticollis. J Int Coll Surg 34:495–505, 1960.)

aggressive technique of postoperative immobilization was devised by Tse and colleagues for treatment of so-called neglected cases. They used a special rigid-head shoulder orthosis to maintain the overcorrected position (Fig. 28–50).[137] Some observers have questioned the benefit of rigid immobilization. Hagen-Torn believed it to be detrimental and recommended early faradic stimulation of the cervical muscles, followed by intensive physical therapy.[95] Macdonald used only physiotherapy postoperatively to achieve his results, which were comparable with most other series.[118]

Complications

There appear to be few if any complications associated with resection of either the mass or the total muscle. Most of the complications arise from the distal myotomy procedure; these include scar formation,

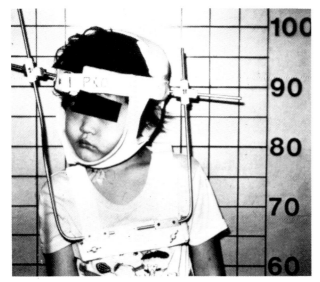

Figure 28–50. The special shoulder cervical orthosis recommended by Tse for treating neglected cases of torticollis. (Reproduced with permission from Tse P, Cheng J, Chow Y, and Leung PC: Surgery for neglected congenital torticollis. Acta Orthop Scand 58:270–272, 1987.)

tethering of the soft tissues to the skin, loss of the V column of the neck, reattachment of the clavicular head, and recurrence of the deformity.

Scar. A scar at the base of the neck is of more concern to females. If the incision is placed distal to or right over the clavicle, the scar has a tendency to hypertrophy and become unsightly. This is usually prevented by placing the incision proximal to the clavicle. A careful subcuticular closure can also decrease the prominence of the scar.

Adherence of Scar. In patients who had a myotomy performed before the age of one year, Ling noticed that the scar tended to adhere to the underlying tissues.[112] This complication was also noted to occur in some patients who were operated on at a later age (Fig. 28–51).

Loss of the Sternomastoid Column. As early as 1930 Hough noticed that when the distal portion of the sternal head was resected, there was a loss of the sternomastoid column, producing asymmetry of the neck.[100] This absence has been widely noticed by many others as well. The many reports in the literature show disagreement over whether this was cosmetically unacceptable.* Ling found that this cosmetic effect was more of a problem in those who underwent surgery in their teenage years (Fig. 28–52). It was his belief that this was the result of the more extensive surgery needed in this age group to correct the deformity.[112]

Ferkel and coworkers thought that this complication could be decreased by performing a Z-plasty lengthening of the sternomastoid portion (Fig. 28–53).[93]

Reattachment of the Lateral Bands. Persistence of a lateral band from the mastoid to the clavicle is one of the most common complications noted in the reported series.[100, 110, 112, 118, 131] In a review of the late results (average 13-year follow-up) of operative management of torticollis, Staheli noticed the development of this persistent lateral band in 85 per cent of his patients (Fig. 28–54). In 64 per cent it resulted in some loss of neck rotation.[131] Macdonald thought that these

*See references 88, 93, 104, 110, 112, 118, 131.

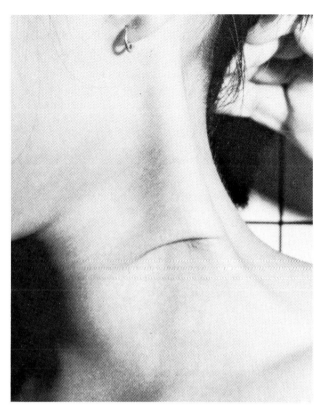

Figure 28–51. This 14-year-old, who had an open tenotomy at the age of six, demonstrates two complications: adherence of the scar and persistence of the lateral band. (Reproduced with permission from Ling CM: The influence of age on the results of open sternomastoid tenotomy in muscular torticollis. Clin Orthop *116*:142–148, 1976.)

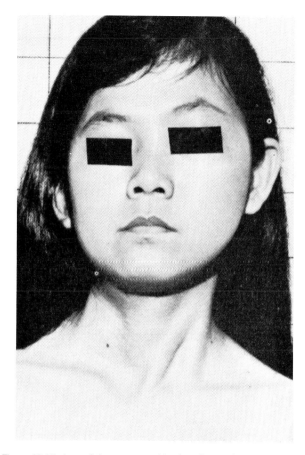

Figure 28–52. Loss of the sternomastoid column in a patient who underwent surgery at the age of 16 years. (Reproduced with permission from Ling CM: The influence of age on the results of open sternomastoid tenotomy in muscular torticollis. Clin Orthop *116*:142–148, 1976.)

bands were also responsible in part for the failure of facial asymmetry to completely resolve.[118] Jahss first noticed this complication in 1936; he believed that in many cases the clavicular portion was more prominent, often extending as a separate band from the mastoid to the midpoint of the clavicle, and did not blend with the sternal portion. He thought that the clavicular head

was the primary offending agent. These patients often had more primary head tilt than rotation; in addition, the neck base appeared wider (Fig. 28–55). Jahss found that in these patients a simple myotomy alone produced a very high recurrence of reattachment of the clavicular

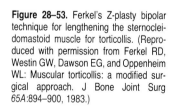

Figure 28–53. Ferkel's Z-plasty bipolar technique for lengthening the sternocleidomastoid muscle for torticollis. (Reproduced with permission from Ferkel RD, Westin GW, Dawson EG, and Oppenheim WL: Muscular torticollis: a modified surgical approach. J Bone Joint Surg *65A*:894–900, 1983.)

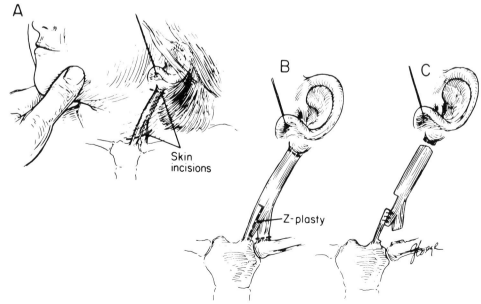

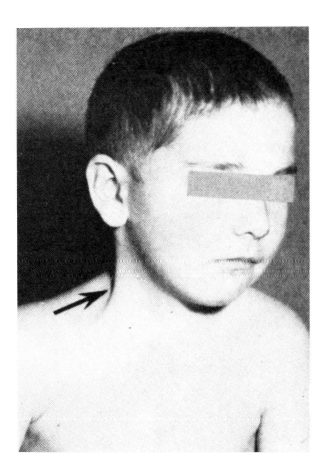

Figure 28–54. Persistence of the lateral band *(arrow)* extending from the mastoid to the clavicle. (Reproduced with permission from Staheli LT: Muscular torticollis: late results of operative treatment. Surgery *69*:469–473, 1971.)

Figure 28–55. The clavicular type of torticollis as described by Jahss, in which the clavicular head is the primary offending agent, produces a widening of the base of the neck. (Reproduced with permission from Jahss SA: Torticollis. J Bone Joint Surg *18*:1065–1068, 1936.)

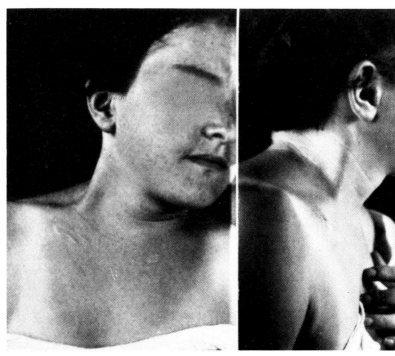

portion with a resultant lateral band. He devised a procedure in which the clavicular head was detached distally and transferred to the undersurface of the sternal head within the fascial compartment. This appeared to eliminate the recurrence of the lateral band. The sternal head was tenotomized only if it was tight and was thought to be a deforming force.[105]

Recurrence of Deformity. Only three of the major series mention any recurrence of the deformities.[93, 112, 131] There was a total of 12 recurrences in 96 cases for a rate of 13 per cent. In all of these patients, function and appearance were improved with second procedures. Two of these authors thought that lack of proper immobilization contributed to recurrence.[93, 131] The other contributing factor appeared to be the persistence of the lateral bands.

Results

The best results for myotomy consistently appear to be in the one- to four-year age group; 60 to 70 per cent of these patients can be expected to achieve good to excellent results.[104, 112, 137] Ippolito and colleagues and Tse believed that this boundary could be extended to six years with equally good results.[104, 137] From five to 11 years, only slightly more than one-third of patients can be expected to achieve the same results. All authors agreed that after the age of 12, none of the patients could be expected to achieve good or excellent results.[104, 110, 112, 137]

Facial Asymmetry

Facial asymmetry seems to be related to the severity of the deformity. Only Ling reported complete resolution of facial asymmetry in his patients who had the release before the age of five years.[112] Staheli, however, in a longer follow-up study, found no difference in loss of facial asymmetry between those done early and those done later.[131] It appears that there is some remodeling of the asymmetry up to the age of 12; after that, very little remodeling can be expected. As stated previously, Macdonald thought that the persistence of the lateral bands appeared to contribute to the lack of resolution of facial asymmetry.[118] If severe facial asymmetry persists, plastic reconstruction of the orbit and mandible may be required.[99, 107]

Author's Preferred Method of Treatment

The Infant

In treating infants one must take into consideration the natural course of sternomastoid tumors. In the series in which aggressive stretching was carried out, 70 to 80 per cent of cases had a successful outcome.[90, 102, 112] It must also be remembered that those cases in which no early treatment is performed probably have an equal rate of success.[86, 90] Thus, one question is whether the success rate of early stretching is dependent on the stretching itself or on the natural course of the disappearance of most tumors. Despite this uncertainty, I think it is important to start an aggressive stretching program when the infant is first seen. I qualify this for infants under the age of six months. I usually have the parents stretch the involved sternomastoid muscle vigorously three or four times a day. It requires two people to stretch the sternocleidomastoid properly. One person holds the child in his or her lap with the head between the knees; this individual stabilizes both shoulders while the other person does the stretching. The sternocleidomastoid is stretched by turning the face toward the shortened side in a slow, gentle manner. The stretching maneuver is performed about 10 times at each session. *It must be emphasized that radiographs must be taken of the cervical spine before beginning the stretching process to ensure that there are no skeletal anomalies.* This must be done even if an obvious sternocleidomastoid tumor is present.

Other mechanisms can be utilized to stimulate those active motions of the cervical spine that stretch the sternocleidomastoid. The bed can be turned so that the infant is forced to turn his or her head in the direction of major activities and, in doing so, actively stretch the sternocleidomastoid. Other games can be played by dangling objects to one side and encouraging the child to actively stretch the involved sternocleidomastoid.

From a practical standpoint I have found that it is difficult to do any effective stretching after about six months of age. By this time the infant is sufficiently large that he or she usually puts up too much resistance. Certainly, after one year stretching is both practically impossible to perform and ineffective.

The Older Child

In the older child with a fixed deformity I prefer to perform a distal myotomy. Three elements must be considered in performing the myotomy. First, the incision must be at least 2 cm cephalad to the clavicle to decrease the chance that it will spread and become unsightly. It also needs to be closed with a meticulous subcuticular closure. Second, the sternal portion should be lengthened by Z-plasty if possible, rather than by a transverse myotomy or distal resection, to try to preserve the contour of the sternomastoid column. Third, if the clavicular portion is prominent it must be transferred under the distal sternal portion to prevent the recurrence of the lateral bands.

Postoperatively I utilize cervical traction for four to six days, followed by a plastizote-lined hard cervical collar for another six to eight weeks. This is coupled with an aggressive program of physical therapy designed to encourage active motion, which strengthens the opposite sternocleidomastoid muscles and continues to stretch the involved side to prevent recurrence.

The Shoulder in Arthrogryposis

PATHOLOGY

The term *arthrogryposis* was introduced in 1923 by Stern in his classic article.[146] It comes from two Greek words that mean "curved joint." Rather than a distinct disease process, it represents a syndrome caused by the failure of muscle development during the early intrauterine period.[145] The syndrome seems to represent two forms, one neurogenic and the other myopathic. Most authors, however, consider the myopathic form a type of congenital muscular dystrophy.[142, 145, 148] Biopsy specimens of the spinal cords of infants who have died with arthrogryposis have revealed a marked decrease or even absence of the anterior horn cells in the major motor center of the cord. There is also an absence of any inflammatory reaction in these areas.[142, 144] For a more complete discussion of the pathology and etiology of arthrogryposis, the reader is referred to the major review articles on this subject.[142, 145, 148]

The pattern of involvement varies considerably. In most patients (46 per cent) all four limbs are involved. However, in some individuals (11 per cent) only the upper extremities are affected and in others (43 per cent) only the lower extremities.[147] Rarely only one upper or lower extremity is involved. As a rule the involvement is symmetrical and bilateral. One rare type of arthrogryposis involves only the distal portion of the upper and lower extremities, with relative sparing of the shoulder. This appears to have an autosomal dominant pattern of inheritance.[143] In the upper extremities the characteristic picture consists of internal rotation of the shoulders, extension contractures of the elbows, and flexion contractures of the wrists and fingers (Fig. 28–56).

TREATMENT

Goals

The upper extremity must be considered as a whole in mapping out a treatment plan. In addition, the function of the lower extremities must be taken into consideration. For example, if the patient requires the aid of a walker or crutches to walk, elbow extension power must be maintained. In general, the lower extremities need to be placed in a position that allows ambulation, i.e., knee and hip extension and plantigrade feet. The upper extremities must be able to perform two important functions—feeding and toileting.[149] Thus, one hand must be able to reach the mouth while the other palm must be able to reach the perineum. The ability to oppose the hands must also be retained.[142] It is best to wait until the patient is independently ambulatory before considering surgery on the upper extremities. Delay often allows the physician and the therapist to better evaluate the overall function of the extremity.[142] Often a very contracted extremity may function quite well owing to trick maneuvers the

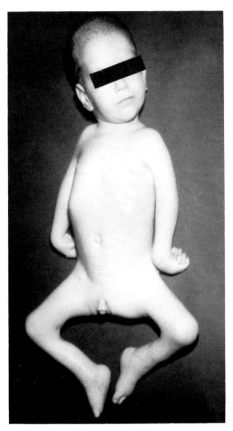

Figure 28–56. A photograph of a young child with arthrogryposis involving all four extremities. The upper extremities demonstrate the typical internal rotation of the shoulders, extension of the elbows, and flexion of the wrists and fingers.

patient has developed. One needs to consider if correcting the deformities will actually improve the function or only improve the appearance. In general, the shoulder and elbow should be considered as a unit. There must be enough external rotation at the shoulder so that the hand can be brought to the mouth rather than the opposite shoulder.

With the shoulders internally rotated, the flexed wrists and hands may face each other by crossing over. This may appear awkward but it does provide some useful function for grasping objects. If shoulder abduction is stronger than shoulder adduction, this crossover grip should be maintained.[148, 149] Externally rotating the shoulders may eliminate this ability to cross-grasp objects and can require secondary procedures to extend the wrists. By the same token, if the wrists are markedly flexed and the shoulders are internally rotated, the dorsum of the hand faces the perineum. Externally rotating the shoulders may allow the palm to be directed toward the perineum, which may improve function. In summary, before undertaking surgery in any one joint of the upper extremities, one must obtain a very thorough occupational therapy evaluation and map out the ultimate functional goals for the patient.

Nonoperative Management

The shoulder rarely responds to an exercise and stretching program.[148, 149] This is probably because there is usually only very little muscle functioning about the shoulder. Often the patient uses substitute motions to make up for absent actions. For example, some abduction may be achieved by laterally bending the spine to the opposite side. Active use of what muscles are present should be encouraged through the use of games and play activities. Repetitive exercises are usually not effective in young children because of their limited attention span.

Special adaptive equipment such as long-handled spoons, special plates, and assistive feeding devices may help the patient perform some activities of daily living. Special adaptations can be made for clothing, as well, to allow the patient to be as independent as possible.

By and large, there are certain limits to the effectiveness of nonoperative treatment. In most instances surgical procedures must be considered.

Operative Management

Although the shoulder is almost always involved to one degree or another in patients with arthrogryposis, surgical procedures on the shoulder are rarely performed. In Bennett and coworkers' series of 25 patients requiring upper extremity procedures, only two required procedures on the shoulder.[141] Adduction con-

tracture is rarely a major problem. There is often enough abduction to allow for hygiene. The primary goal with the shoulder is to allow enough external rotation so that the hand can get to the mouth rather than to the opposite shoulder.

Tenotomy of the pectoralis major and subscapularis tendons has not proved to be effective in the shoulder in these patients.[142] Lloyd-Roberts and Lettin have popularized the use of the humeral osteotomy. The osteotomy can be performed at any location, but it must be stabilized internally with a plate and supported externally in a shoulder spica cast. Use of a simple sling postoperatively tends to perpetuate the internal rotational deformity.[145] Drummond and associates combine the osteotomy with a concomitant division of the subscapularis muscle.[142] This proximal humeral osteotomy seems to be the procedure preferred by most authors reporting on treatment in large series.[141, 142, 145, 149] In planning the incision, it must be remembered that with the extremity internally rotated the radial nerve is more anterior.

Author's Preferred Method of Treatment

It has been my experience that surgery around the shoulder is rarely needed in dealing with the upper extremity in arthrogryposis. More attention is directed

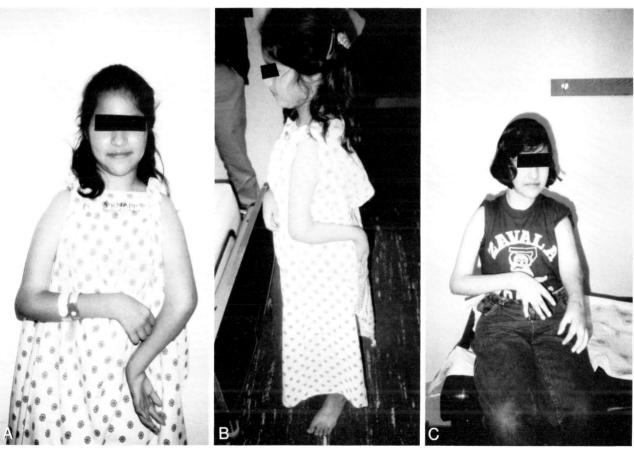

Figure 28–57. *A*, A preoperative view of a young teenager who has upper arthrogryposis primarily involving the upper extremities. The severe internal rotation of the shoulder limits the ability of the hand to reach the face. *B*, Photograph demonstrating the extreme internal rotation of the left upper extremity. *C*, Postoperative view after humeral derotation osteotomy and wrist fusion. The hand can now be brought to a much more functional position.

toward establishing elbow flexion and wrist and finger extension. The criterion I use is whether the patient has so much internal rotation that he or she cannot bring the hand to the mouth (Fig. 28–57).

I perform a simple derotational osteotomy using an anterolateral approach. The osteotomy is usually done at the junction of the middle and proximal thirds. A small plate is used for fixation. Because of the natural tendency of the arm to derotate internally, I usually hold the extremity in a shoulder spica cast postoperatively in as much abduction as possible and with external rotation to at least 75 degrees. One must be careful not to over-rotate the distal fragment. The patient must have at least 30 degrees of internal rotation postoperatively.

Bone and Joint Infections

OSTEOMYELITIS

This discussion will be limited to the acute hematogenous forms of osteomyelitis (AHO) as they occur in the proximal humerus, clavicle, and scapula. This is the area of greatest diagnostic challenge. The contiguous forms resulting from open fractures or surgical procedures are extremely rare in children. In the contiguous types the diagnosis is obvious as a result of the original insult to the bone.

Incidence

With the development of antibiotics it was believed that AHO would disappear as a disease. From 1944 to 1950, an initial happy era, there was a marked decrease in the incidence of AHO; after 1950 this came to an end, however, with a return to the original incidence and the development of antibiotic-resistant organisms.[174] In a more recent study, Vu Quoc and colleagues found that there had been no significant change in the number of cases from 1960 to 1975.[215]

The occurrence of AHO in the shoulder region appears to be reasonably infrequent. In general, the incidence in the lower extremities is six times that of the upper extremities.[174] The best figures for the incidence around the shoulder come from the southern continents. In Australia, Gilmour reviewed 328 cases and found three (less than 1 per cent) occurring in the clavicle, two (less than 1 per cent) occurring in the scapula, and twelve (3 per cent) occurring in the proximal humerus, for a total of a little over 4 per cent occurring around the shoulder.[174] In New Zealand Gillespie and Mayo reviewed 661 cases.[177] Twenty-seven (4 per cent) occurred in the proximal humerus; no mention was made of the occurrence in the clavicle or scapula. Thus it appears that there is a consistent incidence of AHO in the shoulder region in children of less than 5 per cent.

During the ages of skeletal growth there appears to

be no peak age group for the development of AHO.[196] Most large series show a male preponderance.[174, 193, 194, 197, 201, 215] Other series, however, have demonstrated an almost equal male-to-female incidence.[196, 198] The increased incidence in males is thought to be indirect evidence that trauma is a factor in the etiology of AHO.

The mortality rate from AHO has shown a dramatic decrease in the antibiotic era. The most impressive statistics in this regard have been compiled by McHenry in his review of many series totaling 1865 patients.[193] In the preantibiotic era the mortality averaged 20 to 25 per cent; in the postantibiotic era it has decreased to about 1 per cent. The morbidity rate, i.e., recurrences and chronic growth problems, still averages 20 per cent in most series.[155, 176, 177, 194, 218]

Organisms

Staphylococcus aureus is still the predominant organism, ranging from 60 to 95 per cent in the reported series.* McHenry's review of the pre- and postantibiotic eras showed no significant change in the predominance of *Staphylococcus*.[193] *Streptococcus* is the next most common organism, with rates ranging from 5 to 20 per cent depending on the number of infants in the report. In neonates, Group B streptococcus is now the most common organism.[167, 170, 171] Less than 5 per cent of the cases involve gram-negative organisms, with *Haemophilus influenzae* being predominant.[192, 215]

Pathogenesis

The pathogenesis of AHO is well described in the standard textbooks of pediatric orthopedics.[156, 213] Three factors appear to play a part in the development of AHO in the areas of endochondral ossification.

1. Local hemodynamics. The metaphyseal arterioles, which have a relatively high flow rate, abruptly join the venous sinusoids bathing the physis. This area of slow flow allows the blood to sludge. In addition, after one year of age there are no anastomoses through the physeal plate. The capillaries of the metaphysis are inelastic and tortuous, creating easy blockage for the microscopic septic emboli.[158]

2. Altered local resistance in the area of the physis. There are very few phagocytic cells in the metaphyseal sinusoids.

3. Trauma, which appears to play some role in the production of decreased local resistance. In many cases there is a history of trauma. The increased incidence of AHO in males is felt to be indirect evidence of the traumatic factor. Studies in laboratory animals have demonstrated an increased susceptibility to infection when the bone was traumatized prior to infection of bacteria.[216]

Once the infection is established in the bone, the intramedullary pressure increases with thrombosis of

---

*See references 155, 177, 192, 196, 197, 215, 218.

the medullary vessels. This increased pressure by itself can produce necrosis of the bone. Some of the thrombosis within the vessels is also a result of the coagulative enzymes produced by *Staphylococcus*. Once the pressure builds up in the medullary cavity, it seeks release; the metaphysis provides avenues of escape because of its relatively thin cortex, penetrating metaphyseal vessels, and poorly adherent periosteum. As the infection progresses, the purulent material escapes the metaphyseal cortex to elevate the periosteum. This elevation of the periosteum stimulates new bone to produce a proliferative involucrum. The dead bone within the metaphysis remains as a sequestrum.

The key to management of osteomyelitis lies in early recognition and aggressive treatment before there is much development of dead bone or sequestrum. The presence of this sequestrum leads to chronic recurrences.

Specific Sites

Proximal Humerus

The proximal humerus represents the classic picture of AHO in the typical long bone. The infection originates in the juxtaphyseal metaphysis. Because this area is within the articular capsule, when the purulent material escapes from the intramedullary cavity it often penetrates the thin periosteum to enter the glenohumeral joint.

Diagnosis. The clinical picture is still the most important factor in making the diagnosis. The changes occur in the deep soft tissues rather than the superficial tissues; as a result there are few external signs. Rarely is there any superficial erythema unless the primary organism is a streptococcus. At the onset the patient usually demonstrates the characteristic bone pain, i.e., percussion anywhere along the humerus produces pain in the proximal metaphysis. There is a reluctance to move the shoulder. Early in the course there may be a mild sympathetic effusion in the glenohumeral joint; later there may be a true purulent effusion due to breakthrough from the metaphysis. The patient is restless owing to marked pain produced by the increased intraosseous pressure. The patient finds it difficult to relieve this pain by changing positions. In addition, the usual characteristic spiking elevation of the temperature is seen. The patient also appears sick and toxic because of the secondary septicemia.

Early the radiographs demonstrate only deep soft tissue changes. Capitanio and Kirkpatrick have divided the radiographic changes into three stages.[161] Stage I represents deep soft tissue swelling next to the metaphysis. This occurs during the first 72 hours when the infection is still intraosseous. The swelling at this stage is simple periosteal edema. In Stage II there is swelling of the muscles and obliteration of the deep soft tissue planes. This often occurs three to seven days into the infection and represents the presence of purulent material under the periosteum. Stage III presents the classic picture of involucrum and sequestrum, indicating bone death. These signs can occur as early as 10 to 14 days. The diagnosis should be made before this stage.

The advent of radionuclide scans originally was believed to be the answer in making the early diagnosis of AHO. Various nuclides have been used. Technetium diphosphanate (Tc 99m) concentrates primarily in the cement lines at the junctions of the osteoid and mineralized bone.[184, 195] Initially Tc 99m was reported to be highly reliable in localizing AHO.[167, 174, 190, 214] Using an early blood pooling scan, it was helpful also in differentiating AHO from cellulitis.[173] In recent years, however, it has been shown to be less reliable. False-negative results have been reported to occur in as many as 20 to 30 per cent of cases.[153, 186, 211, 212] In addition, it has been shown that Tc 99m scans are not reliable in neonates.[151] Because it requires the production of new osseous material, Tc 99m uptake is delayed until new bone production has ensued; this often means that the infection must be active for three to four days before the scan becomes positive. Thus it may not be helpful in making a very early diagnosis, when treatment is most effective.

Another nuclide, 67 gallium citrate, is taken up by the lysosomes of the leukocytes.[164] Thus these scans may be positive very early in the infection. However, the maximum concentration of gallium may not develop in the focus of infection for at least 48 to 72 hours after the infection. Other disadvantages of gallium are the higher cost and increased radiation exposure.

The accuracy of an early diagnosis may be enhanced by sequential scans. If the technetium scan is negative at four hours it may immediately be followed with the gallium; alternatively, the technetium scan can be repeated in two to three hours.

Another technique involves labeling the patient's leukocytes with radioactive indium.[195] However, this requires much preparation and sophisticated laboratory facilities, and its accuracy is still unproven.

The use of CT is only of limited benefit.[188] The changes with AHO are very nonspecific. There may be increased density in the intramedullary tissue. The major use of CT is to better define the soft tissue planes.

The best diagnostic procedure is actual needle aspiration of the bone. If purulent material is obtained from the subperiosteal plane, surgical evacuation is needed. If there is no infection outside the bone, the needle can then be driven through the thin metaphyseal bone, with cultures being obtained directly from the marrow. In most children this requires anesthesia. Aspiration of the bone alone does not appear to have any effect on the accuracy of a radionuclide scan that may need to be obtained later.[160]

Treatment. There appear to be fewer indications for surgical intervention with present-day treatment modalities. The key to success is to make an early diagnosis while the infection is still within the confines of the cortex. At this stage the infection often responds to antibiotic therapy alone. Major indications for surgical drainage are either the initial finding of purulent material outside the cortex under the periosteum or failure of the patient to respond promptly to intravenous antibiotics.

The initial antibiotics of choice are those effective against coagulase-positive staphylococcus. In the pediatric age group nafcillin is the least toxic semisynthetic penicillin. It should be given at the maximum allowable dose. The cephalosporins have a broader spectrum but are more expensive. Usually the first-generation cephalosporins are more effective against coagulase-positive staphylococcus. In patients highly allergic to penicillin, clindamycin can be given. It produces excellent bone and joint concentrations. Enterocolitis is reported to be a rare complication in children who are given this drug.[168] The choice of antibiotic may change once the cultures have grown and sensitivities have been obtained.

Antibiotic therapy is given initially intravenously until the patient shows an adequate response, i.e., the temperature remains normal for at least 24 to 36 hours. Once this is achieved, adequate blood levels can usually be accomplished with very high levels of oral antibiotics. The recommended drugs are dicloxacillin, 100 mg/kg/day;[157] cefaclor, 150 mg/kg/day;[203] or cephalexin, 100 mg/kg/day.[203] When the original cultures are obtained, it is important that the laboratory be asked to save them so that serumcidal levels can be performed later when the patient is changed over to oral antibiotics. Serumcidal levels of at least 1:8 should be obtained for oral antibiotics to be effective. The sedimentation rate and clinical recovery are the best determinants of how long oral antibiotics should be given. The sedimentation rate should be at least 20 mm/hour or less before the antibiotics are discontinued.

Author's Preferred Method of Treatment. In treating osteomyelitis of the proximal humerus, my decision regarding surgical versus medical management is based on the needle aspirate. Usually the localization of the lesion within the proximal humerus is obvious on clinical grounds alone, and thus there is little need to use radionuclide scans. If the clinical picture is suspicious for acute osteomyelitis of the proximal humerus, I usually aspirate both the glenohumeral joint and proximal humerus with a large-bore needle (18-gauge or larger). In most children this requires general anesthesia. I aspirate the joint first to see if there is any purulent material and then follow with aspiration of the metaphysis. Around the metaphysis, extraosseous tissues are aspirated first. If there is purulent material outside the bone, I usually drain it with an anterior deltopectoral approach. If no purulent material is found outside the bone, I advance the needle through the metaphysis and obtain marrow specimens for cultures. Once these cultures are obtained, I start the patient on very high doses of a first-generation cephalosporin. If a rapid drop in the overall temperature does not occur after 36 to 48 hours of antibiotics, I

reassess the need to either reaspirate or simply drain the bone surgically. Once the temperature remains normal for at least 24 to 36 hours, I usually convert the patient to oral antibiotics. I prefer cefaclor because it is better accepted by the patient, but it is also very expensive. A dosage of 150 mg/kg/day in four doses is used. The less expensive dicloxacillin is equally effective but may not be taken as readily by the patient. I monitor the serumcidal levels to try to obtain at least a 1:8 inhibition. One advantage of dicloxacillin is that the serum levels of this drug can be enhanced by giving probenecid to decrease its excretion by the kidney. The decision to discontinue oral antibiotics is dependent on numerous factors, such as the clinical response, the amount of necrotic or affected bone on the radiographs, and the initial stage of the disease at the onset of treatment. I usually wait until the sedimentation rate is less than 20 mm/hour before considering discontinuation of the antibiotic.

Unusual Organisms. *Streptococcus* is the second most common organism. Its occurrence in the neonate will be discussed later in this chapter. It can occur in the older child as well. Usually there is less purulent reaction and more edema with *Streptococcus* because of the presence of spreading rather than coagulative enzymes. *Streptococcus* usually produces considerable edema in the periosteal adjacent soft tissues. In some cases the skin may be superficially erythematous, with an almost cellulitic appearance. If the periosteum is elevated, it usually contains more of serosanguineous fluid than the thick, purulent material seen with *Staphylococcus*. *Haemophilus influenzae* is only rarely found; it usually also presents with an erythematous soft tissue reaction as well. It is rare to see this organism as a cause of osteomyelitis after the age of four years. *Pneumococcus*, which is also rare, usually presents with a very thick, purulent exudate. If the patient is from the southwest United States, a fungal etiology such as coccidioidomycosis, blastomycosis, or actinomycosis should be suspected, especially if the disease is chronic and there is no response to the usual antibiotics (Fig. 28–58). The best discussions for these unusual fungal and granulomatous infections can be found in the articles by Curtiss[163] and Pritchard[208] and the textbook by Jaffe.[185]

Complications. The most common complication, which fortunately is treatable, is a recurrence. Usually this can be adequately treated with wide surgical debridement of all the necrotic bone. In some cases the use of hyperbaric oxygen may facilitate the healing process postoperatively. Some of the other complications are more difficult to manage. A serious complication is physeal arrest with both angular deformity and shortening of the proximal humerus (Fig. 28–59). Attempts at osseous bridge resection usually are unsuccessful because the remaining physeal cartilage is inadequate to recover and grow.

Another complication is loss of metaphyseal and diaphyseal bone with fracture and chronic nonunion. This usually occurs when the purulent material lies

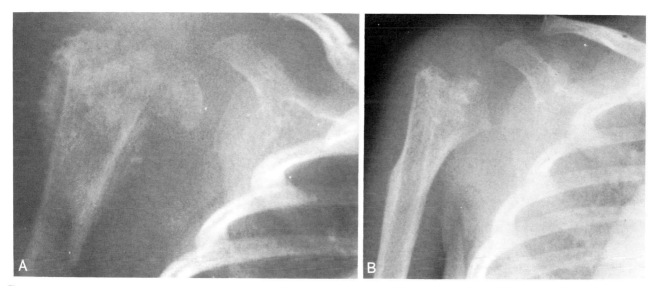

Figure 28–58. A, Radiograph demonstrates considerable involucrum with epiphysiolysis of the proximal humerus in an 18-month-old American Indian infant. The patient had had shoulder pain with minimal systemic signs for at least three months. Open biopsy and culture revealed the organism to be coccidioidomycosis. B, Appearance four months later after appropriate treatment.

under periosteum for a protracted period of time before drainage and the patient's periosteal tissues are destroyed. This eliminates the osteogenic potential for repair, with the resultant persistent defect in the proximal humerus. A pseudarthrosis may develop at the site of the bony defect (Fig. 28–60).

In addition to loss of the metaphyseal or diaphyseal bone, vascular injury can occur to the humeral head. This is more common in neonates and infants but can

occur in the older child as well. It was originally thought that the increased intra-articular pressure within the joint during a septic effusion compresses the epiphyseal vessels on the surface of the bone and renders the head ischemic. This is certainly true in the hip with the blood supply to the femoral head. The shoulder, however, has a less constrictive capsule and thus tolerates a relatively larger effusion than the hip joint without an elevation of the intra-articular pres-

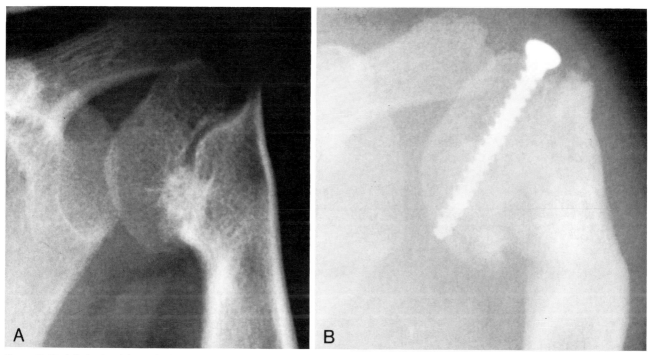

Figure 28–59. A, Deformity of the proximal humerus following an episode of acute hematogenous osteomyelitis in early childhood. B, Although only 30 per cent of the physis was replaced with an osseous bridge, it failed to regrow when the bridge was resected and replaced with Silastic elastomer.

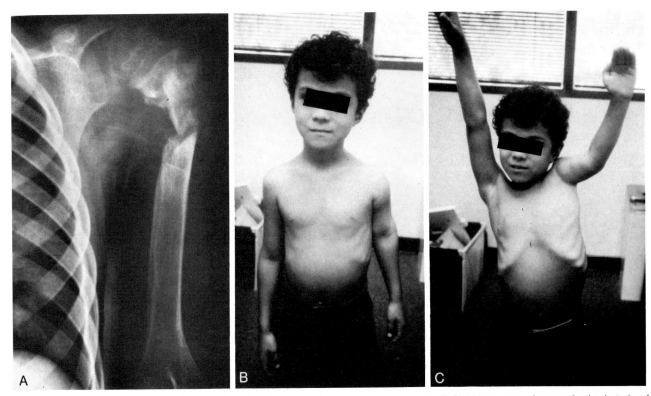

Figure 28–60. A, Nonunion of the proximal left humerus due to bone loss from acute hematogenous osteomyelitis. B, Clinical appearance demonstrating the shortening of the left humerus. C, Despite the nonunion, the patient demonstrated reasonably good ability to abduct and flex the involved shoulder.

sure. It has recently been postulated that compression of the epiphyseal arteries can occur in the inflamed synovium without a significant effusion.[204]

Clavicle

Because of its rarity, osteomyelitis of the clavicle often goes unrecognized initially. In children the incidence ranges from 1 to 3 per cent in selected series.[180, 197, 217] It may occur either as an isolated lesion or as one of multiple sites (Fig. 28–61). Owing to its rarity it often is initially suspected to be a primary neoplasm, with Ewing's sarcoma high on the list.[199] The physis of the clavicle is located medially, making this area more likely to be involved. It has been shown to occur in the midshaft as well.[198] All age groups have been involved; the condition in neonates is more likely to be due to a streptococcus.[189, 198] The diagnosis is made by a combination of local tenderness and the radiographic presence of lysis with or without periosteal new bone formation (usually involving the medial end). A bone scan may be especially helpful in questionable cases.

Treatment consists of aggressive antibiotic management. Again, if purulent material is suspected to be present outside the bone and there is a poor response to medical management, surgical drainage is necessary.[189] In chronic cases the involved portion can be resected without any loss of function and with the expectation of a complete regeneration of the resected area.[198, 199]

Scapula

Osteomyelitis of the scapula is extremely rare; I could not find any isolated cases reported in the literature. Gilmour reported two cases as part of his large series.[174] In the past 15 years I have had only one case, a young girl who had multifocal sites of osteomyelitis as part of a generalized septic process. It appears that the same principles apply to the treatment in this bone as to the clavicle, which is also a flat bone. Most cases can probably be treated medically, but surgical drainage may be necessary if there is accumulation of purulent material.

Neonatal Osteomyelitis

Pathogenesis

Over 50 years ago Green and Shannon noted that osteomyelitis in neonates and infants was a different disease.[180] The fragile bony architecture of neonates is more rapidly and easily injured by the infectious process. In addition, at this age the metaphyseal vessels cross the physeal plate; thus, any infection that settles on the metaphyseal side can travel across to the epiphyseal side and injure the growing cells directly. On the plus side, the rate of repair and osteogenic potential are high in this age group, so recovery is rapid and recurrence is rare. On the minus side, since the epiphyseal side of the physis can be involved with the infection, permanent growth arrest can occur.[206]

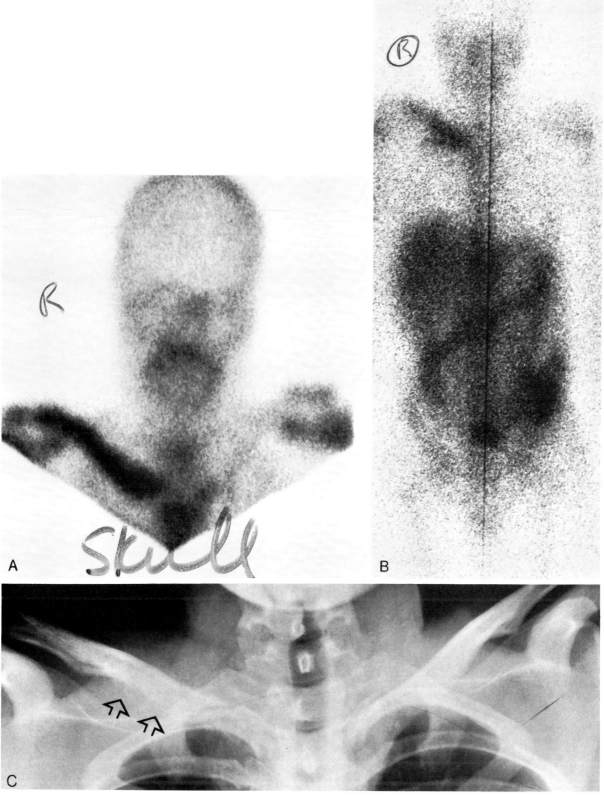

Figure 28–61. A 15-year-old male was suspected initially to have Ewing's sarcoma because of a large mass involving the ileum. *A,* Routine technetium bone scan revealed increased uptake in the area of the right clavicle. *B,* Gallium scan also demonstrated uptake in both the right clavicle and ileum. *C,* Routine radiographs of the chest demonstrated a lytic area in the midshaft of the clavicle *(arrows).* An open biopsy of the clavicle produced tissue consistent with chronic *Staphylococcus* osteomyelitis.

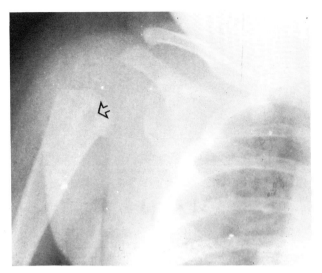

Figure 28–62. The proximal humerus is the typical location for acute hematogenous osteomyelitis due to Group B beta-hemolytic streptococcus in a neonate. Although the lesion (arrows) is in this infant's right humerus, the left is more commonly involved. This infant was treated medically and had a complete recovery.

Finally, the organisms are also different. There is a much higher incidence of *Streptococcus*. In recent years, Group B beta-hemolytic streptococcus has become more predominant.[152, 167, 170] This organism is usually picked up by the infant from the mother's vagina during delivery. It is often a part of a generalized neonatal sepsis.

In streptococcal infections, the proximal humerus, —especially the left one—is most susceptible to localization of the infection (Fig. 28–62). It is theorized that this is because the left shoulder is more likely to be traumatized during delivery. Often the radiographic findings do not become manifest until the medical treatment has been completed. The clinical symptoms associated with these infections are usually minimal.

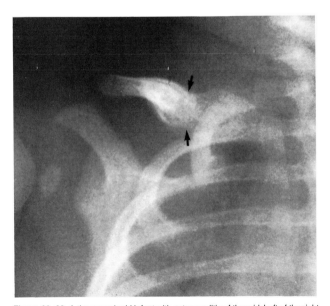

Figure 28–63. A three-week-old infant with osteomyelitis of the midshaft of the right clavicle (arrows). The organism was a Group B beta-hemolytic streptococcus.

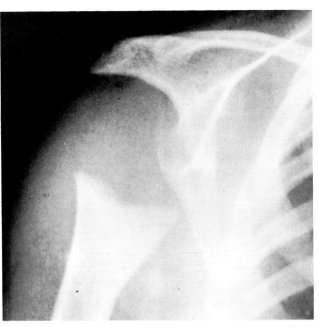

Figure 28–64. Permanent destruction of the proximal humeral physis and epiphysis from staphylococcal osteomyelitis in infancy.

Because there is very little purulent exudate, the incidence of long-term growth arrest appears to be lowered. This organism can involve the clavicle as well (Fig. 28–63).

The other organism seen in this age group is *Staphylococcus*. It is more commonly seen in premature infants or other infants who have altered general resistance. The entrance for this organism is usually through some type of manipulative process, such as the use of an umbilical or indwelling venous catheter. Because it produces a thick, purulent exudate that contains many proteolytic enzymes, destruction of bone is often more extensive. The incidence of growth deformities following this type of infection is much greater (Fig. 28–64).

One condition that may be confused with neonatal osteomyelitis is infantile cortical hyperostosis (Caffey's disease). This usually is manifested by hyperirritability, soft tissue swelling, and cortical hyperostosis of the mandible, clavicles, ribs, skull, scapula, and long bones. It is usually a self-limiting process. Most of the radiographic changes are centered in the diaphysis rather than the metaphysis.[159] One case report exists of an infant with this disorder who also had concurrent osteomyelitis in the same humerus.[158]

SEPTIC ARTHRITIS

Glenohumeral Joint

Incidence

Three-fourths of the cases of septic arthritis in children involve the weight-bearing joints of the lower extremities. In a review of five series involving septic arthritis in children[162, 175, 182, 191, 203] totaling 400 cases, only 21 (5 per cent) involved the glenohumeral joint. As mentioned earlier, osteomyelitis of the humerus may present primarily as a glenohumeral joint infection. In one series of nine shoulders with septic arthritis, five were identified as having concurrent humeral osteomyelitis.[210]

Organisms

In the past, *Staphylococcus* has been considered the primary organism for septic arthritis in children. This remains true for children over the age of three. In the past 20 years, however, an increased predominance of *Haemophilus influenzae* as the major organism in children from 7 to 36 months has been recognized.[150, 191] As in osteomyelitis, there is a preponderance of streptococcal infections in small infants. In one large series from the United States of granulomatous joint infections, especially tuberculosis, no cases were reported in the pediatric age group.[187] These organisms seem to affect the joints of older individuals who have systemic disease. In neonates who have been on long-term antibiotic therapy for other septic processes, arthritis due to the fungus *Candida albicans* may occur.[207] Gonococcal arthritis must also be kept in mind in treating neonates and older children who are likely to have had sexual exposure. Fink reported two cases, one involving the shoulder in a four-year-old girl and the other a seven-year-old boy.[169] In these instances there was an antecedent polyarthritis that migrated before settling in the shoulder. In the female patient, positive cultures were also obtained from the vagina.

Diagnosis

In the older child the diagnosis is usually obvious. Clinically there is local tenderness, warmth, and swelling involving the glenohumeral joint. Any attempt to rotate the shoulder produces severe pain. Radiographically, in the early stages there is only soft tissue swelling, with some widening of the joint if a significant effusion is also present. The key to making the diagnosis rests on aspiration of the joint. If arthrocentesis of the joint produces a purulent fluid, it must be analyzed to see if it meets the criteria for being the product of an infectious agent. Infectious agents usually produce cell counts of at least 50,000 white blood cells (WBC)/mm^3.[181] Certainly, counts above 100,000 WBC/mm^3 should be considered septic. Other keys to the diagnosis include the differential and joint fluid–serum glucose ratios. In septic arthritis, at least 95 per cent of the WBCs will be polymorphonuclear. The normal fluid–serum glucose ratio is between 60 and 70 per cent; if the fluid is produced by an infectious process, the metabolic activity of the leukocytes will cause this ratio to fall to at least 40 per cent or lower.[181] Cultures and smears can also provide valuable assistance in making the diagnosis. Unfortunately, in only about 75 per cent of the cases are the cultures positive. This is thought to be due to the fact that pyogenic joint fluid has natural inhibitors that prevent the growth of the bacteria on culture media. The rate of bacterial growth can be increased by diluting the purulent fluid in blood culture bottles, thereby decreasing the concentration of these natural inhibitors. Griffin recommends that if the WBC count is greater than 50,000/mm^3 with at least 95 per cent of them being polymorphonuclear and the joint fluid–glucose ratio is less than 40 per cent, the patient should be started on the appropriate antibiotic therapy.[181]

Blood cultures have been shown to increase the rate of recovery of organisms in those patients in the age group in which *Haemophilus influenzae* is most common.[191] Because of the relatively high number of negative joint cultures, blood cultures probably should be drawn in all patients who have suspected septic arthritis, especially if they are febrile.

Treatment

Two major decisions must be made in determining the proper treatment of a child with a septic shoulder: (1) the choice of the proper antibiotic and (2) whether to treat the joint with multiple aspirations or incision and drainage.

The initial antibiotic often must be selected before the identity and sensitivities of the organisms are known; thus, the choice is usually based on the most common organism seen in the patient's age group. It must be remembered that *Staphylococcus*, although not always the most common, can be seen in all age groups.

In very small infants who have had a seemingly normal delivery, *Streptococcus* is probably the more common organism. A semisynthetic penicillin such as nafcillin is probably the drug of choice since it provides coverage against both *Streptococcus* and *Staphylococcus*. Once *Streptococcus* has been identified, penicillin will most likely become the drug of choice. If the infant has undergone a manipulative process, i.e., the use of some type of indwelling catheter, then *Staphylococcus* is more likely to be involved; an antistaphylococcal agent such as a semisynthetic penicillin or a first-generation cephalosporin is the proper initial drug.

In patients between 4 and 48 months of age, one must consider *Haemophilus* as the offending organism. Ideally ampicillin is the drug of choice, but many organisms have been shown to be resistant to it. Until the cultures and sensitivities are completed, it is suggested that chloramphenicol be given as the initial drug, along with a semisynthetic penicillin for possible *Staphylococcus*.[181] More recently, the third-generation of cephalosporins, such as cefuroxime, have been found to be effective against ampicillin-resistant strains. These drugs now offer a less toxic choice than chloramphenicol. Once the sensitivities are identified, ampicillin can be utilized as the drug of choice if the organism is sensitive to it.

In patients who are older than four years, a semisynthetic penicillin or a first-generation cephalosporin is probably the drug of choice since the most likely agent in this age group is *Staphylococcus*.

Another area of controversy is whether to aspirate or drain surgically. There are proponents of and indications for either choice. Most orthopedic surgeons prefer to drain the joint surgically, whereas repeated aspirations may be initiated by nonsurgical physicians. The arguments for surgical drainage are that it allows a more complete cleansing and provides more adequate drainage of the joint; it also prevents repeated aspirations, which can be painful. However, the surgical incision results in a scar and increases morbidity slightly.

The need for an incision can be eliminated by needle aspiration. A recent study by Herndon and coworkers demonstrated that when the hip was not considered, aspiration alone can be effective in the treatment of septic arthritis.[182] Thirty-four of 49 joints were effectively managed in this way, with a follow-up of at least three years; 32 of the 34 were treated with a single diagnostic aspiration. In patients who had been symptomatic for longer than six days or who failed to respond promptly to antibiotics and aspiration alone, surgical drainage was performed. Delay in treating the joint surgically after the initial aspiration did not appear to affect the long-term outcome. It must be noted that most of those drained surgically were due to *Staphylococcus*, whereas those treated nonoperatively were due to *H. influenzae*.

Laboratory studies in rabbits have demonstrated that antibiotic therapy combined with surgical drainage results in less thinning of the cartilage, acellularity, and cloning of the chondrocytes than when combined with repeated aspiration.[178]

There are ample experimental and clinical studies to demonstrate that, when given parenterally, most antibiotics achieve adequate levels in the synovial fluids to provide sufficient inhibitory and bactericidal effects.[165, 204] Thus there appears to be no need to instill the antibiotic directly into the joint; similarly, suction irrigation appears to have no advantage over the standard methods of treatment.

As with osteomyelitis, very high doses of oral antibiotics have been shown to achieve adequate levels for treatment after the patient has become afebrile.[205] This is especially useful because it allows the patient to be managed on an outpatient basis postoperatively.

Author's Preferred Method of Treatment

The initial diagnosis depends on a diagnostic aspiration of the shoulder joint. I usually prefer an anterior approach, although if the joint is markedly distended almost any approach usually will yield fluid once the needle enters the joint. The opacity of the fluid and the patient's clinical picture help decide whether to treat this initially as a septic joint. If the patient appears toxic and is febrile and the fluid is very thick and purulent, I usually proceed directly to treating this as a septic joint; if the symptoms are minimal and the fluid is only moderately or slightly purulent, I usually await the results of the joint-fluid analysis. Other factors must also be taken into consideration, such as the patient's age and whether this is an isolated problem or multiple joints are involved. If the patient is toxic and belongs to the age group in which *Staphylococcus* is the most likely organism, I usually proceed with surgical drainage immediately. If the organism is more likely to be *Streptococcus* or *H. influenzae*, I treat the patient initially with aspirations alone. If a prompt response does not occur in 48 to 72 hours, surgical drainage is initiated.

Although I prefer an anterior approach to drain the proximal humerus, the posterior approach appears to be more advantageous in draining the glenohumeral joint. This approach, which has been popularized by Rockwood,[209] involves starting an incision 1 to 2 cm posterior to the lateral corner of the acromion and extending it for a distance of 5 to 6 cm toward the posterior axillary crease (Fig. 28–65*A*). The posterior deltoid is then split distally in line with the incision (Fig. 28–65*B*). The joint capsule is approached between the tendons of the infraspinatus superiorly and the teres minor inferiorly (Fig. 28–65*C*). In the posterior aspect of the axilla, the axillary nerve emerges to enter the undersurface of the deltoid distal to the tendon of the teres minor.

Following surgical drainage, I usually pack the posterior joint and incision with iodoform gauze, which is removed in 24 to 48 hours. Intravenous antibiotics are given until the patient has remained afebrile for at least 24 to 36 hours. He or she is then placed on very high doses of oral antibiotics, which are continued on an outpatient basis until the sedimentation rate is below 20 mm/hour. (See the previous section on treatment of osteomyelitis.)

Sequelae

Because of the relative infrequency of septic arthritis involving the glenohumeral joint, very little information exists regarding its long-term effects. It appears that the multiple complications that occur as a result of septic arthritis in the hip do not develop in the glenohumeral joint. Recently Schmidt and coworkers were able to collect a series of nine patients from two to five years of age with septic glenohumeral joints.[210] Five of them had associated acute osteomyelitis. One required a second arthrotomy to evacuate purulent material that had loculated in the bicipital groove; another had demonstrated a septic rupture of the bicipital tendon. None of the patients exhibited any chronic drainage, recurrent osteomyelitis, or limb length discrepancy or deformity. All regained a satisfactory, painless range of motion. Schmidt and associates emphasized that, when performing an arthrotomy, the bicipital recess must be explored and cleaned out.

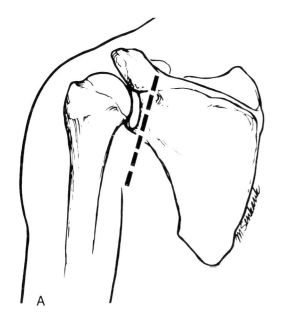

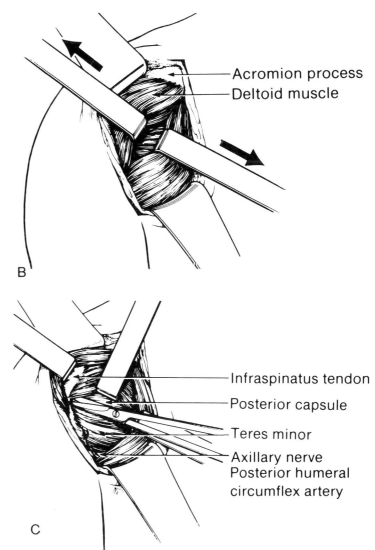

Acromion process
Deltoid muscle

Infraspinatus tendon
Posterior capsule
Teres minor
Axillary nerve
Posterior humeral
circumflex artery

Figure 28–65. Posterior arthrotomy for drainage of the glenohumeral joint. *A,* The incision starts at the scapular spine, 1 to 2 cm medial to the posterior lateral edge of the acromion. *B,* The deltoid fibers are split in the same direction for a distance of 5 to 6 cm. *C,* The joint capsule is entered between the intraspinatus and teres minor tendons. Note: the axillary nerve emerges distal to the teres minor. (Reproduced with permission from Rockwood CA, and Green DP: Fractures (3 vols), 2nd ed. Philadelphia: JB Lippincott, 1984.)

Acromioclavicular and Sternoclavicular Joints

Septic arthritis as an isolated entity involving either the acromioclavicular or sternoclavicular joint is theoretically possible. In the sternoclavicular joint it could be secondary to an osteomyelitis of the metaphysis of the medial clavicle. In reviewing the literature, I was unable to find any case reports of isolated septic arthritis involving either of these joints in children. It appears that the major problem may lie in the diagnosis because of the lack of specific symptoms; this may constitute an ideal indication for the use of radionuclide scans combined with needle aspiration. The decision whether to treat these joints surgically or medically needs to be made on an individual basis.

References

Brachial Plexus Injuries

1. Adams JH, and Cameron HM: Obstetrical paralysis due to ischemia of the spinal cord. Arch Dis Child *40*:93–96, 1965.
2. Adler JB, and Patterson RL: Erb's palsy: long term results of treatment in eighty-eight cases. J Bone Joint Surg *49A*:1052–1064, 1967.
3. Aitken J: Deformity of the elbow joint as a sequel to Erb's obstetrical paralysis. J Bone Joint Surg *34B*:352–365, 1952.
4. Ashurst APC: Birth injuries of the shoulder. Ann Surg *67*:25–50, 1918.
5. Aston JW: Brachial plexus birth palsy. Orthopedics *2*:594–601, 1979.
6. Babbitt DP, and Cassidy RH: Obstetrical paralysis and dislocation of the shoulder in infancy. J Bone Joint Surg *50A*:1447–1452, 1968.
7. Bennett GC, and Harrold AJ: Prognosis and early management of birth injuries to the brachial plexus. Br Med J *1*:1520–1521, 1976.
8. Blount WP: Osteoclasis for supination deformities in children. J Bone Joint Surg *22*:300–314, 1940.
9. Blount WP: Osteoclasis of the upper extremity in children. Acta Orthop Scand *32*:374–382, 1962.
10. Blount WP, and Zuege RC: Drilling osteoclasis for upper extremity deformity. Orthop Rev *7*:53–59, 1978.
11. Bonney G: The value of axon responses in determining the site of lesion in traction injuries of the brachial plexus. Brain *77*:588–609, 1954.
12. Boome RS, and Kaye JC: Obstetric traction injuries of the brachial plexus. J Bone Joint Surg *70B*:571–576, 1988.

13. Boorstein SW: Birth injuries requiring orthopedic treatment. JAMA 85:1866–1869, 1925.

14. Boorstein SW: The use of braces in obstetric brachial paralysis with a report of 211 cases in 200 patients. Am J Dis Child 39:1279–1294, 1930.

15. Bullard WN: Obstetric paralysis. Am J Med Sci 134:93–106, 1907.

16. Brown KLB: Review of obstetrical palsies, nonoperative treatment. In Terzis JK (ed): Microreconstruction of Nerve Injuries. Philadelphia: WB Saunders, 1987, pp 499–511.

17. Chung SM, and Nissenbaum MM: Obstetrical paralysis. Orthop Clin North Am 6:393–400, 1975.

18. Clark LP, Taylor AS, and Prout TP: A study of brachial birth palsy. Am J Med Sci 130:670–707, 1905.

19. Eng GD: Brachial plexus palsy in newborn infants. Pediatrics 48:18–28, 1971.

20. Fairbank HAT: Birth palsy: subluxation of the shoulder joint in infants and young children. Lancet 1:1217, 1913.

21. Gilbert A, and Tassin JL: Obstetrical palsy: a clinical, pathologic, and surgical review. In Terzis JK: Microreconstruction of Nerve Injuries. Philadelphia: WB Saunders, 1987.

22. Gilbert A, Razaboni R, and Amar-Khodja S: Indications and results of brachial plexus surgery in obstetrical palsy. Orthop Clin North Am 19:91–105, 1988.

23. Gilmour J: Notes on the surgical treatment of brachial birth palsy. Lancet 209:696–699, 1925.

24. Gjorup L: Obstetrical lesion of the brachial plexus. Acta Neurol Scand 42(Suppl 18):1–38, 1966.

25. Goddard NJ, and Fixsen JA: Rotation osteotomy of the humerus for birth injuries of the brachial plexus. J Bone Joint Surg 66B:257–259, 1984.

26. Gordon M, Rich H, Deutschberger J, et al: The immediate and long term outcome of obstetric birth trauma. 1. Brachial plexus paralysis. Am J Obstet Gynecol 117:51–56, 1973.

27. Green WT, and Tachdjian MO: Correction of residual deformity of the shoulder from obstetrical palsy. J Bone Joint Surg 45A:1544, 1963.

28. Greenwald AG, Schute PC, and Shiveley JL: Brachial plexus birth palsy: a ten year report on the incidence and prognosis. J Pediatr Orthop 4:689–692, 1984.

29. Gresham EL: Birth trauma. Pediatr Clin North Am 22:317–328, 1975.

30. Hardy AE: Birth injuries of the brachial plexus: incidence and prognosis. J Bone Joint Surg 63B:98–101, 1981.

31. Hentz VR, and Narakas A: Results of microneurosurgical reconstruction in complete brachial plexus palsy. Orthop Clin North Am 19:107–114, 1988.

32. Hoffer MM, Wickenden R, and Roper B: Brachial plexus birth palsies: results of tendon transfers to the rotator cuff. J Bone Joint Surg 60A:691–695, 1978.

33. Jackson ST, Hoffer MM, and Parrish N: Brachial plexus palsy in the newborn. J Bone Joint Surg 70A(8):1217–1220, 1988.

34. Jepson PN: Obstetrical paralysis. Ann Surg 91:724–730, 1930.

35. Johnson EW, Alexander MA, and Koenig WC: Infantile Erb's palsy (Smellie's palsy). Arch Phys Med Rehabil 58:175–178, 1977.

36. Kattan KR, and Spitz HB: Roentgen findings in obstetrical injuries to the brachial plexus. Radiology 91:462–466, 1968.

37. Kawabata H, Masada K, Tsuyuguchi Y, et al: Early microsurgical reconstruction in birth palsy. Clin Orthop 215:233–242, 1987.

38. Kleinberg S: Arthrodesis of the shoulder for obstetrical paralysis. Arch Pediatr 41:252–257, 1924.

39. Kleinberg S: Reattachment of the capsule and external rotators of the shoulder for obstetric paralysis. JAMA 98:294–298, 1932.

40. Leffert R: Brachial plexus injuries. In Congenital Brachial Palsy. New York: Churchill Livingstone, 1985.

41. Leibolt FL, and Furey JG: Obstetrical paralysis with dislocation of the shoulder: a case report. J Bone Joint Surg 35A:227–230, 1953.

42. L'Episcopo JB: Tendon transplantation in obstetrical paralysis. Am J Surg 25:122–125, 1934.

43. L'Episcopo JB: Restoration of muscle balance in the treatment of obstetrical paralysis. NY State J Med 39:357–363, 1939.

44. Levine MG, Holroyde J, Woods JR, et al: Birth trauma: incidence and predisposing factors. Obstet Gynecol 63:792–795, 1984.

45. Manske PR, McCarroll HR Jr, and Hale R: Biceps tendon rerouting and percutaneous osteoclasis in the treatment of supination deformity in obstetrical palsy. J Hand Surg 5:153–159, 1980.

46. Mayer L: Transplantation of the trapezius for paralysis of the abductors of the arm. J Bone Joint Surg 9:412–420, 1927.

47. Mayer L: Operative reconstruction of the paralyzed upper extremity. J Bone Joint Surg 21:377–383, 1939.

48. McFarland LV, Raskin M, Daling JR, and Benedetti TJ: Erb/Duchenne's palsy: a consequence of fetal macrosomia and method of delivery. Obstet Gynecol 68:784–788, 1986.

49. Middleton DS: The pathology of congenital torticollis. Br J Surg 18:188–204, 1930.

50. Moore BH: A new operative procedure for brachial palsy. Erb's paralysis. Surg Gynecol Obstet 61:832–835, 1935.

51. Moore BH: Brachial birth palsy. Am J Surg 43:338–345, 1939.

52. Ober FR: An operation to relieve paralysis of the deltoid muscle. JAMA 99:2182, 1932.

53. Patterson RL Jr: Obstetrical paralysis. Physiother Rev 20:291–296, 1940.

54. Perry J, Hsu J, Barber L, et al: Orthoses in patients with brachial plexus injuries. Arch Phys Med Rehabil 55:134–137, 1974.

55. Platt H: Opening remarks on birth paralysis. J Orthop Surg 2:272–294, 1920.

56. Rogers MH: An operation for correction of the deformity due to "obstetrical paralysis." Boston Med Surg J 174:163–164, 1916.

57. Rubin A: Birth injuries: incidence, mechanisms and end results. Obstet Gynecol 23:218–221, 1964.

58. Scaglietti O: The obstetrical shoulder trauma. Surg Gynecol Obstet 66:868–877, 1938.

59. Sever JW: Obstetric paralysis. A report of 470 cases. Am J Dis Child 12:541–578, 1916.

60. Sever JW: Obstetric paralysis: report of 1,100 cases. JAMA 85:1862–1865, 1925.

61. Sever JW: Obstetrical paralysis. Surg Gynecol Obstet 44:547–549, 1927.

62. Sever JW: Obstetrical paralysis. Pub Health Nurs 32:187–196, 1940.

63. Specht EE: Brachial plexus palsy in the newborn: incidence and prognosis. Clin Orthop 110:32–34, 1975.

64. Suzuki S, Yamamuro T, and Fujita A: The aetiological relationship between congenital torticollis and obstetrical paralysis. Intern Orthop 8:175–181, 1984.

65. Tada K, Tsuyuguchi Y, and Kawai H: Birth palsy: natural recovery course and combined root avulsion. J Pediatr Orthop 4:279–284, 1984.

66. Taylor AS: Results from the surgical treatment of brachial birth palsy. JAMA 48:96–104, 1907.

67. Taylor AS: Conclusions derived from further experience in the surgical treatment of brachial birth palsy (Erb's type). Am J Med Sci 146:836–856, 1913.

68. Taylor AS: Brachial birth palsy and injuries of similar types in adults. Surg Gynecol Obstet 30(5):494–502, 1920.

69. Thomas TT: The relation of posterior subluxation of the shoulder joint to obstetrical palsy of the upper extremity. Ann Surg 59:197–232, 1914.

70. Vassalos E, Prevedourakis C, and Paraschopoulou-Prevedouraki P: Brachial plexus paralysis in the newborn. An analysis of 169 cases. Am J Obstet Gynecol 101:554–556, 1968

71. Wickstrom J, Haslam ET, and Hutchinson RH: The surgical management of residual deformities of the shoulder following birth injuries of the brachial plexus. J Bone Joint Surg 37A:27–36, 1955.

72. Wickstrom J: Birth injuries of the brachial plexus. Treatment of defects in the shoulder. Clin Orthop 23:187–196, 1962.

73. Wolman B: Erb's palsy. Arch Dis Child 23:129–131, 1948.

74. Zachary RB: Transplantation of teres major and latissimus dorsi for loss of external rotation at shoulder. Lancet 2:757–758, 1947.

75. Zalis OS, Zalis AW, Barron KD, et al: Motor patterning following transitory sensory-motor deprivations. Arch Neurol 13:487–494, 1965.

76. Zancolli EA: Classification and management of the shoulder in birth palsy. Orthop Clin North Am 12:433–457, 1981.

Torticollis

77. Anderson W: Clinical lecture on sterno-mastoid torticollis. Lancet 1:9–12, 1893.

78. Armstrong D, Pickrell K, Fetter B, and Pitts W: Torticollis: an analysis of 271 cases. Plast Reconstr Surg 35:14–25, 1965.

79. Balkany TJ, and Mischke RE: Mastoid release for congenital torticollis. Laryngoscope 90:337–338, 1980.

80. Barenfield PA, and Weseley MS: Congenital muscular torticollis: case reports in siblings. Bull Hosp Joint Dis 24:130–134, 1963.

81. Baxter CF, Johnson EW, Lloyd JR, and Clatworthy HW Jr: Prognostic significance of electromyography in congenital torticollis. Pediatrics 28:442–446, 1961.

82. Boisen E: Torticollis caused by infratentorial tumour: three cases. Br J Psychiatry 134:306–307, 1979.

83. Braga MB: Contribucao ao estudo da etiopatogenia do torcicola muscular congenito. Master's Thesis for San Paulo School of Medicine, 1986.

84. Brown JB, and McDowell F: Wry-neck facial distortion prevented by resection of fibrosed sternomastoid muscle in infancy and childhood. Ann Surg 131:721–733, 1950.

85. Campbell CJ, and Peora G: Sternomastoid tumor in identical twins. J Bone Joint Surg 38A:350–352, 1956.

86. Canale ST, Griffin DW, and Hubbard CN: Congenital muscular torticollis: a long term follow-up. J Bone Joint Surg 64:810–816, 1982.

87. Chandler FA: Muscular torticollis. J Bone Joint Surg 30A:566–569, 1948.

88. Chandler FA, and Altenberg A: "Congenital" muscular torticollis. JAMA 125:476–483, 1944.

89. Clarren SK, Smith DW, and Hanson JW: Helmet treatment for plagiocephaly and congenital muscular torticollis. J Pediatr 94:143–146, 1979.

90. Coventry MB, and Harris LE: Congenital muscular torticollis in infancy. J Bone Joint Surg 41A:815–822, 1959.

91. Dubousset J: Torticollis in children caused by congenital anomalies of the atlas. J Bone Joint Surg 68A:178–188, 1986.

92. Dunn PM: Congenital sternomastoid torticollis: an intrauterine postural deformity. Arch Dis Child 49:824–825, 1974.

93. Ferkel RD, Westin GW, Dawson EG, and Oppenheim WL: Muscular torticollis: a modified surgical approach. J Bone Joint Surg 65A:894–900, 1983.

94. Fisher AL: Torticollis: a review. Am J Orthop Surg 14:669, 1916.

95. Hagen-Torn J: Die Loesung des Problems ueber die Entstehung der Schaedelasymmetrie und Skoliose bei Caput Ostipum. Die Beseitigung derselben durch die Operation Nach Meiner Methode. Arch f klin Chir 163:35–54, 1930.

96. Hensinger RN: Orthopedic problems of the shoulder and neck. Pediatr Clin North Am 24:889–902, 1977.

97. Hellstadius A: Torticollis congenita. Acta Chir Scand 62:586, 1927.

98. Holloway LW: Caput obstipum congenitum. South Med J 24:597–601, 1931.

99. Horton CE, Crawford HH, Adamson JE, et al: Torticollis. South Med J 60:953–958, 1967.

100. Hough GD: Congenital torticollis. Surg Gynecol Obstet 58:972–981, 1934

101. Howell BW: The treatment of torticollis. Br Med J 2:714–716, 1929.

102. Hulbert KF: Congenital torticollis. J Bone Joint Surg 32B:50–57, 1950.

103. Hummer CD, and MacEwen GD: The coexistence of torticollis and congenital dysplasia of the hip. J Bone Joint Surg 54A:1255–1256, 1972.

104. Ippolito E, Tudisco C, and Massobrio M: Long term results of open sternocleidomastoid tenotomy for idiopathic muscular torticollis. J Bone Joint Surg 67A:30–38, 1985.

105. Jahss SA: Torticollis. J Bone Joint Surg 18:1065–1068, 1936.

106. Jones PG: Torticollis in Infancy and Childhood. Springfield IL: Charles C Thomas, 1968.

107. Keller EE, Jackson IT, Marsh WR, and Triplett WW: Mandibular asymmetry associated with congenital muscular torticollis. Oral Surg Oral Med Oral Path 60:216–220, 1986.

108. Kiesewetter WB, Neslon PK, Pallidino US, and Koop CE: Neonatal torticollis. JAMA 157:1281–1285, 1955.

109. Kinsbourne M: Hiatus hernia with contortion of the neck. Lancet 1:1058–1061, 1964.

110. Lee EH, Kang YK, and Bose K: Surgical correction of muscular torticollis in the older child. J Pediatr Orthop 6:585–587, 1986.

111. Lidge RT, Bechtol RC, and Lambert CN: Congenital muscular torticollis. J Bone Joint Surg 39A:1165–1182, 1957.

112. Ling CM: The influence of age on the results of open sternomastoid tenotomy in muscular torticollis. Clin Orthop 116:142–148, 1976

113. Ling CM, and Low YS: Sternomastoid tumor and muscular torticollis. Clin Orthop 86:144–150, 1972.

114. Lipson EH, and Robertson WC Jr: Paroxysmal torticollis of infancy: familial occurrence. Am J Dis Child 132:422–423, 1978.

115. Lorenz A: Torticollis. Wein Med Presse 233, 1902.

116. Lyle TK: Practical Orthoptics in the Treatment of Squint. London: Lewis, 1940.

117. McDaniel A, Hirsch BE, Kornblut AD, and Armbrustmacher VM: Torticollis in infancy and adolescence. Ear Nose Throat J 63:478–487, 1984.

118. Macdonald D: Sternomastoid tumour and muscular torticollis. J Bone Joint Surg 51B:432–443, 1969.

119. McKinley LM, and Hamilton LR: Torticollis caused by absence of the right sternocleidomastoid muscle. South Med J 69:1099–1101, 1976.

120. Mickelson MR, Cooper RR, and Ponseti IV: Ultrastructure of the sternocleidomastoid muscle in muscular torticollis. Clin Orthop 110:11–18, 1975.

121. Middleton DS: The pathology of congenital torticollis. Br J Surg 18:188–204, 1930.

122. Mikulicz J: Über die Exstirpation des Kopfsnicjers bein Muskuloren. Schiefhals Neben des Berkungen zur Pathologie diese Leiden. Zbl Chir 1:9, 1895.

123. Morrison DL, and MacEwen GD: Congenital muscular torticollis: observations regarding clinical findings, associated conditions, and results of treatment. J Pediatr Orthop 2(5):500–505, 1982.

124. Moseley TM: Treatment of facial distortion due to wryneck in infants by complete resection of the sternomastoid muscle. Am Surg 28:698–702, 1962.

125. Murphy WJ, and Gellis SS: Torticollis with hernia in infancy: Sandifer syndrome. Am J Dis Child 134:564–565, 1977.

126. Pineyro JR, Yoel J, and Rocco M: Congenital torticollis. J Int Coll Surg 34:495–505, 1960.

127. Reye RDK: Sterno-mastoid tumour and congenital muscular torticollis. Med J Aust 1:867–870, 1951.

128. Sanerkin NG, and Edwards P: Birth injury to sternomastoid muscle. J Bone Joint Surg 48B:441–447, 1966.

129. Sarnat HB, and Morrissy RT: Idiopathic torticollis: sternomastoid myopathy and accessory neuropathy. Muscle Nerve 4:374–380, 1981.

130. Soeur R: Treatment of congenital torticollis. J Bone Joint Surg 22:35–42, 1940.

131. Staheli LT: Muscular torticollis: late results of operative treatment. Surgery 69:469–473, 1971.

132. Steindler A: A Textbook of Operative Orthopedics, 1st ed. New York: D Appleton & Co, 1925.

133. Stevens AE: Congenital torticollis in identical twins. Lancet 2:378, 1948.

134. Sty JR, Wells RG, and Shroeder BA: Congenital muscular torticollis: computed tomographic observations. Am J Dis Child 141:243–244, 1987.

135. Sutcliffe J: Torsion spasms and abnormal postures in children

with hiatus hernia Sandifers Syndrome. Prog Pediatr Radiol 2:190–197, 1969.

136. Suzuki S, Yammamuro T, and Fujita A: The aetiological relationship between congenital torticollis and obstetrical paralysis. Int Orthop 8:175–181, 1984.

137. Tse P, Cheng J, Chow Y, and Leung PC: Surgery for neglected congenital torticollis. Acta Orthop Scand 58:270–272, 1987.

138. Von Lackum HL: Torticollis: removal in early life of the fibrous mass from the sternomastoid muscle. Surg Gynecol Obstet 48:691–694, 1929.

139. Weiner DS: Congenital dislocation of the hip associated with congenital muscular torticollis. Clin Orthop 121:163–165, 1976.

140. Werlin SL, D'Souza BJ, Hogan WJ, et al: Sandifer syndrome: an unappreciated clinical entity. Dev Med Child Neurol 22(3):374–378, 1980.

The Shoulder in Arthrogryposis

141. Bennett JB, Hansen PE, Granberry WM, and Cain TE: Surgical management of arthrogryposis in the upper extremity. J Pediatr Orthop 5:281–286, 1985.

142. Drummond DS, Siller TN, and Cruess RL: Management of arthrogryposis multiplex congenita. AAOS Instr Course Lect 23:79–95, 1974.

143. Kasai T, Oki T, Osuga T, and Nogami H: Familial arthrogryposis with distal involvement of the limbs. Clin Orthop 166:182–184, 1982.

144. Krugliak L, Gadoth N, and Behar AJ: Neuropathic form of arthrogryposis multiplex congenita. Report of 3 cases with complete necropsy, including the first reported case of agenesis of muscle spindles. Neurol Sci 37:179–185, 1978.

145. Lloyd-Roberts GC, and Lettin AWF: Arthrogryposis multiplex congenita. J Bone Joint Surg 52B:494–508, 1970.

146. Stern WG: Arthrogryposis multiplex congenita. JAMA 81:1507, 1923.

147. Swinyard CA, and Mayer V: Multiple congenital contractures. JAMA 183:23, 1963.

148. Williams P: The management of arthrogryposis. Orthop Clin North Am 9:67–88, 1978.

149. Williams PF: Management of upper limb problems in arthrogryposis. Clin Orthop 194:60–67, 1985.

Bone and Joint Infections

150. Almquist EE: The changing epidemiology of septic arthritis in children. Clin Orthop 68:96–99, 1970.

151. Ash JM, and Gilday DL: The futility of bone scanning in neonatal osteomyelitis. J Nucl Med 21:417–420, 1980.

152. Baker CJ: Group B streptococcal infections in neonates. Pediatr Rev 1:5–15, 1979.

153. Berkowitz ID, and Wenzel W: Normal technetium bone scans in patients with acute osteomyelitis. Am J Dis Child 134:828, 1980.

154. Blasier RB, and Aronson DD: Infantile cortical hyperostosis with osteomyelitis of the humerus. J Pediatr Orthop 5:222–224, 1985.

155. Blockey NJ, and Watson JT: Acute osteomyelitis in children. J Bone Joint Surg 52B:77–87, 1970.

156. Bobechko WP: Infections of bones and joints. In Lovell WW, and Winter RB (eds): Pediatric Orthopaedics, 2nd ed. Philadelphia: JB Lippincott, 1984.

157. Bryson JY, Connor JD, LeClerc M, and Giammona ST: High-dose oral dicloxacillin treatment of acute staphylococcal osteomyelitis in children. J Pediatr 94:673–675, 1979.

158. Buchman J: Osteomyelitis. AAOS Instr Course Lect 1959.

159. Caffey J: Infantile cortical hyperostosis: a review of the clinical and radiographic features. Proc R Soc Med 50:347–354, 1956.

160. Canale ST, Harkness RM, Thomas PA, and Massie JD: Does aspiration of bones and joints affect results of later bone scanning? J Pediatr Orthop 5:23, 1985.

161. Capitanio MA, and Kirkpatrick JA: Early roentgen observations in acute osteomyelitis. Am J Roentgenol 108:488–496, 1970.

162. Cole WG, Elliott BG, and Jensen F: Management of septic arthritis in childhood. Aust NZ J Surg 45:178–182, 1975.

163. Curtiss PH Jr: Some uncommon forms of osteomyelitis. Clin Orthop 96:84–87, 1973.

164. Deysine M, Rafkin H, Russell R, et al: The detection of acute experimental osteomyelitis with 67Ga citrate scannings. Surg Gynecol Obstet 141:40–42, 1975.

165. Drutz DJ, Schaffner W, Hillman JW, et al: Penetration of penicillin and other antimicrobiotics into joint fluid. J Bone Joint Surg 49A:1415, 1967.

166. Duszynski DO, Kuhn JP, Afshani E, et al: Early radionuclide diagnosis of acute osteomyelitis. Radiology 117:337–340, 1975.

167. Edwards MS, Baker CJ, Wagner ML, et al: An etiologic shift in infantile osteomyelitis: the emergence of the group B streptococcus. J Pediatr 93:578–583, 1978.

168. Feigin RD, Pickering LK, Anderson D, et al: Clindamycin treatment of osteomyelitis and septic arthritis in children. Pediatrics 55(2):213–223, 1975.

169. Fink CW: Gonococcal arthritis in children. JAMA 194(3):123–124, 1965.

170. Fox L, and Sprunt K: Neonatal osteomyelitis. Pediatrics 62:535–542, 1978.

171. Freedman RM, Ingram DL, Gross I, et al: A half century of neonatal sepsis at Yale: 1928 to 1978. Am J Dis Child 135:140–144, 1981.

172. Ganel A, Horozowski H, Zaltman S, and Farine I: Sequential use of Tc-MDP and Ga imaging in bone infection. Orthop Rev 9(7):73–77, 1981.

173. Gilday DL, Paul DJ, and Paterson J: Diagnosis of osteomyelitis in children by combined blood pool and bone imaging. Radiology 117(2):331–335, 1975.

174. Gilmour WN: Acute haematogenous osteomyelitis. J Bone Joint Surg 44B:841–853, 1962.

175. Gillespie R: Septic arthritis of childhood. Clin Orthop 96:152–159, 1973.

176. Gillespie WJ: Late recurrence following acute haematogenous osteomyelitis. Aust NZ Med J 82:304–305, 1975.

177. Gillespie WJ, and Mayo KM: The management of acute haematogenous osteomyelitis in the antibiotic era. J Bone Joint Surg 63B:126–131, 1981.

178. Goldstein WM, Gleason TF, and Barmada R: A comparison between arthrotomy and irrigation and multiple aspirations in the treatment of pyogenic arthritis. Orthopedics 6:1309–1314, 1983.

179. Green M, Nyhan WL Jr, and Fousek MD: Acute hematogenous osteomyelitis. Pediatrics 17:368–381, 1956.

180. Green WT, and Shannon JG: Osteomyelitis of infants. Arch Surg 332:462–493, 1936.

181. Griffin PP: Septic arthritis in children. Vol I, Lesson 35, Orthopedic Surgery Update Series. Princeton, NJ: Continuing Professional Education Center, 1982.

182. Herndon WA, Knauer S, Sullivan JA, and Gross RH: Management of septic arthritis in children. J Pediatr Orthop 6:576–578, 1986.

183. Howard JB, Highgenboten CL, and Nelson JD: Residual effects of septic arthritis in infancy and childhood. JAMA 236(8):932–935, 1976.

184. Howie DW, Savage JB, Wilson TG, and Paterson D: The technetium phosphate bone scan in the diagnosis of osteomyelitis in childhood. J Bone Joint Surg 65A:431–437, 1983.

185. Jaffe HL: Skeletal lesions caused by certain other infectious agents. In Metabolic, Degenerative and Inflammatory Diseases of Bone and Joints. Philadelphia: Lea & Febiger, 1972.

186. Jones DC, and Cody RB: "Cold" bone scans in acute osteomyelitis. J Bone Joint Surg 63B:376–378, 1981.

187. Kelly PJ, and Karlson AG: Granulomatous bacterial arthritis. Clin Orthop 96:165–167, 1973.

188. Kuhn JP, and Berger PE: Computed tomographic diagnosis of osteomyelitis. Radiology 130:503–506, 1974.

189. Leeson MD, Weiner DS, and Klein L: Osteomyelitis of the clavicle in children. Orthopedics 5:428–432, 1982.

190. Letts RM, Afifi A, and Sutherland JB: Technetium bone scanning as an aid in the diagnosis of atypical acute osteomyelitis in children. Surg Gynecol Obstet 140:899–902, 1975.

191. Martel JR, Ballard A, Scott GB, and Castro A: Hemophilus

influenzae septic arthritis in the pediatric age group. Paper presented at the 27th Annual Meeting of the Society of Military Orthopaedic Surgeons, San Antonio, Texas, December 1985.

192. McAllister TA: Treatment of osteomyelitis. Br J Hosp Med 535–543, October, 1974.

193. McHenry MC: Hematogenous osteomyelitis. Cleve Clin Q 42(1):125–153, 1975.

194. Medlar RC, and Crawford AH: Acute hematogenous osteomyelitis. The long-term follow-up in children. Orthop Rev 7(11):145–150, 1978.

195. Merkel KD, Fitzgerald RH, and Brown M: Scintigraphic evaluation in musculoskeletal sepsis. Orthop Clin North Am 15:401–416, 1984.

196. Mollan RAB, and Piggot J: Acute osteomyelitis in children. J Bone Joint Surg 59B:2–7, 1977.

197. Morrey BF, and Peterson HA: Hematogenous pyogenic osteomyelitis in children. Orthop Clin North Am 6(4):935–951, 1975.

198. Morrey BF, and Bianco AJ Jr: Hematogenous osteomyelitis of the clavicle in children. Clin Orthop 125:24–28, 1977.

199. Morrey BF, Bianco AJ, and Rhodes KH: Hematogenous osteomyelitis at uncommon sites in children. Mayo Clin Proc 53:707–713, 1978.

200. Mortensson W, and Nybonde T: Ischemia of the childhood femoral and humeral head epiphyses following osteomyelitis. Acta Radiol [Diagn] 25:269–272, 1984.

201. Nade S, Robertson FW, and Taylor TK: Antibiotics in the treatment of acute osteomyelitis and acute septic arthritis in children. Med J Aust 2:703–705, 1974.

202. Nade S: Acute haematogenous osteomyelitis. Med J Aust 2:708–711, 1974B.

203. Nelson J, and Krantz WC: Septic arthritis in infants and children. Pediatrics 38:966–971, 1966.

204. Nelson JD: Antibiotic concentrations in septic joint effusions. N Engl J Med 284:349–353, 1971.

205. Nelson JD, Bucholz RW, Kusmiesz H, and Shelton S: Benefits and risks of sequential parenteral-oral cephalosporin therapy for suppurative bone and joint infections. J Pediatr Orthop 2:255–262, 1982.

206. Ogden JA, and Lister G: The pathology of neonatal osteomyelitis. Pediatrics 55:474–478, 1975.

207. Pittard WB, Thullen JD, and Fanaroff AA: Neonatal septic arthritis. J Pediatr 88(4):621–624, 1976.

208. Pritchard DJ: Granulomatous infections of bones and joints. Orthop Clin North Am 6:1029–1047, 1975.

209. Rockwood CA Jr: Fractures and dislocations of the shoulder. In Rockwood CA Jr, and Green DP (eds): Fractures, Vol. I. Philadelphia: JB Lippincott, 1984.

210. Schmidt D, Mubarak S, and Gelberman R: Septic shoulders in children. J Pediatr Orthop 1:67–72, 1981.

211. Sullivan DC, Rosenfield NS, Ogden J, and Gottschalk A: Problems in scintigraphic detection of osteomyelitis in children. Radiology 135:731–736, 1980.

212. Sullivan JA, Vasileff T, and Leonard JC: An evaluation of nuclear scanning in orthopedic infections. J Pediatr Orthop 1:73–79, 1981.

213. Tachdjian MO: Pediatric Orthopedics, Vol 1. Philadelphia: WB Saunders, 1972.

214. Treves S, Khettry J, Broker FH, et al: Osteomyelitis: early scintigraphic detection in children. Pediatrics 57(2):173–186, 1976.

215. Vu Quoc D, Nelson JD, and Haltalin KC: Osteomyelitis in Infants and Children. Am J Dis Child 129:1237-1278, 1975.

216. Whalen JL, Fitzgerald RH Jr, and Morrissy RT: A histological study of acute hematogenous osteomyelitis following physeal injuries in rabbits. J Bone Joint Surg 70A:1383–1392, 1988.

217. White M, and Dennison WM: Acute haematogenous osteitis in childhood: a review of 212 cases. J Bone Joint Surg (Br) 34:608–623, 1952.

218. Winters JL, and Cahen I: Acute hematogenous osteomyelitis. J Bone Joint Surg 42A:691–704, 1960.

The author gratefully acknowledges the assistance provided by Ms. Karen Holder, Mrs. Marizella Boyd, and Mr. Gerald Berg in preparing this manuscript.

Occupational Shoulder Disorders

James V. Luck, Jr., M.D.
Gunnar B. J. Andersson, M.D., Ph.D.

Over the last two decades occupational shoulder problems have increased in frequency to near-epidemic proportions in Australia, Japan, and Scandinavia.[3, 39, 60] Recent data from the United States demonstrate a similar dramatic trend.[63] Surveys in Finland reveal that shoulder complaints exceed back complaints in many groups of workers, such as slaughterhouse workers[95] and large vehicle drivers.[6] Shoulder pain is second to back pain in workers' compensation insurance costs in Australia.[60, 89] Industrial shoulder problems are also second to back problems in the frequency of physician visits in Sweden.[41]

Whether the increase in shoulder complaints is the result of ergonomic changes in industry, brought about by automation and computerization, or merely increased awareness and recognition of an old problem is the subject of much study and debate. It is becoming increasingly apparent that both are true.

Occupational shoulder problems can be separated into three groups: (1) those that are relatively unique to industry, (2) those that are not unique but occur regularly in certain types of work, and (3) those that occur from injury and have no special relationship to industry. An example of the first group is the repetitive strain injury of shoulder and neck muscles, alternately termed cervicobrachial syndrome. These complaints are especially common among workers in light, static occupations, such as keyboard operators and light-assembly workers.

The second group is exemplified by chronic tendinitis, impingement syndrome, and rotator cuff tears; these are seen mostly in moderate to heavy work occupations requiring sustained loads with the shoulder partly abducted and/or forward flexed. These problems are common in certain types of work but are equally prevalent in the nonindustrial setting.

The last group encompasses acute injuries that are the result of direct trauma causing fractures and/or soft tissue injury. The pathology of acute occupational injuries is no different from nonindustrial trauma and is discussed in other chapters in this text. Diagnosis and treatment are also the same and therefore will not be covered here. Special industrial considerations include safety measures and prevention in high-risk occupations, as well as rehabilitation after major industrial trauma. Evaluation of permanent partial disability and appropriate recommendations for work restrictions and job modification will also be discussed.

Occupational Cervicobrachial Disorder

The term *occupational cervicobrachial disorder* (OCD) was first established by the Japan Association of Industrial Health in 1972.[48] It applied to a somewhat vague syndrome of shoulder area pain that included the posterior neck and parascapular musculature, the glenohumeral musculotendinous structures, and also radiating pains to the upper arm. In other words, it is not a pathological or clinical diagnosis but a symptom complex. It was thought to be the result of cumulative trauma from high repetition of simple tasks and was believed to have increased because of automation and computerization of the work environment. The same symptom complex is termed *repetitive stress injury* (RSI) in Australia[14, 60, 89] and is considered part of *cumulative trauma disorders* (CTDs) or *repetitive motion injuries* (RMIs) in the United States.[63]

EPIDEMIOLOGY

Most of the existing epidemiological data on OCD come from Scandinavia, Japan, and Australia. Epidemiological studies are not divided into specific diagnostic categories but instead deal with the incidence of shoulder symptoms as it relates to type of work, physical characteristics of the worker, and work setting. Neck and shoulder symptomatology are often not separated nor is diagnosis such as myositis, tendinitis, or arthritis differentiated. In epidemiological research, it is often not possible to examine the subjects individually; instead a screening method is used, based on questionnaires and sometimes interviews. The choice of diagnostic criteria, then, becomes critical. Sometimes there are no generally accepted criteria, and therefore the diagnosis is based on exclusion of other common causes of pain in the shoulder region. This procedure explains how differences can occur in prevalence and incidence.[56, 95, 96] The later section on etiology will review the extensive experimental studies that attempt to better define specific pathophysiology. Some studies in each section address both epidemiological and etiological issues.

OCD is especially common among keyboard operators and many types of light-assembly workers. Most keyboard operators work with the shoulders in a static posture of slight abduction and forward flexion with fine upper extremity movements at very high frequency, 80,000 keystrokes per day being not uncommon.[60, 63] In 1979, Luopajärvi and coworkers[58a] reported a prevalence among keypunch operators of 16 to 28 per cent. Cash register operators had an incidence of 11 to 16 per cent, light assembly workers 16 per cent, typists 13 per cent, and calculator operators 10 per cent. A 1981 Australian survey of 122 data process workers showed that 78 per cent had some symptoms of OCD.[92] However, only 16 per cent of the whole group had obtained medical treatment. A later study of 52 additional data process workers in the same office showed identical results with 79 per cent symptomatic.[80] The incidence of new reported cases in Australia rose from 2 per cent in 1975–76 to 11 per cent in 1981–82.[60]

Ohara and coworkers reviewed the Japanese literature on OCD and found prevalence rates ranging from 2.4 to 28 per cent for various kinds of employment.[73] Only patients needing medical care or having more severe symptoms were included.

In a Japanese study of 339 cash register operators, 81 per cent reported shoulder stiffness and 49 per cent reported right shoulder pain.[73] Neck pain was differentiated from shoulder pain and was reported in 31 per cent. By comparison, symptoms in the wrist were reported in 13 per cent, in the hand in 19 per cent, and in the fingers in 13 per cent. Other constitutional symptoms included general fatigue (82 per cent), headaches (59 per cent), insomnia (27 per cent), and low back pain (42 per cent). All of these symptoms were significantly more common in cash register operators than in other office machine operators and other office workers. Theoretical explanations for this difference included the standing position with frequent twisting and the inappropriate height of the working surface.

Constitutional symptoms are a common part of OCD. In an article on clinical features of OCD, Miyake and associates suggest that the initial symptoms involve the shoulder and neck and that later, varied constitutional symptoms follow as the condition progresses.[66] Ohara and coworkers' study of cash register operators found that constitutional symptoms of generalized fatigue were about equal to shoulder stiffness and more prevalent than shoulder pain.[73] Some investigators suggest that high levels of stress and subsequent muscle tension predispose to OCD.

Other occupations requiring fine movements in static shoulder postures also cause OCD symptoms. Fry studied a group of 279 musicians, 75 per cent of whom developed pain in their shoulders, neck, and upper extremities severe enough to prevent them from playing their instruments.[29]

Westerling and Jonsson, in a cross-sectional study in Sweden, actually found a negative correlation between heavy work and neck and shoulder problems.[97] Their study included 2537 workers. Females who had to lift weights of 40 kg and males who had to lift 60 kg had significantly less shoulder and neck pain than those who did lighter lifting or did not lift at all. This does not indicate that heavy lifting prevents neck and shoulder problems but results from the fact that OCD is more prevalent among sedentary and light-assembly workers, and that those jobs do not require heavy lifting. Tendinitis, which is more common in jobs requiring higher upper-extremity loads, was lower overall in frequency than OCD.

Westerling and Jonsson also found that people with complaints from the neck and shoulder area took more sick leave for illnesses of all types than did job-matched controls.[97] Very few of the symptomatic individuals sought medical care for neck or shoulder pain. Within this group, women had significantly higher sickness absence than men. This may implicate a constitutional weakness or lack of adequate muscle conditioning. Social factors such as child care may also contribute.

In 1984 Sallstrom and Schmidt in Sweden compared the prevalence of OCD among cash register operators, office workers, and heavy-industry workers.[81] Forty-five per cent of all workers reported symptoms of OCD (60 per cent of all females and 34 per cent of males). This included 28 of 37 cash register operators, all of whom were female. Symptomatic office workers included 14 of 35 female (40 per cent) and 1 of 27 male (4 per cent). Included in these OCD groups were patients with findings attributed to thoracic outlet syndrome (TOS). Such a diagnosis was made in 32 per cent of cash register operators and 10 per cent of office workers. The diagnosis of TOS lacked precision, however, consisting of a history of numbness and paresthesias in one or both arms and a positive abduction–external rotation test.

Patients without findings of TOS followed the typical pattern of OCD described in other studies. It is unclear what proportion of OCD patients in other studies might have demonstrated findings of thoracic outlet syndrome if they had been specifically sought. Sällstrom and

Schmidt found symptoms of TOS in 9.5 per cent of 63 young, healthy subjects used as a control group.[81] Female predominance in TOS is well established; their study showed a female-to-male ratio of 2.5 to 1. Cash register operators had twice the incidence of heavy-industry workers. Symptoms of TOS seem to be more a function of posture than load.

Maeda and coworkers studied 270 female Japanese light-industry workers (cigarette manufacturer); 117 had OCD symptoms, and coldness and numbness of the hands was found in 20 to 40 per cent.[62] The correlation of these symptoms with severity of OCD was very high ($p < 0.05$). This may well implicate a component of TOS.

ETIOLOGY

It seems clear that reports of OCD encompass several disorders, including myositis, tendinitis, arthritis, and TOS. The latter three have fairly distinct physical findings. The most common form of OCD, however, involves intermittent myalgia in response to quite moderate static loading of long duration. Initial attempts to identify pathological changes have been fruitless. Because of this and because of the common association of OCD with "functional" disorders like generalized fatigue, headaches, and insomnia, many investigators have implicated emotional stress as an important etiological factor. The reported incidence of OCD has increased dramatically in the 1980s and has reached epidemic proportions in Australia. This trend has caused some investigators to implicate the patient's belief system, i.e., the worker is taught to consider shoulder girdle pain as a symptom of disease rather than normal fatigue.[5, 60]

The Australian epidemic of RSI has been the subject of much controversy over the last several years.[45, 52, 58, 60, 67] At Telecom Australia, a telecommunications company with 90,000 employees, the rate of RSI began to rise late in 1983, peaked in late 1984 (at a level about 30 times higher than in 1982), and declined in 1985 to reach 1983 levels by 1987.[45] Hocking reviewed different explanations for the rise and decline, including the ergonomic, new technology, and psychosocial theories.[45] He concluded that none of these theories fully explained the epidemic. Little evidence was found of a dose-response relationship of RSI to keystroke rate, age, and job duration. The condition was not related to new technology, and psychosocial factors could not explain the uneven distribution among similar groups of workers and among different states. Kiesler and Finholt postulated that the RSI epidemic in Australia was more indicative of social problems than of workplace factors and that dissatisfaction is a major contributor, as well as social legitimization of RSI complaints.[52]

In essence, two opposing theories exist to explain the rise in incidence of OCD. The *organic* theory relates shoulder pain to overuse caused by static over-

load. The increasing frequency of symptoms, then, is the result of increased automation and computerization, which have created jobs requiring static shoulder postures. These jobs are often sedentary and monotonous, creating a "nonphysiologic, stressful environment." Keyboard operators and many groups of light assembly workers hold the shoulder in a static posture of slight abduction and forward flexion (Fig. 29–1). From that basic posture they perform fine upper-extremity movements at very high frequency—80,000 keystrokes per day are not uncommon. In many instances, a high level of background noise is also a factor causing psychological stress. This stress adds to muscle tension, compounding the problem.

The opposing theory may be termed the *psychosocial*. It contends that shoulder myalgia occurs in jobs in which there is "normal" muscle fatigue and that modern jobs do not result in excessive muscle strain. The increased frequency of worker complaints has nothing to do with overuse but is the result of increased awareness and the belief that shoulder muscle pain is abnormal and indicative of a disease state requiring medical attention. There is also the fear that, if it is ignored, it may progress and become permanently incapacitating. The compensation system certainly can contribute to the psychosocial problem by awarding compensation based on subjective complaints.

Research into the physiological theory is gradually producing supporting evidence. Study techniques include observational techniques, the use of biomechanical models, electromyographic studies of muscle activities with surface and intramuscular electrodes, muscle biopsies, and serum enzyme analyses.

Because static load of the shoulder muscles has been considered such an important etiological factor, the literature on this subject will be reviewed in some detail. Pure static load (continuous unchanged isometric contraction) is rare; usually a superimposed dynamic component is present (Fig. 29–2). The level of activity at which a static contraction can be sustained without negative effects is not specifically known. Rohmert[79] determined that the endurance limit for a muscle in a continuous static contraction was 15 per cent of the maximum voluntary contraction (MVC). The endurance limit was defined as the highest force possible to maintain for an "unlimited" period of time. Other studies have revealed that the endurance limit beyond one hour is about 8 per cent of the MVC.[11] In continuous dynamic contractions, alternating between concentric and eccentric, the endurance limit is about the same.[33] Elevation of an unloaded arm will result in rapid and significant fatigue in several shoulder muscles, as will repetitive arm elevations.[34]

To prevent negative effects of static muscle load, Jonsson suggested that the static load level always be below 5 per cent of the MVC.[47] Although this is an empirical value, it is supported by some recent investigations of the effect of static load on skeletal muscle. Sjogaard and coworkers have demonstrated that muscular fatigue occurs at 5 per cent of the MVC after one hour.[87]

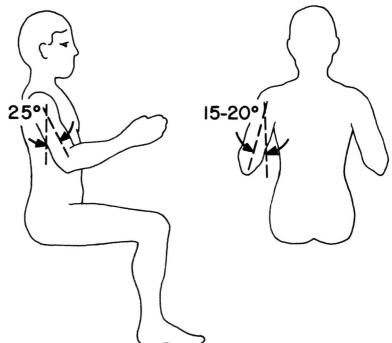

Figure 29–1. Typical shoulder position for keyboard operation requiring slight forward flexion and abduction.

The trapezius muscle is affected by fatigue in many different jobs. These include light electronic assembly,[31a, 47a] floor mopping,[40a, 97c] coffee serving (by flight attendants),[97d] meat cutting,[35b] forwarder operating,[47b] pillar drilling,[18] typewriting,[11a] and sawing, hammering, and nailing.[45a]

Christensen studied 25 electronics assembly workers with surface electromyography of the deltoid, infraspinatus, and trapezius muscles.[18] Of these, 56 per cent reported shoulder pain and 65 per cent reported neck pain. About half (48 per cent) of the subjects had pain in both areas. It is not stated whether any had lost time from work because of these symptoms, but no attempt had been made to change job procedures. The mean power frequency (MPF) was calculated over a two-minute period of sustained contraction at 20 per cent of the MVC. Christensen found no significant difference between morning and afternoon values during an eight-hour work day, indicating that the muscles over the work day did not change their response to a sustained contraction.

The static contraction levels recorded during work were found to exceed currently recommended levels of 2 to 5 per cent of the MVC (deltoid 6.6 per cent, infraspinatus 13.2 per cent, and trapezius 14.9 per cent). It should be mentioned, however, that recommended levels are not well determined, being empirical rather than physiological.

Hagberg and Kvarnstrom studied 10 patients who had shoulder/neck pain of at least one year's duration.[36] Nine of the 10 had been off work for one year. Standard rheumatic and neuromuscular disorders were ruled out. Pain was localized to the shoulder/neck region, and the only objective finding was local tenderness. All 10 were involved in either assembly-line or coil-winding operations that involved high repetition and static shoulder activities. Muscle fatigability (endurance) was evaluated by electromyography in terms of myoelectrical amplitude increase and MPF decrease. Surface electrodes were used on the trapezius, and intramuscular electrodes in the supraspinatus. A standardized work simulation position was utilized with the shoulder held at 30 degrees of forward flexion and the elbow at 90 degrees flexion. Fatigue occurred significantly faster on the painful side than on the pain-free side ($p < 0.01$). The data, therefore, appear to docu-

Figure 29–2. The root mean square (RMS) value of an electromyographic (EMG) signal during static work with superimposed minor dynamic activities. Note that the activity level never drops to zero. There is always a "static" component resulting in muscular activity. (Redrawn with permission from Jonsson B: The static load component in muscle work. Eur J Appl Physiol 57:305–310, 1988.)

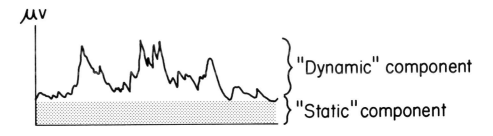

ment the presence of an organic abnormality on the symptomatic side.

Several possible etiologies have been proposed. Awad has theorized that interstitial myofibrositis causes reduced blood flow and more rapid onset of ischemia and muscle fatigue. Degenerated mitochondria and increased glycogen deposits have been demonstrated by Fassbender and Wegner.[26] Increased plasma myoglobin levels have been correlated with muscle tension by Danneskiold-Samsøe and coworkers.[20] The effects of disuse and overprotection may well account for the difference in fatigability found in the group of 9 who had been off work for one year. Eight of the 10 subjects had right-sided symptoms, but dominance is not specified. It is unclear how much they favored or protected their more symptomatic side or in what activities they engaged while on sick leave. Strength testing was not done and age, sex, and anthropometrically matched controls were not evaluated.

Erdelyi and coworkers in Hungary and Sihvonen and associates in Finland[24] studied a group of 14 secretaries using word processors. Eight of the 14 had OCD symptoms, while 6 did not. Surface electrodes were used to measure the mean electrical activity of the trapezius muscles in a controlled work setting. When performing identical tasks, the symptomatic group registered significantly higher levels than the asymptomatic group; within the symptomatic group, higher values were noted on the painful side.

Keyboard work position of the shoulder and arms alone is not sufficient to explain the high static loads of the trapezius that have been measured electromyographically. Chaffin and Andersson calculated the glenohumeral joint torque under average keyboard work conditions at 1 to 2 newton meters.[16] According to Hagberg, glenohumeral joint torque has an almost 1 to 1 relation to the load on the upper trapezius.[32] Given a torque of 1 to 2 newton meters, this would represent only 3 per cent of the MVC. Measured contraction levels, especially in symptomatic individuals, are much higher than this. Hagberg and Sundelin suggest that excessive scapular elevation on the basis of stress may account for some of the increased trapezius load.[38]

Onishi and colleagues measured the static load of the trapezius by electromyographic techniques in 41 keyboard operators.[74] They recorded activity levels of 20 to 30 per cent of the MVC during periods of rapid activity. Sustained contractions were common through nearly the entire operating time. These levels are much higher than those calculated by Chaffin and Andersson.[16] Onishi and coworkers found that, in most instances, the keyboards were too high for the individuals involved.[74] This would result in either increased scapular elevation—substantially increasing the load on the trapezius, as theorized by Hagberg and Sundelin[38]—or increased abduction of the arms, or both. Onishi and coworkers also measured the mean tenderness threshold in the midportion of the trapezius.[74] It was found to substantially decrease during the work week; this

was interpreted as an indication of increased muscle irritability.

Bjelle and associates studied 20 consecutive patients—all assembly line workers—with neck and shoulder pain.[10] Seven were found to have underlying pathology, e.g., cervical ribs, well-defined tendinitis, or arthritis. Of the 13 who had no demonstrable underlying pathology, 8 showed significant elevation of muscle enzymes (creatine phosphokinase and aldolase) that resolved after two to eight weeks of sick leave. All 13 patients had tasks requiring hand elevation above the acromion. Their work required greater frequency and longer duration of abduction and forward flexion than that of 26 asymptomatic controls matched for age, sex, and place of work (Fig. 29–3).

Muscle enzyme elevation and decrease in electromyographic MPF are both thought to occur on the basis of muscle ischemia.

Both Z-disc ruptures in muscle fibers and hydroxyproline elevation have been reported after heavy exercise. Proper training reduces these effects. Disc ruptures may cause muscle pain by release of metabolites, causing edema and pain-receptor stimulation. This mechanism of pain is probably quite uncommon in the workplace. Work rarely requires exertions at the levels studied; it is possible, of course, that this mechanism could apply to occasional high-level workload situations.[35]

Hagberg and colleagues studied serum creatine kinase (SCK) levels in controlled exercises and work settings.[37] They found significant elevations lasting for 24 to 48 hours after "lifting work" but not after bicycle ergometry, despite the fact that the latter involved four times as much work. Six of 10 subjects developed shoulder pain with the lifting task. During work, elevated SCK levels were found among welders, cash register operators, and assemblers but not among controllers and fork-lift drivers.

The mechanism of SCK release is theorized to result from sustained high load, especially static, which results in severe adenosine triphosphate depletion, increased permeability, and release of SCK. After complete depletion, replacement of glycogen stores requires 24 to 48 hours.[39]

In a recent review article, Edwards proposed that occupational myalgia results from an imbalance in the use of muscles for postural activity (holding or supporting fine movements) compared with phasic use in dynamic work.[23] This would tend to move the emphasis away from the muscle itself to an alteration in central motor control, resulting in the imbalance between recruitment and relaxation of muscle motor units. This would explain the apparent importance of mental stress to the occurrence of these disorders, and also why a more skilled worker seems to have less risk of symptoms than an unskilled worker. Edwards' theory does not contradict the almost general agreement on muscle load as a major etiological factor.[85]

Several different methods have been developed to analyze the workplace with respect to shoulder loads.

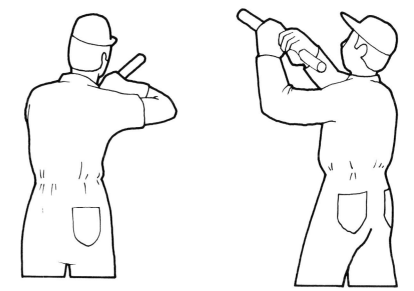

Figure 29-3. Typical shoulder position for much heavy industry requiring acromion-level upper-arm position. This example is from an automobile assembly line.

It is beyond the scope of this chapter to review all of them. The interested reader is referred to the works by Chaffin and Andersson,[16] Corlett and associates,[18a] Hagberg,[35a] and Westgaard.[97a] Measurements using electromyography can be used, as discussed frequently in this chapter; different biomechanical model approaches are also currently used and evaluated. Usually these mesurement methods and more sophisticated analyses are more suitable for research than for routine work analysis. To the latter purpose a number of observational methods have emerged, usually employing video technique. Two of these methods are mentioned here as examples of current development.

Persson and Kilbom developed a video recording technique to study work movements.[75] Workers were recorded from two angles and the data subjected to microcomputer analysis in terms of movement pattern for shoulders and neck. Melin utilized this Video Registration and Analysis (VIRA) in the telephone industry in Sweden to compare symptomatic and asymptomatic individuals.[64] Subjects with OCD were found to have "significantly higher loading resulting from moving their arms forward and outward in their work than those in the problem-free control group."

Keyserling from the Center for Ergonomics at the University of Michigan has developed a simplified modification of VIRA.[51] The trunk, left shoulder, and right shoulder are analyzed on separate replays of a video recording made from a single angle and replayed in real time. Microcomputer analysis is similar to VIRA.

Shoulder Tendinitis

Tendinitis about the shoulder is common in industry and usually is much more distinct than OCD. Physical findings of focal tenderness, subacromial crepitation, pain with specific motions, and, sometimes, palpable tissue thickening often make the diagnosis quite straightforward. As discussed elsewhere in this text, other studies can then be done to confirm the diagnosis. Degenerative changes in the rotator cuff may be evident on magnetic resonance imaging, arthrography, or ultrasonography. Eventual rupture of the supraspinatus, infraspinatus, or long head of the biceps tendon may occur as a result of chronic peritendinous inflammation, hypovascularity, fiber degeneration, and impingement; the mechanisms have been well described.[7, 78] Shoulder tendinitis and rotator cuff tears tend to occur under different occupational demands than does OCD.

EPIDEMIOLOGY

Herberts and coworkers in 1981 compared the frequency of supraspinatus tendinitis in welders with that in office clerks.[43] Shoulder pain was reported by 27 per cent of the former compared with 2 per cent of the latter. On examination, 8 per cent of the welders were diagnosed as having supraspinatus tendinitis. The average age of the office workers was greater than that of the welders, but the prevalence of supraspinatus tendinitis in the latter was not age dependent.

Further investigation of the problem of rotator cuff tendinitis in shipyard workers was published by Herberts and coworkers in 1984.[44] Supraspinatus tendinitis was present in 18.3 per cent of welders and 16.2 per cent of plate workers. Both of these occupations involve heavy manual labor. Hagberg and Wegman[39] reviewed the literature and calculated odds ratios for the shipyard welders in these studies. The odds ratio is an estimate of the incidence rate ratio of exposed to nonexposed, and in the welders it was found to be 13. In another industrial group exposed to work tasks above the shoulder level, the odds ratio was 11.[10]

ETIOLOGY

Requirements common to all the jobs discussed in the above studies are frequent arm elevation and the use of heavy hand tools (Fig. 29–4). These two load factors cause high shoulder muscle loads, especially of the supraspinatus and infraspinatus muscles. Increased load can cause pain by energy depletion, ultrastructural rupture,[44] and tendon ischemia. Sustained strain reduces blood flow to the subacromial segment of the supraspinatus tendon, which is marginal under normal circumstances. Subacromial and coracoacromial arch impingement compounds the problem.[69] Chronic inflammation, tendon degeneration, reactive hyperplasia, and shoulder-girdle muscle atrophy may follow with eventual rupture of the rotator cuff. Rathbun and Macnab found microruptures and degeneration of the supraspinatus, biceps, and infraspinatus tendons in areas of relative avascularity, which were present in all these tendons.[78] These changes reduce the strength of the tendon and therefore increase the risk of failure (tear). The degenerative changes increase with advancing age.[13] Any shoulder activity that contributes to increasing the avascularity for periods of time is a potential accelerator of the degenerative process and increases the risk of failure. Such ischemic effects can be due to constant tension on the supraspinatus tendon from working with abducted and flexed arms.[42a, 83] Other mechanisms include direct compression of the tendon from the humeral head[78] and the presence of acromioclavicular osteophytes.[77]

Rupture of the long head of the biceps tendon and acromioclavicular arthritis can also result from static and frequent dynamic loading of the shoulder. In the general population these problems occur most frequently in the 40- to 50-year age range, when "natural" degeneration of the rotator cuff is thought to begin.[61]

Many investigators have studied the effect of upper extremity position and hand load on shoulder girdle musculature. Sigholm and coworkers used electromyographic signals to determine the contraction force of the deltoid (three parts), infraspinatus, supraspinatus, and trapezius.[86] Hand loads of 0, 1, and 2 kg had little effect on deltoid activity. Infraspinatus activity was particularly influenced by the hand load, whereas the trapezius and supraspinatus muscles were moderately affected.

As expected, the anterior deltoid is very active in forward flexion and the mid-deltoid in abduction. The trapezius is more active in abduction than in forward flexion. The supraspinatus and infraspinatus muscles behave in a very similar way in forward flexion and abduction; their activity increases with increasing flexion and abduction up to 45 degrees and then plateaus. Higher flexion angles had a negligible effect on shoulder muscle activity. It was concluded that shoulder muscle strain could be best reduced by keeping the upper arm as close to the side of the body as possible and by reducing the weight of hand tools. This is hardly surprising, based on mechanical theory.

Herberts and coworkers used electromyography to document muscle strain and fatigue.[44] The root-mean-square (RMS) value of the myoelectric signal, which is a measure of the amount of electrical activity in the muscle, was found to be largely proportional to muscle force output. Muscle fatigue was found to be associated with lower muscle-fiber firing frequency. This is probably the result of a decreased velocity of the depolarization wave, which is caused by metabolic changes resulting from ischemia due to sustained contraction of the muscle fibers.

Welders with shoulder pain were categorized by age and experience.[43, 44] As expected, the greatest shoulder muscle fatigue occurred in overhead work with the arm elevated and abducted; inexperienced workers showed fatigue more frequently than those with more experience, indicating learning effects. There was no evidence of fatigue when work was performed at shoulder level with the arm in less than 30 degrees of forward flexion. However, impingement becomes a greater problem when the shoulder is lightly extended and the arm is supported on the elbow. Welders who

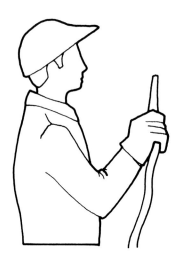
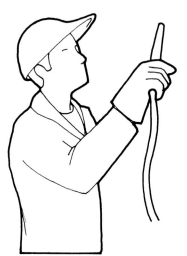

Figure 29–4. Work with the hand near eye level, typical for ship welders and much assembly line work. The mass of the hand tool is critical.

work with the shoulder in static positions were found to develop supraspinatus tendinitis earlier than plate workers, whose work was more dynamic.

As mentioned previously, the infraspinatus muscle is more influenced by hand load than any other shoulder muscle. For each kilogram of hand load, the RMS value increased 35 per cent in flexion and 41 per cent in abduction. The supraspinatus muscle showed increases of 22 per cent in flexion and 20 per cent in abduction for each additional kilogram; similar increases were found in the anterior deltoid (21 per cent and 16 per cent, respectively).[86]

Some studies have used intramuscular pressure measurements to determine muscle force. This is valid since it has been found that a near-linear relationship exists between muscle pressure and external load. Herberts and coworkers found that the supraspinatus intramuscular pressure levels are much higher than those in any other skeletal muscles tested.[44]

Although less common than rotator cuff disease, bicipital tendinitis can also result from certain work positions and repeated load. The long head of the biceps tendon differs from the rotator cuff in that it is completely surrounded by a synovial sheath within the intertubercular groove and is a truly intra-articular structure. As in the rotator cuff, chronic inflammation can predispose to rupture. Neviaser has shown that bicipital tendinitis can result from rubbing of the synovial sheath against the lesser tuberosity, which occurs with overhead work. Frequent contraction of the biceps has also been shown to cause peritendinitis of the tendon to the long head.

Degenerative Arthritis

The relationship between osteoarthritis of the shoulder and occupational factors other than direct trauma is unclear. A few studies lend support to the theory that specific occupations increase the risk of osteoarthritis of the glenohumeral joint.

Katevuo and coworkers compared farmers and dentists in Finland.[47c] Of 40 dentists over 49 years of age, 46 per cent had radiographic evidence of osteoarthritis, with 44 per cent showing bilateral changes. In contrast, of 83 farmers only 11 (13 per cent) showed findings of osteoarthritis.

Cervical and lumbar spine changes were also evaluated. Fifty-two per cent of the dentists showed cervical spine changes compared with 19 per cent of the farmers. In the lumbar spine, the findings were reversed; spondylosis occurred in 22 per cent of the dentists and 43 per cent of the farmers.

Dentists' work requires sustained static load on the shoulder and cervical spine with the shoulder in moderate forward flexion and abduction. Moderate scapular elevation is required, resulting in high sustained static loads on the glenohumeral joint. This ergonomic situation may well result in progressive degenerative arthritis, but the data at this time are limited and can only generate hypotheses. The high but dynamic loads of farm work appear to result in less shoulder and cervical spine arthritis. The increased loads in lifting, however, take their toll on the lower back.

Bovenzi and colleagues in Italy found radiographic changes of shoulder osteoarthritis in 12 per cent of 67 shipping and grinding operators and in 24 per cent of heavy manual laborers.[12] Both groups had an average age of 39 years. These values are similar to those of the Finnish farmers.

Arthritis of the glenohumeral joint is comparatively rare. Sternoclavicular arthritis is more common and not infrequently symptomatic according to Yood and Goldenberg.[99] Worchester and Green found no relationship between sternoclavicular osteoarthritis and occupation.[98]

Acromioclavicular joint changes are more common than osteoarthritis in the glenohumeral joint. DePalma found changes in almost all subjects after age 50,[21] whereas Petersson frequently observed changes in 30- to 50-year-old individuals and regularly in people 60 years and older.[77] Degeneration occurred as often in women as in men and with the same severity in the left and right shoulders, again making occupation an unlikely cause.

Kellgren and Lawrence and later Lawrence found that the prevalence of degeneration of the glenohumeral joint in men was influenced by occupation.[49, 57a] Petersson, on the other hand, did not find a correlation and, in addition, found degeneration to be more prevalent in women.[76] Cartilage degeneration and rotator cuff degeneration were found to occur at the same time in 76 per cent of shoulders and were usually bilateral, making work factors less likely as causes. Not a single shoulder exhibited degeneration before age 60.

Prevention

There are four basic approaches to the prevention of shoulder disorders in industry: (1) workplace design, (2) work method design, (3) worker selection, and (4) worker training. The first two fit the job to the worker; the second two fit the worker to the job. Each of these approaches has advantages and drawbacks. Although workplace and work method designs require little participation on the part of the worker, they will influence every worker, and sometimes they require major investments. Worker selection is inexpensive but is not developed to a point where it presents an ethically and legally viable option, and therefore it is rarely used for shoulder disorders. Worker training is theoretically attractive but requires active participation on the part of the worker.

WORKPLACE DESIGN

How the work is designed determines the stress imposed on the worker's shoulder. The overall work layout, the muscle forces needed to perform a job, the static component of the work task, the body movements required, and the design of the work tools all require consideration.

The overall layout is critical in a processing industry because the flow of materials determines when and how the worker is involved. The equipment used must not only be able to do the job but must also fit the worker. Dimensions and space requirements often influence the way work can be performed and therefore also dictate the load on the shoulder.

Shoulder loads occur primarily from three sources: the position of the arm, the external load handled, and the movements of the arm. The effect of holding the arm in different positions has been discussed previously in this chapter. The weight of the arm and the location of its center of mass relative to the shoulder determine the external shoulder moment that must be balanced by the shoulder muscles. The weight of the arm is about 5 per cent of the total body weight; its center of mass is about halfway between the shoulder and the wrist joints. The moment created by holding the arm straight out is about 15 to 20 per cent of the maximum

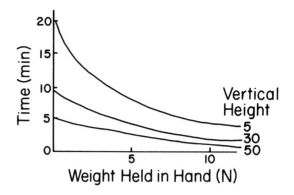

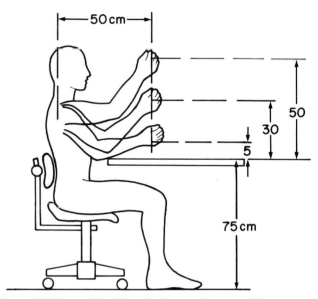

Figure 29–6. Expected time before significant shoulder muscle fatigue develops for different arm flexion postures. (Redrawn with permission from Chaffin DB: Localized muscle fatigue—definitions and measurement. J Occup Med 15:346–354, 1973.)

strength for women and 10 to 15 per cent for men (Fig. 29–5). Chaffin's studies of the average time that the arm can be held in various elevated positions are illustrated in Figures 29–6 and 29–7 as examples of the influence of flexion and abduction, respectively, on the shoulder muscle.[15] The larger the flexion angle and/or abduction angle, the higher is the load moment and the earlier fatigue will develop. This effect also occurs from forward-reach arm postures (Fig. 29–8).

A load held in the hand will increase the moment acting on the shoulder in proportion to its weight and its perpendicular distance to the shoulder joint. Large moments can occur on the shoulder from such activities. For example, if the arm is held nearly horizontal and reaching forward and a 5-kg (10-pound) load is lifted, the load moment at the shoulder will be equivalent to the flexor muscle strength of an average female worker.[16] The equivalent load for a male is about 11 kg (24 pounds). Essentially, this means that even small loads cannot be supported for long periods by the shoulder muscles. To aid in work requiring such activities, therefore, forearm supports or arm slings should be used and tools should be suspended from a tool

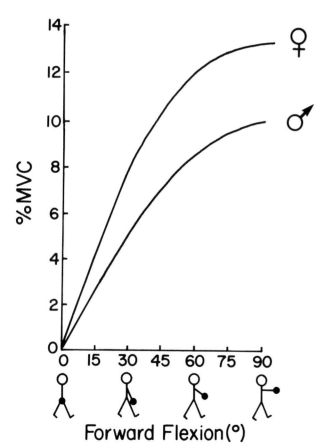

Figure 29–5. The shoulder-moment in percent of the maximum voluntary contraction as a function of forward flexion of the arm. (Modified from Hagberg M: The importance of the work environment to painful conditions of the shoulder joint and cervical spine. Stockholm: Swedish Work Environment Fund, 1988.)

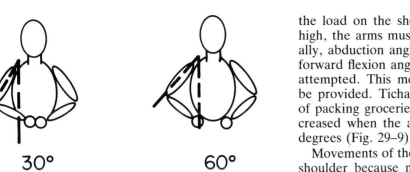

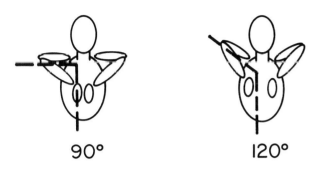

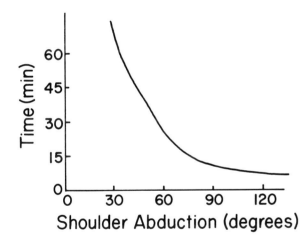

Figure 29–7. Expected time before significant shoulder muscle fatigue develops for different arm abduction angles. (Modified from Chaffin DB: Localized muscle fatigue—definitions and measurement. J Occup Med 15:346–354, 1973.)

the load on the shoulder. If the work surface is too high, the arms must be elevated or abducted. Generally, abduction angles of 15 to 20 degrees or less and forward flexion angles of 25 degrees or less should be attempted. This means that adjustable tables should be provided. Tichauer found that the metabolic cost of packing groceries increased while performance decreased when the arm abduction angles exceeded 20 degrees (Fig. 29–9).

Movements of the arm contribute to the load on the shoulder because muscle contractions are needed to accomplish them. As discussed previously, rapid movements have a similar effect on the shoulder muscles as continuous static loading. Generally, the larger the movement, the faster it is, and the farther away from the shoulder the center of mass, the more the shoulder will be loaded.

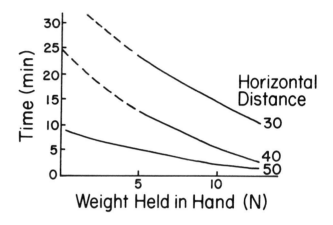

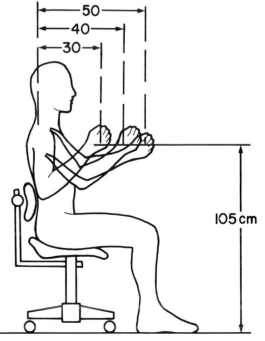

Figure 29–8. Expected time before significant shoulder muscle fatigue develops for different forward-reach arm postures. (Redrawn with permission from Chaffin DB: Localized muscle fatigue—definitions and measurement. J Occup Med 15:346–354, 1973.)

balancer whenever possible. Arm and forearm postures, and therefore shoulder loads, are influenced by the orientation of the hand. If the hand is supinated, the arm will usually be adducted and close to the trunk; if pronated, the arm will be more abducted and elevated. Therefore, if a screw is to be turned clockwise (supination), the elbow flexion angle should be 90 degrees or more and the shoulder adducted.[94]

Abduction seems to be particularly damaging to the shoulder because the rotator cuff muscles provide the main counterbalancing moment. This is also true when working in sitting postures. The vertical height of the work surface or the work piece is crucial in determining

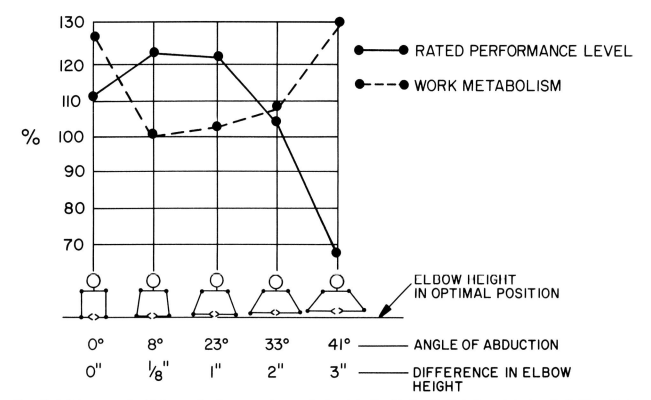

Figure 29–9. Performance and metabolic expenditure in grocery packers as a function of shoulder abduction. (Modified with permission from Chaffin DB, and Andersson GBJ: Occupational Biomechanics. New York: John Wiley, 1984.)

Table 29–1 illustrates different parameters influencing the shoulder load and examples of how to reduce those loads. Keyserling and coworkers[51a] have reviewed different occupational risk factors for shoulder disorders and suggest the following guidelines for preventing "awkward" shoulder postures caused by reach requirement. Generally, the lower the reach target, the better is the posture. As illustrated in Figure 29–10, there is an area of joint reach limits between males and females. The work station design should satisfy the reach limits of a small female. By keeping the reach target below the shoulder height of a small female, most cases of severe shoulder flexion and abduction can be avoided. This means that objects should not be stored above 126 cm. The maximum reach radius for the small female is 66.5 cm.

WORK METHOD DESIGN

Because static loading of the shoulder appears to be such an important factor in the etiology of occupational shoulder disorders, and because the task may require static postures to be maintained for long periods of time, the work method is an important tool in reducing the negative effects of such loads on the shoulder. Two principal methods exist—rest breaks and job rotation.

The issue of rest breaks has been particularly controversial in Video Display Terminal (VDT) work. Zwalen and coworkers found advancing musculoskeletal discomfort over a day's VDT work, even though the physical environment was ergonomically sound.[100] Although there is some agreement that rest breaks are helpful, the information is insufficient to specify the optimum length and frequency of such breaks. The National Institute of Occupational Safety and Health (NIOSH) recommended a 15-minute rest break after one or two hours of VDT work.[67] The Swedish National Board of Occupational Safety and Health suggested an upper limit of one to two hours of continuous VDT work.[91] Break frequency, duration, and content are all important factors in preventing shoulder disorders arising from static or highly repetitive work activities.

Hourly or more frequent work breaks have been

Table 29–1. PARAMETERS INFLUENCING SHOULDER LOAD AND METHODS TO REDUCE LOADS

Influencing Parameter	Load-reducing Factor	Examples
Moment arm	Reduce horizontal distance	1. Move work piece, etc. closer 2. Stand or sit close to the workplace 3. Slope the work surface
	Adjust vertical height	1. Adjust table height, etc. 2. Adjust chair height 3. Slope the work surface
External load	Reduce load magnitude	1. Divide into several loads 2. Choose light tools 3. Use tool balancer, etc.
	Provide arm support	1. Armrests 2. Balance slings

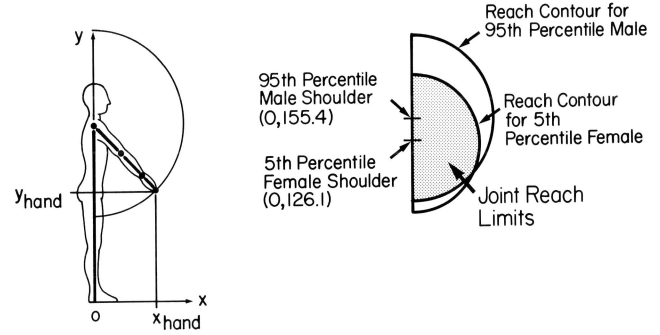

Figure 29–10. Maximum reach limits and the reach envelope for upright standing men and women. (Redrawn from Keyserling WM, Punnett L, and Fine LJ: Postural stress of the trunk and shoulders. *In* Ergonomic Interventions to Prevent Musculoskeletal Injuries in Industry. Chelsea, MI: Lewis Publishers, 1987, pp 11–26.)

found to increase productivity.[9, 19] Too-frequent breaks may interfere with work rhythms, however,[90] and regular breaks are preferable to irregular.[9] When considering muscle fatigue with respect to rest breaks in work characterized by constrained postures and static efforts, short rest breaks may be needed as often as every 10 to 20 minutes.[11, 46, 55, 82] The optimum length of the rest break depends on the length of a work spell and on the physical work load. A total break length of 5 to 10 per cent of the work day is often suggested,[17] preferably in several short breaks rather than a few long ones. Recovery from muscle fatigue is quite rapid except for the last few per cent up to full recovery.[31]

Sundelin and associates did not find effects of 14-second micropauses either on musculoskeletal discomfort or electromyographic recordings.[90] Active rest breaks have been the subject of considerable recent interest.[3a, 57b, 57c] The idea is to counteract stresses occurring from the work activity.

On the basis of a rather extensive literature on breaks, the following suggestions can be made: (1) regular, scheduled breaks of 5 to 10 minutes should be allowed at least on an hourly basis; (2) micropauses should be allowed every 10 to 15 minutes; and (3) breaks preferably should be active.

Job rotation can be an effective method to prevent static loading of select muscles. This requires, of course, that the jobs are sufficiently different to involve different groups of muscles and to alter the main posture. This solution can be more easily accomplished in assembly line work than in, for example, office work. The main disadvantages of job rotation are organizational, but workers also need to be trained to perform different activities, which can increase the initial cost. In a predominantly static work setting such

as the office, job rotation is a less attractive alternative than a well-planned rest break schedule simply because there is not often enough variation in work tasks, with respect to load on the shoulders.

WORKER SELECTION

To fit a worker to a job or to screen workers for job placement is a frequently used prevention method in industry but its reliability in preventing most shoulder injuries has not been established. Our present knowledge of the sensitivity, specificity, and predictive value of different screening methods is incomplete; consequently, we cannot advocate this method of prevention for all industrial shoulder problems. Clearly, the worker's dimensions should be suited to the work if the workplace cannot be changed, and the worker's strength should be adequate to perform the job. Workers with already existing shoulder problems are at higher risk of recurrence and may require modifications of their work places, tools, and tasks.

Pre-employment screening may help to identify the individual who is at high risk for OCD. This is especially important for entry-level employees. Most experienced workers have already undergone a natural selection process and proved that they can perform high-repetition work with sustained static load of shoulder girdle muscles without significant problems. However, poor ergonomic and environmental conditions in a new job may cause OCD even in an experienced worker with no history of it.

Kitayama divides screening criteria into "absolutely unsuitable" and "relatively unsuitable" categories.[53] Criteria that render an individual absolutely unsuitable include a history of OCD, sequelae of a whiplash syndrome, uncorrectable visual acuity problems, and upper-extremity functional disorders. It seems reasonable that a history of Grade I OCD (Table 29–2) that responded well to ergonomic changes, followed by an adequate asymptomatic period, would not disqualify an individual from the type of work in question; in fact, such a person might be less prone to OCD by virtue of learned adaptive work patterns and sensitivity to early signs of muscle fatigue. Relative unsuitability is based on mental conditions resulting in high external stress, extremely cold fingers and hands, and loose-jointedness. Cold hands may be functional or indicative of serious underlying disease, and a cause must be sought before work suitability can be determined. Raynaud's phenomenon qualifies an individual for Grade IV OCD in the Japanese classification and would render him or her a poor candidate for keyboard or high-repetition work if it occurred during such activity. Cold hands may be a sign of autonomic overload or thoracic outlet syndrome, either of which, if uncorrectable, is a strong negative factor for this type of work. Other literature does not substantiate loose-jointedness as a risk factor. Recurrent subluxation or dislocation of the shoulder, however, would seem to be a relative risk factor.

WORKER TRAINING

The simple biomechanical principles of safe work techniques should be explained to all workers. For the shoulder they include working with the arms in as little abduction and flexion as possible; handling loads close to the body; using both hands whenever possible; avoiding excessive and fast arm movements; taking breaks from static work activities; and supporting the arms, work pieces, and tools as much as possible. Shoulder education for patients in the form of "shoulder schools" are commercially available, as are "active rest break programs." The value of these has yet to be determined—certainly the shoulder school concept makes sense as secondary prevention.

DOES PREVENTION WORK?

In 1973, the Japanese Ministry of Labor issued guidelines about cash register work. They included job rotation, limitation of continuous time spent on keyboard work, and periodic medical examinations. Follow-up studies indicate that, at least in the short perspective, these changes did result in fewer complaints.[66a]

Spilling and coworkers[88a] have performed a cost-benefit analysis of improvements made in an electronics plant to reduce predominantly neck and shoulder disorders. The average sick leave for a musculoskeletal disorder was reduced from 5.3 to 3.1 per cent and long-term sick leave from 9.9 to 9.4 per cent. Further,

the labor turnover was reduced from 30.1 to 7.6 per cent.[97b] The economic savings turned out to be 10 times the investment in ergonomic improvements.

These are two examples of successful prevention efforts. Unfortunately, the literature is not very complete regarding this type of information. There is a fundamental need to develop follow-up analysis techniques to truly evaluate intervention effects.

Treatment

The discussion of treatment of occupational shoulder problems, following the same diagnostic classification as the prior sections on epidemiology and etiology, is divided into three anatomical groups: muscles (OCD), tendons (tendinitis), and joints (degenerative arthritis). The basic treatment of the latter two are discussed in detail in other chapters of this text. For the purpose of treatment as well as scientific study, it is important to separate these diagnoses because both etiology and treatment are different. Some patients will manifest involvement of more than one of these structures. As in all areas of medicine, treatment must be individualized. Detailed knowledge of the pathology and basic treatment is not enough in this patient group. Successful rehabilitation of the injured worker requires special understanding of workplace ergonomics so that residual impairment may be matched to job requirements. The unique psychosocial and economic aspects of occupational injuries are recognized as a crucial component, but one in which formal education is lacking; most musculoskeletal specialists are largely self taught.

The differential diagnosis of OCD is quite broad in addition to tendinitis and arthritis and must be considered at the time of initial evaluation. Neurological and vascular causes of shoulder girdle pain must be ruled out. A common component of cervical radiculopathy is interscapular pain. As described earlier, thoracic outlet syndrome is common and often presents with shoulder and upper extremity pain and paresthesias. Subscapular bursitis is not uncommon and can often be identified by subscapular popping or crepitation with resistive motion. Shoulder girdle osteochondromas can also cause this finding. Congenital or developmental deformities of the cervical spine or shoulder girdle can certainly predispose to OCD. The shoulder is a favored site of musculoskeletal neoplasms, both primary and metastatic, which, although rare, must be considered. Pain may also be referred to the shoulder girdle from other organ systems, especially gastrointestinal and pulmonary.

MYOGENIC PAIN IN OCD

Demonstrable pathology may be very elusive in the patient with mild OCD who presents with a complaint of shoulder girdle pain that resolves overnight. The

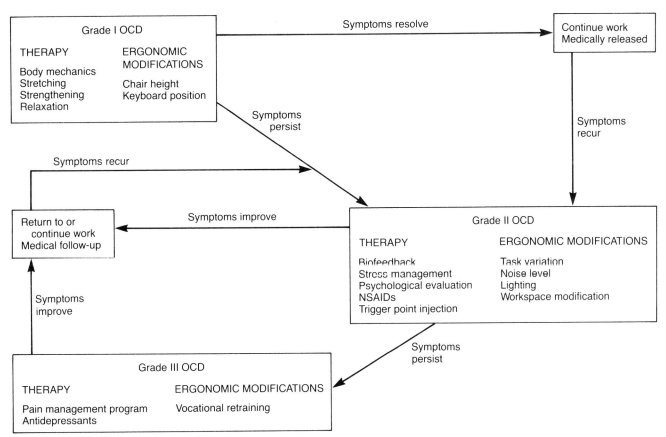

Figure 29–11. Sample algorithm for the treatment of occupational cervicobrachial disorders (OCD). Modifications should be made by the physician to include treatment preferences and methodologies of the workers' compensation system involved.

only physical finding may be mild focal tenderness over the upper trapezius or supraspinatus or along the vertebral border of the scapula at the attachment of the rhomboids or levator scapulae.

Under such circumstances, the examining physician is unable to document objective evidence of organic pathology. This frustrating scenario is all too familiar to the physicians and administrators who deal with industrial injuries. A patient management protocol or algorithm based on current knowledge is helpful in approaching such problems (Fig. 29–11). It provides consistency and quality assurance and reduces the frustration inherent in this situation.

A classification of disease severity is an essential element in the development of a treatment protocol. The OCD committee of the Japan Association of Industrial Health developed a five-grade classification, which included tendinitis and a broad range of neurological and vascular functional symptoms that accompany shoulder girdle muscle pain in some patients (Table 29–2). The Occupational Repetition Strain Advisory Committee in Australia developed a simplified three-stage system based on symptom persistence and interference with work (Table 29–3). We propose a modification of the Australian classification that focuses on the myogenic pain and attempts to relate it to a scientific model on the basis of the pathophysiological research performed to date (Table 29–4). Ten-

Table 29–2. JAPANESE GRADING SYSTEM

Grade I	Subjective complaints without clinical findings
Grade II	Subjective complaints with induration and tenderness of the neck, shoulder, and arm muscles
Grade III	Includes Grade II plus any of the following: 1. Increasing tenderness and/or enlargement of affected muscles 2. Positive neurological tests (Addison's test, Morley's test, and others) 3. Paresthesia 4. Decrease of muscle strength 5. Tenderness of spinous processes of the vertebrae 6. Tenderness of paravertebral muscles 7. Tenderness of nerve plexus 8. Tremor of hand and/or eyelid 9. Cinesalgia of the neck, shoulder, and upper extremity 10. Functional disturbance of peripheral circulation 11. Severe pain or subjective complaints of the neck, shoulder, or upper extremity

Grade IV	Divided into two groups:
	 1. Severe type of Grade III
	 2. Direct development from Grade II without passing through Grade III, but having specific findings as follows:
	   a. Orthopedic diagnosis of the neck-shoulder-arm syndrome
	   b. Organic disturbances such as tendinitis or tenosynovitis
	   c. Autonomic nervous disturbances such as Raynaud's phenomenon, passive hyperemia, or dysequilibrium
	   d. Mental disturbance such as anxiety, sleeplessness, thinking dysfunction, hysteria, or depression

Grade V	Disturbances not only at work but also in daily life

Table 29–3. AUSTRALIAN STAGING SYSTEM

Stage I	Aching and tiredness of the affected limb that occurs during the work shift but subsides overnight and during days off work. There is no significant reduction in work performance, and there are no physical signs. This condition can persist for months and is reversible.
Stage II	Symptoms fail to settle overnight, cause sleep disturbance, and are associated with a reduced capacity for repetitive work. Physical signs may be present. The condition usually persists for months.
Stage III	Symptoms persist at rest, sleep is disturbed, and pain occurs with nonrepetitive movement. The person is unable to perform light duties and experiences difficulty with nonoccupational tasks. Physical signs are present. The condition may persist for months to years.

dinitis and arthritis are separated from OCD. Constitutional or functional symptoms, which are often part of more severe OCD, are a manifestation of stress and indicate the need for appropriate evaluation and treatment of that component of the disease.

Treatment of Grade I or early OCD is based on the pathophysiological model that sustained static load causes metabolic changes that resolve gradually over 12 to 24 hours.[32, 35] A methodology for the measurement of the tenderness threshold using a strain gauge pressure sensor has been developed. In symptomatic individuals, this measurement improved (increased) overnight but gradually worsened (decreased) during the work week.[74] This is a subjective parameter. Test validity requires patient cooperation, and results are subject to conscious or unconscious control. Consistency is an important indicator of validity. This test, if validated, would be especially useful in the monitoring of progress with treatment.

In Grade I OCD, ergonomic modification that includes changes in work position and the insertion of frequent breaks or task variation may be all that is required for symptom resolution. Instruction in shoulder girdle range-of-motion and stretching exercises and muscle relaxation techniques, including surface electrode biofeedback training when available, is valuable in treatment and helps to prevent recurrence. Muscle relaxation training increases awareness of static muscle tension, allowing the patient to change his or her position and relax involved muscles earlier. This may prevent sustained static load from reaching a level that

Table 29–4. PATHOPHYSIOLOGICAL GRADING SYSTEM

Grade I (Mild)	Shoulder girdle muscle pain that occurs during work or similar activities and resolves a few hours later. No finding on physical examination.
Grade II (Moderate)	Shoulder girdle muscle pain that persists for several days after work. Muscle belly and insertional tenderness on examination.
Grade III (Severe)	Shoulder girdle muscle pain that is constant for weeks or longer. Multiple tender areas. Palpable induration indicative of muscle fibrosis. Muscle belly contracture. Reduced range of motion of myogenic origin.

causes metabolic changes and pain that are slow to reverse.

Grade II OCD is manifested by symptoms that do not resolve after a few hours off work. The theoretical pathophysiological model is one of low-grade inflammatory reaction and early interstitial fibrosis. At this time, muscle biopsy is only used for research and is not recommended as a diagnostic tool. Furthermore, because of local muscle damage and scar formation, it may actually compound the problem. Focal tenderness along the upper margin of the trapezius over the first rib may indicate a "trigger point" that will respond to injection with local anesthetic and a depositing cortisone acetate preparation. In some cases, this will give lasting relief and can be repeated every few months. More frequent injections should not be utilized because of the potential for local inflammation and fibrosis. Whereas patients in Group I do not require time off work, this group often does. Most can be treated by the methods described for Group I and returned to their prior occupation with ergonomic modifications. Some individuals in high-risk occupations will require vocational retraining for a different type of work.

Another research methodology that may be useful in the evaluation and treatment of OCD is electromyographic measurement of muscle fatigability. As described earlier, many investigators have correlated a decrease in MPF and an increase in myoelectrical amplitude with muscle fatigue. Hagberg and Kvarnstrom found a significant difference between symptomatic and asymptomatic sides in patients with long-standing OCD symptoms.[36] The test was done with surface electrodes on the trapezius and needle electrodes in the supraspinatus and was performed under conditions of a standardized static load. Subjects held the shoulders in 30 degrees of forward flexion with elbows flexed 90 degrees for as long as possible. Endurance time was correlated with the electromyographic changes. This technique is much more objective than the tenderness threshold and may have some use in the evaluation of Grades II and III OCD. As documented by Christensen, patients with mild OCD symptoms that do not require work modification will probably not demonstrate these electromyographic changes.[18]

Grade III OCD is the most advanced stage; the pathophysiological model is one of permanent myopathy with interstitial fibrosis, as described by Fassbender and Wegner.[26] Patients in this group have long-standing symptoms and can be expected to demonstrate a low tenderness threshold and rapid fatigability on the electromyographic static stress test. They will require placement in a type of work in which static load of shoulder girdle musculature is minimal. Dynamic loads may be better tolerated. Recommended levels could be best determined by preplacement functional testing.

A wide variety of constitutional or functional complaints have been associated with OCD.[73] The most common of these include generalized fatigue, headache, sleeplessness, and gastrointestinal upset. Coldness and paresthesias of the upper extremity may be functional and related to autonomic overload but may also be an indication of thoracic outlet syndrome causing either neurological or vascular encroachment; this is relatively common and must be ruled out.[81] Functional complaints have been associated with advanced grades of OCD in terms of the duration of symptoms and work incapacity, but they are not necessarily indicative of advanced pathophysiological changes of shoulder musculature. As mentioned earlier, we prefer a classification based on myopathy. Thoracic outlet syndrome is treated as an entity separate from OCD. The functional complaints listed above are treated as a manifestation of stress. Origins of stress may be classified into three groups with reference to the workplace: (1) external, (2) internal, and (3) physiological.

External stress is the result of personal factors outside the workplace. Individuals who have high levels of external stress are believed to be at greater risk of developing OCD when placed in high-repetition, static load positions. Increased baseline shoulder girdle muscle tension and a reduced ability to relax muscles, especially the upper trapezius, during high-repetition work are the theoretical reasons for this predisposition. Pre-employment screening is recommended in the Japanese literature; individuals with functional symptoms of the upper extremities or mental disturbances are considered unsuitable candidates for this type of work.[53]

Internal stress refers to factors in the workplace that increase worker stress levels. High background noise, suboptimal lighting, cramped work space, job dissatisfaction, inadequate work breaks, and excessive productivity demand have all been associated with OCD. Modification of these factors has resulted in a reduction in the incidence of OCD.

Physiological stress is secondary to the myalgia itself. A painful muscle is more difficult to relax, setting up a cycle that increases sustained static load levels and duration. Working in pain is stressful and may inhibit concentration, performance, and productivity. Grades II and III OCD are manifested by persistent pain that interrupts sleep, further increasing stress levels.

Evaluation of Impairment

The evaluation of musculoskeletal impairment is an almost inescapable part of today's orthopedic practice. Treatment of occupational shoulder problems includes evaluation and rating of permanent partial disability in patients who do not completely recover from their injuries. It is important that the evaluator clearly understands the difference between impairment and disability and is familiar with the various methods for the evaluation of physical impairment.

Disability is a broad term encompassing not only medical impairment but also educational level, work experience, motivation, emotional and psychological factors, age, socioeconomic background, and financial status. Medical impairment includes all medical disciplines, both physical and psychiatric. Physical impairment refers to an anatomical or physiological defect that hinders the individual's ability to perform certain functions in a standard fashion. He or she may be able to do any task but require modified techniques or assistive devices. Disability, on the other hand, refers to a performance incapacity—some activity or task that the individual cannot do. Many individuals have physical impairments for which they compensate and thus avoid disability. A dramatic example is the amputee skier. Kessler reported a paraplegic who continued working in high steel construction, climbing girders by the great strength in his arms.[50]

The disability evaluation process is both medical and administrative. Only a physician is qualified to determine medical impairment. In most states, the primary purpose of the orthopedic evaluation is to accurately and objectively determine impairment of the musculoskeletal system. Rating scales or guides assign values to specific anatomical defects or diseases that are estimated to represent an average percentage loss of potential function to that body segment and to the total body without reference to age, occupation, or other factors. Impairment rating is somewhat arbitrary and artificial because it does not consider the individual as a whole. Such a rating is only one step in the disability evaluation process. Functional evaluation and work restriction recommendations go beyond impairment rating into the realm of disability evaluation.

Many different systems for the evaluation of physical impairment and disability have been developed. Requisites for such a methodology include accuracy, objectivity, reproducibility, and, whenever possible, simplicity. No system perfectly fulfills all of these criteria. Impairment rating systems may be classified by orientation into (1) anatomical, based on physical examination findings; (2) pathological, based on diagnosis; and (3) functional, based on activity or work capacity.

ANATOMICAL SYSTEMS

The earliest disability systems were anatomical in their orientation and based on amputation or ankylosis, such as those used by the medieval guilds and some of the better organized 17th-century pirates. Esquemeling's journal, originally published in 1678, describes such a system in which a right arm was worth 600 pieces of eight, a right leg 500, and an eye 100.[8, 25] These disability schedules were simple, accurate, objective, and reproducible, but they were very limited in scope and covered only a small part of musculoskeletal pathology. They were gradually expanded to include partial loss of motion, weakness, and loss of sensation; this included much more musculoskeletal pathology but at the expense of objectivity, accuracy, and reproducibility.

Currently the most widely used evaluation guide is one developed in 1958 by the American Medical Association (AMA) and published as *Guides to the Evaluation of Permanent Impairment*. The third edition was released in 1988.[2] About half of the states in the United States suggest, and a few mandate, the use of the AMA *Guides* for the rating of permanent partial impairment. The musculoskeletal section is anatomical in its orientation and has evolved from those based on amputation and ankylosis. More recent editions have included more diagnosis-based impairment ratings to cover situations in which anatomical evaluation is not adequate.

Examination parameters include almost exclusively range of motion in the orthopedic section and sensation and muscle strength in the extremity part of the neurological section. These are "soft" rather than "hard" findings and are subject to conscious or unconscious control. Other, more objective parameters such as swelling, reflex changes, atrophy, radiographic changes, and laboratory abnormalities are not included.

The extremity section of the AMA *Guides* does not include a rating for non-neurological weakness or pain. Under such a system, a patient with a flail shoulder following a proximal humeral resection with severe muscle atrophy receives a minimal impairment rating because a good range of motion is preserved. By comparison, a patient with a fused shoulder in optimal position who can lift heavy objects and functions much better receives a much higher impairment rating because of loss of motion. A less extreme example is the patient with significant rotator cuff pathology in which weakness occurs through a certain arc of the total range. This weakness may not be very evident if only antigravity range is tested with resistance only at the end of the range, as is recommended in the extremity neurological section of the latest AMA *Guides*. Nevertheless, this patient may have a significant impairment that prevents him or her from performing many jobs that require frequent or sustained shoulder forward flexion and abduction. Cases like this obviously require a physician's judgment for proper rating; this is why the AMA text is termed a guide rather than a system. Several court decisions have supported the concept that no system, even if state mandated, can include all situations and that a physician's judgment is an essential component. It is also evident that combining elements of anatomical, diagnostic, and functional methods allows the greatest range of clinical situations to be covered.

In 1962, the American Academy of Orthopaedic Surgeons (AAOS) published the *Manual for Orthopaedic Surgeons in Evaluating Permanent Physical Impairment*, a condensed modification of the AMA *Guides*.[1] The committee responsible for the *Manual* included two of the most noted pioneers in disability evaluation: Earl D. McBride (chairman), who published his first of many works on the subject in 1936, and Henry H. Kessler, whose first book on the subject appeared in 1931.[50, 59] The *Manual* included a scale for pain that was in line with documented organic pathology and also gave impairment ratings for some orthopedic conditions and procedures not included in the AMA system. The AAOS *Manual* is currently undergoing extensive revision into a full-sized didactic and methodological text.

DIAGNOSTIC SYSTEMS

Physical impairment based on pathology or diagnosis has the advantages of objectivity, simplicity, and reproducibility. However, as both Kessler and McBride have clearly documented, the degree of impairment and the resultant disability for a given diagnosis are highly variable.[50, 59] In some instances, the diagnosis may be in question and vary from one evaluator to another. This is often the case when pain complaints are not specifically and directly attributable to clearly evident organic pathology. Therefore, a pathological basis for impairment rating has drawbacks and, in our opinion, is best used as an adjunct to other methodologies. Both the AMA *Guides* and the AAOS *Manual* use diagnoses for some conditions. Two current examples of systems more extensively based on diagnosis are the Social Security Administration's *Disability Evaluation Under Social Security*[88] and the Minnesota Medical Association's *Worker's Compensation Permanent Partial Disability Schedule*.[65]

Musculoskeletal disability qualifying for Title II or XVI of the Social Security system is based principally on diagnosis supported by specific criteria of the history, physical examination, radiography, and laboratory evaluation. This system requires total disability that must be expected to last for at least 12 months and is much more oriented to disease than to residuals of trauma. The Minnesota system was developed for the evaluation of permanent partial disability and utilizes diagnosis as an adjunct to the history, physical findings, and x-ray evaluation. In areas of the musculoskeletal system where range of motion is not a reliable evaluation method, such as the spine, documented pathology is used instead.

FUNCTIONAL SYSTEMS

Many scholars in this field have emphasized the desirability of a system based on function.[30, 50, 59] Function is the "bottom line" in the process of disability evaluation; administrators for worker's compensation want to know what the patient can do and what work restrictions are recommended. The California Division of Industrial Accidents developed a rating scale based in part on the work restrictions recommended by the physician.[22] In these cases the physician does not estimate the percentage of permanent physical impairment but instead submits a comprehensive report outlining subjective and objective factors of disability as well as recommended work restrictions. This report, along with other documents, is reviewed by a court-appointed administrator (a Disability Evaluation Specialist), who arrives at a partial permanent disability percentage. The schedule to which he or she refers includes anatomical, pathological, and functional factors as well as a pain scale and an age-factoring system.

As part of this process, the physician is provided with detailed job profiles and may be requested to estimate the length of time a patient can stand, sit, walk, bend, and stoop, as well as lifting capacity and postural considerations. This is the closest any system has come to a functional orientation. However, the answers to most of these questions represent intuitive estimates on the physician's part. In order for this type of system to be accurate and reproducible, we need objective methodologies of evaluating physical performance independent of motivation. Modern technology is developing tools that promise to improve our capacity to measure the strength and function of the spine and extremities.[30] Larger physical therapy units often include work capacity evaluation programs. These include a variety of function assessment methods, ranging from simple static and dynamic lifting tasks to costly computerized isokinetic testing. Currently these methods are best developed for evaluation of the hand and knee. The more central musculoskeletal sections, including the spine, hip, and shoulder, are more difficult to isolate and reliably assess. Because of the social and economic importance of disability evaluation, there is tremendous interest in and support for the study and development of functional assessment. If accuracy, reproducibility, and availability can be established, functional evaluation will play an increasing role in the estimation of musculoskeletal impairment and resultant disability.

APPORTIONMENT

In addition to rating permanent physical impairment, the physician is often called upon to determine what portion of the worker's problem is related to nonindustrial factors such as aging and the normal progression of degenerative processes. The 57-year-old dentist with degenerative arthritis of the shoulder and the 60-year-old ship welder with a rotator cuff tear are good examples of this dilemma. To what degree is the condition related to a claimed industrial injury? How much is the result of continuous trauma? How much should be apportioned to normal aging?

Deciding such questions is especially difficult when there is no history or prior medical record of a previous problem of this type, yet radiographs and physical findings suggest a long-standing condition. Epidemiological studies are sometimes helpful in resolving the question of apportionment. In both examples described above, we know that strong evidence exists relating these conditions to the work involved. In the absence of predisposing factors outside the job, such as previous

injury or involvement in a sport associated with shoulder problems, it seems likely that the condition is work related. In individuals for whom other factors do exist, such as a welder who played baseball for years, the assignment of apportionment percentages is, at best, a rough estimate lacking any scientific basis.

Some apportionment determinations should be legal rather than clinical constructs. An example would be a welder whose cuff degeneration is work related but who has worked for several employers over the span of his career. The physician should not hesitate to defer the rating of apportionment when there is no adequate clinical or scientific basis. When values are recommended by a medical evaluator, they must be supported by clinical and/or scientific evidence.

CONCLUSIONS

Each impairment rating system has its strengths and weaknesses. The optimal method would combine anatomical, pathological, and functional evaluations in a way most suitable to each part of the musculoskeletal system. Accuracy, objectivity, and reproducibility must be balanced against simplicity. No system can ever cover all clinical situations. Medical evaluation will always contain an element of judgment that reflects the physician's education and experience. The value of this essential component is in direct proportion to the physician's ability to support his or her opinion by comprehensive knowledge of the patient's problem and thorough understanding of the disability evaluation process.

References

1. American Academy of Orthopaedic Surgeons. Manual for Orthopaedic Surgeons in Evaluating Permanent Physical Impairment. Chicago: AAOS, 1962.
2. American Medical Association. Guides to the Evaluation of Permanent Impairment, 3rd ed. Chicago: AMA, 1988.
3. Aoyama H, O'Hara H, Oze Y, and Itani T: Recent trends in research on occupational cervicobrachial disorder. J Hum Ergol 8:39–45, 1979.
3a. Austin D: Tone Up at the Terminals. Sunnyvale, CA: Verbatim, 1984.
4. Awad EA: Interstitial myofibrosis: hypothesis of mechanism. Arch Phys Med Rehabil 54:449–453, 1973.
5. Awerbach M: RSI or "Kangaroo paw." Med J Aust 412:337–338, 1985.
6. Backman AL: Health survey of professional drivers. Scand J Work Environ Health 9:30–35, 1983.
7. Bateman J: The Shoulder and Neck. Philadelphia: WB Saunders, 1978.
8. Beals RK: Compensation and recovery from injury. West J Med 140(2):234–235, 1984.
9. Bhatia N, and Murrell KFH: An industrial experiment in organized rest pauses. Hum Factors 11:167–174, 1969.
10. Bjelle A, Hagberg M, and Michaelson G: Occupational and individual factors in acute shoulder-neck disorders among industrial workers. Br J Ind Med 38:356–363, 1981.
11. Bjorksten M, and Jonsson B: Endurance limit of force in long term intermittent static contractions. Scand J Work Environ Health 3:23–27, 1977.
11a. Bjorksten M, Itani T, Jonsson B, and Yoshizawa M: Evalu-

ation of muscular load in shoulder and forearm muscles among medical secretaries during occupational typing and some non-occupational activities. *In* Jonsson B (ed): Biomechanics X. Baltimore: University Park Press, 1987.

12. Bovenzi M, Fiorito A, and Volpe C: Bone and joint disorders in the upper extremities of chipping and grinding operators. Int Arch Occup Environ Health *59*:189–198, 1987.

13. Brewer JB: Aging of the rotator cuff. Am J Sports Med *7*:102–110, 1979.

14. Browne CD, Nolan B, and Faithful D: Occupational repetition strain injuries. Med J Aust *140*:329–332, 1984.

15. Chaffin DB: Localized muscle fatigue—definitions and measurement. J Occup Med *15*:346–354, 1973.

16. Chaffin DB, and Andersson GBJ: Occupational Biomechanics. New York: John Wiley, 1984.

17. Chapman LJ: Work Rest Schedules in Light Industrial and Office Work (Contract No. 86-71383). Cincinnati OH: National Institute of Occupational Safety and Health, 1986.

18. Christensen H: Muscle activity and fatigue in the shoulder muscles of assembly-plant employees. Scand J Work Environ Health *12*:582–587, 1986.

18a. Corlett N, Wilson J, and Manenica I: The Ergonomics of Working Postures. London: Taylor & Francis, 1986.

19. Dainoff MJ: Ergonomic Comparison of Video Display Terminal Work Stations. II: Effects of Work-rest Breaks. Cincinnati OH: National Institute of Occupational Safety and Health, 1985.

20. Danneskiold-Samsøe B, Christiansen E, Lund B, and Andersen R: Regional muscle tension and pain ("fibrositis"). Scand J Rehabil Med *15*:17–20, 1983.

21. DePalma AF: Degenerative Changes in the Sternoclavicular and Acromioclavicular Joints in Various Decades. Springfield IL: Charles C Thomas, 1957.

22. Division of Industrial Accidents of the State of California: Schedule for Rating Permanent Disabilities. Sacramento, 1978, p 13A.

23. Edwards RHT: Hypothesis of peripheral and central mechanisms underlying occupational muscle pain and injury. Eur J Appl Physiol *57*:275–281, 1988.

24. Erdelyi A, Sihvonen T, Helin P, and Hänninen O: Shoulder strain in keyboard workers and its alleviation by arm supports. Int Arch Occup Environ Health *60*:119–124, 1988.

25. Esquemeling J: The Buccaneers of America. New York: Dorset Press, 1987.

26. Fassbender H, and Wegner K: Morphologie und Pathogenese des Weichteilrheumatismus. Z Rheumaforsch *32*:355–374, 1973.

27. Foster CVL, Harman J, Harris RC, and Snow DH: ATP distribution in single muscle fibers before and after maximal exercise in the thoroughbred horse. J Physiol *378*:64P, 1986.

28. Friden J, Segar J, and Ekblom B: Sublethal muscle fiber injuries after high-tension anaerobic exercise. Eur J Appl Physiol *57*:360–368, 1988.

29. Fry HJH: Overuse injury in musicians—pathology, treatment, and prevention. Proceedings of Seminar of Repetition Strain Injury and Musicians, Melbourne, Australia, May 11, 1985. The Arts Health Advisory Committee of the Victorian Ministry of the Arts.

30. Frymoyer JW, and Mooney V: Occupational orthopaedics. J Bone Joint Surg *68A*:469–474, 1986.

31. Funderbunk CF, Hipskind SG, Welton RC, and Lind AR: Development and recovery from fatigue induced by static efforts at various tensions. J Appl Physiol *37*:392–396, 1974.

31a. Granstrom B, Kvarnstrom S, and Tiefenbacher F: Electromyography as an aid in the prevention of excessive muscle strain. Appl Ergonomics *16*:49–54, 1985.

32. Hagberg M: Work load and fatigue in repetitive arm elevations. Ergonomics *24*:543–555, 1981a.

33. Hagberg M: Muscular endurance and surface electromyogram in isometric and dynamic exercise. J Appl Physiol *51*:1–7, 1981b.

34. Hagberg M: Electromyographic signs of shoulder muscular fatigue in two elevated arm positions. Am J Phys Med *60*:111–121, 1981c.

35. Hagberg M: Occupational musculoskeletal stress and disorders of the neck and shoulder: a review of possible pathophysiology. Int Arch Occup Environ Health *53*:269–278, 1984.

35a. Hagberg M: Occupational Shoulder and Neck Disorders. Stockholm: The Swedish Work Environment Fund, 1987.

35b. Hagberg M, Jonsson B, Brundin L, et al: Musculoskeletal pain in butchers: an epidemiologic, ergonomic and electromyographic study [In Swedish]. Work and Health *12*:6–52, 1983.

36. Hagberg M, and Kvarnstrom S: Muscular endurance and electromyographic fatigue in myofascial shoulder pain. Arch Phys Med Rehabil *65*:522–525, 1984.

37. Hagberg M, Michaelson G, and Ortelius A: Serum creatine kinase as an indicator of local muscular strain in experimental and occupational work. Int Arch Occup Environ Health *50*:377–386, 1982.

38. Hagberg M, and Sundelin G: Discomfort and load on the upper trapezius muscle when operating a wordprocessor. Ergonomics *29*:1637–1645, 1986.

39. Hagberg M, and Wegman DH: Prevalence rates and odds ratios of shoulder-neck diseases in different occupational groups. Br J Ind Med *44*:602–610, 1987.

40. Hagg G, Suurkula J, and Liew M: A worksite method for shoulder muscle fatigue measurements using EMG, test contractions and zero crossing technique. Ergonomics *30*:1541–1551, 1987.

40a. Hagner IM, Hagberg M, Hammerstrom U, et al: Physical load when cleaning floors using different techniques [In Swedish]. Work and Health *29*:7–27, 1986.

41. Hammond G, Torgerson W, Dotter W, and Leach R: The painful shoulder. Instr Course Lect *20*:83–90, 1971.

42. Henriksson KC: Muscle pain in neuromuscular disorders and primary fibromyalgia. Eur J Appl Physiol *57*:348–352, 1988.

42a. Herberts P, and Kadefors R: A study of painful shoulder in welders. Acta Orthop Scand *47*:381–387, 1976.

43. Herberts P, Kadefors R, Andersson G, and Petersen I: Shoulder pain in industry: an epidemiological study of welders. Acta Orthop Scand *52*:299–306, 1981.

44. Herberts P, Kadefors R, Högfors C, and Sigholm G: Shoulder pain and heavy manual labor. Clin Orthop *191*:166–178, 1984.

45. Hocking B: Epidemiological aspects of "repetition strain injury" in Telecom Australia. Med J Aust *147*:218–222, 1987.

45a. Itani T, Yoshizawa M, and Jonsson B: Electromyographic evaluation and subjective estimation of the muscular load in shoulder and forearm muscles during some leisure activities. *In* Jonsson B (ed): Biomechanics X-A. Champaign: Human Kinetics Publishers, 1987, pp 241–247.

45b. Jones DA, Newham DJ, Round JM, and Tolfree SEJ: Experimental human muscle damage: morphological changes in relation to other indices of damage. J Physiol *375*:435–448.

46. Jonsson B: Kinesiology. With special reference to electromyographic kinesiology. Electroencephalogr Clin Neurophysiol [Suppl]*34*:417–428, 1978.

47. Jonsson B: The static load component in muscle work. Eur J Appl Physiol *57*:305–310, 1988.

47a. Jonsson B, Hagberg M, and Sima S: Vocational electromyography in shoulder muscles in an electronics plant. *In* Morecki A, Fidelus K, Kedzior K, and Wit A (eds): Biomechanics VII-B. Baltimore: University Park Press, 1981, pp 10–15.

47b. Jonsson B, Brundin L, Hagner IM, et al: Operating a forwarder: an electromyographic study. *In* Winter DA, Nouman RW, Wells RP, et al (eds): Biomechanics IX-B. Champaign: Human Kinetics Publishers, 1985, pp 21–26.

47c. Katevuo K, Aitasalo K, Lehtinen R, and Pietilä J: Skeletal changes in dentists and farmers in Finland. Commun Dent Oral Epidemiol *13*:23–25, 1985.

48. Keikenwan SI: Report of the Committee on Occupational Cervicobrachial Disorder of the Japan Association of Industrial Health, 1973.

49. Kellgren JH, and Lawrence JS: Rheumatism in miners. Part II: X-ray study. Br J Ind Med *9*:197–207, 1952.

50. Kessler H: Disability Determination and Evaluation, Philadelphia: Lea and Febiger, 1970.

51. Keyserling WM: Postural analysis of the trunk and shoulders in simulated real time. Ergonomics *29*:569–583, 1986.

51a. Keyserling WM, Punnett L, and Fine LJ: Postural stress of the trunk and shoulders: identification and control of occupational risk factors. In Ergonomic Interventions to Prevent Musculoskeletal Injuries in Industry. Chelsea, MI: Lewis Publishers, 1987, pp 11–26.

52. Kiesler S, and Finholt T: The mystery of RSI. Am Psychol 43:1004–1015, 1988.

53. Kitayama T: Health care relating to the occupational cervicobrachial disorder. J Hum Ergol 11:119–124, 1982.

54. Kivi P: Rheumatic disorders of the upper limbs associated with repetitive occupational tasks in Finland in 1975–1979. Scand J Rheumatol 13:101–107, 1984.

55. Kogi K: Finding appropriate work-rest rhythm for occupational strain on the basis of electromyographic and behavioural changes. In Buser PA, Cobb WA, and Okuna T (eds): Kyoto Symposia: Electromyography and Clinical Neurophysiology. Amsterdam: Elsevier, 1982.

56. Kuorinka I, and Viikari-Juntura E: Prevalence of neck and upper limb disorders (NLD) and work load in different occupational groups. Problems in classification and diagnosis. J Hum Ergol 11:65–72, 1982.

57. Kvarnstrom S: Occupational cervico-brachial disorders in an engineering company. Scand J Rehab Med [Suppl]8:77–100, 1983.

57a. Lawrence JS: Rheumatism in coal miners. Part III. Occupational factors. Br J Indust Med 12:249–261, 1955.

57b. Lee KS, and Oh YG: An alternative to reduce the physical stress of VDT operators. In Proceedings of the Human Factors Society, 29th Annual Meeting, Santa Monica, CA, 1985, pp 932–936.

57c. Lee KS, Mangum M, Waikas A, and Carver S: Evaluation of identified exercises and development of exercises for VDT operators. Cincinnati, OH: National Institute for Occupational Safety and Health, Contract No 87-12182, 1987.

58. Lucire Y: Neurosis in the work place. Med J Aust 145:323–327, 1986.

58a. Luopajärvi T, Kuorinka I, Virolainen M, and Holmberg M: Prevalence of tenosynovitis and other injuries of the upper extremities in repetitive work. Scand J Work Environ Health [Suppl] 3:48–55, 1979.

59. McBride ED: Disability Evaluation, 6th ed. Philadelphia: JB Lippincott, 1963.

60. McDermott F: Repetition strain injury: a review of current understanding. Med J Aust 144:196–200, 1986.

61. Maeda K: Occupational cervicobrachial disorder and its causative factors. J Hum Ergol 6:193, 1977.

62. Maeda K, Harada N, and Takamatsu M: Factor analysis of complaints of occupational cervicobrachial disorder in assembly lines of a cigarette factory. Kurume Med J 27:253–261, 1980.

63. Mallory M, and Bradford H: An invisible work place hazard getting harder to ignore. Business Week, Jan. 30, 1989, pp 92–93.

64. Melin E: Neck-shoulder loading characteristics and work technique. Ergonomics 30:281–285, 1987.

65. Minnesota Medical Association: Worker's Compensation Permanent Partial Disability Schedule. Minneapolis: Minnesota Medical Association, 1984.

66. Miyake S, Himeno J, and Hosokawa M: Clinical features of occupational cervicobrachial disorder (OCD). J Hum Ergol 11:109–117, 1982.

66a. Nakaseko M, Tokunaga R, and Hosokawa M: History of occupational cervicobrachial disorders in Japan. J Hum Ergol 11:7–16, 1982.

67. National Institute of Occupational Safety and Health: Potential Health Hazards of Video Display Terminals (DHSS Publication No. 81-129). Cincinnati OH: National Institute of Occupational Safety and Health, 1981.

68. National Occupational Health and Safety Commission (Worksafe Australia): Repetition Strain Injuries (RSI): A Report and Model Code of Practice. Canberra, Australia: Australian Government Publishing Service, 1986.

69. Neer C: Anterior acromioplasty for the chronic impingement syndrome of the rotator cuff of the shoulder. J Bone Joint Surg 54A:41–50, 1972.

70. Neviaser R: Lesions of the biceps and tendinitis of the shoulder. Orthop Clin North Am 11:343–348, 1980.

71. Newham DJ: The consequences of eccentric contractions and their relation to delayed onset muscle pain. Eur J Appl Physiol 57:353–359, 1988.

71a. Newham DJ, Jones DA, and Tolfree SEJ: Skeletal muscle damage: a study of isotope uptake enzyme efflux and pain after stepping. Eur J Appl Physiol 55:106–112, 1986.

72. Newham DJ, Mills KR, Quigley BM, and Edwards RHT: Pain and fatigue after concentric and eccentric muscle contractions. Clin Sci 64:55–62, 1983.

73. Ohara H, Aoyama H, and Itani T: Health hazard among cash register operators and the effects of improved working conditions. J Hum Ergol 5:31–40, 1976.

74. Onishi N, Sakai K, and Kogi K: Arm and shoulder muscle load in various keyboard operating jobs of women. J Hum Ergol 11:89–97, 1982.

75. Persson J, and Kilbom A: VIRA, a simple videofilm technique for registration and analysis of work positions and movements. Invest Rep Ed J 10:23, 1983.

76. Petersson CJ: Degeneration of the gleno-humeral joint. Acta Orthop Scand 54:277–283, 1983.

77. Petersson CJ: Degeneration of the acromioclavicular joint. Acta Orthop Scand 54:434–438, 1983.

78. Rathbun J, and Macnab I: The microvascular pattern of the rotator cuff. J Bone Joint Surg 52B:540–553, 1970.

79. Rohmert W: Problems in determining rest allowances. Appl Ergonomics 4:91–95, 1973.

80. Ryan G, Mullerworth J, and Pimble J: The prevalence of repetition injury in data process operators. Proceedings of the 21st Annual Conference of Ergonomics Society of Australia and New Zealand, Sidney, 1984, pp 279–288.

81. Sällstrom J, and Schmidt H: Cervicobrachial disorders in certain occupations, with special reference to compression in the thoracic outlet. Am J Ind Med 6:45–52, 1984.

82. Sato H, Ohashi J, Iwanaga K, et al: Endurance time and fatigue in static contractions. J Hum Ergol 13:147–154, 1984.

83. Schatzker J, and Branemark PI: Intravital observations on the microvascular anatomy and microcirculation of the tendon. Acta Orthop Scand [Suppl]126:80, 1965.

84. Schuldt K, Ekholm J, Harms-Ringdahl K, et al: Effects of changes in sitting work posture on static neck and shoulder muscle activity. Ergonomics 29:1525–1537, 1986.

85. Sejerstedt OM, and Westgaard RH: Occupational muscle pain and injury. Eur J Appl Physiol 57:271–274, 1988.

86. Sigholm G, Herberts P, Almström C, and Kadefors R: Electromyographic analysis of shoulder muscle load. J Orthop Res 1:379–386, 1984.

87. Sjogaard G, Kiens B, Jorgensen K, and Saltin B: Intramuscular pressure, EMG and blood flow during low-level prolonged static contraction in man. Acta Physiol Scand 128:475–484, 1986.

88. Social Security Administration: Disability Evaluation Under Social Security (DHEW Publication No. (SSA) 05-10089). Washington DC: U.S. Government Printing Office, 1979, pp 1–22.

88a. Spilling S, Eitrheim J, and Aaras A: Cost-benefit analysis of work environment investment at STK's Telephone Plant at Kongsvinger. In Corlett N, Wilson J, and Manenica I (eds): The Ergonomics of Working Posture. London: Taylor & Francis, 1986, pp 380–397.

89. Stone WE: Repetitive strain injuries. Med J Aust 2:616–618, 1983.

90. Sundelin G, Hagberg M, and Hammarstrom U: The effects of pauses on muscular load and perceived discomfort when working at a VDT word processor. Presented at Work with Display Units, Stockholm, 1985.

91. Swedish National Board of Occupational Safety and Health: Ordinance (ASF 1985:12) Concerning Work With Visual Display Units (VDUS). Stockholm, 1985.

92. Taylor R, and Pitcher M: Medical and ergonomic aspects of an industrial dispute concerning occupational related conditions in data process operators. Community Health Stud 8:172–180, 1984.

93. Tichauer ER: Potential of Biomechanics for Solving Specific Hazard Problems: Proceedings of ASSE 1968 Conference. Park Ridge IL: American Society of Safety Engineers, 1968, pp 149–187.

94. Tichauer ER: The Biomechanical Basis of Ergonomics. New York: Wiley-Interscience, 1978.

95. Viikara-Juntura E: Neck and upper limb disorders among slaughterhouse workers. Scand J Work Environ Health 9:283–290, 1983.

96. Waris P, Kuorinka I, Kurppa K, et al: Epidemiologic screening of occupational neck and upper limb disorders. Methods and criteria. Scand J Work Environ Health 5(Suppl 3):25–38, 1979.

97. Westerling D, and Jonsson B: Pain from the neck-shoulder region and sick leave. Scand J Soc Med 8:131–136, 1980.

97a. Westgaard RH: Measurement and evaluation of postural load in occupational work situations. Eur J Appl Physiol 57:291–304, 1988.

97b. Westgaard RH, and Aaras A: The effect of improved workplace design on the development of work-related musculoskeletal illnesses. Appl Ergonomics 16:91–97, 1985.

97c. Winkel J, Ekblom B, Hagberg M, and Jonsson B: The working environment of cleaners. Evaluation of physical strain in mopping and swabbing as a basis for job redesign. In Ergonomics of Workstation Design. London: Butterworth, 1983, pp 35–44.

97d. Winkel J, Ekblom B, and Tillberg B: Ergonomics and medical factors in shoulder/arm pain among cabin attendants as a basis for job redesign. In Malsvi H, and Kobayashi K (eds): Biomechanics VIII-A. Champaign, IL: Human Kinetics Publishers, 1983, pp 563–567.

98. Worchester JN, and Green DP: Osteoarthritis of the acromioclavicular joint. Clin Orthop 58:69–73, 1968.

99. Yood RA, and Goldenberg DL: Sterno-clavicular joint arthritis. Arthritis Rheum 23:232–239, 1980.

100. Zwalen HT, Hartman AL, and Kothari N: Effects of rest breaks in continuous VDT work on visual and musculoskeletal comfort/discomfort and on performance. In Salvendi G (ed): Human-Computer Interaction. Amsterdam: Elsevier, 1984, pp 315–319.

Index

C

H

I

J

U

Y

Z